Fundamentals of Mathematical Evolutionary Genetics

Mathematics and Its Applications (*Soviet Series*)

Volume 22

Yuri M. Svirezhev and Vladimir P. Passekov

Department of Mathematical Modeling in Ecology and Medicine, U.S.S.R. Academy of Sciences, Moscow, U.S.S.R.

Fundamentals of Mathematical Evolutionary Genetics

Kluwer Academic Publishers

Dordrecht / Boston / London

Library of Congress Cataloging in Publication Data

Svirezhev, I͡U. M.
Fundamentals of mathematical evolutionary genetics.

(Mathematics and its applications. Soviet series ; 22)
Translation of: Osnovy matematicheskoĭ genetiki.
Includes index.
1. Population genetics--Mathematical models.
2. Genetics--Mathematical models. I. Pasekov, V. P.
II. Title. III. Series: Mathematics and its applications (D. Reidel Publishing Company). Soviet series ; 22.
QH438.4.M3S9413 1989 575.1'5'0724 88-12798
ISBN 90-277-2772-4

Published by Kluwer Academic Publishers,
P.O. Box 17, 3300 AA Dordrecht, The Netherlands.

Kluwer Academic Publishers incorporates
the publishing programmes of
D. Reidel, Martinus Nijhoff, Dr W. Junk and MTP Press

Sold and distributed in the U.S.A. and Canada
by Kluwer Academic Publishers,
101 Philip Drive, Norwell, MA 02061, U.S.A.

In all other countries, sold and distributed
by Kluwer Academic Publishers Group,
P.O. Box 322, 3300 AH Dordrecht, The Netherlands.

Translated from Russian by
Alexey A. Voinov and Dmitriĭ O. Logofet

printed on acid-free paper

Printed in The Netherlands

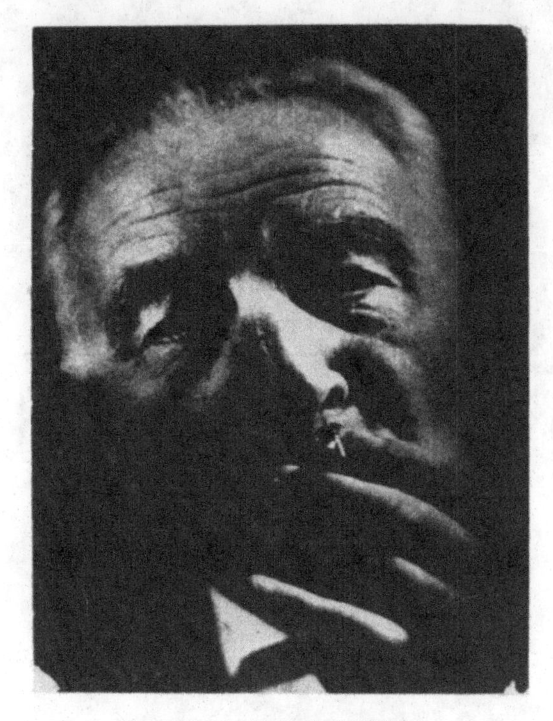

N. V. TIMOFEEFF–RESSOVSKY

To the Teacher

Table of Contents

SERIES EDITOR'S PREFACE

'Et moi, ..., si j'avait su comment en revenir, je n'y serais point allé.'

Jules Verne

The series is divergent; therefore we may be able to do something with it.

O. Heaviside

One service mathematics has rendered the human race. It has put common sense back where it belongs, on the topmost shelf next to the dusty canister labelled 'discarded non-sense'.

Eric T. Bell

Mathematics is a tool for thought. A highly necessary tool in a world where both feedback and non-linearities abound. Similarly, all kinds of parts of mathematics serve as tools for other parts and for other sciences.

Applying a simple rewriting rule to the quote on the right above one finds such statements as: 'One service topology has rendered mathematical physics ...'; 'One service logic has rendered computer science ...'; 'One service category theory has rendered mathematics ...'. All arguably true. And all statements obtainable this way form part of the raison d'être of this series.

This series, *Mathematics and Its Applications*, started in 1977. Now that over one hundred volumes have appeared it seems opportune to reexamine its scope. At the time I wrote

> "Growing specialization and diversification have brought a host of monographs and textbooks on increasingly specialized topics. However, the 'tree' of knowledge of mathematics and related fields does not grow only by putting forth new branches. It also happens, quite often in fact, that branches which were thought to be completely disparate are suddenly seen to be related. Further, the kind and level of sophistication of mathematics applied in various sciences has changed drastically in recent years: measure theory is used (non-trivially) in regional and theoretical economics; algebraic geometry interacts with physics; the Minkowsky lemma, coding theory and the structure of water meet one another in packing and covering theory; quantum fields, crystal defects and mathematical programming profit from homotopy theory; Lie algebras are relevant to filtering; and prediction and electrical engineering can use Stein spaces. And in addition to this there are such new emerging subdisciplines as 'experimental mathematics', 'CFD', 'completely integrable systems', 'chaos, synergetics and large-scale order', which are almost impossible to fit into the existing classification schemes. They draw upon widely different sections of mathematics."

By and large, all this still applies today. It is still true that at first sight mathematics seems rather fragmented and that to find, see, and exploit the deeper underlying interrelations more effort is needed and so are books that can help mathematicians and scientists do so. Accordingly MIA will continue to try to make such books available.

If anything, the description I gave in 1977 is now an understatement. To the examples of interaction areas one should add string theory where Riemann surfaces, algebraic geometry, modular functions, knots, quantum field theory, Kac-Moody algebras, monstrous moonshine (and more) all come together. And to the examples of things which can be usefully applied let me add the topic 'finite geometry'; a combination of words which sounds like it might not even exist, let alone be applicable. And yet it is being applied: to statistics via designs, to radar/sonar detection arrays (via finite projective planes), and to bus connections of VLSI chips (via difference sets). There seems to be no part of (so-called pure) mathematics that is not in immediate danger of being applied. And, accordingly, the applied mathematician needs to be aware of much more. Besides analysis and numerics, the traditional workhorses, he may need all kinds of combinatorics, algebra, probability, and so on.

In addition, the applied scientist needs to cope increasingly with the nonlinear world and the extra mathematical sophistication that this requires. For that is where the rewards are. Linear models are honest and a bit sad and depressing: proportional efforts and results. It is in the non-linear world that infinitesimal inputs may result in macroscopic outputs (or vice versa). To appreciate what I am hinting at: if electronics were linear we would have no fun with transistors and computers; we would have no TV; in fact you would not be reading these lines.

There is also no safety in ignoring such outlandish things as nonstandard analysis, superspace and anticommuting integration, p-adic and ultrametric space. All three have applications in both electrical engineering and physics. Once, complex numbers were equally outlandish, but they frequently proved the shortest path between 'real' results. Similarly, the first two topics named have already provided a number of 'wormhole' paths. There is no telling where all this is leading - fortunately.

Thus the original scope of the series, which for various (sound) reasons now comprises five subseries: white (Japan), yellow (China), red (USSR), blue (Eastern Europe), and green (everything else), still applies. It has been enlarged a bit to include books treating of the tools from one subdiscipline which are used in others. Thus the series still aims at books dealing with:

- a central concept which plays an important role in several different mathematical and/or scientific specialization areas;
- new applications of the results and ideas from one area of scientific endeavour into another;
- influences which the results, problems and concepts of one field of enquiry have, and have had, on the development of another.

The present volume concerns mathematical biology: quite possibly the fastest growing area of applied mathematics. For this last fact several reasons can, with some hindsight, be discerned. For one thing, the potential applications are great and important. Think, for instance, of the harvesting of microbial (and other) biological populations. For another, the subject is good at generating new kinds of mathematical problems. Thus, after a somewhat slow and tentative start, mathematization of (parts of) biology is in full swing.

This book is on what is perhaps the most mathematical (for the moment) part of mathematical biology: the subject of mathematical genetics and population dynamics including the modern topic of age-structured populations. Both deterministic and stochastic models are considered.

As one referee replied, now several years ago, this volume is a nice solid, thorough, complete book in the justly famous USSR tradition of high level workmanlike monographs and textbooks. It is also by two top experts in the field and thus very welcome in this series.

Perusing the present volume is not guaranteed to turn you into an instant expert, but it will help, though perhaps only in the sense of the last quote on the right below.

The shortest path between two truths in the real domain passes through the complex domain.

J. Hadamard

La physique ne nous donne pas seulement l'occasion de résoudre des problèmes ... elle nous fait pressentir la solution.

H. Poincaré

Never lend books, for no one ever returns them; the only books I have in my library are books that other folk have lent me.

Anatole France

The function of an expert is not to be more right than other people, but to be wrong for more sophisticated reasons.

David Butler

Bussum, March 1989

Michiel Hazewinkel

Preface

Mathematical genetics is one of the most formalized fields of biology. It is concerned both with speculations aimed at a better understanding of the evolutionary process and with purely practical aspects used, say, in animal and plant breeding plans, in artificial selection, etc. It would be difficult to cover all possible applications of mathematical methods to problems of genetics within the limits of one book, therefore this book is mainly devoted to the evolutionary aspect of genetical problems. The first part is concerned with deterministic models of mathematical genetics and the second part – with the stochastic ones. Some basic facts from genetics are included, sufficient to understand the problems considered. It is assumed that the reader is familiar with fundamentals of integral and differential calculus, the qualitative theory of differential equations, and probability theory. The authors have tried to make the chapters independent. To understand Chapters 3–9 of Part 1, which ignore the age-structure of populations, the reader may restrict him- or herself to Sections 15 and 16 of Chapter 2. The Chapters of Part 2 can be read independently if the results of Chapter 10 are known; if the reader is familiar with diffusion equations, he may read only Sections 4–6 and 9 of this Chapter.

Every chapter is concluded with references and comments, given in such a way that the reader finds information not only about sources of the presented results and methods, but also about the directions of their further research and generalization.

A word about the numbering of formulas and sections in the book is in order. Numbers of formulas within one chapter are made up of two figures – the section number and the number of a formula itself. If we refer to a formula from another chapter, the first number presents the number of the chapter; the second one, of the section, the third one, of the formula. Similarly, references to sections within one chapter contain only its number, references to sections from other chapters also have the chapter number.

We have failed to give only a unique meaning to symbols, since a lot of variables had to be introduced. However, within sections, and to a great extend within chapters, each symbol represents one variable.

Chapters 1–8 have been written by Yu. M. Svirezhev. Chapters 9–13 – by V. P. Passekov.

In conclusion we would like to say some words about how the book has been written. In the mid-1960's our teacher, the outstanding biologist of today Nikolai Vladimirovich Timofeeff-Ressovsky formulated a grand program for the mathematization of population genetics and evolution theory. Realizing this program we prepared chapters of the book. Each of them was discussed in much detail. Timofeeff-Ressovsky suggested a conceptual scheme, and we tried to translate it into the language of mathematics. Next came the stage of interpretation of the results; here again his role was also great.

Unfortunately, Timofeeff-Ressovsky did not live to see the appearance of this book. We wish to dedicate the book to his memory.

YU. M. SVIREZHEV
V. P. PASSEKOV

PART 1

DETERMINISTIC MODELS IN MATHEMATICAL GENETICS

Chapter 1

Brief Outline of Microevolution Theory with Some Facts from Genetics

1.1. History and Personalia

At present general population genetics is the conceptual basis of modern, so-called 'synthetic', evolution theory. The fundamental principle of natural selection as the main evolutionary principle has been formulated by C. Darwin long before the discovery of genetical mechanisms. Ignorant of the basic hereditary principles, Darwin hypothesized fusion or blending inheritance, supposing that parental qualities mix together like fluids in the offspring organism. His selection theory arose serious objections, first stated by F. Jenkins: crossing quickly levels off any hereditary distinctions, and there is no selection in homogeneous populations (the so-called 'Jenkins nightmare').

It was not until 1865, when G. Mendel discovered the basis principles of transferrence of hereditary factors from parent to offspring, which showed the discrete nature of these factors, that the 'Jenkins nightmare' could be explained, since because of this discreteness there is no 'dissolution' of hereditary distinctions.

Mendelian laws became known to the scientific community after they had been independently rediscovered in 1900 by H. de Vries, K. Correns and K. von Tschermak. Genetics was further developed by T. Morgan and his collaborators, who proved experimentally that chromosomes are the main carriers of hereditary information and that genes, which present hereditary factors, are lined up on chromosomes. Later on, accumulated experimental facts showed Mendelian laws to be valid for all sexually reproducing organisms.

However, Mendel's laws, even after they had been rediscovered, and Darwin's theory of natural selection remained independent, unlinked concepts. And moreover, they were opposed to each other. Not until the 1920's (see, for instance, the classical work by S. S. Četverikov, "On Some Aspects of the Evolutionary Process from the Viewpoint of Modern Genetics") was it proved that Mendel's genetics and Darwin's theory of natural selection are in no way conflicting and that their happy marriage yields modern evolutionary theory.

As the fundamental system of concepts in general population genetics was making its appearance, and as they were verified under field and laboratory conditions, the science of mathematical population genetics was becoming well established. One pioneer of the new science was the well-known English mathematician G. H. Hardy (1908). His early work triggered an "explosion" in publications on mathematical population genetics. (At present the bibliography in mathematical genetics amounts to many hundreds of titles.)

At the same time two fundamental approaches evolved in population genetics. The first, so-called 'deterministic', approach is mainly due to J. B. S. Haldane and R. A. Fisher. This approach assumes that populations are large enough, it neglects fluctuations of phase variables and describes the population evolutionary process by time variations of these variables. The phase variables are usually the concentrations or frequencies both of the genes and of some combinations of them (gametes or zygotes) in the population. The model usually characterizes these concentrations or frequencies depending on such factors as selection, migration, deviation from random mating, etc. The factors are specified by certain parameters on the right-hand sides of the difference or differential equations of the model. For instance, the selection coefficients are the parameters specifying the selection pressure on different genotypes. As a matter of fact, deterministic models are dynamic models with populations presented by a dynamical system; its behavior is affected by various changes in the workings of the system and is described by a trajectory in the phase space of frequencies, which is a unit simplex in the positive orthant.

The second approach to population genetics, the so-called 'stochastic' one, originates with S. Wright and R. A Fisher. This approach considers the variation of gene numbers or of the combinations in a population as a Markov process. The assumption of large population size is no longer needed, and stochastic models may be successfully applied to genetic processes in small populations (to be more exact, to finite populations), where fluctuations due to random sampling (the so-called 'genetic- automatic processes' or 'random genetic drift') may be significant.

These two approaches differ markedly both in model structure and in the mathematics used. While the deterministic approach uses the qualitative theory of integral, differential and difference equations and stability theory, the stochastic one uses methods of the theory of random processes (mostly Markov chains and diffusion approximation).

For this reason our book consists of two more or less independent parts, which are rather different with respect to the mathematics applied. But, to a great extent, this difference is formal, since the two basic approaches in population genetics by no means oppose each other; they only reflect two aspects of the same phenomenon – evolution of populations of organisms. If populations are large enough, if the selection pressure is quite well manifested, and if the effect of other factors is also rather pronounced, then over a long enough period (many generations) the behavior of a population may be viewed as the behavior of a dynamical system and described by a deterministic model. But if the pressures of selection, mutations, migration and other factors are weak and have practically no effect upon gene concentrations during one generation and the population itself is small, then its behavior over sufficiently short periods (several generations) is largely defined by random factors. Actually, stochastic models should be used when it is hard to detect typical rates of directional evolutionary variations; then random effects come to the fore (for example, fluctuations in population numbers).

Generally, the problem of the relation between the deterministic and the stochastic in evolution is one of the basic problems in modern evolutionary theory. Extreme points of view are voiced, often being supported by rather 'learned' and modernistic speculations. The problem itself seems to be as old as the history of humanity. As soon as man began to wonder about his place in the changing world and about his own evolution, two points of view immediately appeared. The first point of view, the one connected with Eastern philosophy, its fatalism and faith in predetermination, considered Chance to be the motive force of development. "Again I saw that under the sun the race is not to the swift, nor the battle to the strong, nor bread to the wise, nor riches to the intelligent, nor favor to the men of skill; but time and chance happen to them all".*

The other viewpoint, closely related to the Hellenist, Aristotelian philosophy of life, was deterministic in principle (it seems that no other one could even appear in the ordered Graeco-Roman society in its prime).

> Multaque tum interiisse animantum saecla necessest
> Nec potuisse propagando procudere prolem.
> Nam quaecumque vides vesci vitalibus auris,
> Aut dolus, aut virtus, aut denique mobilitas est
> Ex ineunte aevo genus id tutata reservans.**

The mathematical theory of microevolution and mathematical population genetics are the branches of biology in which quantitative methods struck the deepest roots, and so one may even consider them branches of applied mathematics. Because of the algebraic nature of Mendelism, the modern theory of microevolution and population genetics are greatly formalized systems.

Before we turn to these system, however, we would like to present a kind of biological introduction to microevolution and population genetics. This introduction seems to be very important both in terms of the essence of the problem (i.e. in which way and from which natural phenomenon emerge the formal problems to be considered below) and in terms of terminology, since even formal problems abound in purely biological nomenclature. Moreover, the book contains descriptions of biological experiments meant to test our mental constructs and to remind us that there really exists an object of modeling.

In conclusion, we would like to quote the well known English biologist C. H. Waddington***. He seems to have given an appreciation of works like ours, and their place among other studies concerned with evolution.

I should remind you that the mathematico-genetical theory of natural selection is largely inapplicable in practice, in that it is expressed in terms of variables, such as effective population number, which are almost impossible to measure. But no one could possibly deny the enormous importance which these

* The Bible. Ecclesiastes, 9.

** Lucreti. *De Rerum Natura*. Liber 5, 855.

*** Waddington, C. H.: 1962, *New Patterns in Genetics and Development*, Columbia Univ. Press, N.Y., London, 271 p. page 50.

theoretical development have had in providing a general framework of concepts within which our thoughts about evolutionary processes can move without so much danger of drifting off into mere cloudy verbalizations.

1.2. Conceptual Model of Microevolution

No quantitative theory based on mathematical models can develop without conceptual schemes, which are, in fact, the same models but formulated in terms of everyday, rather than formal language. Our task is much simplified by the fact that such a theory has been created by the 1930's – the theory of microevolution. In what follows we give just a brief account of the theory, following the ideas set forth by the outstanding Russian biologist N. V. Timofeeff-Ressovsky.

Microevolution deals only with starting mechanisms of evolution. The final stage of microevolution is the beginning of species formation, the macroevolution. Processes of micro- and macroevolution have different rates and specific time scales. We already know a lot about microevolutional phenomena and factors and can give a sufficiently reliable quantitative interpretation of the process. Unfortunately, we cannot say the same about macroevolution and we therefore leave it beyond the framework of our book.

1.3. Elementary Evolutionary Structure and Elementary Evolutionary Phenomenon

Life on our planet can be represented by an hierarchical system of discrete forms. Those species at the lowest level are combined more or less naturally according to both the similarity of some characters, considered to be essential, and the similarity of origin (phylogenesis) to form categories of higher order (genera, families, orders, classes, types). Being the basic category of this system, the species in natural conditions is practically in complete biological isolation from other species, even similar ones, i.e. individuals of two different species either cannot cross, or their offspring is inviable or sterile. Individuals with species are free to cross and produce quite viable offspring. Every species inhabits a certain territory or water body, which is the *area* of its prevalence. Within the area individuals of one species are never distributed homogeneously; they always form groups of different numbers, separated from each other by spaces either with no individuals of this species at all, or with considerably lower densities of these individuals. Such groups are usually termed populations. A *population* is a group of individuals occupying a certain area for many generations, with a certain extend of isolation from identical neighboring groups and with a certain extent of *panmixia* (random mating) occurring with this group. Obviously, this definition is rather loose and general. At the same time, populations in this sense are actually and historically existing communities of organisms within the limits of each species, which in no reasonable way may be further subdivided. They are the elementary reproductive groups and in this sense they are the *elementary structures of evolution*: no evolutionary process can take place without changing the hereditary content of populations.

Because of the continually occurring hereditary variations and crossings, all populations are heterogeneous in the hereditary content of individuals. Consequently, at any one time the genotype population content may be characterized by the total population size and the distribution of frequencies for its various genotypes. If the environment is constant, the population may be at the state of relative dynamic equilibrium, so that during many generations both the average number and the genotypic population content will not change. But sufficiently strong or prolonged variations in environment conditions may disturb such a dynamic equilibrium switching the population into another state, and changing the genotype distribution. A change in genotypic population content such that the population is switched from one rather prolonged state of dynamic equilibrium to another, will be termed *elementary phenomenon of evolution* (or, for short, the evolution of population).

1.4. Elementary Evolutionary Material

For any evolutional variations to occur populations need to be hereditary heterogeneous. It may well be asked: "What are the elementary units of hereditary variability that may serve as the elementary material of evolution?" Such hereditary variations should primarily affect all those characters and features, which can vary in a particular species; these variations are to occur in different directions, representing the 'indefinite variability', which C. Darwin postulated as one of the basic premises of his evolution theory. These variations are to appear constantly in all living organisms and they are to be present in all natural populations. And finally, those hereditary distinctions between taxons existing in nature (variaties, races, subspecies) that are due to crossing must be reduced to combinations of these elementary hereditary variations.

From a large body of experimental evidence we know the only type of hereditary variability that complies with all these conditions, namely the mutations. Spontaneous mutations in living organisms are further inherited according to Mendel's laws. Therefore, we may think that the elementary material of evolution is represented by different types of mutations, quite well known from experimental genetics.

The number of various mutations types in all living organisms, even in simply organized ones, is very large (due to the great number of different genes); therefore, the probabilities of some special types of mutations are fairly low ($10^{-5}-10^{-7}$). Most of mutations that appear are rejected by selection, very few of them have a chance to take root in the population. This suggests that genotypes of living organisms are very stable, being apparently stabilized at a certain optimal level (from the evolutionary viewpoint) as a result of a prolonged natural selection. If genotypes were too labile structures responding to all variations in natural conditions, no directional evolutionary process could be possible: inherited features of organisms would constantly change together with different varying factors and conditions.

1.5. Elementary Evolutionary Factors

We distinguish four elementary factors of evolution: mutation process, populational waves ('waves of life'), isolation, and selection.

The mutation process is characterized by the average rate of mutations and their qualitative spectrum. An essentially random undirectional process, it just supplies the elementary material of evolution.

Populations of all living organisms oscillate with amplitudes that may be very high (for instance, populations of species with short life-cycles). So in insects the ratio between maximum and minimum may be as high as 10^6. When populations sharply decline random (i.e. independent of genotype features) selection takes place. The randomly changed distribution of genotypes in the population, serving as the reproductive stock for a new population peak, is subjected to the rapid and intensive effect of difectional selection. As a result, the population acquires mutations and genotypes, which were originally present in negligible concentrations. Consequently, population waves, though quite different in their nature from the mutation process, are also a factor supplying the material of evolution. By a random mechanism this factor destroys a part of mutations in the population, transferring the rest of them into other conditions of selection; this all makes the fixation of relatively rare mutations and genotypes more probable.

The third elementary factor of evolution is isolation. By isolation we mean any extent or form of deviation from panmixia (random mating). Isolation fixes all sorts of genotypic distinctions within one population or between different populations. Without isolation all fresh intra- and interpopulational distinctions are leveled off by crossing and mixing. Isolation is, therefore, the factor that hastens the differentiation of populations, thus creating new forms. There may be many forms of isolation, but all of them may be broadly divided into types – territorial and biological isolations. Territorial forms are very diverse and they are determined by external conditions (for instance, the isolation of insular floras and faunas). All the forms of biological isolation are eventually caused by genetic distinctions between the corresponding individuals, i.e., by reasons intrinsic to, rather than independent of the organisms themselves (for example, the offspring of interspecific hybrids are sterile or inviable). Isolation by itself cannot serve as the directional factor of evolution, though it works towards the appearance of distinctions and maintains them.

Finally, the last but the most important elementary factor of evolution is natural selection. It was Darwin and Wallace who formulated the principle of natural selection and showed that it really exists in nature. The necessity of natural selection is premised by the following basic features of living organisms. All organisms, though to a different extent, overproduce their offspring. It is clear that in order to maintain constant population a pair of organisms of the previous generation is to produce on the average only one pair of offspring. However, organisms of all species produce far more offspring per pair (some plants, insects and fish produce thousands, tens or hundreds of thousands or even millions of 'children' per parential pair). Struggle for existence is the inevitable result of the overproduction of offspring. Another feature of living organisms is their hereditary variability, which was considered above. Inevitably, this makes organisms non-identical and consequently unequal in certain conditions. This, in turn, inevitably implies that in conditions of tough competition the probability for different organisms to attain the reproductive age should be different. In the general form the selection pressure (quantitative aspect of the effect) may be measured, for instance, by the difference between the probabilities for two different genetically specified forms to reach the reproductive age. It is known that mutations and their combinations may have very different relative viabilities (with respect to the original form) in different genotypic, populational and biogeocenotic environment. This greatly increases the potential for selection. The principle that the fittest survive defines the 'movement' of the population genotypic structure towards the improvement of the whole population. This principle indicates that natural selection is the only directional elementary factor of evolution, which, in combination with the three other ones, can provide adaptation, differentiation, specialization and coordination of parts and organs in ontogenesis, thus creating the so-called directedness and progress in evolution of living organisms.

Interestingly enough, the principle of selecting from a certain set (of trajectories, combinations, speciments, etc.) a subset that satisfies some criterion, and 'moving' further on within this subset is a general principle for all systems in evolution. Principles of selection (variational principles) lie at the base of mechanics and physics. From all the set of trajectories only one is left, the 'best' one by a certain criterion. In biology each set of admissible trajectories (possible ways of evolution) is associated with a certain optimal distribution, and to a certain extent the choice of the further way is made by chance. In other words, at any one time a biological system, a population, has several different opportunities for its further evolution, but only one way is realized.

These four elementary factors of evolution may be classed into three groups according to their effect: the mutation process and population waves are 'suppliers' of evolutionary material, isolation is the 'initiator and fixing agent' of inter- and intrapopulational group distinctions (the main factor of form differentiation), while natural selection is the 'directing and creative' factor of evolution (it constructs adaptations, transfers to higher levels of relationships between organisms and environment and, as a result, creates evolutionary progress).

1.6. An Introduction to Principles of Inheritance

All modern genetics has developed from the laws introduced by Mendel in 1865. These quite simple and explicit laws are formulated in terms of frequencies and they are essentially stochastic. Since for our purposes some very general facts from genetics will do, the following account will be very schematic, greatly simplifying the actual picture of such a complex natural phenomenon as hereditary.

Each cell of every organism of a given species carries a certain number of *chromosomes* – the material bearers of hereditary information. Man, for instance, has 46 of them. Chromosomes of diploid organisms appear in pairs: each chromosome is associated with a homologous one. All chromosomes are made of elementary units – *genes* – arranged in linear succession; every gene controls the inheritance of one or several characters. Homologous chromosomes have similar sequences of genes. Genes of certain characters are located at certain places of the chromosome, which are called *loci*. Any character of individuals (for example, the color of eyes) can manifest itself differently; the gene is said to be in several states, called *alleles*. Sometimes these states of a gene are also called genes.

The process of reproduction consists of two stages: the formation of sex cells – gametes, and fertilization. The constant number of chromosomes is ensured by the *meiosis* process, which occurs when gametes mature; in meiosis the cell divides twice in succession, halving the number of chromosomes. As a result, gametes have half as many chromosomes (*haploid* set) as other cells (*diploid* set). For simplicity, suppose that a cell contains only one chromosome pair: ♂ $\{Aa\}$ for males and ♀ $\{Aa\}$ for females, where A is a chromosome and a is a homologous chromosome.

At the beginning of meiosis each chromosome doubles to form a *tetrad* (Figure 1a), made of four linear structural units, the *chromatids*. The doubled chromosome is called a *dyad*, and the chromatids it consists of are said to be sister ones. At the next stage chromatides twist together and, as a result, homologous chromatides may break up at the same places. Breaking up might occur at any place of a chromatide between loci (with a certain probability) (Figure 1b). A chromatide may break into any number of parts not more than $m-1$, where m is the number of loci. Figure 1b presents the simplest case of breaking into two parts. After breaking up chromatides recombine but not necessarily in the previous order. For example, in our case one of the two events takes place: either the two parts reconnect in the same order as before (Figure 1c, the scheme for females), or a part of one chromatide unites with the other part of the second chromatide (Figure 1c, the scheme for males). This is the *recombination* process. As a result, homologous chromosomes exchange segments, the exchange is known as *crossing-over*. Next the homologous chromosomes, each presented by a pair of sister chromatides, are pulled apart towards the opposite poles. This completes the first division of meiosis. The result is two daughter cells with a halved number of chromosomes.

In the second division each of the daughter nuclei divides again, separating the chromosomes presented by sister chromatides. Consequently, each cell in the meiosis process, after two successive divisions produces four cells with a halved (haploid) set of chromosomes, these cells are called *gametes*. This process is presented in Figure 1d.

In the process of fertilization two randomly chosen gametes – one from the father and one from the mother – merge to form one cell, the *zygote*, which originates a new organism, the offspring of the parental pair (Figure 1e). Notice that the recombination process for the paternal and maternal gametes may proceed differently (see Figure 1b, c). When there is no crossing-over, only two types of gametes are formed, each containing one of the homologous chromosomes, and the entire process described above may be presented by a simpler scheme.
In Figure 2 we have:

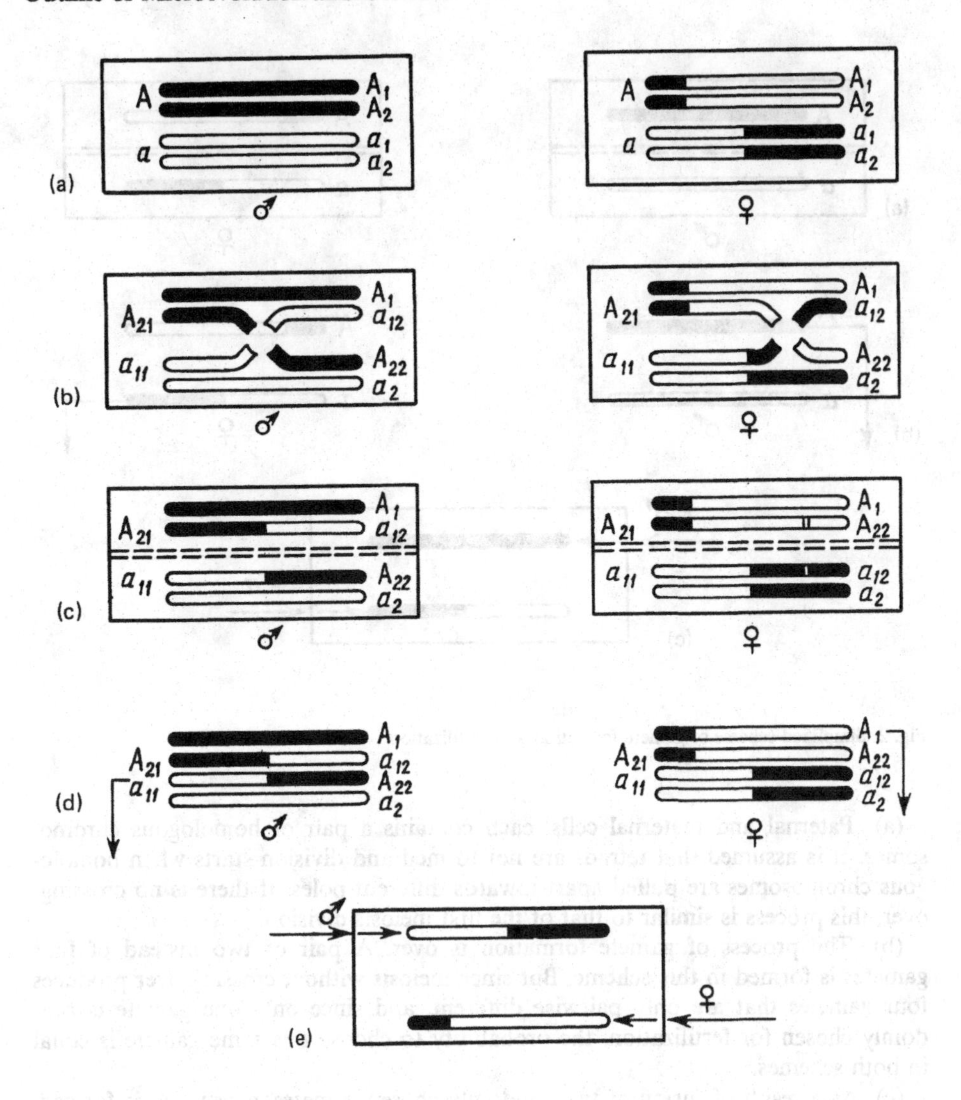

Fig. 1. Process of meiosis and fertilization. (a) Male and female cells with two chromosomes A and a. Tetrads are already formed: each chromosome is presented by two sister chromatids: $A(A_1, A_2)$, $a(a_1, a_2)$. (b) The same cells but with chromatids pulled apart. Chromatids A_2 and a_1 twisted together and broke at the crossing. The new parts a_{11}, a_{12}, A_{21}, A_{22} start to move more or less independently. (c) A first division of meiosis begins. While male homologous chromatides exchanged segments, there was no exchange between the female ones and they remained unchanged. (d) A second division of meiosis is over and four gametes are formed. While all male gametes are different, the female ones are of two types only. (e) As a result of fusion of two randomly chosen gametes a new cell, the zygote, is formed.

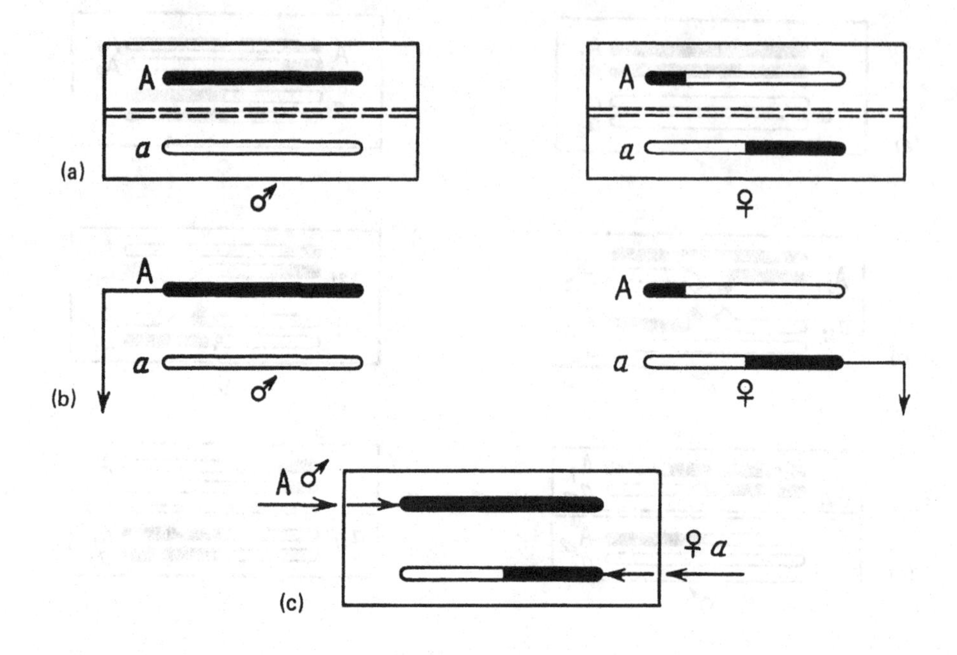

Fig. 2. Simplified scheme of gamete formation and fertilization

(a) Paternal and maternal cells, each contains a pair of homologous chromosomes. It is assumed that tetrads are not formed and division starts when homologous chromosomes are pulled apart towards different poles. If there is no crossing-over, this process is similar to that of the first meiosis division.

(b) The process of gamete formation is over. A pair of two instead of four gametes is formed in this scheme. But since meiosis without crossing-over produces four gametes that are only pairwise different, and since only one gamete is randomly chosen for fertilization, the probability to choose this same gamete is equal in both schemes.

(c) As a result of fusion of two randomly chosen gametes, a new cell is formed, the zygote.

Though this scheme does not represent the actual process, its final result is similar to that of the more correct but more complex scheme. In what follows we shall widely make use of the model schemes of the second type.

Suppose now a chromosome has only one locus and the gene localized in it is in one of the two states: G and g, corresponding to the two possible ways in which a character may manifest itself. If two organisms with such a chromosome pair are crossed, the offspring can have zygotes of the following four genotypes: $\{♂G\,♀G\}$, $\{♂G\,♀g\}$ or $\{♂g\,♀G\}$, $\{♂g\,♀g\}$. Zygotes (and the organisms they develop) with two identical alleles, say $\{♂G\,♀G\}$ or $\{♂g\,♀g\}$, are called *homozygous* with respect to a given locus, those with two different alleles, say {♂*G*♀*g*} or {♂*g*♀*G*}, are called *heterozygous*, or simply homozygotes and heterozygotes (hybrids).

It should be noted that the total action of two genes (alleles) manifested in a zygote is not always additive (moreover, it is nearly always non-additive). If a given character is manifested in the heterozygotes {♂*G*♀*g*} or {♂*g*♀*G*} in the same way as in the homozygote {♂*G*♀*G*}, the gene (allele) *G* is said to be *dominant*, while gene (allele) *g* is said to be *recessive*. In intermediate cases the dominance is said to be incomplete. Quite often a heterozygote may manifest a given character (for instance, the intensity of coloring) even better than both homozygotes. In this case we speak about overdominance.

Throughout the book, in those models that account for only one locus in a chromosome the chromosome notations, *A* and *a*, will be also used to denote various alleles of the gene localized in this chromosome. This means that in the aforesaid we would have to substitute *A* for *G* and *a* for *g*.

This concludes our brief outline of some facts from genetics and evolution theory, which are surely quite known to all biologists, but hardly known to members of other professions.

1.7. Notes and Bibliography

To 1.1.

Četverikov, S. S.: 1926, 'O nekotoryh momentah evolucionnovo processa s točki zrenija sovremennoi genetiki (On some Aspects of the Evolutionary Process From the Viewpoint of Modern Genetics. In Russian)', *J. Exper. Biol.* **2**, 1, 3–54

(the paper has been reprinted in Bulletin of the Moscow Society of Naturalists, *Biological Series*, 1965, **79**, 4, 33–74).

This paper was the first to give a clear and accurate formulation of the tasks of population genetics, and to bring together the evolutionary theory and genetics.

One of the first papers in mathematical genetics seems to be: Hardy, G. H.: 1908, 'Mendelian Proportions in a Mixed Population', *Science* **28**, 49–50.

The notions of panmixia and panmictic population were first strictly formulated, and it was shown that without selection in an infinite panmictic population with inheritance of a character defined by one diallele gene, the ratio between genotype frequencies equilibrates immediately after the first generation and stays the same for all further generations. This statement is usually called the Hardy theorem or even the Hardy principle. Often the name Hardy is accompanied by another one, and the Hardy principle becomes the Hardy-Wienberg principle, which is not without reason since at the same time there appeared a paper by

Weinberg, W.: 1908, 'Über den Nachwies der Verebung beim Menschen', *Jahresh. Verein f. vater. Naturk. in Wurtenberg*, **61**, 368–382,

that contained a similar statement.

In 1924-1932 the journal Proceedings of Cambridge Philosophical Society published some papers of J. Haldane under the general heading:

Haldane, J. B. S.: 1924-1932, 'A Mathematical Theory of Natural and Artificial Selection', *Proc. Cambridge Philosophical Society*, **23**, 19–41, 158–163, 363–372, 607–615; **26**, 220–230; **27**, 232–242; **28**, 24–248.

Many problems of population genetics were given clear mathematical formulations and elegant solutions. Even now these works are far from being obsolete. Unfortunately, some of these problems deal with too special cases, and there is no general concept in them. To some extent this drawback is,

compensated in the book by the same author:
Haldene, J. B. S.: 1932, *The Causes of Evolution*, Harper, London, 234 p.
Papers by Haldane continued to appear until 1964. They were noted for originality of problem formulation and elegancy of the solutions, which usually found very apt biological interpretations.
Another classical work in this field is the still significant book by R. Fisher, a well known English mathematician and statistician:
Fisher, R. A.: 1930, *The Genetical Theory of Natural Selection*, Clarendon Press, Oxford, 272 p.
While Haldane's models were mostly deterministic frequency models, among Fisher's models we also find stochastic ones.
Since 1921 works by S. Wright, one of the pioneers of mathematical population genetics, keep appearing. We list only some of the fundamental ones:
Wright, S.: 1921, 'Systems of Mating, I-V', *Genetics* **6**, N1-2, 111-178;
Wright, S.: 1931, 'Evolution of Mendelian Populations', *Genetics* **16**, 2, 97-159;
Wright, S.: 1939, *Statistical Genetics in Relation to Evolution*, Herman et Cie, Paris; 63 p.
Wright, S.: 1951, 'The Genetical Structure of Populations', *Ann. Eugenics* **15**, 323–354;
Wright, S.: 1955, 'Classification of the Factors of Evolution', *Cold Spring Harbor Symp. Quant. Biol.* **20**, 16–24.
Quite recently the four fundamental volumes by S. Wright were published: 1968, 1969, 1977, 1978. Evolution and the Genetics of Population. University Press, Chicago.
They summarize the many years of his research in genetics of populations.
A number of classical papers by J. Haldene, R. Fisher, S. Wright are collected in the book:
Papers on Quantitative Genetics: 1962, Raleigh, USA.
Among modern books on mathematical genetics we can name the following ones:
Crow, J. F., Kimura, M.: 1970, *An Introduction to Population Genetics Theory*, Harper and Row, New York; 591 p.
Kojima, K. (ed.): 1970, *Mathematical Topics in Population Genetics*, Springer-Verlag, Berlin; 400 pp.
Poluektov, R. A. (ed.): 1974, *Dinamičeskaja teorija biologičeskih populjatsiy* (*Dynamical Theory of Biological Populations*. In Russian), Nauka, Moscow; 455 pp.
Nagylaki T.: 1977, *Selection in One- and Two-Locus Systems*, Springer-Verlag, Berlin, 208 pp.
While the last two books consider deterministic models, the book by
Maruyama, T.: 1977, *Stochastic Problems in Population Genetics*, Springer-Verlag, Berlin, 245 p.
deals only with stochastic ones.
We conclude the list by mentioning two books of educational character, which can serve as good introductions to the problem:
Ratner, V. A.: 1976, *Matematičeskaja populjatsionnaja genetika* (*Mathematical Populational Genetics*. In Russian), Nauka, Novosibirsk; 126 p.
Li, C. C.: 1976, First Course in Population Genetics. Pacific Grove, California: The Boxwood Press, VII, 631 p.

To 1.2 – 1.5.
When describing the processes of microevolution we exactly followed the paper by
Timofeeff-Ressovsky, N. W.: 1958, 'Mikroevolucija, elementarnyi jevlenija, material i faktory evolucionnova processa (Microevolution, Elementary Phenomena, Material and Factors of Evolutionary Process. In Russian)', *Botanical Journal* **43**, 317-336,
which clearly outlines the logical structure of this theory. The methodological principles, formulated in this work, can be successfully applied to other fields of biology, expanding the significance applied to other fields of biology, expanding the significance of this paper beyond the limits set by its title.
An elementary introduction to the evolutionary theory is given by
Ayala, F. J.: 1982, *Population and Evolutionary Genetics: a Primer*, The Benjamin/Cummings Publ. Co., Menlo Park, California, Davis.
Among other books we mention the following one:
Schmalhausen, I. I.: 1949, *Factors of Evolution: The Theory of Stabilizing Selection*, Blackiston Co., Dodrick, New York.

The book

Mayr, E.: 1963, ***Animal Species and Evolution***, Belknap press of Harvard Univ. Press, Cambridge (Mass), XIV, 797 p.

is useful mostly because it contains a large body of factual material and a review of current achievements in evolutionary theory.

Various aspects of evolutionary theory, quite unexpected sometimes, and the relationship between this theory and other branches of biology, are covered in the books:

Huxley, J.: 1955, ***Evolution. The Modern Synthesis***, G. Allen & Unwin LTD, London; 645 p.

Dobzhansky, Th.: 1970, ***Genetics of Evolutionary Process***, Columbia Univ. Press, N.Y.; 505 pp.

Dobzhansky, Th., Hecht, M. K. and Steere, W. C. (eds.): 1967, ***Evolutionary Biology***, v. 1, North-Holland, Amsterdam.

To 1.6.

The book

Auerbach, S.: 1961, ***The Science of Genetics***, Harper and Row, New York, Evanston, London, 273 p.

is a good introduction to genetics. More serious textbooks are:

Lobashev, M. E.: 1979, ***Genetika*** (***Genetics***. In Russian), Leningrad Univ. Press, Leningrad, 750 p.

Dubinin, N. P.: 1976, ***Obshaja genetika*** (***General Genetics***. In Russian), Nauka, Moscow

Chapter 2

Basic Equations of Population Genetics

2.1. Description of a Population

We regard a population as a group of individuals that can cross and produce viable offspring. Individuals within population may differ with respect to genotype, age and sex. Let a population be made of N genotypic groups with numbers $x_i(t, \tau_x)$ and $y_i(t, \tau_y)$, $i=\overline{1, N}$, where $x_i(t, \tau_x)$ is the number of males of age τ_x with the genotype denoted by index $\{i\}$ at time t, $y_i(t, \tau_y)$ is the number of females of age τ_y with the genotype denoted by index $\{i\}$ at time t. Naturally, $\tau_x, \tau_y \geqslant 0$. The distributions of $x_i(t, \tau_x)$ and $y_i(t, \tau_y)$ with respect to non-negative τ are called *age distributions* of the corresponding genotypes, and the time variation of these variables is called the *evolution* of population.

The evolution of population is the result of two processes: *reproduction* and *death*.

The reproduction process may be split into two stages: mating (formation of reproductive pairs) and production of offspring. Consider each of them separately.

(a) *Mating*. Suppose at time t mating takes place between a male of age τ_x with genotype $\{i\}$ and a female of age τ_y with genotype $\{j\}$. We denote the number of such pairs in the population by $m_{ij}(t, \tau_x, \tau_y, \mathbf{X}, \mathbf{Y})$, where $\mathbf{X}(t, \tau_x)$ and $\mathbf{Y}(t, \tau_y)$ are vectors with components $x_i(t, \tau_x)$ and $y_i(t, \tau_y)$, respectively, $i=\overline{1, N}$.

The *system of mating* is specified either by the concrete form of these functions, or by some rules, which the entries of matrix $\| m_{ij} \|$ are to satisfy.

*Panmixia**, or random mating is one of the most simple (and most widespread in nature) systems of mating. The term 'panmixia' was introduced already by Galton. By his definition, under panmixia the probability of pairing is independent of the male and female genotypes (just as it should follow from the definition for random mating). But in our case, when we take into account the age of mating individuals, this probability depends upon the relation between ages. Therefore we expand this definition to make difference between the *genotypic* (Galtonian) *panmixia,* when for a priori fixed ages of a female and a male, their genotypes in the mating process are independent, and the *age panmixia,* when for a priori fixed genotypes of partners the choice of their ages is also independent. When the choice of a male with genotype $\{i\}_{\tau_x}$ is independent of the choice of a female with genotype $\{j\}_{\tau_y}$ at fixed ages τ_x, τ_y and vice versa, and this is so for all ages and genotypes, then panmixia is said to be *global*.

* A more strict definition of a panmixia will be presented in Section 2.5.

(b) *Production of offspring*. We assume that each pair produces $F_{ij}(t, \tau_x, \tau_y)$ of male offspring and $G_{ij}(t, \tau_x, \tau_y)$ of female offspring. We call F_{ij} and G_{ij} the *fecundity functions* for appropriate pairs. In the general case they may as well depend upon X and Y. This dependence comes into play, for instance, when fertility is considered to be affected by both competition between genetic groups and competition within them.

As it was shown above, due to Mendelism pairs can produce not only those akin to themselves, but also offsprings of other genotypes. For this reason we introduce the values $\omega_{ij}^k(♂)$ and $\omega_{ij}^k(♀)$, which stand for the *proportions* of genotype $\{k\}$ in the offspring of the pair $♂\{i\}_{\tau_x}$, $♀\{j\}_{\tau_y}$ among the female and male offsprings, respectively. Obviously,

$$\sum_k \omega_{ij}^k(♂) = \sum_k \omega_{ij}^k(♀) = 1, \quad i, j, k = \overline{1, N}. \tag{1.1}$$

The appropriate *principle of inheritance* is defined by the particular set of constants $\Omega\{\omega_{ij}^k\}$.

Taking into account all the foregoing, the number of newborns with genotypes $\{k\}$ and $♀\{k\}$ at time t will be

$$x_k(t, 0) = \sum_{i,j} \omega_{ij}^k(♂) \cdot \int_{a_y}^{b_y} d\tau_y \int_{a_x}^{b_x} F_{ij}(t, \tau_x, \tau_y, \mathbf{X}, \mathbf{Y}) m_{ij}(t, \tau_x, \tau_y, \mathbf{X}, \mathbf{Y})\, d\tau_x,$$

$$y_k(t, 0) = \sum_{i,j} \omega_{ij}^k(♀) \cdot \int_{a_y}^{b_y} d\tau_y \int_{a_x}^{b_x} G_{ij}(t, \tau_x, \tau_y, \mathbf{X}, \mathbf{Y}) m_{ij}(t, \tau_x, \tau_y, \mathbf{X}, \mathbf{Y})\, d\tau_x, \tag{1.2}$$

$$i, j, k = \overline{1, N}.$$

Here $[a_x, b_x]$ and $[a_y, b_y]$ are the reproductive intervals for males and females, that is the ages when they can reproduce. It is clear that, defining the fecundity functions in an appropriate way (say, assuming they vanish outside the reproductive intervals), we can set $a_x = a_y = 0$ and $b_x = b_y = \infty$ in (1.2). Equations (1.2) we will call *birth equations*.

Another process, that defines the evolution of population together with the reproduction process, is mortality. If we denote by D_k and E_k the *proportions* of those individuals with genotypes $♂\{k\}$ and $♀\{k\}$, that die off over a unit period of time, then the death rates for these genotypes will be $D_k x_k$ and $E_k y_k$. Naturally, D_k and E_k, which we term *mortality functions*, depend upon both t, τ and the populations themselves. For instance, competition, which in turn is a function of the numbers in competing groups, enhances the mortality functions.

2.2. Sexless Population

The process of mating between higher organisms already assumes that the population is characterized by sexual dimorphism, i.e. that it contains two subpopulations: males and females. Suppose that males and females in a population are indistinguishable neither with respect to the considered genotypic features, nor with respect to the ecologically physiological ones. Consequently we may assume that $D_k \equiv E_k$ for all $k=\overline{1, N}$.

The genetic sex determination stipulates equal proportions of sexes in the offspring, so that $F_{ij} \equiv G_{ij}$ for all $i, j=\overline{1, N}$. Besides, suppose that the offspring distribution in genotypes is also independent of the offspring sex. Whence it follows that $\omega_{ij}^k(♂)=\omega_{ij}^k(♀)=\omega_{ij}^k$ for all $i, j, k=\overline{1, N}$.

Birth and death are the only processes, that define the time variations in populations, therefore, if initially $x_i(0, \tau) \equiv y_i(0, \tau)$ for all $i=\overline{1, N}$, then $x_i(t, \tau) \equiv y_i(t, \tau)$ for any $t>0$. Such a population is said to be *sexless*. Since the subpopulations of males and females evolve absolutely alike in this case, the evolution of one of them totally characterizes the evolution of the whole population.

2.3. Equations for Populations in Evolution

Application of various conservation principles (for mass, energy, etc.) is a widely used method in mechanical and physical modeling. The universality of these principles makes quite natural their application to modeling in biology. Here we use one such principle – the principle of conservation of the number of particles (individuals).

Let each individual with genotype $\{k\}$ be characterized by a set of n parameters: $\eta_1, \eta_2, \ldots, \eta_n$, depending upon the age τ of the individual. These may be the sizes of individuals, their biomass, mobility, and so on. Naturally, the biological time (age) for each individual may differ from the astronomical time (same for the whole population), already since individuals have different birth dates. Let the variations of these parameters be specified by a dynamical system, with the individual age as time:

$$\frac{d\eta_i}{d\tau} = \phi_i(\eta_1, \ldots, \eta_n, t), \quad \eta_i(\tau=0) = \xi_i, \quad i=\overline{1, n}. \tag{3.1}$$

Unlike the astronomical time t, age is a phase variable, since it is an individual characteristic of an organism. Let us accept the simplest assumption about the relationship between age and time: $d\tau/dt=1$, that is, the rate of age variations equals the rate of time variations. Then expanding our n-dimensional phase space to the $(n+1)$-dimensional one by introducing the coordinate τ, we get the following system for the state of individual in the expanded phase space $\{\eta_1, \eta_2, \ldots, \eta_n, \tau\}$:

$$\frac{d\eta_i}{dt} = \phi_i(\eta_1, \ldots, \eta_n, \tau), \quad \frac{d\tau}{dt} = 1, \quad i=\overline{1, n}. \tag{3.2}$$

Define the functions $x_k(t, \tau, \eta_1, \ldots, \eta_n)$ and $y_k(t, \tau, \eta_1, \ldots, \eta_n)$ as the distribution densities for males and females with genotype $\{k\}$ in the phase space. These functions determine the numbers of individuals with appropriate characteristics. Mortality may be regarded as a number of sinks with intensities D_k and E_k, distributed over the phase space. All the newborn individuals are to lie on the phase hyperplane $\tau=0$, therefore any operator that specifies the process of birth ((1.2), for instance) should be the operator of projection onto this plane.

Let us look at some volume V in the phase space, such that the boundary $\tau=0$ lies outside of it. Because of the obvious fact that inside the phase space no new individuals can appear (all new individuals come only from the boundary $\tau=0$), the total number of individuals in V (those living at present plus those who have died by this time) should remain constant, i.e.

$$\int_V x_k(t, \tau, \eta_1, \ldots, \eta_n)\,dv + \int_{t_0}^{t}\int_V D_k x_k(t, \tau, \eta_1, \ldots, \eta_n)\,dv\,dt = \text{const.} \tag{3.3}$$

If we differentiate (3.3) with respect to t and insert the differentiation under the integral sign in the first term, we get

$$\int_V \left[\frac{\partial x_k}{\partial t} + \operatorname{div}(\phi_{n+1} x_k)\right] dv + \int_V D_k x_k\,dv = 0. \tag{3.4}$$

Here $\phi_{n+1} = \{\phi_1, \ldots, \phi_n, 1\}$. And finally, due to the arbitrariness in the choice of the phase volume V, we get

$$\frac{\partial x_k}{\partial t} + \operatorname{div}(\phi_{n+1} x) = -D_k x_k, \quad k = \overline{1, N}. \tag{3.5}$$

Similar equations may be derived for $y_k(t, \tau, \eta_1, \ldots, \eta_n)$.

In this book we treat only one special case of equations (3.5), that is when an individual of each genotype is characterized by only one phase variable – its age τ. In this case system (3.2) is made up of only one equation: $d\tau/dt = 1$ and $\phi_{n+1} = 1$. Then from (3.5) we readily get

$$\frac{\partial x_k}{\partial \tau} + \frac{\partial x_k}{\partial t} = -D_k x_k, \quad k = \overline{1, N}. \tag{3.6}$$

These are the well known equations widely used in demography. Similar will be the equations for $y_k(t, \tau)$:

$$\frac{\partial y_k}{\partial \tau} + \frac{\partial y_k}{\partial t} = -E_k y_k, \quad k = \overline{1, N}. \tag{3.6'}$$

System (3.6), (3.6') with boundary conditions (1.2) and initial conditions $x_k(0, \tau) = x_k^0(\tau)$, $y_k(0, \tau) = y_k^0(\tau)$ completely define the evolution of a population.

2.4. Evolution of Populations and Integral Renewal Equations

Assuming nothing special about the birth functions, let us assume that the mortality functions can depend upon τ, t and the *total* sizes of genotypic groups $\bar{x}_i(t)$ and $\bar{y}_i(t)$. The total sizes are defined as

$$\bar{x}_i(t) = \int_0^\infty x_i(t, \tau)\,d\tau, \quad \bar{y}_i(t) = \int_0^\infty y_i(t, \tau)\,d\tau, \quad i = \overline{1, N}. \tag{4.1}$$

Then the general solution to system (3.6), (3.6') can be presented in the form

$$x_k(t, \tau) = S_k(t-\tau)\Phi_k(\ ),\ y_k(t, \tau) = R_k(t-\tau)\Phi_k(\ ), \tag{4.2}$$

where S_k and R_k are certain functions with an evident biological meaning, which will be clarified somewhat later.

As to the functions Φ_k the situation is more complicated. Let $D_k = D_k(t, \tau, \overline{\mathbf{X}}, \overline{\mathbf{Y}})$, $E_k = E_k(t, \tau, \overline{\mathbf{X}}, \overline{\mathbf{Y}})$. Here $\overline{\mathbf{X}}$ and $\overline{\mathbf{Y}}$ are vectors with components $\overline{x}_i(t)$ and $\overline{y}_i(t)$, $i = \overline{1, N}$. Then

$$\Phi_k(♂) = \exp\left\{-\int_0^\tau D_k[t-\tau+\xi, \xi, \overline{\mathbf{X}}(t-\tau+\xi), \overline{\mathbf{Y}}(t-\tau+\xi)]\,d\xi\right\},$$

$$\Phi_k(♀) = \exp\left\{-\int_0^\tau E_k[t-\tau+xi, \xi, \overline{\mathbf{X}}(t-\tau+\xi), \overline{\mathbf{Y}}(t-\tau+\xi)]\,d\xi\right\}. \tag{4.3}$$

If the functions D_k and E_k are 'good' enough (and this is the common case in these problems), the integrals in (4.3) have no singularities and $\Phi_k(♂) = \Phi(♀) = 1$ when $\tau \to 0$. Then from the boundary conditions (1.2) it follows that $x_k(t, 0) = S_k(t)$, $y_k(t, 0) = R_k(t)$, i.e. functions $S_k(t)$ and $R_k(t)$ are nothing else but the numbers of the newborn.

On substituting the solutions (4.2) into the boundary conditions (1.2) and the initial conditions, we get

$$S_k(t) = \sum_{i,j} \omega_{ij}^k(♂) \int_{a_y}^{b_y} d\tau_y \int_{a_x}^{b_x} F_{ij}(t, \tau_y, \tau_x, \mathbf{X}, \mathbf{Y}) m_{ij}(t, \tau_y, \tau_x, \mathbf{X}, \mathbf{Y})\,d\tau_x, \tag{4.4}$$

$$R_k(t) = \sum_{i,j} \omega_{ij}^k(♀) \int_{a_y}^{b_y} d\tau_y \int_{a_x}^{b_x} G_{ij}(t, \tau_y, \tau_x, \mathbf{X}, \mathbf{Y}) m_{ij}(t, \tau_y, \tau_x, \mathbf{X}, \mathbf{Y})\,d\tau_x,$$

$$S_k(-\tau) = \left.\frac{x_k^0(\tau)}{\Phi_k(♂)}\right|_{t=0},\quad R_k(-\tau) = \left.\frac{y_k^0(\tau)}{\Phi_k(♀)}\right|_{t=0}. \tag{4.5}$$

Here, according to (4.2) and (4.3) the components of vectors $\mathbf{X}$ and $\mathbf{Y}$ depend on $S_i(t-\tau)$ and $R_i(t-\tau)$, $i = \overline{1, N}$, and on the integrals of the already known functions. Apparently, if $t < a_x, a_y$, then the arguments of functions S_i and R_i under the integral signs will be negative, and by (4.5) we get the values that S_i and R_i take on over the interval $[0, \min\{a_x, a_y\}]$. If $t > \min\{a_x, a_y\}$, the integrals in (4.4) may be presented as a sum

$$\int_{a_y}^{b_y}\int_{a_x}^{b_x} = \int_{a_y}^{t}\int_{a_x}^{t} + \int_{t}^{b_y}\int_{a_x}^{t} + \int_{a_y}^{t}\int_{t}^{b_x} + \int_{t}^{b_y}\int_{t}^{b_x}.$$

Then in the last summand $t - \tau \leqslant 0$ and consequently the integrals

$$Q_k(t) = \sum_{i,j} \omega_{ij}^k(♂) \int_t^{b_y} d\tau_y \int_t^{b_x} F_{ij} m_{ij}\,d\tau_x,$$

$$P_k(t) = \sum_{i,j} \omega_{ij}^k(♀) \int_t^{b_y} d\tau_y \int_t^{b_x} G_{ij} m_{ij}\,d\tau_x. \tag{4.6}$$

will depend only on the initial conditions and known functions. And finally system (4.4) may be written in the form

$$S_k(t) = \sum_{i,j}\omega_{ij}^k(\male)\left\{\int_{a_y}^{t}\int_{a_x}^{t} + \int_{a_y}^{t}\int_{t}^{b_x} + \int_{t}^{b_y}\int_{a_x}^{t}\right\} + Q_k(t),$$

$$R_k(t) = \sum_{i,j}\omega_{ij}^k(\female)\left\{\int_{a_y}^{t}\int_{a_x}^{t} + \int_{a_y}^{t}\int_{t}^{b_x} + \int_{t}^{b_y}\int_{a_x}^{t}\right\} + P_k(t). \qquad (4.7)$$

These integral equations completely describe the evolution of a population. They are known as the renewal equations. The existence and uniqueness proof for the solutions to these equations is no difficult problem. In fact, it is easy to show that if the difference between male and female reproductive periods is biologically reasonable, then the current value of the variable in these equations can be found by integration of either the unknown or the initial conditions over a certain preceding time period. If the known functions and the initial conditions contained in the equations are 'good' enough (say, integrable), then the integrals always exist, and therefore exists the solution. And this solution is unique, since for each initial value the corresponding solution is uniquely 'renewed' (by integrating). Moreover, by their biological meaning all the mortality, fecundity, mating functions and the initial numbers are non-negative. Consequently, the solution will be non-negative as well.

From (4.6) and (4.7) it follows that if t exceeds the length of the reproductive period, $t>b_x, b_y$, then $Q_k(t)$, $P_k(t)$, as well as the second and third integrals in (4.7), become indentically zero. Therefore, for sufficiently large t (greater than the length of the reproductive period) instead of (4.7) we can write

$$S_k(t) = \sum_{i,j}\omega_{ij}^k(\male)\int_{a_y}^{b_y}\mathrm{d}\tau_y\int_{a_x}^{b_x}F_{ij}m_{ij}\mathrm{d}\tau_x, \quad t>b_x, b_y,$$

$$R_k(t) = \sum_{i,j}\omega_{ij}^k(\female)\int_{a_y}^{b_y}\mathrm{d}\tau_y\int_{a_x}^{b_x}F_{ij}m_{ij}\mathrm{d}\tau_x, \quad i, j, k=\overline{1, N}. \qquad (4.8)$$

As it follows from the aforesaid, the initial conditions tell only when time does not exceed the reproductive period. The specific time of evolution is measured in dozens and hundreds of generations, therefore, when looking at processes of evolution, instead of the exact equations (4.7) we are free to use the asymptotic equations (4.8), which coincide with the exact ones provided that zero initial conditions are taken. From (4.5) it readily follows that zero initial conditions are equivalent to the assumption about zero values of S_i and R_i for negative arguments.

In what follows only the asymptotic equations (4.8) will be considered as the equations of evolution.

2.5. Panmixia and Other Systems of Mating

Suppose that at any time t the population is characterized by bilateral monogamy, i.e. each female pairs only with one male and each male fertilizes only one female. Suppose a matrix $\| m_{ij}(t, \tau_x, \tau_y) \|$, $i, j=\overline{1, N}$ is given with the entry m_{ij} presenting the number of pairs of the type $♂\{i\}_{\tau_x}$, $♀\{j\}_{\tau_y}$. The unconditional probability of a male of age τ_x to have the genotype $\{i\}$, is

$$P\left\{♂\{i\}_{\tau_x}\right\} = \sum_j \int \frac{m_{ij} d\tau_y}{M(t)}.$$

Here $M(t)=\sum_{i,j} \int\int m_{ij}\, d\tau_y\, d\tau_x$ is the total amount of pairs in the population at time t; the integral is taken with respect to all reproductive ages. Likewise, the unconditional probability of a female of age τ_y to have the genotype $\{j\}$ is

$$P\left\{♀\{j\}_{\tau_y}\right\} = \sum_i \int \frac{m_{ij}\, d\tau_x}{M(t)}.$$

Global panmixia is a system of mating such that the choices of the male $♂\{i\}_{\tau_x}$ and the female $♀\{j\}_{\tau_y}$ are mutually independent, and this is so for all genotypes and all fixed ages.

In order to check this condition we are to calculate the conditional probability that a partner has the given genotype and age, knowing a priori the age and genotype of the second partner. For example,

$$P\left\{♂\{i\}_{\tau_x} \middle| ♀\{j\}_{\tau_y}\right\} = \frac{m_{ij}}{\sum_i \int m_{ij} d\tau_x},$$

$$P\left\{♀\{j\}_{\tau_y} \middle| ♂\{i\}_{\tau_x}\right\} = \frac{m_{ij}}{\sum_j \int m_{ij} d\tau_y}.$$

If now

$$\frac{m_{ij}}{\sum_i \int m_{ij}\, d\tau_x} = \sum_j \frac{\int m_{ij} d\tau_y}{M(t)},$$

$$\frac{m_{ij}}{\sum_j \int m_{ij} d\tau_y} = \sum_i \frac{\int m_{ij} d\tau_x}{M(t)} \tag{5.1}$$

for all ages and genotypes, then the conditional probabilities are equal to the unconditional ones, male and females are chosen independently, and the mating system, characterized by matrix $\| m_{ij} \|$ with elements complying with conditions (5.1), is a global panmixia. Conditions (5.1) can be presented in the form

$$m_{ij}=\frac{\sum_i\int m_{ij}\,\mathrm{d}\tau_x\sum_j\int m_{ij}\,\mathrm{d}\tau_y}{\sum_{i,j}\int\int m_{ij}\,\mathrm{d}\tau_y\,\mathrm{d}\tau_x},\quad i,j=\overline{1,N}.$$

Less restricting is the *genotypic* (or local) panmixia. It is defined with respect to a priori fixed male or female ages. The system of mating is considered to be a local panmixia if for ages τ_x and τ_y the choice of male and female genotypes is mutually independent. To check this condition we are to make sure that elements of matrix $\| m_{ij} \|$ satisfy the equations

$$m_{ij}=\frac{\sum_i m_{ij}\sum_j m_{ij}}{\sum_{i,j} m_{ij}} \tag{5.3}$$

for all $i, j=\overline{1,N}$, and for prefixed ages τ_x and τ_y.

In a similar way we define the *age* panmixia, for which the choice of ages of the a priori fixed male and female genotypes is mutually independent. Under age panmixia the elements of $\| m_{ij} \|$ should comply with the conditions

$$m_{ij}=\frac{\int m_{ij}\,\mathrm{d}\tau_x\int m_{ij}\,\mathrm{d}\tau_y}{\int\int m_{ij}\,\mathrm{d}\tau_x\,\mathrm{d}\tau_y} \tag{5.4}$$

for all reproductive ages and given genotypes of the male ♂$\{i\}$ and the female ♀$\{j\}$.

The fact that conditions (5.3) and (5.4) simultaneously hold does not necessarily mean that conditions (5.2) holds. In other words, combined local and age panmixia do not ensure the existence of the global one.

In case condition (5.2) fails to hold, we can speak about 'deviations' from panmixia or about an *assortative* system of mating. For instance, if

$$\frac{m_{ij}}{\sum_i\int m_{ij}\,\mathrm{d}\tau_x}>\frac{\sum_j\int m_{ij}\,\mathrm{d}\tau_y}{M(t)},$$

that is $P\{♂\{i\}_{\tau_x}\mid ♀\{j\}_{\tau_y}\}>P\{♂\{i\}_{\tau_x}\}$, we can say that males of age τ_x with genotype $\{i\}$ prefer to mate with females of age τ_y with genotype $\{j\}$. Let us then define the function $\theta_{ij}(t,\tau_x,\tau_y)\geqslant 0$ such that

$$\theta_{ij}m_{ij}=\frac{\sum_i\int m_{ij}\,\mathrm{d}\tau_x\sum_j\int m_{ij}\,\mathrm{d}\tau_y}{\sum_{i,j}\int\int m_{ij}\,\mathrm{d}\tau_y\,\mathrm{d}\tau_x}. \tag{5.5}$$

$\theta_{ij}(t,\tau_x,\tau_y)$ will be called *preference functions*. When $\theta_{ij}\equiv 1$, individuals mate at random, i.e. panmixia takes place. For $\theta_{ij}>1$ males $\{i\}_{\tau_x}$ prefer to mate with females $\{j\}_{\tau_y}$, and for $\theta_{ij}<1$ males $\{i\}_{\tau_x}$ avoid these females. If

$\theta_{ij}(t, \tau_x, \tau_y) = \theta(t, \tau_x, \tau_y)$ for all $i, j = \overline{1, N}$, only age preferences come into play; when θ_{ij} is independent of τ_x and τ_y, only genotypic preferences affect mating. Functions θ_{ij} cannot be picked arbitrarily. Evident relations follow from (5.5):

$$\sum_j \int [m_{ij}(\theta_{ij} - 1)]\, d\tau_y = \sum_i \int [m_{ij}(\theta_{ij} - 1)]\, d\tau_x = 0. \tag{5.6}$$

These restrictions result from the assumption about bilateral monogamy, since preference between certain individuals immediately reduces the number of other kinds of couples.

Let us look at the following principle of mating. Let ♂$\{i\}_{\tau_x}$ be picked at random from the set of all males. Then its chance to be picked is $x_i(t, \tau_x)/\bar{x}(t)$, where $\bar{x}(t) = \sum_i \int x_i(t, \tau_x)\, d\tau_x$. Let ♀$\{j\}_{\tau_y}$ be also picked at random from the set of all females with probability $y_j(t, \tau_x)/\bar{y}(t)$, $\bar{y}(t) = \sum_j \int y_j(t, \tau_y)\, d\tau_y$. If in both cases the choice is independent, then the probability of a pair ♂$\{i\}_{\tau_x}$♀$\{j\}_{\tau_y}$ is $x_i(t, \tau_x) y_j(t, \tau_y)/\bar{x}(t)\bar{y}(t)$. If the sex-ratio in the reproductive part of the population is 1:1, then the number of possible couples is in proportion to $\bar{x}(t) = \bar{y}(t)$. But if the 1:1 sex ratio is disturbed, the number of couples will be determined either by the number of females or by the number of males. With most animals, males usually manage to fertilize all females, even though females are more numerous. In this case the number of reproductive pairs is in proportion to the number of females, and assuming that all females mate at the reproductive age, this number is simply equal to the number of females. This is the case considered hereafter. Then

$$m_{ij}(t, \tau_x, \tau_y) = x_i(t, \tau_x) \frac{y_j(t, \tau_y)}{\bar{x}(t)}, \quad i, j = \overline{1, N}. \tag{5.7}$$

However, note that there exist species such that males can fertilize only once. Then the number of reproductive pairs will be determined by the number of males.

It is easy to see that the system of mating given by matrix (5.7) is a global panmixia. Moreover, it complies with the conditions of both local and age panmixia.

An even more general statement is correct: if elements of matrix $\| m_{ij} \|$ can be presented in the form

$$m_{ij}(t, \tau_x, \tau_y) = \mu_i(t, \tau_x)\mu_j(t, \tau_y)\phi(t), \tag{5.8}$$

then the system of mating is a global panmixia. Moreover, in this case for any pair of genotypes age panmixia takes place, and local panmixia takes place for any pair of ages. This is easy to check, substituting (5.8) into the appropriate conditions.

Likewise one can show that if we have

$$m_{ij}(t, \tau_x, \tau_y) = \mu_{ij}(t, \tau_x)\mu_{ij}(t, \tau_y)\phi(t), \tag{5.9}$$

then the corresponding system of mating is age panmixia, and it will be local panmixia if

$$m_{ij}(t, \tau_x, \tau_y) = \mu_i(t, \tau_x, \tau_y)\mu_j(t, \tau_x, \tau_y)\phi(t). \tag{5.10}$$

In what follows almost always (unless otherwise stipulated) the mating system will be regarded as global panmixia with matrix $\| m_{ij} \|$ given by (5.7).

2.6. Principles of Inheritance

As it was already mentioned in Chapter 1, the rules that determine the offspring genotype will be markedly different depending on whether the organisms carry a single or a double set of homologous chromosomes. As a rule, haploid organisms (those with the single set of chromosomes) cannot reproduce sexually, they reproduce by fission, gemmation, sporulation, and consequently they can produce only those similar to themselves (if we exclude mutations). Bacteria, algae, yeast, fungae are haploids. If $x_i(t, \tau)$ is the number of genotype $\{i\}$ of age τ, then for haploids the equations of evolution will take the form

$$\frac{\partial x_i}{\partial t} + \frac{\partial x_i}{\partial \tau} = -D_i x_i,$$

$$x_i(t, 0) = \int_a^b F_i x_i \, d\tau, \quad i = \overline{1, N}, \tag{6.1}$$

$$x_i(0, \tau) = x_i^0(\tau).$$

This is the Lotka equations and nothing else. They are widely used in demography and their theory is developed fairly well. For this reason we do not dwell upon them in this book.

Diploid organisms (with the double chromosome set), as a rule, reproduce sexually, and the offspring, combining the parental chromosome sets, not at all necessarily belongs to the same genotype as one of the parents. Higher plants and animals are diploids, so diploidy and sexual reproduction seem to be evolutionally 'younger' systems.

There exist organisms with chromosome sets with multiplicity higher than two (polyploids). But since they are much more rare in nature than haploids and diploids, we also give no consideration to them in this book.

Let us look at the simplest case, when inheritance of the only character, that makes organisms different in the population, is determined by one autosomal gene, that can be in several states $A_1, A_2, \ldots, A_n$, $n \geqslant 2$. This gene is located at one locus of a chromosome, unrelated to the genetic sex determination. Since organisms contain a double set of chromosomes, n^2 genotypes A_iA_j may be possibly formed. A zygote is formed by two fusing gametes – one from the male, another from the female. Therefore it would be more correct to denote the genotype by $\{♂A_i \, ♀A_j\}$ and from this viewpoint genotypes $\{♂A_i \, ♀A_j\}$ and $\{♂A_j \, ♀A_i\}$ should differ. But actually for the given scheme of inheritance, these genotypes are indistinguishable (the so-called "principle of equality of sexes in inheritance"), and practically populations can produce only $n(n+1)/2$ different genotypes. However, we will distinguish these genotypes (for purely formal reasons).

Consider how organisms of the new generation are produced by a mating pair $♂\{A_iA_k\}$, $♀\{A_sA_j\}$. Each of the partners with probability $1/2$ produce one of the gametes that make up their genotypes: gametes ♂A_i and ♂A_k from ♂$\{A_iA_k\}$, gametes ♀A_s and ♀A_j from ♀$\{A_sA_j\}$. Fusion of these gametes produces a zygote, originating an organisms of the next generation. Consequently with probabilities 1/4 the offspring of the pair ♂$\{A_iA_k\}$, ♀$\{A_sA_j\}$ contains genotypes $\{$♂A_i♀$A_s\}$, $\{$♂A_i♀$A_j\}$, $\{$♂A_k♀$A_s\}$, $\{$♂A_k♀$A_j\}$ or, dropping the symbols ♂ and ♀, $A_iA_s, A_iA_j, A_kA_s, A_kA_j$. (Recall that for purely formal reasons we distinguish genotypes A_iA_j, A_jA_i, etc.).

To reflect the principal action of diploidy, we introduce a new numeration for all quantities related to genotypes: we use two indices instead of one. Then the genotype A_iA_j will be denoted by $\{ij\}$, the number of males of age τ_x with genotype A_iA_{jj} – by $x_{ij}(t, \tau_x)$ and so on.

Since $\{is\}$, $\{ij\}$, $\{ks\}$, $\{kj\}$ are the only genotypes that can appear with equal frequencies in the offspring of the pair ♂$\{ik\}$, ♀$\{sj\}$, the offspring sex being independent of its genotype, the concrete expressions for the components of Ω may be presented in the form

$$\omega_{ik,sj}^{lm} = \frac{1}{4}\left[\delta_i^l+\delta_k^l\right]\left[\delta_s^m+\delta_j^m\right], \quad i, k, s, j, l, m=\overline{1, n}. \tag{6.2}$$

Here

$$\delta_i^l = \begin{cases} 1, & i = l, \\ 0, & i \neq l, \end{cases}$$

is the Kronecker symbol.

A similar transmission mechanism for the hereditary material is implied in Mendel's laws, and therefore the heredity principle presented by (6.2) (the principle of offspring distribution with respect to genotypes), we will call the *Mendelian law*.

More complicated situations are also possible, for instance, when the genotype determines the offspring sex; or when inheritance is determined by several genes localized either on different chromosomes segments, or on different chromosomes; or when normal gamete segregation is disturbed, that is when gametes are produced with different probabilities, etc. However, we give no consideration to these cases here, postponing it to those chapters that specially deal with these situations.

2.7. Multi-Allele Autosomal Gene: Equations of Evolution

Suppose a sufficiently large population is given, with inheritance determined by one n-allele autosomal gene.

We will look at two systems of mating: one, defined by equations (5.7), or in new notations

$$m_{ik,sj} = \frac{x_{ik}(t, \tau_x)y_{sj}(t, \tau_y)}{x(t)}, \quad i, k, s, j=\overline{1, n},$$

$$x(t) = \sum_{i,j}\int_{a_x}^{b_x} x_{ij}(t, \tau_x)\, d\tau_x, \tag{7.1}$$

and the other one, defined by the equations

$$m_{ik,sj} = \frac{x_{ik}(t, \tau_x) y_{sj}(t, \tau_y) \delta(\tau_x - \tau_y)}{x(t)}, \quad i, k, s, j = \overline{1, n}, \tag{7.2}$$

$$x(t, \tau_x) = \sum_{i,j} x_{ij}(t, \tau_x), \quad \delta\text{--delta}-\text{function.}$$

While the first mating system, being global panmixia (as well as local and age panmixia), describes random mating both between genotypes and between all reproductive ages, the second one, being only local panmixia, implies that mating takes place only between individuals of one and the same age.

As for the functions of fecundity and mortality, we will assume, firstly, that they depend only on age, and, secondly, that the fecundity functions may be presented in either of the two forms:

$$F_{ik,sj}(\tau_x, \tau_y) = F_{ik}(\tau_x) F_{sj}(\tau_y),$$

$$G_{ik,sj}(\tau_x, \tau_y) = G_{ik}(\tau_x) G_{sj}(\tau_y), \tag{7.3}$$

or

$$F_{ik,sj}(\tau_x, \tau_y) = \frac{1}{2}[F_{ik}(\tau_x) + F_{sj}(\tau_y)],$$

$$G_{ik,sj}(\tau_x, \tau_y) = \frac{1}{2}[G_{ik}(\tau_x) + G_{sj}(\tau_y)]. \tag{7.4}$$

In other words, fecundity of a couple is either a multiplicative or an additive function of the fecundities of constituting individuals.

It follows from the condition of equality of sexes in inheritance, that

$$F_{ik,sj} = F_{ki,sj} = F_{ki,js} = F_{ik,js},$$

$$G_{ik,sj} = G_{ki,sj} = G_{ki,js} = G_{ik,js}, \quad i, k, j = \overline{1, n}, \tag{7.5}$$

and that quantities with two-letter indices are symmetric with respect to these indices $F_{ik} = F_{ki}$, $D_{ij} = D_{ji}$, etc. Relations (7.3), (7.4) impose even more stringent conditions on the fecundity functions:

$$F_{ik,sj} = F_{sj,ik}, \quad G_{ik,sj} = G_{sj,ik}.$$

Suppose that the 1:1 ratio between sexes is maintained in the population and mortality is independent of the organism's sex. Since the gene is autosomal (with no sex linkage), the population may be considered 'sexless' (in the sense of the definition from Section 2.2). Therefore we will consider only the evolution of x_{ij}, thinking that $y_{ij} = x_{ij}$.

Substituting the concrete expressions for $m_{ik,sj}$, $F_{ik,sj}$ (formula (7.1), (7.3)) into the birth equation (1.2), making use of the hereditary principle, specified by equation (6.2), and taking into account the order of genotype indices, we get

$$x_{lm}(t, 0) = \frac{1}{x(t)} \sum_{i,k,s,j} \left[\delta_i^l + \delta_k^l\right] \left[\delta_s^m + \delta_j^m\right] \times$$

$$\times \int_a^b \int_a^b F_{ik}(\tau_x) x_{ik}(t, \tau_x) F_{sj}(\tau_y) x_{sj}(t, \tau_y)\, d\tau_y\, d\tau_x, \tag{7.6}$$

$$x(t) = \sum_{i,j} \int_a^b x_{ij}(t, \tau_x)\, d\tau_x, \quad i, k, s, j, l, m = \overline{1, n}.$$

Summing up and taking into account the form of the integrand, we can rewrite (7.6) in the following way

$$x_{lm}(t, 0) = \frac{\sigma_l(t)\sigma_m(t)}{x(t)}, \quad l, m = \overline{1, n}, \tag{7.7}$$

where

$$\sigma_i = \sum_k \int_a^b F_{ik}(\tau) x_{ik}(t, \tau)\, d\tau, \quad i, k = \overline{1, n}.$$

In accord with the theory set forth in Section 2.4, we can write the integral equations of evolution for $S_{lm}(t) = x_{lm}(t, 0)$ (the special case of system (4.8)):

$$S_{lm}(t) = \frac{\sigma_l(t)\sigma_m(t)}{x(t)}, \quad l, m = \overline{1, n}, \tag{7.8}$$

where

$$\sigma_i(t) = \sum_k \int_a^b K_{ik}(\tau) S_{ik}(t-\tau)\, d\tau, \tag{7.9}$$

$$K_{ik}(\tau) = F_{ik}(\tau)\Phi_{ik}(\tau), \quad i, k = \overline{1, n}, \quad \tau \in [a, b], \tag{7.10}$$

$$\Phi_{ik}(\tau) = \exp\left\{-\int_0^\tau D_{ik}(\xi)\, d\xi\right\}, \tag{7.11}$$

$$x(t) = \sum_{l,m} \int_a^b \Phi_{lm}(\tau) S_{lm}(t-\tau)\, d\tau. \tag{7.12}$$

From (7.8) it follows that symmetry of functions F_{ij}, D_{ij} and $S_{ij}(t-\tau)$ with respect to indices implies that $S_{ij}(t)$ is also symmetric, so that $S_{ij}(t) = S_{ji}(t)$.

Suppose now that mating is again specified by formula (7.1), but fecundity is additive, that is the fecundity function may be represented as (7.4). Then going through the same operations as in the previous case, we get the following evolutionary equations for $S_{lm}(t)$:

$$S_{lm}(t) = \frac{\sigma_l(t)x_m(t) + \sigma_m(t)x_l(t)}{2x(t)}, \quad l, m = \overline{1, n}, \tag{7.13}$$

where

$$x_i(t) = \sum_k \int_a^b \Phi_{ik}(\tau) S_{ik}(t-\tau)\, d\tau, \quad i, k = \overline{1, n}, \tag{7.14}$$

and the variables σ_l, σ_m, $x(t)$ are defined by (7.9)–(7.12). Note that here again $S_{ij}(t)=S_{ji}(t)$.

If the system of mating is given by (7.2), then the evolutionary equations may be written in the following form (for multiplicative fecundity):

$$S_{lm}(t) = \int_a^b \frac{\eta_l(t, \tau)\eta_m(t, \tau)}{x(t, \tau)}, \quad l, m=\overline{1, n}, \tag{7.15}$$

where

$$\eta_i(t, \tau) = \sum_k K_{ik}(\tau)S_{ik}(t-\tau), \quad i, k=\overline{1, n}, \tag{7.16}$$

$$x(t, \tau) = \sum_{l,m} \Phi_{lm}(\tau)S_{lm}(t-\tau). \tag{7.17}$$

And eventually, for additive fecundity the evolutionary equations can be represented in the form

$$S_{lm}(t) = \int_a^b \frac{\eta_l(t, \tau)x_m(t, \tau)+\eta_m(t, \tau)x_l(t, \tau)}{2x(t, \tau)}\, d\tau, \tag{7.18}$$

$$l, m=\overline{1, n}.$$

Here

$$x_i(t, \tau) = \sum_k \Phi_{ik}(\tau)S_{ik}(t-\tau), \quad i, k=\overline{1, n}, \tag{7.19}$$

and η_l, η_m, $x(t, \tau)$ are specified by (7.16), (7.17). Obviously, in these two models, just like in the two previous ones, $S_{ij}(t)=S_{ji}(t)$.

The obtained equations of evolution, being non-linear and integral, are rather hard to study, and there is only a vague resemblance with the widely known Fisher–Haldane–Wright equations of population genetics. Naturally questions arise: "Under what conditions do these equations turn into the classic ones?" "What other types of equations, besides the classic ones, may be obtained?"

2.8. Equations of Evolution with Specific Demographic Functions

2.8.1. *Global Panmixia, Multiplicative Fecundity*

In this Section we look at those situations, when demographic functions (functions of fecundity and mortality) are independent of age.

Let the evolutionary equations be given in the form (7.8) – (7.12). Introduce new variables: $s_i=\sum_j S_{ij}$ for the number of alleles among the newborn, and $u_{ij}=S_{ij}/\sum_{i,j} S_{ij}$ and $p_i=s_i/\sum_i s_i$ for the frequencies of genotypes and alleles, respectively. Then from (7.8) it follows that

$$u_{ij} = p_i p_j, \quad i, j=\overline{1, n}. \tag{8.1}$$

The relations (8.1) are widely known in genetics as the *Hardy–Weinberg principle.* Besides, from (7.8) we immediately get

$$p_i = \frac{\sigma_i}{\sigma}, \quad \sigma = \sum_i \sigma_i, \tag{8.2}$$

$$S(t) = \sum_{i,j} S_{ij}(t) = \frac{\sigma^2}{x(t)}. \tag{8.3}$$

Then to describe evolution instead of using (7.8) we can consider the equations for frequencies p_i and the total population size S:

$$p_i(t) = \frac{\left\{\sum_j \int_a^b K_{ij}(\tau) p_i(t-\tau) p_j(t-\tau) S(t-\tau)\, d\tau\right\}}{\sigma(t)}, \tag{8.4}$$

$$\sigma(t) = \sum_{i,j} \int_a^b K_{ij}(\tau) p_i(t-\tau) p_j(t-\tau) S(t-\tau)\, d\tau, \tag{8.5}$$

$$S(t) = \frac{\sigma^2}{\left\{\sum_{i,j} \int_a^b \Phi_{ij}(\tau) p_i(t-\tau) p_j(t-\tau) S(t-\tau)\, d\tau\right\}}. \tag{8.6}$$

Substituting $\xi = t - \tau$, all integrals in our equations may be rewritten in a somewhat different form. For instance,

$$I = \int_a^b K_{ij}(\tau) p_i(t-\tau) p_j(t-\tau) S(t-\tau)\, d\tau =$$

$$= \int_{t-b}^{t-a} K_{ij}(t-\xi) p_i(\xi) p_j(\xi) S(\xi)\, d\xi.$$

Let us think that the reproductive interval starts from the zero age, that is, $a = 0$, and that $b = \infty$. Deriving the asymptotic equations of evolution, we assumed that $S_{ij} = 0$ for negative values of the argument (see Section 2.4). Therefore the lower limit $t - b$ can be replaced by zero. And finally,

$$I = \int_0^t K_{ij}(t-\xi) p_i(\xi) p_j(\xi) S(xi)\, d\xi. \tag{8.7}$$

Integrals presented in this form are apt to be differentiated with respect to the parameter t. Differentiating (8.4) with respect to t, we get

$$\frac{dp_i(t)}{dt} = \frac{1}{\sigma(t)} \left\{ \int_0^t [v_i'(t, \xi) p_i(\xi) - v'(t, \xi) p_i(t)] S(\xi)\, d\xi \right\} + \tag{8.8}$$

$$+ \frac{S(t)}{\sigma(t)} \left\{ p_i(t) \left[\sum_j K_{ij}(0) p_j(t) - \sum_{i,j} K_{ij}(0) p_i(t) p_j(t) \right] \right\},$$

where

$$v_i'(t, \xi) = \sum_j K_{ij}'(t-\xi)p_j(\xi), \quad v' = \sum_{i,j} K_{ij}'(t-\xi)p_i(\xi)p_j(\xi),$$

K_{ij}' is the derivative of K_{ij} with respect to $t-\xi$, which can be presented in the form

$$K_{ij}' = \left[\frac{F_{ij}'}{F_{ij}} - D_{ij}\right]K_{ij}. \tag{8.9}$$

Suppose the fecundity and mortality functions are independent of age, their genotypes being indistinguishable with respect to mortality, i.e. $D_{ij} = D = \text{const}$. Then, by (8.9), $K_{ij}' = -DK_{ij}$ and the first term in (8.8) vanishes. In fact,

$$\frac{1}{\sigma(t)}\int_0^t \sum_j K_{ij}'(t-\xi)p_i(\xi)p_j(\xi)S(\xi)\,d\xi =$$

$$= -\frac{D}{\sigma(t)}\int_0^t \sum_j K_{ij}(t-\xi)p_i(\xi)p_j(\xi)S(\xi)\,d\xi = -Dp_i(t),$$

$$\frac{p_i(t)}{\sigma(t)}\int_0^t \sum_{i,j} K_{ij}'(t-\xi)p_i(\xi)p_j(\xi)S(\xi)\,d\xi =$$

$$= -\frac{Dp_i(t)}{\sigma(t)}\int_0^t \sum_{i,j} K_{ij}(t-\xi)p_i(\xi)p_j(\xi)S(\xi)\,d\xi = -Dp_i(t).$$

Consequently, only the second term remains, and we come to the evolutionary equation in the form

$$\frac{dp_i(t)}{dt} = \frac{S(t)}{\sigma(t)}p_i(t)[w_i(t) - w(t)],$$

$$w_i = \sum_j w_{ij}p_j, \tag{8.10}$$

$$w = \sum_i w_i p_i = \sum_{i,j} w_{ij}p_ip_j, \quad i, j = \overline{1, n},$$

where $w_{ij} = K_{ij}(0) = F_{ij}$. Let us look more attentively at the coefficient $S(t)/\sigma(t)$. Under our assumptions

$$\frac{S(t)}{\sigma(t)} = \frac{\sigma(t)}{x(t)} = \frac{\sum_{i,j} F_{ij}\int_0^t \Phi(t-\xi)S(\xi)p_i(\xi)p_j(\xi)\,d\xi}{\sum_{i,j}\int_0^t \Phi(t-\xi)S(\xi)p_i(\xi)p_j(\xi)\,d\xi}$$

or, taking into account the normalization $\sum_i p_i = 1$ and substituting $w = \sum_{i,j} F_{ij}p_ip_j$, we get

$$\frac{S(t)}{\sigma(t)} = \frac{\int_0^t \Phi(t-\xi)S(\xi)w(\xi)\,d\xi}{\int_0^t \Phi(t-\xi)S(\xi)\,d\xi}. \tag{8.11}$$

By definition the function $\Phi(t-\xi)S(\xi)$ does not change its sign over the interval $[0, t]$, therefore using the mean-value theorem, we can get

$$\frac{S(t)}{\sigma(t)} = w(T), \quad 0 \leqslant T \leqslant t.$$

Obviously $w(T) \geqslant \min_{i,j} F_{ij} > 0$ when $F_{ij} > 0$. (It can be proved that w is positive even under weaker restrictions, $F_{ij} \geqslant 0$, but here we skip it.) Consequently, in (8.10) we can change over to the new time

$$\theta = \int_0^t \frac{S(\xi)}{\sigma(\xi)} \mathrm{d}\xi \tag{8.12}$$

and rewrite (8.10) in the form

$$\frac{\mathrm{d}p_i}{\mathrm{d}\theta} = p_i(w_i - w), \quad i = \overline{1, n}. \tag{8.13}$$

System (8.13) is nothing else than the classical Fisher–Haldane–Wright equations, well known in population genetics. The variables w_{ij} (which coincide with fecundities in our case) are known as the *Malthusian parameters* of the appropriate genotypes. Evidently, systems (8.10) and (8.13) have identic phase portraits – the only difference is in the rate with which the representing point moves along phase trajectories.

The equations derived above characterize the evolution only of the genetic structure of the population. To describe evolution completely we are to supplement them with the evolutionary equations for the total population number $S(t)$ or for variables related to it – $\sigma(t)$, $x(t)$. Differentiating the expressions for $\sigma(t)$ and $x(t)$ with respect to t (see formulas (8.5) and (7.12)), we get

$$\frac{\mathrm{d}\sigma}{\mathrm{d}t} = wS - D\sigma, \quad \frac{\mathrm{d}x}{\mathrm{d}t} = S - Dx, \tag{8.14}$$

or, taking into account that $S = \sigma^2/x$,

$$\frac{\mathrm{d}\sigma}{\mathrm{d}t} = \frac{w\sigma^2}{x} - D\sigma, \quad \frac{\mathrm{d}x}{\mathrm{d}t} = \frac{\sigma^2}{x} - Dx, \tag{8.15}$$

$$\frac{\mathrm{d}S}{\mathrm{d}t} = \frac{S}{\sigma}\left[2wS - D\sigma - \frac{S^2}{\sigma}\right].$$

From (8.15) we can easily derive the equation for the ratio $z = S/\sigma$:

$$\frac{\mathrm{d}z}{\mathrm{d}t} = z^2(w - z), \tag{8.16}$$

or in terms of the new time

$$\frac{\mathrm{d}z}{\mathrm{d}\theta} = z(w - z). \tag{8.17}$$

Let $p_i(\theta)$, $i = \overline{1, n}$ be a solution to system (8.13). Then $w[p_i(\theta), \ldots, p_n(\theta)] = w(\theta)$. Suppose there exists the limit $\lim_{\theta\to\infty} w(\theta) = w^*$. Then $z \to w^*$ for $\theta \to \infty$, and as it follows from the third equation in (8.15), $\dot{S}=[(w^*)^2-D]S=cS$, where $c=$const. In other words, over the course of a significant period of time the total population number will vary exponentially according to the Malthusian principle.

In conclusion let us note that a similar form of evolutionary equations is obtained, if we assume that K_{ij} is independent of age. Then $K'_{ij}=0$, the first term in (8.8) vanishes and we get the evolutionary equation in the form of (8.10). The equations (8.14) for the total population become:

$$\frac{d\sigma}{dt} = wS,$$

$$\frac{dx}{dt} = S-\sum_{i,j}\int_0^t D_{ij}(t-\xi)\Phi_{ij}(t-\xi)p_i(\xi)p_j(\xi)S(\xi)\,d\xi, \tag{8.18}$$

and the equation for $z=S/\sigma$ becomes:

$$\frac{dz}{dt} = z^2(w-z+\frac{I_D}{\sigma}), \tag{8.19}$$

where I_D is the integral from the second equation in (8.18). Hence we immediately see, that though the phase portraits of these two systems are identic in the space $\{p_i\geqslant 0, \sum_i p_i=1, i=1,n\}$, the rates of evolution differ.

From the condition that

$$K_{ij} = F_{ij}(\tau)\exp\left\{-\int_0^\tau D_{ij}(\xi)\,d\xi\right\}$$

be independent of age, immediately follows that $F_{ij}(\tau)=K_{ij}\exp\{\int_0^\tau D_{ij}(\xi)\,d\xi\}$, i.e. that fecundity is to increase with age in inverse proportion to the chance to live up to this age (the function $\Phi_{ij}(\tau)=\exp\{-\int_0^\tau D_{ij}(\xi)\,d\xi\}$ defines this probability). In this case individuals are already fertile at the zero age. We may argue which of the two hypotheses is more biologically grounded – this one or the one that demographic functions are independent of age, but this discussion lies beyond the scope of this book. Since both these hypotheses result in approximately similar results, in the subsequent Sections we will make use of only one hypothesis, namely that F_{ij} and D_{ij} are independent of age.

2.8.2. *Global Panmixia, Additive Fecundity*

Let us now look at the evolutionary equations for a population with global panmixia and additive fecundity function (see (7.13)). Passing to the frequencies of genotypes and alleles, u_{ij} and p_i, and substituting the new frequencies: $\pi_i=\sigma_i/\sum_i\sigma_i$ and $\rho_i=x_i/\sum x_i$, from (7.13) we get

$$u_{ij} = \frac{1}{2}(\pi_i\rho_j+\pi_j\rho_i),\quad p_i = \frac{1}{2}(\pi_i+\rho_i). \tag{8.20}$$

Just like in the preceeding case, suppose that F_{ij} and D_{ij} are independent of age and that $D_{ij}=D=\text{const}$. Then applying the same methods as in subsection 2.8.1., we come to the following system of equations:

$$\frac{d\pi_i}{dt} = \frac{1}{2}\left[\pi_i \sum_j F_{ij}\rho_j + \rho_i \sum_j F_{ij}\pi_j\right] - \pi_i \sum_{i,j} F_{ij}\pi_i\rho_j,$$

$$\frac{d\rho_i}{dt} = \frac{S(t)}{2x(t)}(\pi_i - \rho_i), \quad i, j = \overline{1, n}, \tag{8.21}$$

$$\frac{S(t)}{x(t)} = \frac{\sum_{i,j} F_{ij} \int_0^t \Phi(t-\xi) S(\xi) \pi_i(\xi) \rho_j(\xi)\, d\xi}{\int_0^t \Phi(t-\xi) S(\xi)\, d\xi}, \tag{8.22}$$

$$\Phi(t-\xi) = \exp\{-D\cdot(t-\xi)\}.$$

Evidently, for S/x we have the same estimate as in the previous subsection:

$$\frac{S(t)}{x(t)} = \sum_{i,j} F_{ij}\pi_i(T)\rho_j(T) = w_1(T), \quad 0 \leqslant T \leqslant t, \tag{8.23}$$

that is $w_1(T) \geqslant \min_{i,j} F_{ij} > 0$, and the evolution of ρ_i may be treated in terms of new time $T = \int_0^t w_1(T)\, dT$.

Consider new the equations for the evolution of the total population. From (7.13), summing over all indices, we have

$$S(t) = \sigma(t) = \sum_{i,j} \int_0^t K_{ij}(t-\xi)\rho_i(\xi)\rho_j(\xi) S(\xi)\, d\xi, \tag{8.24}$$

or if we differentiate with respect to parameter t,

$$\frac{dS}{dt} = (w_1 - D)S. \tag{8.25}$$

The dynamics of the ratio $z_1 = S/x$, characterizing the rate of the genetic evolution, can be represented by the equation

$$\frac{dz_1}{dt} = z_1(w_1 - z_1). \tag{8.26}$$

System (8.21) together with the Equation (8.26) completely describe the evolution of the genetic structure of the population.

2.8.3. *Local Panmixia*

Let us now look at the models with local panmixia. For multiplicative fecundity of a pair (Equations (7.15)), under the same assumptions concerning the fecundity and mortality functions (independence of age and equal mortality for all genotypes), the equations of evolution will be

$$\frac{d\tilde{p}_i}{dt} = V(t)\tilde{p}_i(\tilde{w}_i - \tilde{w}),$$
$$\tilde{w}_i = \sum_i w_{ij}\tilde{p}_j, \quad \tilde{w} = \sum_{i,j} w_{ij}\tilde{p}_i\tilde{p}_j, \quad i, j=\overline{1, n}. \tag{8.27}$$

Here again $w_{ij}=F_{ij}$, but frequencies $\tilde{p}_i$ are no longer allele frequencies. They are expressed in terms of S_{ij} by the formulas

$$\tilde{p}_i = \sum_j \frac{F_{ij}S_{ij}}{\sum_{i,j} F_{ij}S_{ij}}, \quad i, j=\overline{1, n}. \tag{8.28}$$

The function $V(t)=\sum_{i,j} F_{ij}u_{ij}$, where u_{ij} are the genotype frequencies, is positive when $F_{ij}>0$. Therefore, we can introduce the new time $\theta=\int_0^t V(\xi)\,d\xi$ and represent (8.27) in the form of classical equations:

$$\frac{d\tilde{p}_i}{d\theta} = \tilde{p}_i(\tilde{w}_i - \tilde{w}), \quad i=\overline{1, n}. \tag{8.29}$$

Obviously, the phase portraits of systems (8.27) and (8.29) are identic.

Equations for the total population and the factor V will have the form

$$\frac{dS}{dt} = (V^2 - D)S, \quad \frac{dV}{dt} = V^2(\tilde{w} - V). \tag{8.30}$$

In the case of additive fecundity, when F_{ij} and $D_{ij}=D$ are independent of age, Equations (7.18) take the form similar to that of (8.21) but with π_i substituted by $\tilde{p}_i$, ρ_i – by p_i, and the factor $S(t)/x(t)$ by $V(t)=\sum_{i,j} F_{ij}u_{ij}$.

Thus, we can see that the classical equations of population genetics can be derived from the general evolutionary equations under very unnatural assumptions, namely that fecundity and mortality are independent of age, and moreover that mortality is equal for all genotypes. Of course, we did not prove that these assumptions are unique, maybe other assumptions can provide the same result. However, we failed to find them. The results obtained should make us alert: "Is everything O.K. in the fundamentals of the classical theory if they turn out to be based on assumptions absurd from the biological viewpoint?" Nevertheless, we will widely use models of this kind; partly due to their relative simplicity, and partly since in spite of the fact that they are derived under artificial assumptions, they still reflect the basic mechanisms of the microevolutionary process.

2.9. Equations of Evolution: Fecundity of a Couple is Determined by that of the Female

Quite frequently it is assumed that the number of offspring of a reproductive couple depends only on the female age and genotype, that is

$$F_{ik,sj}(\tau_x, \tau_y) = F_{sj}(\tau_y), \quad F_{sj} = F_{js},$$
$$G_{ik,sj}(\tau_x, \tau_y) = G_{sj}(\tau_y), \quad G_{sj} = G_{js}. \tag{9.1}$$

We do not discuss here whether this assumption is biologically correct or not, we only note that a hypothesis of this kind is rather popular in papers on mathematical population genetics.

Obviously this hypothesis (unlike the hypotheses of Section 7) immediately breaks the symmetry between $S_{ij}(t)$ and $R_{ij}(t)$, that stand for numbers of genotypes $\{ij\}$ and $\{ji\}$, that is, $S_{ij} \neq S_{ji}$ and $R_{ij} \neq R_{ji}$, though actually genotypes $\{ij\}$ and $\{ji\}$ are identic. To prove this statement write out the evolutionary equations for the 'sexless' population with global panmixia. Just as in Section 7, the birth equations are

$$x_{lm}(t, 0) = \frac{1}{x(t)} \sum_{i,k,s,j} \left[\delta_i^l + \delta_k^l\right] \left[\delta_s^m + \delta_j^m\right] \times$$
$$\times \int_a^b \int_a^b x_{ik}(t, \tau_x) F_{sj}(\tau_y) x_{sj}(t, \tau_y) \, d\tau_y \, d\tau_x, \tag{9.2}$$
$$x(t) = \sum_{i,j} \int_a^b x_{ij}(t, \tau_x) \, d\tau_x.$$

Summing over i, j, k, s, we get

$$x_{lm}(t, 0) = \frac{x_l(t) \chi_m(t)}{x(t)}, \quad l, m = \overline{1, n}, \tag{9.3}$$

where

$$x_i(t) = \sum_k \int_a^b x_{ik}(t, \tau) \, d\tau,$$
$$\chi_i(t) = \sum_k \int_a^b F_{ki}(\tau) x_{ki}(t, \tau) \, d\tau, \quad i, k = \overline{1, n}. \tag{9.4}$$

Passing to integral equations for $S_{lm}(t)$, instead of (9.3) we will have

$$S_{lm} = \frac{x_l(t) \sigma_m(t)}{x(t)}, \quad l, m = \overline{1, n}, \tag{9.5}$$

where

$$\sigma_i(t) = \sum_k \int_a^b K_{ki}(t, \tau) S_{ki}(t - \tau) \, d\tau,$$
$$x_i(t) = \sum_k \int_a^b \Phi_{ik}(\tau) S_{ik}(t - \tau) \, d\tau, \quad i, k = \overline{1, n}. \tag{9.6}$$

Functions K_{ki} and Φ_{ik} have the same meaning as in Section 7. That $S_{ij}(t)$ is asymmetric with respect to indices immediately follows from (9.5). This result is quite natural since by such a hypothesis about fecundity we assume that partners play unequal roles in the reproductive process. However, if we now define the number of the genotype $\{ij\}$ as $\tilde{S}_{ij}=1/2(S_{ij}+S_{ji})$, we get $\tilde{S}_{ij}=\tilde{S}_{ji}$, this bringing us back to the model with additive fecundity (see Equation (7.13)). Therefore, there is no use to give any special consideration to this case.

2.10. Equal Fecundity, Different Mortality: Another Form for Evolutionary Equations

Up till now we assumed that genotypes are different only with respect to the age-independent fecundity; mortality was the same for all genotypes. Let us now treat the inverse situation: fecundities of all genotypes are the same and equal to F, but genotypes differ with respect to mortality D_{ij}. Like before let us think that F and D_{ij} are independent of age.

Since fecundities are the same, there is no use in studying multiplicative and additive fecundities separately: the results will be the same. The only difference (related to the definition of fecundity) is that the constant that appears, is F^2 in the first case, and F – in the second. Therefore, we restrict ourselves to the case of multiplicative fecundity.

Suppose that there is global panmixia in the population. Then for our assumptions from (7.8) – (7.12) it follows that

$$S_{ij}(t) = \frac{F^2 x_i(t) x_j(t)}{x(t)}, \quad S(t) = F^2 x(t),$$
$$x(t) = \sum_i x_i(t), \quad x_i(t) = \sum_j x_{ij}(t), \tag{10.1}$$
$$x_{ij}(t) = \int_a^b \Phi_{ij}(\tau) S_{ij}(t-\tau)\, \mathrm{d}\tau, \quad i,j=\overline{1,n}.$$

Differentiating x_{ij} with respect to t, we get (for $a=0$)

$$\frac{\mathrm{d}x_{ij}}{\mathrm{d}t} = -D_{ij}x_{ij}+S_{ij}, \quad i,j=\overline{1,n}, \tag{10.2}$$

or in frequencies $u_{ij}=S_{ij}/S$ and $\tilde{u}_{ij}=x_{ij}/x$,

$$\frac{\mathrm{d}\tilde{u}_{ij}}{\mathrm{d}t} = \tilde{u}_{ij}\left[\sum_{i,j} D_{ij}\tilde{u}_{ij} - D_{ij}\right] + F^2(u_{ij}+\tilde{u}_{ij}), \quad i,j=\overline{1,n}. \tag{10.3}$$

From (10.1) it immediately follows that

$$u_{ij} = \tilde{p}_i\tilde{p}_j, \quad \tilde{p}_i = \frac{\sum_j x_{ij}}{x} = \sum_j \tilde{u}_{ij}. \tag{10.4}$$

The Equations (10.3) together with the relations (10.4) completely define the evolution of the population genotypic structure. Since $S=F^2x$, by summing in (10.2) we get the equation for the population size:

$$\frac{dS}{dt} = S\left[F^2 - \sum_{i,j} D_{ij}\tilde{u}_{ij}\right]. \tag{10.5}$$

Equations for gene frequencies result from summation of (10.3) over j, since $p_i = \sum_j u_{ij} = \tilde{p}_i$, we have

$$\frac{dp_i}{dt} = p_i \sum_{i,j} D_{ij}\tilde{u}_{ij} - \sum_j D_{ij}\tilde{u}_{ij}, \quad i, j = \overline{1, n}. \tag{10.6}$$

The right-hand sides in these equations depend on $\tilde{u}_{ij}$, which do not satisfy the relationships of the Hardy–Weinberg type. Therefore to close system (10.6) we are to write the equations for $\xi_{ij} = p_i p_j - \tilde{u}_{ij}$:

$$\frac{d\xi_{ij}}{dt} = -F^2\xi_{ij} + (p_i p_j + \xi_{ij})(W + D_{ij}) -$$

$$-(p_i W_j + p_j W_i), \quad i, j = \overline{1, n}, \tag{10.7}$$

where $W_i = \sum_j D_{ij}(p_i p_j + \xi_{ij})$, $W = \sum_i W_i$. For sufficiently large $F \gg \max D_{ij}$ these equations can be written in the form

$$\frac{d\xi_{ij}}{dt} = -F^2\xi_{ij} + \epsilon\phi_{ij}(p_1, \ldots, p_n, \xi_{11}, \ldots, \xi_{nn}). \tag{10.8}$$

ξ_{ij} tends to zero for small ϵ and $t \to \infty$, hence we can carry on from (10.6) to its asymptotic analogy

$$\frac{dp_i}{dt} = p_i\left[\sum_{i,j} D_{ij} p_i p_j - \sum_j D_{ij} p_j\right]. \tag{10.9}$$

We easily see that setting $w_{ij} = 1 - D_{ij}$, we come to the equations of population genetics in their classical form.

Consider the case of local panmixia. From (7.15) – (7.17) we find

$$S_{ij}(t) = F^2 \int_a^b \frac{x_i(t, \tau)x_j(t, \tau)}{x(t, \tau)}\, d\tau,$$

$$x(t, \tau) = \sum_i x_i(t, \tau), \quad x_i(t, \tau) = \sum_j x_{ij}(t, \tau), \tag{10.10}$$

$$x_{ij}(t, \tau) = \Phi_{ij}(\tau)S_{ij}(t - \tau), \quad i, j = \overline{1, n}.$$

Let us introduce the variable

$$x_{ij}(t) = \int_a^b \Phi_{ij}(\tau)S_{ij}(t - \tau)\, d\tau, \quad i, j = \overline{1, n}. \tag{10.11}$$

Differentiating $x_{ij}(t)$ with respect to t for $a = 0$ we get

$$\frac{dx_{ij}}{dt} = -D_{ij}x_{ij} + S_{ij}, \quad i, j = \overline{1, n}. \tag{10.12}$$

These equations coincide with Equations (10.2) which were derived for the case of global panmixia.

Let $p_i = \sum_j S_{ij} / S$, $\tilde{u}_{ij} = x_{ij}(t) / \sum_{i,j} x_{ij}(t)$. Summing up in (10.10) over j, differentiating with respect to t and changing over to frequencies p_i and $\tilde{u}_{ij}$, we get

$$\frac{dp_i}{dt} = p_i \sum_{i,j} D_{ij}\tilde{u}_{ij} - \sum_j D_{ij}\tilde{u}_{ijj}, \quad i, j = \overline{1, n}. \tag{10.13}$$

Equations (10.13) coincide with Equations (10.6). Likewise, we get Equation (10.5) for $S(t)$. Hence, the hypothesis of local panmixia results in the same equations of evolution as the hypothesis of global panmixia. This result is quite natural, because different types of mating affect the evolution of a population only if the fecundity functions are different.

2.11. Semelparity: Models with Discrete Time

Suppose the population can reproduce only once, at a fixed age τ^*. This property is known as semelparity. Already this assumption implies that if the mating system is panmixia, then it can be only the local one. With this reason in mind we will use only models (7.15) or (7.18). Semelparity may be modelled by fecundity functions of the form

$$F_{is,kl}(\tau) = F_{is,kl}\delta(\tau - \tau^*), \tag{11.1}$$

where $\delta(\tau - \tau^*)$ is a delta-function.

If fecundity is multiplicative, that is, if $F_{is,kl} = F_{is} \cdot F_{kl}$, then the evolution of the population will be characterized as follows

$$S_{lm}(t) = \frac{\eta_l(t, \tau^*)\eta_m(t, \tau^*)}{x(t, \tau^*)}, \quad l, m = \overline{1, n}, \tag{11.2}$$

$$\eta_i(t, \tau^*) = \sum_k F_{ik}\Phi^*_{ik}S_{ik}(t - \tau^*), \quad i, k = \overline{1, n},$$

$$x(t, \tau^*) = \sum_{l,m} \Phi^*_{lm}S_{lm}(t - \tau^*), \tag{11.3}$$

$$\Phi^*_{ik} = \exp\left\{ -\int_0^{\tau^*} D_{ik}(\xi)\, d\xi \right\}.$$

These equations represent a special case of Equations (7.15) for $F_{ik}(\tau)F_{sj}(\tau) = F_{ik}F_{sj}\delta(\tau - \tau^*)$.

Let $w_{ij} = F_{ij}\Phi^*_{ij}$ stand for the Malthusian parameter of the $\{ij\}$th genotype. Then $\eta_i(t, \tau^*) = \sum_k w_{ik}S_{ik}(t - \tau^*)$. If in (11.2) we now pass to genotype frequencies $u_{ij} = S_{ij} / S$, where $S = \sum_{i,j} S_{ij}$, we get

$$u_{ij}(t) = \tilde{p}_i(t-\tau^*)\tilde{p}_j(t-\tau^*), \quad i, j=\overline{1, n}. \tag{11.4}$$

Here

$$\tilde{p}_i(t-\tau^*) = \frac{\eta_i(t, \tau^*)}{\sum_i \eta_i(t, \tau^*)} = \frac{\sum_j w_{ij}S_{ij}(t-\tau^*)}{\sum_{i,j} w_{ij}S_{ij}(t-\tau^*)} = \frac{\sum_j w_{ij}u_{ij}(t-\tau^*)}{\sum_{i,j} w_{ij}u_{ij}(t-\tau^*)}.$$

Obviously, $p_i = \sum_j u_{ij}$ is the frequency of the allele A_i. Then summing up in (11.4) over j, we obtain $p_i(t) = \tilde{p}_i(t-\tau^*)$. Whence immediately follows that

$$u_{ij}(t) = p_i(t)p_j(t), \quad i, j=\overline{1, n}. \tag{11.5}$$

The relations (11.5) are nothing else but the Hardy–Weinberg principle. From the condition that $p_i(t) = \tilde{p}_i(t-\tau^*)$ and from the definition of $\tilde{p}_i(t-\tau^*)$ we get

$$p_i(t) = \frac{\sum_j w_{ij}u_{ij}(t-\tau^*)}{\sum_{i,j} w_{ij}u_{ij}(t-\tau^*)},$$

or substituting (11.5)

$$p_i(t) = p_i(t-\tau^*)\frac{\sum_j w_{ij}p_j(t-\tau^*)}{\sum_{i,j} w_{ij}p_i(t-\tau^*)p_j(t-\tau^*)}, \quad i, j=\overline{1, n}. \tag{11.6}$$

Equations (11.6) are the classical equations of population genetics for populations with no overlapping generations (model with discrete time). If τ^* is taken as the average period of one generation, these equations describe the evolution of gene (allele) frequencies in the sequence of generations. Let the prime indicate that the corresponding value of the variable belongs to the subsequent generation. Then (11.6) can be rewritten in the form

$$p_i' = \frac{p_i w_i}{w}, \quad w_i = \sum_j w_{ij}p_j,$$

$$w = \sum_{i,j} w_{ij}p_i p_j, \quad i, j=\overline{1, n}. \tag{11.7}$$

From (11.2) we can readily find the equation for the total population $S = \sum_{i,j} S_{ij}$

$$S' = \frac{Sw^2}{\Phi^*}, \quad \Phi^* = \sum_{i,j} \Phi^*_{ij}p_i p_j. \tag{11.8}$$

If we now assume that fecundity is additive, that is, $F_{is,kl} = 1/2(F_{is} + F_{kl})$, from Equations (7.18), recalling (8.27), we easily get

$$S_{lm}(t) = \frac{\eta_l(t, \tau^*)x_m(t, \tau^*) + \eta_m(t, \tau^*)x_l(t, \tau^*)}{2x(t, \tau^*)}, \quad l, m=\overline{1, n}, \tag{11.9}$$

where η_l and x are defined by (11.3) and

$$x_i(t, \tau^*) = \sum_k \Phi^*_{ik} S_{ik}(t-\tau^*), \quad i, k = \overline{1, n}. \tag{11.10}$$

Carrying on to frequencies, from (11.9) we obtain

$$u_{ij}(t) = \frac{1}{2}\{\tilde{p}_i(t-\tau^*)\rho_j(t-\tau^*)+\tilde{p}_j(t-\tau^*)\rho_i(t-\tau^*)\}, \tag{11.11}$$

where the frequency $\tilde{p}_i$ is defined just like before, and $\rho_i = x_i/x$. Summing up in (11.11) over j we immediately get

$$p_i(t) = \frac{1}{2}\{\tilde{p}_i(t-\tau^*)+\rho_i(t-\tau^*)\}. \tag{11.12}$$

Taking into account that

$$\tilde{p}_i = \frac{\sum_j w_{ij}u_{ij}}{\sum_{i,j} w_{ij}u_{ij}}, \quad \rho_i = \frac{\sum_j \Phi^*_{ij}u_{ij}}{\sum_{i,j} \Phi^*_{ij}u_{ij}},$$

and making use of (11.11) we come to the following equations of evolution

$$\tilde{p}_i' = \frac{[\tilde{p}_i w_i(\rho)+\rho_i w_i(\tilde{p})]}{(2w)},$$

$$\rho_i' = \frac{[\tilde{p}_i \Phi^*_i(\rho)+\rho_i \Phi^*_i(\tilde{p})]}{2\Phi^*},$$

$$w_i(\rho) = \sum_j w_{ij}\rho_j, \quad w_i(\tilde{p}) = \sum_j w_{ij}p_j, \quad w = \sum_{i,j} w_{ij}\tilde{p}_i\rho_j, \tag{11.13}$$

$$\Phi^*_i(\rho) = \sum_j \Phi^*_{ij}\rho_j, \quad \Phi^*_i(\tilde{p}) = \sum_j \Phi^*_{ij}\tilde{p}_j\rho_j, \quad \Phi^* = \sum_{i,j} \Phi^*_{ij}\tilde{p}_i\rho_j,$$

$$i, j = \overline{1, n}.$$

Here, as above, the subsequent generation is primed. The equation for the total size S, which we get by summing up in (11.9) can be written in the form

$$S' = wS. \tag{11.14}$$

It is easy to see that if $F_{ij} = F$, i.e. if fecundities are the same for all genotypes, then the right-hand sides in the equations for $\tilde{p}_i$ and ρ_i coincide and for equal initial conditions $\tilde{p}_i = \rho_i$. Then $p_i = \tilde{p}_i$, $u_{ij} = p_i p_j$ and Equations (11.13) acquire the classical form (11.7).

2.12. More Realistic Assumptions About the Particular Form of Fecundity and Mortality Functions

Though semelparity is specific of many populations of insects and fish (a typical representative of the latter are the salmonidae), nature is multiformed and it provides an abundance of examples which by no means comply neither with the hypothesis of the age- independent fecundity and mortality, nor with the hypothesis of semelparity. Let us study some more realistic hypothesis about the particular form of demographic functions.

(a) Above we assumed that the reproductive period starts at the zero age. The assumption that $a>0$ is more natural. As concerns the rest, we will still think that F_{ij} and D_{ij} are independent of age when $\tau>a$, and that $D_{ij}=D$. Evidently $F_{ij}(\tau)\equiv 0$ for $0\leqslant\tau<a$.

Consider the case of global panmixia and multiplicative fecundity. We can then use the model (8.4)–(8.6), but when differentiating with respect to t we are to substitute the upper limit t in the appropriate integrals by $t-a$. Therefore, instead of (8.10) we are to get

$$\frac{dp_i(t)}{dt} = \frac{S(t-a)}{\sigma(t)}\{p_i(t-a)w_i(t-a)-p_i(t)w(t-a)\},$$
$$w_i(t) = \sum_j w_{ij}p_j(t), \quad w(t) = \sum_{i,j} w_{ij}p_i(t)p_j(t), \quad i,j=\overline{1,n}, \tag{12.1}$$

where

$$w_{ij} = F_{ij}(a) = F_{ij}.$$

Likewise, for the equations of population dynamics

$$\frac{d\sigma(t)}{dt} = w(t-a)S(t-a)-D\sigma(t),$$
$$\frac{dx(t)}{dt} = S(t-a)-Dx(t), \quad S(t) = \frac{\sigma^2(t)}{x(t)}. \tag{12.2}$$

Thus, we describe the evolution by a system of differential equations with a time-lag. Solutions to this system demonstrate much more complex behavior than those of the corresponding system of differential equations with $a=0$.

(b) Making no assumptions about the particular form of the relationships between demographic functions and age, we adopt only one hypothesis of a qualitative character, namely, we assume that mortality is high, that is, $D_{ij}(\tau)=\mu\tilde{D}_{ij}(\tau)$ where μ is a large parameter, $\mu>>1$, and $\tilde{D}_{ij}\sim 1$. As before we consider the case of global panmixia and multiplicative fecundity.

Note that the appropriate evolutionary equations (8.4)–(8.6) contain the integral of the following form (for $a=0$)

$$I_{ij} = \int_0^b K_{ij}(\tau)p_i(t-\tau)p_j(t-\tau)S(t-\tau)\,d\tau,$$

which can be rewritten as

$$I_{ij} = \int_a^b Z_{ij}(t,\tau)\exp\left\{-\mu\int_0^\tau \tilde{D}_{ij}(\xi)d\xi\right\}d\tau, \tag{12.3}$$

$$Z_{ij}(t,\tau) = F_{ij}(\tau)p_i(t-\tau)p_j(t-\tau)S(t-\tau).$$

Suppose that functions F_{ij} and $\tilde{D}_{ij}$ in the vicinity of $\tau=0$ can be represented in the form

$$F_{ij}(\tau) = f_{ij}\tau^{\lambda-1}, \quad \tilde{D}_{ij}(\tau) = \tilde{d}_{ij}\nu^{-1}, \tag{12.4}$$

where $\lambda>1$, $\nu>0$. Imposing the condition $\lambda>1$, we take into account the fact that actually $F_{ij}(0)=0$. Moreover, at first $F_{ij}(\tau)$ may grow very slowly with τ so that both $F'_{ij}=0$ and $F''_{ij}(0)=0$. On the other hand, mortality among the newborn can be very high, this being usually presented by the term d_{ij}/τ^α, where $0<\alpha<1$. The condition $\alpha<1$ provides the existence of the zero limit

$$\lim_{\tau\to 0}\int_0^\tau \frac{d_{ij}}{\tau^\alpha}d\tau = 0 \quad \text{for} \quad \alpha<1,$$

thus satisfying the condition that the probability for the newborn to live till the age τ, $\Phi_{ij}(\tau)$, should approach unity as $\tau\to 0$.

Suppose that $p_i(t)\neq 0$, $S(t)\neq 0$. Then the expansion of function $Z_{ij}(t,\tau)$ in the vicinity of $\tau=0$ should begin with the same powers of τ, as the one for function $F_{ij}(\tau)$. For integrals of the (12.3)-type, Laplace method gives an asymptotic evaluation of the form

$$I_{ij} = \int_0^T Z_{ij}(t,\tau)\exp\left\{-\mu\int_0^\tau \tilde{D}_{ij}(\xi)\,d\xi\right\}d\tau \simeq$$

$$\simeq \frac{f_{ij}p_i(t)p_j(t)S(t)}{\nu}\Gamma\left[\frac{\lambda}{\nu}\right]\left[\frac{\nu}{\mu\tilde{d}_{ij}}\right]^{\lambda/\nu}. \tag{12.5}$$

Here $\Gamma(...)$ is the Euler gamma-function. Using (12.5) to estimate the integrals in (8.4) – (8.6), we get

$$p_i(t) = \frac{p_i(t)w_i(t)}{w(t)} + o(1), \quad i,j=\overline{1,n},$$

$$w_i = \sum_j w_{ij}p_j, \quad w = \sum_{i,j} w_{ij}p_ip_j. \tag{12.6}$$

But unlike the preceeding sections, here Malthusian parameters are complicated functions of demographic characteristics:

$$w_{ij} = \frac{f_{ij}}{(\mu\tilde{d}_{ij})^{\lambda/\nu}} = \frac{f_{ij}}{(d_{ij})^{\lambda/\nu}}. \tag{12.7}$$

This asymptotic evaluation shows that the population quickly equilibrates with respect to gene frequencies. (Equation (12.6) is nothing else but the equation for steady-state solutions to system (8.13) for for the fixed points of system (11.7).)

It should be noted that the asymptotic (12.5) is not unique. Other asymptotics may exist, resulting in other expressions for Malthusian parameters, and, moreover, in other evolutionary equations. Consider a concrete example. Let functions $K_{ij}(\tau)$

have the form

$$K_{ij}(\tau) = k_{ij}\tau^m e^{-d\tau}, \tag{12.8}$$

where m is large enough. This is quite a good approximation of real demographic curves.

In Figure 3 we compare the demographic function $K(\tau)= F(\tau)\exp\{-\int_0^\tau D(\xi)d\xi\}$ for a beetle population (*Calandra oryzae*) with its approximation $K(\tau)=k\tau^m e^{-d\tau}$. The function $K(\tau)$ was derived from the data published by L. C. Birch (The intrinsic rate of natural increase of insect population. *J. Anim. Ecol.*, 1948, **17**, No. 1, pp. 15-26). In $K(\tau)$ the parameters are $m=7$, $d=1.4$ ($\circ$ are the values of $K(\tau)$ for the considered ages).

Here we accepted a similarity hypothesis, that the demographic genotype functions are distinguished only by the age-independent factors k_{ij}. Then the integral I_{ij} can be written in the form

$$I_{ij} = k_{ij}\int_a^b P_{ij}(t-\tau)\tau^m e^{-d\tau}\, d\tau,$$

where $P_{ij}(t-\tau)=p_i(t-\tau)p_j(t-\tau)S(t-\tau)$. Since $K_{ij}\to 0$ as $\tau\to\infty$, the upper limit in these integrals can be considered to be infinite. Substituting $\tau=m\theta$ we get

$$I_{ij} = k_{ij}m^{m+1}\int_0^\infty P_{ij}(t-m\theta)\exp\{m(-d\theta+\ln\theta)\}\, d\theta. \tag{12.9}$$

The function $h(\theta)=-d\theta+\ln\theta$ has a maximum at $\theta^*=1/d$. Therefore, we can apply the Laplace formula to (12.9) to get the following asymptotic evaluation for I_{ij}:

$$I_{ij} \simeq \sqrt{2\pi m}\, e^{-m}m^m P_{ij}(t-\tau^*)\frac{k_{ij}}{d^{m+1}}, \quad \tau^* = \frac{m}{d}. \tag{12.10}$$

Just like before, using (12.10) to estimate the integrals in (8.4) – (8.6), we arrive at the following asymptotic relationships

$$p_i(t) \approx \frac{p_i(t-\tau^*)w_i(t-\tau^*)}{w(t-\tau^*)}, \quad i, j=\overline{1, n}, \tag{12.11}$$

$$w_i(t-\tau^*) = \sum_j w_{ij}p_j(t-\tau^*),$$

$$w(t-\tau^*) = \sum_{i,j} w_{ij}p_i(t-\tau^*)p_j(t-\tau^*),$$

where Malthusian parameters are $w_{ij}=k_{ij}$. System (12.11) coincides in form with (11.6), that is with the discrete model derived for the case of semelparity. However, practically these models are different: firstly, their Malthusian parameters w_{ij} (or selection coefficients) are defined differently; secondly, they incorporate different time-lags τ^* (or time steps). While in the model of semelparity τ^* is the reproductive age, in model (12.11) τ^* is the age when $K_{ij}(\tau)$ attains maximum. Usually the latter is less.

Here we approached a very important (and a very delicate) problem in mathematical genetics. It is the problem of the meaningful definition of Malthusian parameters or selection coefficients. From the aforesaid it is already clear that their values are functionals of the demographic functions, and various hypotheses about their definite form result in different values of the Malthusian parameters. We will go into details concerning this problem in Section 3.7.

2.13. Some Generalizations of Classical Equations in Population Genetics. Another Way to Derive these Equations

In the preceeding sections of this chapter we showed that under sufficiently stringent assumptions about demographic functions, the general equations of evolution can be reduced to the classical Fisher–Haldane–Wright equations. Here for the same assumptions concerning the demographic functions we will somewhat generalize these equations.

Under global panmixia and multiplicative, age-independent function of fecundity the number of newborn genotypes $\{ij\}$ is presented by (7.7). Suppose now $a=0$ and $b=\tau_{\max}$, which is the maximal age of individuals. Integrating the Equation (3.6) with respect to $\tau\in[0, b]$, with the age-independent mortality functions being equal for all genotypes, and the single-index genotype notations being substituted by the double-index ones, we get

$$\frac{dx_{ij}(t)}{dt} = x_{ij}(t, 0) - Dx_{ij}(t), \quad i, j = \overline{1, n}, \tag{13.1}$$

where

$$x_{ij}(t) = \int_0^b x_{ij}(t, \tau)\, d\tau$$

is the number of individuals with genotype $\{ij\}$ over all ages. Clearly, nothing will change in Equation (13.1) if we suppose that $D=D[x(t)]$, that is, mortality is a function of the total population size.

A similar conclusion holds for formula (7.7), where we can think that $F_{ij}=F_{ij}[x(t)]$. Substituting the expression for $x_{ij}(t, 0)$ from (7.7) with age-independent $\{F_{ij}\}$, into (13.1) we find

$$\frac{dx_{ij}(t)}{dt} = \frac{1}{x(t)} \sum_s F_{is}x_{is}(t) \sum_k F_{kj}x_{kj}(t) - Dx_{ij}(t), \quad i, j, k, s = \overline{1, n}. \tag{13.2}$$

The equation for the total population $x(t)$ is derived by summing up in (13.2) over i and j:

$$\frac{dx(t)}{dt} = \frac{\left[\sum_{k,s} F_{ks}x_{ks}(t)\right]^2}{x(t)} - Dx(t), \quad k, s = \overline{1, n}. \tag{13.3}$$

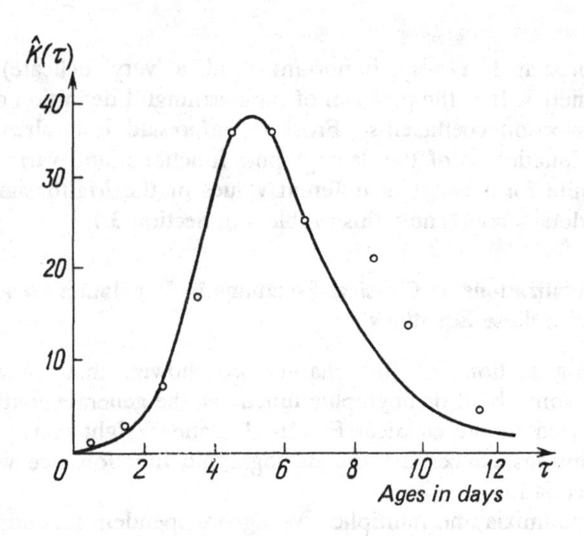

Fig. 3.

Define a new variable $n_i = \sum_s F_{is} x_{is}$ which is the mean number of alleles A_i, weighted with respect to fecundity. Then multiplying (13.2) by F_{ij} and summing over j, we have

$$\frac{dn_i}{dt} = \frac{n_i}{x(t)} \sum_j F_{ij} n_j - D n_i, \quad i, j = \overline{1, n}, \tag{13.4}$$

and for $N = \sum_i n_i$,

$$\frac{dN}{dt} = \frac{1}{x(t)} \sum_{i,j} F_{ij} n_i n_j - DN, \quad i, j = \overline{1, n}. \tag{13.5}$$

Let us introduce the frequency of allele A_i by the formula $p_i = n_i / N$. Then from (13.4) and (13.5) we get

$$\frac{dp_i}{dt} = \left[\frac{N}{x(t)}\right] p_i (w_i - w),$$

$$w_i = \sum_j F_{ij} p_j, \tag{13.6}$$

$$w = \sum_i w_i p_i = \sum_{i,j} F_{ij} p_i p_j, \quad i, j = \overline{1, n}.$$

In addition, write out the equations for N, x and $z = N / x$:

$$\frac{dN}{dt} = N(zw - D), \quad \frac{dx}{dt} = x(z^2 - D),$$

$$\frac{dz}{dt} = z^2(w-z). \tag{13.7}$$

One of the frequently used hypotheses (which was implicitly applied in Section 2.10) is the so-called hypothesis of 'weak selection'. The gist of it is as follows. Assumed is that Malthusian parameters, which are the fecundities in this case, can be represented in the form

$$F_{ij} = F+\epsilon f_{ij}, \text{ where } 0 < \epsilon << 1, \tag{13.8}$$

Substituting these expressions into (13.5) and (13.6) we get

$$\begin{aligned}\frac{dp_i}{dt} &= \epsilon z p_i(\hat{w}_i-\hat{w}), \quad i=\overline{1, n},\\ \frac{dN}{dt} &= N(zF-D+\epsilon\hat{w}z),\\ \frac{dx}{dt} &= x(z^2-D),\\ \frac{dz}{dt} &= z^2(F-z+\epsilon\hat{w}), \quad \hat{w} = \sum_{i,j} f_{ij}p_ip_j.\end{aligned} \tag{13.9}$$

Accepting the hypothesis of weak selection and assuming that $|F^2-D|=0(\epsilon)$, we immediately split the system variables into 'slow' ones, which are the allele frequencies x, N and the 'fast' one which is the ratio $z=N/x$. z quickly approaches F when ϵ is sufficiently small, thus bringing the further system evolution into the vicinity of the plane $z=F$. Therefore over sufficiently long periods of time we can replace the full equations of system evolution (13.9) by the 'truncated' one, with $z=F$:

$$\begin{aligned}\frac{dp_i}{dt} &= Fp_i(w_i-w), \quad i=\overline{1, n},\\ \frac{dN}{dt} &= N(Fw-D),\\ \frac{dx}{dt} &= x(F^2-D).\end{aligned} \tag{13.10}$$

In what follows we will assume that $F\equiv 1$, and only the mortality function depends on the total 'population size' N. In this case the equations for frequencies completely coincide with the classical ones:

$$\begin{aligned}\frac{dp_i}{dt} &= p_i(w_i-w), \quad w_i = \sum_j w_{ij}p_j,\\ w &= \sum_i p_iw_i, \quad i, j=\overline{1, n}\end{aligned} \tag{13.11}$$

(here we denoted $F_{ij}=w_{ij}$), and the equation for the total population N becomes

$$\frac{dN}{dt} = N[w-D(N)]. \tag{13.12}$$

If $p_i(t)\to p_i^*$ for $t\to\infty$, so that $w(t)\to w^*$ and $D'(N^*)>0$, where N^* is the unique positive solution to the equation $D(N^*)=w^*$, then $N(t)\to N^*$.

We derived these equations from the general evolutionary equations under the assumptions, which are practically equivalent to the disregard of the population age structure. Below we derive these same equations not so strictly but much more obviously, for the case when the population age structure is totally neglected.

Let $x_{ij}(t)$, $i, j=\overline{1,n}$ be the number of genotype $\{ij\}$ (we consider a 'sexless' population). Suppose the fecundities of all pairs are the same and equal to F. Mortalities will be considered to be of two types: $w_{ij}\delta t$, presenting the genotype-dependent probability to survive over the interval δt, and $D(N)\delta t$, presenting the genotype-independent competitive mortality. Here $N=\sum_{i,j}x_{ij}$ is the total population size.

Let now $m_{ik,sj}=m_{ik,sj}(x_{11}, x_{12}, \ldots, x_{nn})$, $i, j, k, s=\overline{1,n}$ be the number of $\{ij\}$, $\{sj\}$-pairs. If the principle of inheritance is specified by the operator $\Omega\{\omega_{ik,sj}^{lm}\}$, the equations of population dynamics for genotypic groups can be written as follows

$$\frac{dx_{lm}}{dt} = Fw_{lm}\sum_{i,k,s,j}\omega_{ik,sj}^{lm}m_{ik,sj}-D(N)x_{lm}, \quad i, k, s, j, l, m=\overline{1,n}. \tag{13.13}$$

When inheritance is determined by one gene with multiple alleles, and the system of mating is panmixia, then $\omega_{ik,sj}$ is given by formulas (6.2), $m_{ik,sj}=x_{ik}x_{sj}/N$, and (13.13) becomes

$$\frac{dx_{ij}}{dt} = \frac{Fw_{ij}}{N}\sum_k x_{ik}\sum_s x_{sj}-D(N)x_{ij}, \quad i,k, s, j=\overline{1,n}. \tag{13.14}$$

Carrying on from numbers in genotypic groups to numbers of alleles $x_i=\sum_j x_{ij}$, we get

$$\frac{dx_i}{dt} = \frac{Fx_i}{N}\sum_j w_{ij}x_j-D(N)x_i, \quad i, j=\overline{1,n}. \tag{13.15}$$

If we now use the scheme $Fw_{ij}\Rightarrow w_{ij}$ to introduce new Malthusian parameters, changing over to frequencies, we get the standard Fisher–Wright–Haldane equations, but with an unusual equation of the (13.12) form for the total population size of the species.

In what follows we will often substitute the strict deduction of evolutionary equations by the method set forth above. And finally, along with the name 'Malthusian parameter for genotype $\{ij\}$' the value w_{ij} will be also termed 'fitness of genotype $\{ij\}$'.

2.14. Discrete-time Equations of Evolution

The deduction scheme for evolutionary equations that we have just set forth, can be used for the case of discretely changing time, say, if it is measured in generations. We represent the evolution of population as a sequence of the following events: formation of reproductive couples, reproduction of individuals of the new generation and death of parents at the end of a generation, differential survival of offspring throughout the next generation.

Let the number of individuals with genotype $\{ij\}$ at the end of the $(t-1)$st generation be $x_{ij}(t-1)$. (The value of a variable before the change of generations will be indexed '-', after – '+'.) Let us denote the number of $\{ik\}$, $\{jk\}$-pairs by $m^-_{ik,sj}=m^-_{ik,sj}[x^-_{11}(t-1),\ldots,x^-_{nn}(t-1)]$, $i, k, s, j=\overline{1, n}$. Suppose each such pair produces the same number of offspring, which is F. The distribution of offspring among genotypic groups is again characterized by the operator $\Omega\{\omega^{lm}_{ik,sj}\}$, $l, m=\overline{1, n}$.

If now w_{lm} is the proportion of individuals with genotype $\{lm\}$ that live to the end of the generation and are engaged in mating, then

$$x^-_{lm}(t) = w_{lm}x^+_{lm}(t), \quad l, m=\overline{1, n}. \tag{14.1}$$

Taking into account that $x^-_{lm}(t)$ are the offspring of individuals of the preceeding generation, we get

$$x^-_{lm}(t) = Fw_{lm} \sum_{i,k,s,j} \omega^{lm}_{ik,sj} m^-_{ik,sj}, \quad i, j, k, s, l, m=\overline{1, n}. \tag{14.2}$$

Supposing that inheritance is determined by one gene with multiple alleles and that the mating system is panmixia, Equations (14.2) may be written in the form $(N=\sum_{i,j} x_{ij})$:

$$x^-_{ij}(t) = \frac{Fw_{ij}}{N^-(t-1)} \sum_k x^-_{ik}(t-1) \sum_s x^-_{sj}(t-1), \quad i, j, k, s, l, m=\overline{1, n}. \tag{14.3}$$

These recurrence relations correlate the numbers in genotypic groups at the end of two successive generations. Changing over to allele frequencies $p_i=\sum_j x_{ij}/N$ from (14.3) we get

$$p^-_i(t) = \frac{p^-_i(t-1)w^-_i(t-1)}{w^-(t-1)},$$

$$w^-_i = \sum_j w_{ij}p^-_j, \quad w^- = \sum_{i,j} w_{ij}p^-_i p^-_j, \quad i, j=\overline{1, n}. \tag{14.4}$$

Obviously the relation between the numbers in genotypic groups at the end of the preceeding generation and at the beginning of the next one can be given by the equation

$$x^+_{ij}(t) = \frac{F}{N^-(t-1)} \sum_k x^-_{ik}(t-1) \sum_s x^-_{sj}(t-1). \tag{14.5}$$

Changing over to allele frequencies in (14.5), we have $p^+_i(t)=p^-_i(t-1)$. That is, carrying on from one generation to another, gene frequencies remain continuous.

Therefore in (14.4) we can drop the index '-' and rewrite these equations as follows

$$p_i' = \frac{p_i w_i}{w}, \quad w_i = \sum_j w_{ij} p_j,$$

$$w = \sum_{i,j} w_{ij} p_i p_j, \quad i, j = \overline{1, n}. \tag{14.6}$$

(Here the prime indicates that the variable corresponds to the subsequent generations.)

Summing up in (14.3) over subscripts, we get the equation for the total population size

$$N^-(t) = Fw^-(t-1)N^-(t-1). \tag{14.7}$$

But since $N^+(t) = FN^-(t-1)$ and $p_i^+(t) = p_i^-(t-1)$, the equations for numbers at the end and at the beginning of a generation will be similar, and therefore we can write

$$N' = FwN, \quad w = \sum_{i,j} w_{ij} p_i p_j. \tag{14.8}$$

Clearly, system (14.6) does not change if we suppose that $F = F(N)$ and $w_{ij} = w_{ij}\phi(N)$. Besides, without changing (14.6), we can substitute $Fw_{ij} \Rightarrow w_{ij}$, which is equivalent to the assumption $F \equiv 1$. In this case only the rate of the total population variations will be altered, the rate of evolution of the gene structure will remain unchanged.

And in conclusion we will go into the concept of the so-called 'gamete pool'. Let us represent the formation of new zygotes (of individuals of the new generation) as a sequence of the following stages:

1. Each of the parents produce an equal number of gametes, the frequency of each type of gametes, produced by heterozygotes, being 1/2; all gametes make up a new population of gametes (the 'gamete pool').

2. Out of the gamete population a random sample of two is picked; these samples make up the population of zygotes- offspring.

Clearly, if there is no correlation between gametes, the probability that a zygote $\{ij\}$ is produced (which can be presented by the frequency of this zygote u_{ij} in large populations) is given by

$$u_{ij}^+(t) = p_i^-(t-1)p_j^-(t-1), \quad i, j = \overline{1, n}. \tag{14.9}$$

Selection in the course of the subsequent generation modifies these frequencies so that

$$u_{ij}^-(t) = \frac{w_{ij} u_{ij}^+(t)}{\sum_{i,j} w_{ij} u_{ij}^+(t)}, \quad i, j = \overline{1, n}. \tag{14.10}$$

Substituting (14.9) into (14.10) and taking into account that $\sum_j u_{ij} = p_i$, we get the equation for p_i in the form of (14.6).

From (14.9) it follows that there is an equivalence between the assumption that gametes are incorrelated and the assumption about panmixia.

The concept of 'gamete pool', which reduces the relationships at the genotype level to those at the gamete level, is a very handy method to make evolutionary equations much more simple. Naturally, accepting this concept, we discard many mechanisms of evolution, which actually go at the level of genotypes rather than gametes; however, this happens to be simply inevitable in order to get some kind of a final result without being lost in formal difficulties.

2.15. On the Relationship Between Continuous and Discrete Models

It should be noted that formally we can consider Equations (14.6) and (14.8) as a finite difference scheme with a step $h=1$, approximating the differential equations

$$\frac{dp_i}{dt} = \frac{p_i(w_i - w)}{w}, \quad \frac{dN}{dt} = N(Fw-1), \quad i=\overline{1,n}, \tag{15.1}$$

where $\dot{p}_i = p(t) - p(t-1)$. These equations seem to be the simplest ones among the set of differential equations, such that (14.6), (14.8) are their difference approximation with $h=1$. However, while in the theory of difference schemes we can show that for $h \to 0$ the difference between the solutions to Equations (14.6), (14.8) and Equations (15.1) is arbitrarily small (under certain restrictions imposed on the right-hand side of the differential equation), in our case there is no meaning in such a passage to the limit.

Let us evaluate the error, which we get when we replace the difference equations (14.6), (14.8) by the differential ones (15.1). Their solutions will be compared over sufficiently long time intervals, containing many generations.

Let us study the behavior only of the errors $\epsilon_i = p_i - \hat{p}_i$ ($\hat{p}_i$ is the solution to the discrete system). The analysis for the total population size is similar. From (15.1) for one generation we get

$$p_i(t+1) = p_i(t) + \int_t^{t+1} f_i[\mathbf{p}(\xi)]\, d\xi = p_i(t) + f_i[\mathbf{p}(t)] + \sum_j \left[\frac{\partial f_i}{\partial p_j} f_j\right]\Bigg|_{t+\theta_j}, \tag{15.2}$$

$$\theta_j \in [0, 1], \quad i, j = \overline{1, n}.$$

Here f_i are the right-hand sides of the Equations (15.1). Subtracting (15.2) from (14.6) we get

$$\epsilon_i(t+1) = \sum_j \left[\frac{\partial \phi_i}{\partial p_j}\right]\Bigg|_t \epsilon_j(t) + \sum_j \left[\frac{\partial f_i}{\partial p_j} f_j\right]\Bigg|_{t+\theta_j} + o[\epsilon_j(t)]. \tag{15.3}$$

Here ϕ_i are the right-hand sides of (14.6). Introducing the following norms

$$\|\epsilon\| = \max_i |\epsilon_i|, \quad \|\Phi\| = \max_i \left|\sum_j \frac{\partial \phi_i}{\partial p_j}\right|, \quad p_i \in [0, 1],$$

$$\| M \| = \max_{p_i \in [0,\,1]} \left\{ \left| \sum_j \frac{\partial f_i}{\partial p_j} f_j \right| \right\}, \quad i, j = \overline{1, n},$$

from (15.3) we get

$$\| \epsilon(t+1) \| \leqslant \| \Phi \| \, \| \epsilon(t) \| + \| M \|. \tag{15.4}$$

Therefore when $\| \Phi \| < 1$ we will have

$$\lim_{t \to \infty} \| \epsilon(t) \| \leqslant \frac{\| M \|}{1 - \| \Phi \|}. \tag{15.5}$$

For the error to be bounded it is necessary and sufficient that $\| \Phi \| < 1$. We can also see that the error will be small for small values of

$$\| M \| = \max_i \left\{ \left| \sum_j \frac{\partial f_i}{\partial p_j} f_j \right| \right\}.$$

Therefore, while the first condition is nothing else but the requirement that alterations in gene frequencies over one generation be small, the second one implies that the curve of gene frequency is to be sufficiently smooth (the curvature of the diagram for the relationship between gene frequency and time is to be small). Since $\ddot{p}_i = \sum_j f_j \partial f_i / \partial p_j$, the second condition automatically holds if the first one is satisfied and the derivatives $\partial f_i / \partial p_j$ are bounded.

The final result of these speculations may be stated as follows: if the variables p_i are only slightly changed over one step, then we can replace the difference equations (14.6) by the differential ones (15.1) with no significant mistakes. The variations in p_i are small either when the values of p_i, $i = \overline{1, n}$ are close to the fixed point of the operator $\phi = \{\phi_i(\mathbf{p})\}$ acting on $\mathbf{p}$, or if weak selection takes place, for example, when fitnesses are close to unity ($F \equiv 1$). In the latter case, from (15.1) we have

$$\frac{dp_i}{dt} = p_i(w_i - w) + o(\epsilon), \quad i = \overline{1, n}. \tag{15.6}$$

Here $\epsilon = \max_{i,j} | w_{ij} - 1 | << 1$. Equations (15.6) to within $o(\epsilon)$ coincide with the equations of the continuous model (13.10).

2.16. Notes and Bibliography

To 2.1.

Birth equations in a somewhat different form were proposed in the paper:

Cornette, J. L.: 1975, 'Some Basic Elements of Continuous Selection Models', *Theor. Pop. Biol.*, **8**, 3, 301–313.

As birth equations the author takes

$$\eta_{ij}(t, 0) = \sum_k \sum_l \int_0^d \int_0^d Y_{ik,lj}(t, x, y) a_{ik,lj}(t, x, y) \, dy \, dx,$$

where $Y_{ik,lj}$ is the 'density of mating pairs', $a_{ik,lj}$ is the fecundity of a pair with genotypes $\{ik\}$ and $\{lj\}$.

To 2.3.

In a similar way the survival equation is derived (from the Liouville equation) in the paper:

Svirezhev, Yu. M.: 1975, 'O matematičeskih modeljah biologičeskih soobshestv i svjazannyh s nimi zadačah upravlenija i optimizacii (On Mathematical Models of Biological Communities and Related Problems of Control and Optimization), In: *Matematiceskoje modelirovanije v biologii* (*Mathematical Modelling in Biology*), Nauka, Moscow, 30–55.

The survival equations in the form (2.8) are differently derived in the works:

Von Förster, H.: 1959, 'Some Remarks on Changing Populations', The Kinetics of Cellular Proliferation, Crune and Stratton, N.Y., London, 382–388;

Poluektov, R. A. (Ed.): 1974, *Dinamičeskaja teorija biologičeskih populjatsiy* (*Dynamical Theory of Biological Populations*), Nauka, Moscow, 455 p.,

and in the monograph:

Nagylaki, T.: 1977, *Selection in One- and Two-Locus Systems*, Springer-Verlag, Berlin, 208 p.

which also includes an extensive bibliography on models of population genetics, among them those that take into account the age structure.

To 2.12.

Asymptotic evaluations, used in this selection are taken from the book:

Erdelyi, A.: 1956, *Asymptotic Expansions*, Dover, N.Y., 108 p.

To 2.13.

The hypothesis of 'weak selection' is used by B. Charlesworth in the paper:

Charlesworth, B.: 1974, 'Selection in Populations with Overlapping Generations. VI. Rates of Change of Gene Frequence and Population Growth Rate', *Theor. Pop. Biol.* **6**, 1, 108–133.

Assuming that demographic parameters of all genotypes are close to each other, the author also assumes that variations in gene frequencies over a certain time interval are small and makes use of the approximation

$$p(t-x) = p(t) - x\frac{dp}{dt},$$

that is, *a priori* certain restrictions are imposed on the solutions to the system.

From the monograph

Vasiljeva, A. B., Butuzov, V. F.: 1973, *Asimptotičeskije razloženija resheniy singuljarno vozmushennyh uravneniy* (*Asymptotic Solutions to Singularly Perturbed Equations.* In Russian), Nauka, Moscow, 272 p.

we can find out how to distinguish fast and slow variables for the analysis of solutions on finite time intervals.

The approximation of systems of equations with fast and slow variables over semi-infinite time intervals is studied in the paper:

Butuzov, V. F.: 1963, *Asimptotičeskije formuly dlja reshenija sistemy differencialnyh uravneniy s malym parametrom pri proivodnoi na polubeskonečnom promežutke* ($0 \leq t < \infty$) (*Asymptotic Formulae for the Solution of a System of Differential Equations with a Small Parameter in the Derivative over Semi-Infinite Interval* ($0 \leq t < \infty$). In Russian), Vestnik MGU (Bulletin of the Moscow State Univ., 4, 3–14.

Chapter 3

Simplest Population Models

3.1. Introduction

In this chapter we will show how even simple models, describing the most elementary populational genetic processes, bring us to conclusions, which are interesting due to their biological clearness. Simple models are still better since they are readily verified in experiments, clearly demonstrating their merits and drawbacks and showing to what extent mathematical models may be applied to the analysis of populational genetic processes. A complex model of great generality is hard to apply to concrete biological situations. The arising mathematical complications can totally shade the biological origin of the problem, shifting the basic accent of the study onto the lines of their overcoming.

Here we will look at one of the most simple objects in population genetics: a sufficiently large panmictic population of organisms, with inheritance of a character determined by one two-allele gene. The population is thought to be 'sexless', that is both sexes are equal in both the inheritance and the selection.

If we denote alleles by A and a, then the population contains only three genotypic groups: AA, Aa and aa. Our task will be to describe the population dynamics in these groups as a factor of demographic functions. Occasionally, the population dynamics of two alleles, or even one allele, can well represent the evolution.

3.2. Equations of Evolution

Obviously, the equation of evolution for a two-allele gene is a special case of the equations, derived in the preceeding chapter, for $n=2$. Let us suppose that the population features global panmixia and that fecundity is multiplicative. Like before let us think that the reproduction in the population takes place over an age interval $[a, b]$, where $0 \leqslant a < b \leqslant \infty$. Besides suppose that $F_{ij}(x) = F_c = \text{const}$. Equations (8.4) – (8.6) of the preceeding chapter in this case become more simple:

$$p(t) = \frac{\int_a^b p(t-\tau)S(t-\tau)[K_1(\tau)p(t-\tau) + K_2(\tau)q(t-\tau)]\, d\tau}{S(t)},$$

$$q(t) = \frac{\int_a^b q(t-\tau)S(t-\tau)[K_2(\tau)p(t-\tau) + K_3(\tau)q(t-\tau)]\, d\tau}{S(t)}, \tag{2.1}$$

$$p(t) + q(t) = 1,$$

where by p and q we denoted the frequencies of alleles A and a among the newborn, and subscripts 1, 2, 3 correspond to the double subscripts 11, 12, 22 used before. Functions $K_i(\tau)$ now have the form $K_i(\tau)=F_c^2 \exp\{-\int_0^\tau D_i(\xi)\,d\xi\}$, where the presence of the coefficient F_c^2 is due to our assumption about multiplicative fecundity. Denoting $F\equiv F_c^2$, we return to the previous form of these function. The equations for frequencies (2.1) can be rewritten in terms of new variables $S_i(t)$, standing for the numbers of the newborns of the ith genotype ($i=1, 2, 3$):

$$S_1(t)+S_2(t) = \int_a^b K_1(\tau)S_1(t-\tau)\,d\tau+\int_a^b K_2(\tau)S_2(t-\tau)\,d\tau, \tag{2.2}$$

$$S_3(t)+S_2(t) = \int_a^b K_3(\tau)S_3(t-\tau)\,d\tau+\int_a^b K_2(\tau)S_2(t-\tau)\,d\tau,$$

$$S_2^2=S_1S_3.$$

In what follows we will sometimes use this equivalent form for Equations (2.1), bearing in mind that $S_1+2S_2+S_3=S$. And if before we derived the well-known equations of population genetics completely neglecting the characteristics of age distributions, here we try to keep the demographic functions at least minimally dependent on age.

3.3. Existence Conditions for Polymorphism

One of the most interesting steady states of the population is the state of a stable coexistence of all three genotypes, the so-called genetic polymorphism. In terms of alleles this means that both alleles, A and a, are present.

Therefore to analyze the existence conditions for polymorphism, we will seek for conditions such that for $t\to\infty$ the population evolves towards the state $p^*=\text{const}$, $0<p^*<1$, that is, $p(t)\to p^*$. Substituting the limiting value p^* for $p(t)$ in (2.1), we get

$$S(t) = \int_a^b S(t-\tau)[K_1(\tau)p^*+K_2(\tau)q^*]\,d\tau, \tag{3.1}$$

$$S(t) = \int_a^b S(t-\tau)[K_2(\tau)p^*+K_3(\tau)q^*]\,d\tau, \quad q^*=1-p^*.$$

Here $S(t)$ is the value S takes on for sufficiently large t. The equation of the form

$$x(t) = \int_a^b K(\tau)x(t-\tau)\,d\tau$$

is the well-known renewal equation.* We have already come across equations of

* Bellman, R. and Cooke, K. L.: 1963, *Differential-Difference Equations*, Acad. Press, New York, 500 p.

this type (more complex ones) in Chapter 2, when deriving the equations of evolution. This equation has the solution of the form

$$x(t) = \sum_{i=1}^{\infty} C_i e^{z_i t},$$

where z_i are roots of the equation

$$\int_a^b K(\tau) e^{-z\tau} d\tau = 1,$$

with $\lambda = z_1 > \mathrm{Re}\, z_i$, $i=2, 3, \ldots$ (we suppose that the roots are numerated in such a way that their real parts are non-increasing).

Since $K_1(\tau)p^* + K_2(\tau)q^*$ is never less than zero (being not identically zero), the equation $\int_a^b [K_1(\tau)p^* + K_2(\tau)q^* e^{-z\tau} d\tau = 1$ has one root λ^* on the real axis. Since this root exceeds the real parts of all other roots, the asymptotics of $S(t)$ will be determined by the term $ce^{\lambda^* t}$, while other terms contribute to the oscillatory effect, its relative influence falling away with time.

Substituting the expression $ce^{\lambda^* t}$ for $S(t)$ in (3.1), we get

$$p^* \omega_1(\lambda^*) + q^* \omega_2(\lambda^*) = 1, \quad (3.2)$$

$$p^* \omega_2(\lambda^*) + q^* \omega_3(\lambda^*) = 1,$$

where $\omega_i(\lambda^*) = \int_a^b K_i(\tau) e^{-\lambda^* \tau} d\tau$, $i=1, 2, 3$. Let us introduce the numbers λ_i which are the only real roots of equations $\omega_i(z)=1$, $i=1, 2, 3$. Obviously, (3.2) is satisfied, if $\omega_i(\lambda^*)=1$, i.e. $\lambda_i = \lambda^*$, $i=1, 2, 3$. The values of p^* and q^* can be arbitrary in this case. Such a situation corresponds to the state of neutral population equilibrium, which is of little interest to us. Therefore we will seek for the non-trivial solution to system (3.2), considered as a λ-dependent system of linear algebraic equations with respect to p^* and q^*:

$$p^*(1-\omega_1) + q^*(1-\omega_2) = 0, \quad (3.3)$$

$$p^*(1-\omega_2) + q^*(1-\omega_3) = 0.$$

The existence condition for a non-trivial solution is

$$\begin{vmatrix} 1-\omega_1 & 1-\omega_2 \\ 1-\omega_2 & 1-\omega_3 \end{vmatrix} = 0. \quad (3.4)$$

Besides, the positiveness of p^* and q^* implies that

$$\omega_1(\lambda^*) > 1, \ \ \omega_3(\lambda^*) > 1, \ \ \omega_2(\lambda^*) < 1, \quad (3.5)$$

or

$$\omega_1(\lambda^*) < 1, \ \ \omega_3(\lambda^*) < 1, \ \ \omega_2(\lambda^*) > 1.$$

Since the functions $\omega_i(\lambda)$ are strictly monotone, the inequalities (3.5) may be replaced by the inequalities

$$\lambda^* < \lambda_1, \ \lambda^* < \lambda_3, \ \lambda^* > \lambda_2, \tag{3.6}$$
$$\lambda^* > \lambda_1, \ \lambda^* > \lambda_3, \ \lambda^* < \lambda_2.$$

The Equation (3.4) has a unique root λ^*, complying with one of the conditions (3.6). Let us prove it.

Suppose that $\lambda_2 > \lambda_1, \lambda_3$ and to make it definite let $\lambda_1 \geqslant \lambda_3$. Consider the function

$$f(\lambda) = \frac{[1-\omega_1(\lambda)][1-\omega_3(\lambda)]}{[1-\omega_2(\lambda)]^2}.$$

Obviously $f(\lambda_1)=0$. Besides, $f(\lambda)\to+\infty$, for $\lambda\to\lambda_2$, because from the monotonicity of $\omega_i(\lambda)$ it follows that $\omega_1(\lambda_2)<\omega_1(\lambda_1)=1$, and moreover, $\omega_3(\lambda_2)<1$. $f(\lambda)$ is continuous on $[\lambda_1, \lambda_2)$ and it may be easily checked that $f(\lambda)$ grows steadily on $[\lambda_1, \lambda_2)$, therefore there exists only one point λ^* such that $f(\lambda^*)=1$, indicating that the equality (3.4) holds. Similar will be the analysis of the case $\lambda_2 < \lambda_1, \lambda_3$.

For p^* and q^* we get the following expressions:

$$p^* = \frac{\omega_2(\lambda^*)-\omega_3(\lambda^*)}{2\omega_2(\lambda^*)-\omega_1(\lambda^*)-\omega_3(\lambda^*)}, \quad q^* = \frac{\omega_2(\lambda^*)-\omega_1(\lambda^*)}{2\omega_2(\lambda^*)-\omega_1(\lambda^*)-\omega_3(\lambda^*)}. \tag{3.7}$$

Let us formulate the basic results of this section. If under the pressure of selection the population evolves towards the state of polymorphism, then:

1) the numbers of the genetic groups that make up the population will be changing exponentially with one and the same exponent λ^*;

2) the exponent λ^* is the only solution to Equation (3.4), taking into account one of the inequalities (3.6), i.e. the possible state of polymorphism is unique;

3) the equilibrium allele frequencies among the newborn are defined by formulas (3.7);

4) the necessary existence conditions for polymorphism are

$$\lambda_1, \lambda_3 < \lambda_2 \tag{3.8}$$

or

$$\lambda_2 < \lambda_1, \lambda_3. \tag{3.9}$$

Thus we found, that the necessary existence conditions for polymorphism are defined only by the relationships between parameters λ_i or, which is the same, between the real roots of the equations $\int_a^b K_i(\tau)e^{-z\tau}\,d\tau=1$, $i=1, 2, 3$. In the following section we are to derive a kind of sufficient conditions for a population to attain a certain state, namely the conditions of stability for limiting trajectories under small (in the sense of the further defined metric) deviations from the initial equilibrium age distribution.

3.4. Sufficient Conditions for Stability of Limiting States of a Population

Since in stability analysis we cannot do without taking account of the effect of initial perturbations, here we will use the full (rather than asymptotic) equations of evolution, which are the special case of the Equations (4.5) – (4.7) of Chapter 2. The Equations (2.4.5) in our case will have the form

$$S_i(-\tau) = g_i(\tau)\exp\left[\int_0^{\tau} D_i(\xi)\,\mathrm{d}\xi\right], \quad i=1,2,3,$$

where $g_i(\tau)$ are the given functions for the initial age distribution (for $t=0$) of the genotypic groups in the population. If we take into account the initial conditions, the full Equations (2.2), which are written out in Section 3.2, can be presented in the form

$$\begin{aligned} S_1(t)+S_2(t) &= \int_0^t K_1(\tau)S_1(t-\tau)\,\mathrm{d}\tau+\\ &\quad+\int_0^t K_2(\tau)S_2(t-\tau)\,\mathrm{d}\tau+G_1+G_2,\\ S_3(t)+S_2(t) &= \int_0^t K_3(\tau)S_3(t-\tau)\,\mathrm{d}\tau+\\ &\quad+\int_0^t K_2(\tau)S_2(t-\tau)\,\mathrm{d}\tau+G_2+G_3,\\ S_2^2(t) &= S_1(t)S_3(t), \end{aligned} \tag{4.1}$$

where

$$G_i \equiv G_i(t) = \\ = \int_t^{\infty} K_i(\tau)g_i(\tau-t)\exp\left\{\int_0^{\tau-t} D_i(\xi)\,\mathrm{d}\xi\right\}\mathrm{d}\tau, \quad i\neq 1,2,3.$$

For the sake of simplicity let us consider an infinite reproductive interval, starting from zero. It can be proved that all further speculations hold for an arbitrary reproductive interval $[a, b]$.

Dividing the first two equations in (4.1) by $e^{\lambda^* t}$ and the third one – by $e^{-2\lambda^* t}$ (λ^* is the root of (3.4), satisfying one of the conditions (3.6)), we will get a new system for the functions $\Omega_i(t)=S_i(t)e^{-\lambda^* t}$, which has the same form as the system (4.1), but with functions $K_i(\tau)$ substituted by the functions $K_i^0(\tau)=K_i(\tau)e^{-\lambda^*\tau}$, and with $G_i(t)$ substituted by $f_i(t)=G_i(t)e^{-\lambda^* t}$.

For the real roots θ_i of the equations

$$\int_0^{\infty} K_i^0(\tau)e^{-z\tau}\,\mathrm{d}\tau = 1, \quad i=1,2,3,$$

the equality $\theta_i = \lambda_i - \lambda^*$ holds, which can be easily proved by direct substitution. Since

$$p(t) = \frac{S_1(t)+S_2(t)}{S_1(t)+2S_2(t)+S_3(t)} = \frac{S_1(t)+\sqrt{S_1(t)S_3(t)}}{S_1(t)+2\sqrt{S_1(t)S_3(t)}+S_3(t)} = \frac{\sqrt{S_1(t)}}{\sqrt{S_1(t)}+\sqrt{S_3(t)}},$$

it follows that as the population tends towards polymorphism

$$S_i(t) \underset{t-\infty}{\rightarrow} c_i S(t) = c_i e^{\lambda^* t}, \quad i=1, 2, 3,$$

and, hence, $\Omega_i(t) \rightarrow C_i$, where $c_1 = p^{*2}$, $c_2 = p^* q^*$, $c_3 = q^{*2}$. Suppose $e_i(t) = \Omega_i(t) - c_i$, $i=1, 2, 3$. Then the equations for $e_i(t)$ (to within $o(e_i)$) will have the form

$$e_1(t)+e_2(t) = \int_0^t K_1^0(\tau) e_1(t-\tau)\, d\tau + \int_0^t K_2^0(\tau) e_2(t-\tau)\, d\tau + h_1(t) + h_2(t),$$

$$e_3(t)+e_2(t) = \int_0^t K_3^0(\tau) e_3(t-\tau)\, d\tau + \int_0^t K_2^0(\tau) e_2(t-\tau)\, d\tau + h_3(t) + h_2(t), \tag{4.2}$$

$$e_2(t) = \alpha e_1(t) + \beta e_3(t), \quad h_i(t) = \int_t^\infty K_i^0(\tau)[g_i(\tau-t) e^{\lambda^*(\tau-t)} - c_i] e^{\int_0^{\tau-t} D_i(\xi)\, d\xi}\, d\tau,$$

where

$$\alpha = \frac{q^*}{2p^*}, \quad \epsilon = \frac{p^*}{2q^*}.$$

The initial condition of a solution to (4.1) will be said to lag behind the initial condition of another solution by no more than δ if

$$\left| \int_0^\infty \left[G_i^1(t) - G_i^2(t) \right] dt \right| \leqslant \delta, \quad i=1, 2, 3. \tag{4.3}$$

Here $G_i^k(t) = \int_t^\infty K_i(\tau) g_i^k(\tau - t) \exp\{\int_0^{\tau-t} D_i(\xi)\, d\xi\}\, d\tau$ are the functions defined by the initial distributions $g_i^k(t)$ where $k=1, 2$ are the numbers of two different distributions. It should be noted, that in case of a finite reproductive interval $[a, b]$ $G_i^k(t) \equiv 0$ for $t > b$, and consequently the integrals in (4.3) are surely convergent.

Applying the Laplace transformation and excluding one of the variables, we have

$$\tilde{e}_1(z)\left[1-\tilde{K}_1^0(z)+\alpha\left[1-\tilde{K}_2^0(z)\right]\right]+\tilde{e}_3(z)\beta\left[1-\tilde{K}_2^0(z)\right] = \tilde{H}_{12}(z), \tag{4.4}$$
$$\tilde{e}_1(z)\alpha\left[1-\tilde{K}_2^0(z)\right]+\tilde{e}_3(z)\left[1-\tilde{K}_3^0(z)+\beta\left[1-\tilde{K}_2^0(z)\right]\right] = \tilde{H}_{32}(z),$$

where

$$\tilde{H}_{12}(z) = \tilde{h}_1(z)+\tilde{h}_2(z) = \int_0^\infty [h_1(t)+h_2(t)]e^{-zt}\,dt,$$
$$\tilde{H}_{32}(z) = \tilde{h}_3(z)+\tilde{h}_2(z).$$

Here we applied the well known property of a convolution of two functions:

$$F\left[\int_0^t f(\tau)g(t-\tau)\,d\tau\right] = F(f)F(g),$$

where F is the Laplace transformation. In what follows the Laplace transform of a function will be denoted by a wavy line above as in (4.4).

For $\tilde{e}_1(z)$ and $\tilde{e}_3(z)$ we get the following expressions:

$$\tilde{e}_1(z) = \frac{\Delta_1(z)}{\Delta(z)}, \quad \tilde{e}_3(z) = \frac{\Delta_3(z)}{\Delta(z)},$$

where

$$\Delta_1(z) = \begin{vmatrix} \tilde{H}_{12}(z) & \beta\left[1-\tilde{K}_2^0(z)\right] \\ \tilde{H}_{32}(z) & 1-\tilde{K}_3^0(z)+\beta\left[1-\tilde{K}_2(z)\right] \end{vmatrix},$$

$$\Delta_3(z) = \begin{vmatrix} 1-\tilde{K}_1^0(z)+\alpha\left[1-\tilde{K}_2^0(z)\right] & \tilde{H}_{12}(z) \\ \alpha\left[1-\tilde{K}_2^0(z)\right] & \tilde{H}_{32}(z) \end{vmatrix},$$

$$\Delta(z) = \begin{vmatrix} 1-\tilde{K}_1^0(z)+\alpha\left[1-\tilde{K}_2^0(z)\right] & \beta\left[1-\tilde{K}_2^0(z)\right] \\ \alpha\left[1-\tilde{K}_2^0(z)\right] & 1-\tilde{K}_3^0(z)+\beta\left[1-\tilde{K}_2^0(z)\right] \end{vmatrix}.$$

It can be shown that the transforms of functions e_1 and e_3 comply with the second expansion theorem* and, consequently, the functions themselves will have the form

$$e_i(t) = \sum_{j=1}^{\infty} \gamma_i^j e^{z_j t}, \quad i=1,2,3,$$

* Lavrentiev, M. A. and Shabat, B. V.: 1958, *Metody teorii funkciy kompleksnovo peremennovo* (*Methods of the Theory of Functions of a Complex Variable.* In Russian), Nauka, Moscow, p. 483.

where z_j are roots of function $\Delta(z)$, and γ_i^j are the residues of functions $\Delta_i(z)/\Delta(z)$ at the poles z_j. Thus our problem is reduced to the localization of zeros of $\Delta(z)$ on the complex plane.

In Section 3.3 we showed that polymorphism can be reached either if $\lambda_2>\lambda_1, \lambda_3$ or if $\lambda_2<\lambda_1, \lambda_3$. Obviously similar inequalities are to take place for θ_i, and if λ^* is a root of the equation

$$[1-\omega_1(z)][1-\omega_3(z)] = [\omega_2(z)-1]^2,$$

then $\theta^*=0$ will be the root of

$$\left[1-\omega_1^0(z)\right]\left[1-\omega_3^0(z)\right] = \left[\omega_2^0(z)-1\right]^2, \tag{4.5}$$

where $\omega_i^0(z)\equiv\tilde{K}_i^0(z)$.

Suppose now that $\lambda_2>\lambda_1\geqslant\lambda_3$ (since subscripts 1 and 3 are symmetric, with no less generality we can assume that $\lambda_1\geqslant\lambda_3$). Let us represent the determinant $\Delta(z)$ in the form

$$\Delta(z) = \det[\mathbf{I}-\mathbf{A}(z)],$$

where $\mathbf{I}$ is a unit matrix and $\mathbf{A}(z)$ is a matrix of the form

$$\mathbf{A}(z) = \left\|\begin{matrix} \omega_1^0(z)+\alpha\left[\omega_2^0(z)-1\right] & \beta\left[\omega_2^0(z)-1\right] \\ \alpha\left[\omega_2^0(z)-1\right] & \omega_3^0(z)+\beta\left[\omega_2^0(z)-1\right] \end{matrix}\right\|.$$

Obviously, for θ_i the following inequalities hold: $\theta_3<\theta_1<0<\theta_2$.

Let us look at $\mathbf{A}(z)$ over the interval $[\theta_1, \theta_2]$. Since $\omega_2^0(z)>1$ for $z<\theta_2$, on this interval $\mathbf{A}(z)$ will be made up of positive monotone decreasing entries.

Consequently, this matrix complies with the Perron–Frobenius theory*. Using this theory, let us evaluate the Perron root (the maximal eigenvalue of matrix $\mathbf{A}(\theta_1)$). Since $\omega_2^0(\theta_1)>1$, we have

$$a_{11}(\theta_1)\equiv\omega_1^0(\theta_1)+\alpha\left[\omega_2^0(\theta_1)-1\right] = 1+\alpha\left[\omega_2^0(\theta_1)-1\right] > 1.$$

Here a_{11} is the left upper element of matrix $\mathbf{A}$. Then by the well-known property of matrices with positive elements**, the Perron root $r[\mathbf{A}(\theta_1)]$ will be greater than 1. Besides, direct calculations show that $r[\mathbf{A}(\theta_2)]<1$. Consequently, by the well-known theorem***), there exists a positive number θ^* on the interval $[\theta_1, \theta_2]$, such that $r[\mathbf{A}(\theta^*)]=1$, whence $\Delta(\theta^*)=0$.

Let us show that $\theta^*=0$. Recalling that $\alpha=q^*/(2p^*)$ and $\beta=p^*/(2q^*)$ represent $\Delta(z)$ in the form

* Bellman, R. and Cooke, K. L.: 1963, *Differential-Difference Equations*, Acad. Press, New York, p. 258–263

** *ibid.*, p. 259

*** *ibid.*, p. 259 (Theorem 8.3).

$$\left|\begin{matrix} 1+p^*\left[1-\omega_1^0\right]-\left[p^*\omega_1^0(z)+q^*\omega_2^0(z)\right] & p^*\left[1-\omega_1^0(z)\right] \\ q^*\left[1-\omega_2^0(z)\right] & 1+q^*\left[1-\omega_3^0(z)\right]-\left[p^*\omega_2^0(z)+q^*\omega_3^0(z)\right] \end{matrix}\right|.$$

By (3.2) $p^*w_1^0(0)+q^*\omega_2^0(0)=p^*\omega_1(\lambda^*)+q^*\omega_2(\lambda^*)=1$ and $p^*\omega_2^0(0)+q^*\omega_3^0(0)=1$, hence, calculating the determinant $\Delta(z)$, we get

$$\Delta(0) = p^*q^*\left[\left[1-\omega_1^0(0)\right]\left[1-\omega_3^0(0)\right]-\left[1-\omega_2^0(0)\right]^2\right].$$

In the state of polymorphism $p^*, q^*\neq 0$, and since $\theta^*=0$ is a root to Equation (4.5), it follows that $\Delta(\theta^*=0)=0$, Q.E.D.

Thus over the interval $[\theta_1, \theta_2]$ function $\Delta(z)$ has a unique real root, which is zero, while the real parts of all complex-valued roots (by the same theorem) are less than zero. Besides, writing the equation

$$\Delta(z) = \left[1-\omega_1^0(z)\right]\left[1-\omega_3^0(z)\right]+\alpha\left[1-\omega_2^0(z)\right]\left[1-\omega_3^0(z)\right]+ \\ +\beta\left[1-\omega_1^0(z)\right]\left[1-\omega_2^0(z)\right], \tag{4.6}$$

we can easily find, that $\omega_i^0(z)<1$, $i=1,2,3$ for real z, greater than θ_2, and consequently, $\Delta(z)>0$.

Clearly, $\Delta(z)$ has no complex-valued roots, such that $\mathrm{Re}\,z>0$. Otherwise, applying the above mentioned theorem to the interval (θ_2, ∞), we would derive that $\Delta(z)$ is to have a real root greater than θ_2, which is impossible.

Thus, we proved that the maximal real root of the function $\Delta(z)$ is zero, and that real parts of all complex-valued roots are negative. Consequently, the function $e_1(t)$ can be represented in the form

$$e_1(t) = \gamma_1^1+\eta(t), \tag{4.7}$$

where

$$\gamma_1^1 = \operatorname*{Res}_{z=0}\left[\frac{\Delta_1(z)}{\Delta(z)}\right] = \left.\frac{\Delta_1(z)}{\left[\frac{d\Delta}{dz}\right]}\right|_{z=0}, \tag{4.8}$$

$$\Delta_1(0) = \tilde{H}_{12}(0)\left[1-\omega_3^0(0)+\beta\left[1-\omega_2^0(0)\right]\right]-\beta\tilde{H}_{32}(0)\left[1-\omega_2^0(0)\right] = \\ = \frac{1}{2}\left[1-\omega_3^0(0)\right]\left[\tilde{H}_{12}(0)+\tilde{H}_{32}(0)\right].$$

Note that $0<1-\omega_3^0(0)<1$ and $(d\Delta/dz)\big|_{z=0}>0$. The function $\eta(t)$ approaches zero as $t\to\infty$ and, consequently, starting from some time $\bar{t}$ we have $\eta(t)<|\gamma_1^1|$ for all $t>\bar{t}$.

Likewise we can represent $e_2(t)$ and $e_3(t)$.

Let us now formulate the basic statement of this section, proved above.

THEOREM. *If the numbers* λ_i, *being the only real roots of the equations* $\omega_i(z)=1$, $i=1,2,3$, *satisfy the inequality*

$$\lambda_2 > \lambda_1, \lambda_3,$$

then for any arbitrarily small $\epsilon>0$ *there exists a* $\delta = 1/3\epsilon(\mathrm{d}\Delta/\mathrm{d}z)\big|_{z=0}$ *such that as soon as*

$$|\tilde{h}_i(0)| = \left| \int_0^\infty \int_t^\infty K_i^0(\tau)\left[g_i^0(\tau-t)-c_i\right] \exp\left\{\int_0^{\tau-t} D_i(\xi)\,\mathrm{d}\xi\right\} \mathrm{d}\tau \right| < \delta,$$

the inequality

$$|S_i(t)e^{-\lambda^* t} - c_i| < \epsilon, \quad i=1,2,3,$$

holds (maybe starting from some time $\bar{t}$*).*

In other words, for small (in terms of the introduced metrics) deviations of the initial age distributions from the equilibrium ones the deviation between the solution to our problem and the steady state age distribution at equilibrium, corresponding to polymorphism, will be less than ϵ. It is only natural to call this statement theorem about polymorphism stability for a system, evolving according to system (4.1).

Suppose $\lambda_1 > \lambda_3 > \lambda_2$ and accordingly $\theta_1 > \theta_3 > 0 > \theta_2$, that is, θ_2 and the pair θ_1 and θ_3 are separated by zero. Then $\Delta(\theta_1)\Delta(\theta_3)<0$ and since $\Delta(z)$ is continuous, there should exist a root θ such that $0<\theta_3<\theta<\theta_1$. In this case clearly $|e_i(t)| \to \infty$ for $t\to\infty$, i.e. the state of polymorphism is unstable. A similar statement holds for $\lambda_3 > \lambda_1 > \lambda_2$. Thus the second alternative condition (out of the necessary ones) of the polymorphism existence (condition (3.9)) actually corresponds to the state of unstable polymorphism.

Using this method, in a similar way we can prove that for $\lambda_1 \geqslant \lambda_2$ the state with $p^*=1$ will be stable, with no effect of λ_3 upon the stability of this state, provided that the evolution of the population originates sufficiently close to the point $p^*=1$. In case $\lambda_3 \geqslant \lambda_2$ the state $p^*=0$ will be stable, being independent of λ_1. Unfortunately, here we cannot make any global conclusions about stability and cannot indicate the domains of attraction for stable steady states. For instance, we know that for $\lambda_2 < \lambda_1, \lambda_3$ polymorphism is unstable. However, we cannot say the vicinity of which of the two states, $p^*=0$ or $p^*=1$, the trajectories will approach.

3.5. Population Without Age Structure. Continuous Model

Giving no consideration to the population age structure we can simplify the model to the utmost, however keeping some of the basic features of the genetic structure evolution in the population affected by differential selection. The independent analysis of the evolution of allele frequencies and of the total population number further simplifies the study, actually reducing it to the solution analysis for one first-order differential equation.

From (2.15.11) with $n=2$ we get

$$\frac{dp}{dt} = p(1-p)[(\beta-\gamma)-(2\beta-\alpha-\gamma)p]. \tag{5.1}$$

Here we used new notations: $p_1=p$, $p_2=1-p$, $w_{11}=\alpha$, $w_{12}=w_{21}=\beta$, $w_{22}=\gamma$. The phase portrait of this equation on the plane $\{\dot{p}, p; p\in[0,1]\}$ will depend upon the relation between α, β, γ. The following situations may occur:

1. Suppose $\alpha>\beta\geqslant\gamma$, that is, the homozygote AA is most fit. The phase portrait for this case is presented in Figure 4a. Since $\dot{p}\geqslant 0$, there is only one stable state $p^*=1$, corresponding to the complete replacement of allele a.

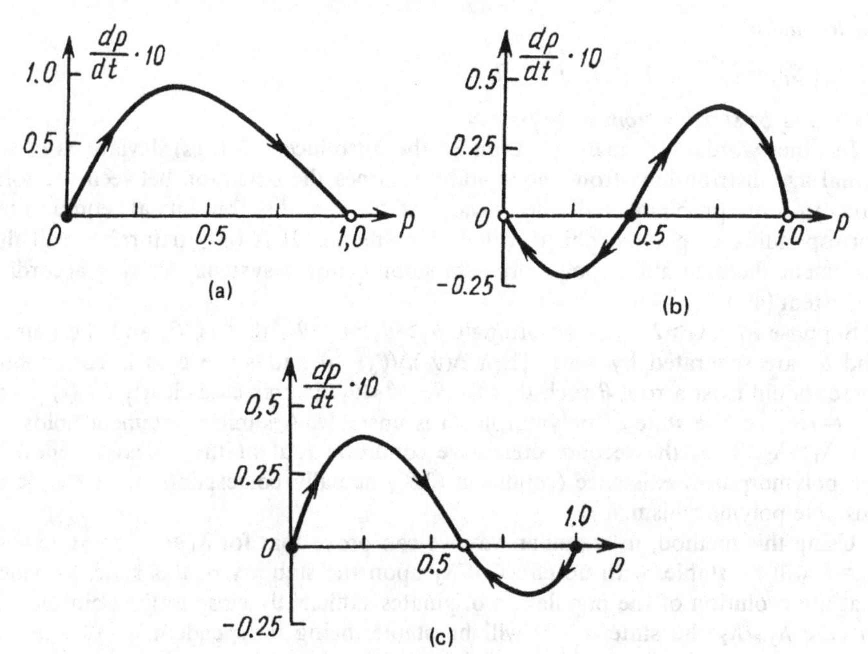

Fig. 4. Phase trajectories of the system, generated by (5.1) (O stable state, ● unstable state). (a) $\alpha=1$, $\beta=0.9$, $\gamma=0.5$, (b) $\alpha=1$, $\beta=0.5$, $\gamma=0.9$, (c) $\alpha=0.8$, $\beta=1$, $\gamma=0.7$.

2. Suppose $\beta<\alpha,\gamma$. Then $\dot{p}<0$ for $p\in(0,\hat{p})$ and $\dot{p}>0$ for $p\in(\hat{p},1)$, $\hat{p}=(\beta-\gamma)/(2\beta-\alpha-\gamma)$. Hence, the population has two stable states: $p_1^*=0$ and $p_2^*=1$, the first one attained for $p(t_0)<\hat{p}$ and the second one – for $\hat{p}(t_0)>\hat{p}$. The phase portrait for this case is shown in Figure 4b.

3. Suppose $\beta>\alpha,\gamma$, that is, the heterozygote Aa is most fit. Then $\dot{p}>0$ for $p\in(0,\hat{p})$ and $\dot{p}<0$ for $p\in(\hat{p},1)$. Consequently there exists only one stable state $p^*=\hat{p}$, which is the polymorphism. Figure 4c displays the phase portrait for this

population.

4. Suppose $\alpha \leqslant \beta < \gamma$, that is, the homozygote *aa* is most fit. Substituting *A* for *a* we reduce this case to the first one, where all the statements for allele *a* are to be replaced by similar ones, but for allele *A*, and vice versa. For instance, this is the case when allele *A* is completely replaced.

5. Suppose $\alpha = \beta > \gamma$, that is, the homozygote *AA* and the heterozygote *Aa* have the same fitnesses, which are maximal. In this case $p^* = 1$, the system behavior is similar to the one considered in 1.

6. Suppose $\alpha < \beta = \gamma$, that is, *Aa* and *aa* have the same fitnesses. Substituting *A* for *a* we reduce this case to 5.

7. Both homozygotes are equally fit, so that $\alpha = \gamma$. In this case, if the viability of the heterozygote is higher than that of the homozygote, then the system behavior is similar to the one considered in 2; otherwise – to the one considered in 1.

8. All three genotypes are equally fit, that is, $\alpha = \beta = \gamma$. Consider the case, when $\dot{p} \equiv 0$ for all p. Clearly, the necessary and sufficient conditions for this are as follows:

$$2\beta - \gamma - \alpha = 0, \quad 3\beta - 2\gamma - \alpha = 0, \quad \beta - \gamma = 0$$

This system has the non-trivial solution: $\alpha = \beta = \gamma$. Hence, without differential pressure of selection on genotypes, the genetic structure of a population does not change – quite an obvious conclusion. This case corresponds to the neutral genetic equilibrium.

What will happen to the total number of the population, characterized by the equation

$$\frac{dN}{dt} = N[w - d(N)], \tag{5.2}$$

$$w = (\alpha + \gamma - 2\beta)p^2 + 2(\beta - \gamma)p + \gamma?$$

Since $p(t) \to p^*$, when $t \to \infty$, its non-zero number at equilibrium is a root to the equation $d(N^*) = w(p^*)$, which is unique, if $d(N)$ is a steadily growing function. Moreover, this equilibrium will be stable, since for stability of N^* it is necessary and sufficient that $d'(N^*)$ be positive. Consequently, $N(t) \to N^*$ for $t \to \infty$, and if $N(t_0) < N^*$ then $N(t) < N^*$ for any $t_0 < t < \infty$. In fact, if at some point $N(t)$ is greater than N^*, due to continuity there should necessarily exist a point at which $\dot{N} = 0$ and $\ddot{N} < 0$. But at this point, by (5.2), $\ddot{N} = N\dot{w}$. And since $\dot{w} = (\partial w / \partial p)\dot{p} = p(1-p)^2[(\beta - \gamma) - (2\beta - \alpha - \gamma)p]^2 \geqslant 0$, it immediately follows that no such point can exist. The proved statement implies that no oscillations of numbers occur in the population.

3.6. Population Without Age Structure. Discrete Model

From (2.14.6) for $n = 2$, using the same notations as in Section 3.5, we can get

$$p' = \frac{p[(\alpha - \beta)p + \beta]}{(\alpha + \gamma - 2\beta)p^2 + 2(\beta - \gamma)p + \gamma}, \tag{6.1}$$

and the equation for the total population size:

$$N' = Nw, \quad w = (\alpha+\gamma-2\beta)p^2+2(\beta-\gamma)p+\gamma. \tag{6.2}$$

As mentioned above, fitnesses α, β and γ can depend upon the total population N. Obviously, if these fitnesses are modified by a common factor $F(N)$, the Equation (6.1) does not change and accordingly the gene frequency evolution can be studied independently of the total population evolution, which will be characterized by the equation $N'=NF(N)w(p)$.

It is readily seen that the points $p^*=0$, $p^*=1$ and $p^*=\hat{p}=(\beta-\gamma)/(2\beta-\alpha-\gamma)$ will be the fixed points of the differentiable mapping (6.1), transforming the interval [0, 1] into itself. It is known* that if there exists a point $p_s\in[0, 1]\,(p_s\neq p^*)$, at which $df/dp=0$, $d^2f/dp^2\neq 0$, then the equation $p'=f(p)$ can have either periodic or 'chaotic' trajectories. Checking directly we make sure that for $f(p)$, specified by formula (6.1), no such point exists, $df/dp=0$ only at the points $p^*=0, 1, \hat{p}$. The only regimes that can exist in this system, is $p\to p^*$. Moreover, always $p'\leqslant p$ or $p'\geqslant p$ (the identity takes place only for $p=p^*$). These statements become especially vivid if we use the so- called 'Lamerey diagram' to solve (6.1)**. It goes as follows.

Let us plot the functions $p'=f(p)$ and $p'=p$ on the plane $\{p',p;p',p\in[0, 1]\}$ (Figure 5).

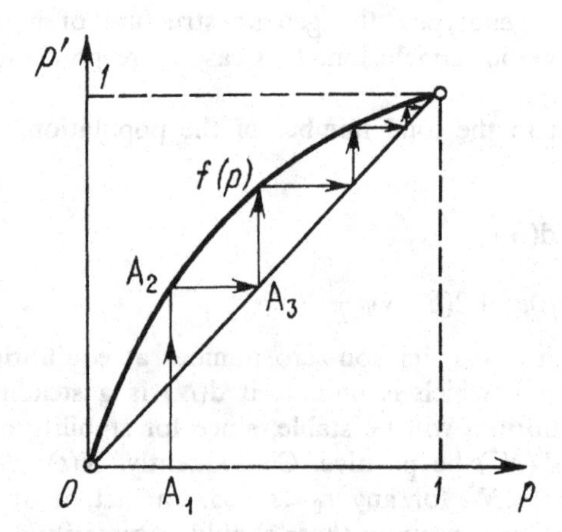

Fig. 5. Graphic solution to Equation (6.1) for $\alpha>\beta\geqslant\gamma$. (Allele *a* is steadily replaced.)

Next, let us take a point p_0 on the axis p (let it be A_1) and let us draw a straight

* Yakobson, M. V.: 1975, *O svoistvakh dinamicheskykh system porozhdayamykh otobrazheniyami vida* $x\to Axe^{-\beta x}$ (On properties of dynamical systems, generated by the mapping $x\to Axe^{-\beta x}$). In: *Modelirovaniye biologicheskykh soobshestv* (Modeling of biological communities). Vladivostok, DVNC AS U.S.S.R., p. 141–162.

** Andronov, A. A., Vitt, A. A., and Khaiken, S. E.: 1966, *Theory of Oscillations*, Pergamon Press, London.

line through this point, parallel to the p' axis, till it intersects the curve $f(p)$ (interval A_1A_2 in the figure). Then from the intersection point we draw a line, parallel to the p axis, till it intersects the line $p'=p$ (A_2A_3 in the figure). From the new intersection we draw a line parallel to the p' axis, till it intersects $f(p)$ and so on, until a limit point or a limit cycle is attained. It might sometimes happen that this process never converges to a specific set, and then the regime is said to be 'chaotic'. Such a situation is exampled in Figure 6.

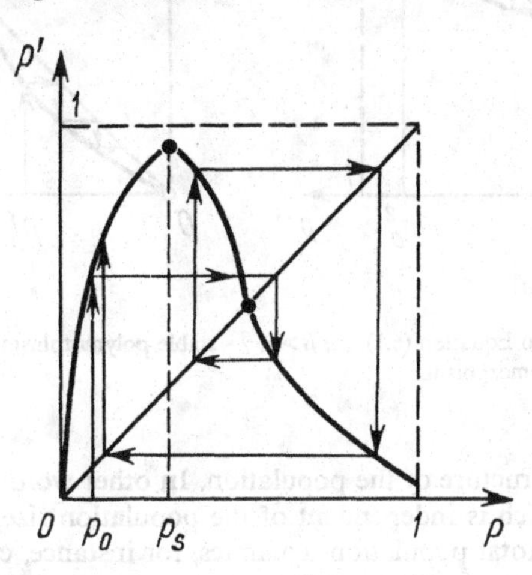

Fig. 6. Graphic solution of the hypothetical equation $p'=f(p)$ with 'chaotic' trajectories. In reality this can be the case when fitnesses are certain functions of the frequency p.

One can see that there exists the point p_s, where $f(p)$ peaks. It should be noted, however, that this condition is only necessary.

Above we studied the case when $\alpha>\beta\geqslant\gamma$ and allele a is eliminated. Suppose now $\beta>\alpha, \gamma$. Then the graphic solution of (6.1) shows (Figure 7a) that polymorphism is established in the population – trajectories tend to the point p^*. If $\beta<\alpha, \gamma$, then polymorphism is unstable and depending on the initial frequency either allele A, or allele a is elminated (Figure 7b).

And lastly let us look at the total population dynamics. The equation $N'=Nf(N)$, where $f(N)$ is a monotone decreasing function and $f(0)=r>0$, has been studied fairly well*. It was shown that, depending upon r and the rate of decrease of f, the behavior spectrum of the trajectories of this equation includes stable equilibria, stable cycles of any length and even 'chaotic' solutions, which are determined by the initial conditions. In our case $f(N)=F(N)w(p)$, i.e. the behavior of the trajectories depends not only on the form of the function, which characterizes how the chance to survive falls with the growth of the total population, but

* Svirezhev, Yu. M. and Logofet, D. O.: 1983, *Stability of Biological Communities*, Moscow, Mir, 320 p.

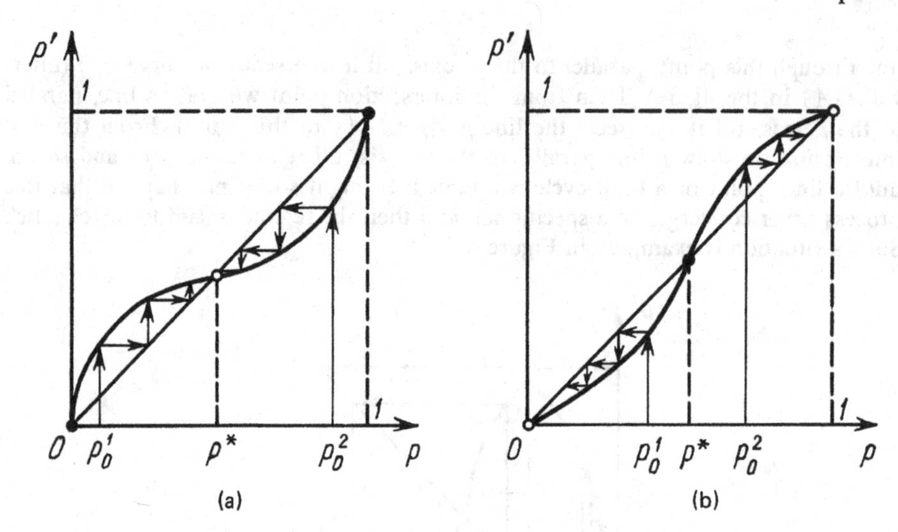

Fig. 7. Graphic solution to Equation (6.1). (a) $\beta>\alpha, \gamma$ - stable polymorphism; (b) $\beta<\alpha, \gamma$ - unstable polymorphism.

also on the genetic structure of the population. In other words, the evolution of the genetic structure, which is independent of the population size, can result in principal variations of the total population dynamics, for instance, cyclic oscillations may appear in the population*. The problem is not yet studied, but is undoubtedly very interesting.

Note that while the evolution of the genetic structure is more or less regular (tendency towards a stable equilibrium, either 'pure' or 'polymorphic'), the total population can demonstrate a fair variety of behaviors.

3.7. Polymorphism. Experiments and Theory. What Are the Malthusian Parameters or Genotype Fitnesses?

The problem of existence of genetic polymorphism is one of the most serious problems of today's population genetics. Numerous observations in natural populations show that all of them are polymorphic to a certain extent. However, up till now we cannot understand the mechanisms, that provide the existence of polymorphism. In this chapter by purely theoretical means we showed that one such mechanism, the advantage of heterozygotes compared to homozygotes, can result in the existence of polymorphism. But in this situation we still have no idea, what are the Malthusian parameters of genotypes (or their fitnesses) and how can they be measured.

* Asmussen, M. A.: 1979, 'Regular and Chaotic Cycling in Models of Ecological Genetics', *Theor. Pop. Biol.*, **16**, 2, 172–190.

Comparing the results of Sections 3.3–3.6, we can see that in all models the necessary and sufficient condition for polymorphism is provided by the advantage of heterozygotes. However, while in models with age structure this advantage was measured by λ_i, the maximal real roots of the equations

$$F_c \int_a^b \exp\left\{\int_0^\tau D_i(\xi)\,d\xi - \lambda\tau\right\} d\tau = 1, \quad i=1,2,3, \tag{7.1}$$

which actually defined some maximal growth rate for each genotypic group, in models with no age structure it was measured by fitnesses α, β and γ. And these parameters are characterized either by differential fecundity, or by the probability of survival. Naturally, in each of the above listed variants in order to evaluate these parameters various observations are to be made and different experiments are to be performed. For instance, in the first case we need the so-called 'life tables'.

This short 'biological' excursus shows that the definition of Malthusian parameters or fitnesses remains to be a very uncertain and obscure problem. This obstacle makes some workers call in question the value of mathematical models in genetics. They may be right speaking about *quantitative* prediction of genetic evolution. Note, however, that in spite of different definitions of Malthusian parameters, *qualitatively* all these models have something in common: for polymorphism it is necessary and sufficient that heterozygotes have advantage, no matter how it is evaluated or measured. And this is the result, which gives us some ground for a more optimistic point of view. Another argument, favoring our optimism, results from the following classical experiment of N. V. Timofeeff-Ressovsky, which we felt necessary to quote in our book.

Model populations of *Drosophila melanogaster* were engaged in the experiment (the fruit-fly is a classical experimental object in genetics). Each such population contained three genotypes: the normal one *AA* and those of the heterozygote *Aa* and the homozygote *aa* with respect to the *ebony* mutation. Direct genetic analysis showed that this mutation affects only one locus. To eliminate such a factor as the dependency of the selection pressure on total population number, the latter has been kept constant (about 15–16 thousand, which corresponds to the level of maximal density) during the whole experimental period (about 650 days) by a special system of alternating feeding regimes. At zero time the quantitatively stable *ebony* populations were infected by 50 pairs of normal flies. Every 50 days (3 generations) flies of different genotypes were counted. The results of the experiment are contained in Figure 8. It is seen, that in spite of a relatively fast initial replacement of the *ebony* flies by the normal ones, the former are not eliminated from the population and stabilize at a certain level (8–9%). A stable state of polymorphism is observed, three different forms coexist in the population.

In order to evaluate the Malthusian parameters or the genotype fitnesses additional experiments needed to be staged. Let us note that in Drosophila populations, which are usually highly panmicitic, selection mostly affects the stage of larva, which most intensively compete for food. The experiments were as follows. An equal number of eggs, layed by heterozygotes, were put in test-tubes with food

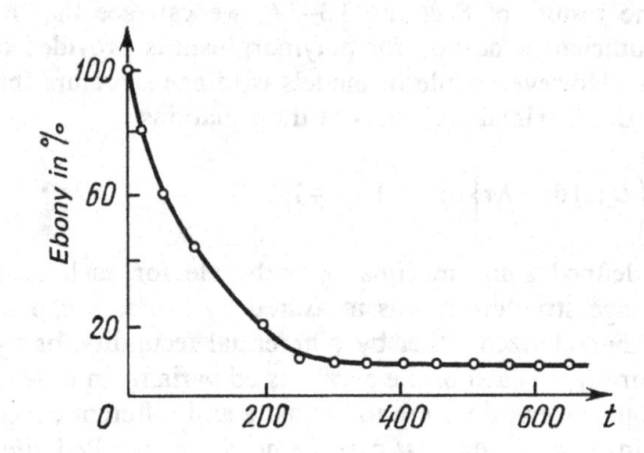

Fig. 8. Replacement of Drosophila melanogaster flies by normal specimens in model populations (O - experimental values).

and then the number of emerging flies with different genotypes was counted. If selection acted with no differentiation, the ratio of genotype numbers should have been 1:2:1. And this was observed in sparsely populated test-tubes. However in overpopulated tubes (the extent of over population corresponding to the model populations) this ratio was equal to 0.815:1:0.518. The emerging flies practically always live up till their reproductive age and produce offspring. Therefore if we accept that a heterozygote reaches its reproductive age with unit probability, then the appropriate probabilities for the normal and mutant homozygotes will be 0.815 and 0.518, respectively. Obviously, these quantities may be taken for the Malthusian parameters or genotype fitnesses:

$$\alpha = 0.815, \quad \beta = 1, \quad \gamma = 0.518.$$

At equilibrium we can think that the genotype frequency $aa - u_3^* \simeq (1-p^*)^2$. Taking $u_3^* \simeq 0.085$, we get $p^* \simeq 0.71$. On the other hand, from theory we know that $p^* = (\beta - \gamma)/(2\beta - \alpha - \gamma) = 0.72$. Comparison of these two values presents a fairly unique (for biological experiments) agreement between the experimentally deduced and theoretically predicted polymorphism levels. It should be also noted that unlike most experiments, with fitnesses defined by the evolutionary trajectories of the genotypic content, here these parameters were derived from other additional experiments.

Comparing the theoretical and experimental curves over the non- stationary regions, we come across two obstacles: firstly, it is hard to define the initial frequency of the normal allele, secondly, it is hard to define the time scale (mean generation length) and to choose the model type (discrete or continuous). To overcome the first obstacle we took the values at $t_0 = 50$ days as the common initial point of the theoretical and experimental curves. As to the model type, our choice fell upon the discrete one, since the Drosophila populations demonstrate quite high synchronization of generations. And lastly, our choice of the mean generation length fell upon two values: 16 and 25 days. Actually this factor is very sensitive to ambient temperature, as well as to other environmental factors. Usually in experimental studies this value varies from 12 to 26 days. Obviously, the inaccurate definition of the generation length tells only on the non-stationary part of the curve; the steady-state value attained for $t \to \infty$ is independent of the chosen time-scale.

Figure 9 displays the curves for the frequency of allele *A*, calculated from experimental results and computed by (6.1). The measurements of the frequency of genotype *aa* were quite scarce, at intervals exceeding the generation length. Therefore we may think that at the moments of counts the population satisfies the Hardy–Weinberg relation and $p(t) = 1 - \sqrt{u_3(t)}$.

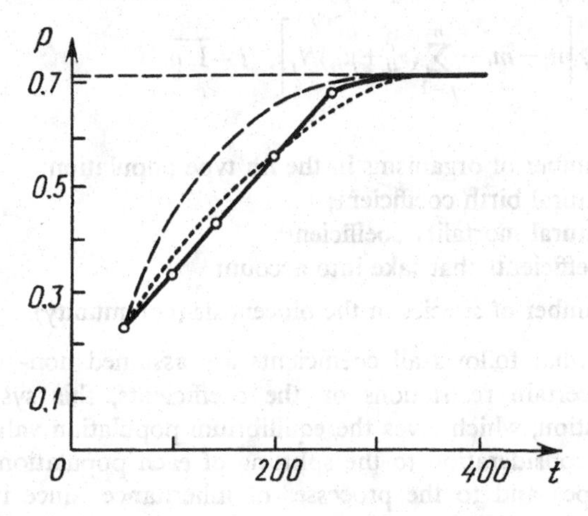

Fig. 9. Theoretical and experimental curves presenting the replacement of the mutant allele: (-) experimental curve; (---) theoretical curve (generation length = 16 days); (....) theoretical curve (generation length = 25 days).

Comparing the curves in Figure 9 we see that on the non-stationary section the agreement between theory and experiment is worse; however, if the model makes use of the generation length enhanced to 25 days, then the fit becomes much better.

Nevertheless, taking into account how hard it is to get the experimental data of this kind, we can say that the obtained agreement between the theoretical and experimental data for the dynamics of the population gene content is good enough. This implies that in spite of the very strict constraints the model is based upon, the actual biological system, the population, is modelled quite well.

3.8. Genetico-Ecological Models

There is still another class of genetic models, orginating from the Volterra type models of mathematical ecology – the Kostitzin models.

The frequency models of Fisher–Wright–Haldane (the classical models of population genetics) operate with the most primitive description of selection in terms of Malthusian parameters or fitnesses. In this case the selection pressure on the genotype depends only upon the genotype itself, and is in no way related to the interaction between genotypes. However, as we know from population ecology, the leading role in population dynamics of species is played by relationships of competition, that is pair intersections between organisms of different species or intraspecific groups (say, genotypic groups). Models, taking account of this effect, are the Volterra equations widely known in mathematical ecology:

$$\frac{dN_i}{dt} = N_i\left[n_i - m_i - \sum_{j=1}^{n}(\nu_{ij} + \mu_{ij})N_j\right], \quad i=\overline{1,n}, \tag{8.1}$$

where

N_i = number of organisms in the ith type population;
n_i = natural birth coefficient;
m_i = natural mortality coefficient;
ν_{ij}, μ_{ij} = coefficients that take into account
n = number of species in the biocenosis (community).

Here and in what follows all coefficients are assumed non- negative. One can show that for certain restrictions on the coefficients, this system has a stable steady-state solution, which gives the equilibrium population values. However, this model gives no consideration to the splitting of each population into groups with different genotypes and to the processes of inheritance, since it is assumed that organisms of one population can produce only their likes. If we consider N_i to be the numbers of different genotypes, competing with one another, the situation becomes much more complicated, since organisms of the ith population can produce organisms of other groups in addition to those of the same group. On the other hand, the population age structure is by no means present in these equations. Therefore, drawing out models, which consider both competition and genetic processes (in what follows they will be termed 'genetico-ecological' models), we neglect the age structure and suppose that processes of birth and death occur simulaneously.

Let

N_i = the number of organisms with genotype $AA - \{1\}$;
N_2 = the number of organisms with genotype $Aa - \{2\}$;
N_3 = the number of organisms with genotype $aa - \{3\}$.

The total population number is $N = N_1 + N_2 + N_3$. Organisms are assumed to mate at random (panmixia) and produce equal proportions of male and female offspring. In this case the probability that a couple ♀{i}, ♂{j}, $i, j = 1, 2, 3$, will be formed is equal to $N_i N_j / N^2$ (similarly for the couple ♀{j}, ♂{i}). With no regard of competition let each such pair produce offspring in unit time. For instance, the couple ♀{Aa}, ♂{Aa} in favorable conditions with no competition produces n_{22} offspring with $n_{22}/2$ male and $n_{22}/2$ female organisms among them.

n_{ij} is not necessarily equal to n_{ji}. Actually n_{ij} is the coefficient of natural birth or the fecundity coefficient, which is dependent on both the male and female genotypes.

Suppose competition affects the females in such a way that natality falls so that the birth-rate coefficient declines by the value $\sigma_{,i} = \sigma_{,i}(N_j, t)$. Likewise, competition affects males so that the birth coefficient declines by the value $\tau_{i,} = \tau_{i,}(\mathrm{N}_j, t)$, $i, j = 1, 2, 3$. (Subscripts with a comma before them belong to females, those with a comma after – to males; in two-index notations the first index is related to the male genotype, the second one – to the female genotype). Under these assumptions the birth coefficient for a couple made with the ith genotype and a female with the jth genotype ($i, j = 1, 2, 3$) can be written in the form

$$F_{ij} = n_{ij} - \tau_{i,} - \sigma_{,j}. \tag{8.2}$$

Let us call F_{ij} the *generalized* birth-rate coefficient for the couple ♀{i}, ♂{j}. Counting the total amount of different couples and taking into account that these couples have different birth-rate coefficients, one can calculate the increase of the total population due to the birth of organisms of a new generation over the time period δt:

$$\delta N_F = \left[\frac{F_{11} N_1^2}{2N} + \frac{F_{12} + F_{21}}{2N} N_1 N_2 + \frac{F_{13} + F_{31}}{2N} N_1 N_3 + \right. \tag{8.3}$$

$$\left. + \frac{F_{22} N_2^2}{2N} + \frac{F_{23} + F_{32}}{2N} N_2 N_3 + \frac{F_{33} N_3^2}{2N} \right] \delta t.$$

Here we took advantage of the fact, that if a couple, say ♀{AA}, ♂{Aa}, is formed with a probability $N_1 N_2 / N^2$ then $N_1 N_2 / (2N)$ such couples can be formed in a population of individuals with equal proportions of sexes, and each such pair produces F_{12} offspring in unit time.

By Mendel's laws the couples ♀{AA}, ♂{AA} will produce offspring with genotypes AA only; the offspring of the couples ♀{aa}, ♂{aa} will have genotype aa; that of the couples ♀{AA}, ♂{aa} and ♀{aa}, ♂{AA} will have genotype Aa, the offspring of the couples ♀{AA}, ♂{Aa} and ♀{Aa}, ♂{AA} will be made of genotypes AA and aa, occurring with a frequency $1/2$; the offspring of ♀{Aa}, ♂{aa} and ♀{aa}, ♂{Aa} will be made of genotypes Aa and aa with a frequency $1/2$; and eventually, the offspring of ♀{Aa}, ♂{Aa} will be made of genotypes AA, aa, Aa with frequencies $1/4$, $1/4$, $1/2$, respectively. Therefore, the total increment δN_F will be split between genotypic groups, as follows:

$$\delta N_{1F} = \left[\phi_{11}N_1^2+\phi_{12}N_1N_2+\frac{1}{4}\phi_{22}N_2^2\right]\frac{\delta t}{N},$$

$$\delta N_{2F} = \left[\phi_{12}N_1N_{12}+\frac{1}{2}\phi_{22}N_2^2+2\phi_{13}N_1N_3+\phi_{23}N_2N_3\right]\frac{\delta t}{N}, \tag{8.4}$$

$$\delta N_{3F} = \left[\phi_{32}N_2N_3+\frac{1}{4}\phi_{22}N_2^2+\phi_{33}N_3^2\right]\frac{\delta t}{N}.$$

Here we introduced new notations: $2\phi_{ij}=(F_{ij}+F_{ji})/2$ so that $\phi_{ij}=\phi_{ji}$, $i, j=1, 2, 3$.

Let us again turn to our good old model (8.1) and rewrite it in the form

$$\frac{dN_i}{dt} = P_i-M_i,\ \ P_i = N\left[n_i-\sum_{j=1}^{n}\nu_{ij}N_j\right], \tag{8.5}$$

$$M_i = N_i\left[m_i+\sum_{j=1}^{n}\mu_{ij}N_j\right],\ \ n=3;\ i=1, 2, 3.$$

The variable P_i characterizes the increase of the ith population due to birth, M_i stands for the decrease of the population due to mortality. Naturally, m_i and μ_{ij} being independent of reproductive relations between groups of different genotypes, depend only on genotypes of individuals. In our case we treat the mating process between organisms of different groups, and processes in which organisms of one group produce organisms of other groups. Consequently, in (8.5) we are to substitute P_i by a term of (8.4) type. Then the equations for the dynamics of genotypic groups can be written in the form

$$\frac{dN_1}{dt} = \frac{1}{4N}(4\phi_{11}N_1^2+4\phi_{12}N_1N_2+\phi_{22}N_2^2)-N_1\left[m_1+\sum_{j=1}^{3}\mu_{ij}N_j\right], \tag{8.6}$$

$$\frac{dN_2}{dt} = \frac{1}{2N}(2\phi_{21}N_1N_2+\phi_{22}N_2^2+4\phi_{13}N_1N_3+2\phi_{23}N_2N_3)-$$

$$-N_2\left[m_2+\sum_{j=1}^{3}\mu_{2j}N_j\right],$$

$$\frac{dN_3}{dt} = \frac{1}{4N}(4\phi_{32}N_2N_3+\phi_{22}N_2^2+4\phi_{33}N_3^2)-N_3\left[m_3+\sum_{j=1}^{3}\mu_{3j}N_j\right].$$

We still have not specified how the variables ϕ_{ij} actually depend on N_k. Most simple is the assumption that these variables are constant or depend linearly on N_k. Say,

$$F_{ij} = n_{ij}-\tau_{i,}-\sigma_{,j} = n_{ij}-\sum_{k=1}^{3}\lambda_{ik}N_k-\sum_{k=1}^{3}\rho_{kj}N_k, \tag{8.7}$$

$$\phi_{ij} = \frac{1}{4}(F_{ij}+F_{ji}),\ \ i, j=1, 2, 3,$$

where λ_{ik}, ρ_{kj} are coefficients which may be explicit functions of time, being independent of N_k, $k=1, 2, 3$. λ_{ik} present the competition effects on males resulting in declines of natality, ρ_{kj} are the same for females.

This model, formulated for numbers of different genotypes, brings into focus the effects of various ecological factors of selection upon the genotypic population dynamics.

3.9. Special Cases of Genetico-Ecological Models

To make it more clear let us attend to some special cases of the general model (8.6).

(a) Let genotypes be different only with respect to natural mortality. Then $\phi_{ij}=\phi$, $\mu_{ij}=\mu$ for all $i, j=1, 2, 3$. This is equivalent to assuming that fecundity is constant and independent of male and female genotype, modified by competition, which depends on the total population number. Then from (8.6) it follows

$$\begin{aligned} \frac{dN_1}{dt} &= \frac{\phi}{N}\left[N_1+\frac{N_2}{2}\right]^2 - m_1N_1-\mu N_1N, \\ \frac{dN_2}{dt} &= \frac{2\phi}{N}\left[N_1+\frac{N_2}{2}\right]\left[\frac{N_2}{2}+N_3\right]-m_2N_2-\mu N_2N, \\ \frac{dN_3}{dt} &= \frac{\phi}{N}\left[\frac{N_2}{2}+N_3\right]^2-m_3N_3-\mu N_3N. \end{aligned} \tag{9.1}$$

It is a simple matter to prove that for positive parameters and non-negative initial values the solutions to this system will be non-negative. Summing up (9.1) we get the equation for the total population size:

$$\frac{dN}{dt} = \phi N-\mu N^2-\sum_{i=1}^{3} m_iN_i. \tag{9.2}$$

If $\phi<m=\min\{m_1, m_2, m_3\}$, then $\dot{N}<0$ for all positive N. Hence, the total population steadily declines till extinction (when $N=0$, $\dot{N}=0$). Since N_1, N_2, N_3 are non-negative by their biological meaning, when $N=N_1+N_2+N_3=0$ the genotype numbers N_1, N_2 and N_3 are to be also zero. In other words, when the fecundity coefficient is less than the coefficient of natural mortality, all genotypes die off, which is quite an obvious result.

The steady state points for (9.1) can be found from the equations

$$\begin{aligned} \frac{\phi}{N^*}\left[N_1^*+\frac{N_2^*}{2}\right]^2 &= N_1^*(m_1+\mu N^*), \\ \frac{2\phi}{N^*}\left[N_1^*+\frac{N_2^*}{2}\right]\left[\frac{N_2^*}{2}+N_3^*\right] &= N_2^*(m_2+\mu N^*), \\ \frac{\phi}{N^*}\left[\frac{N_2^*}{2}+N_3^*\right]^2 &= N_3^*(m_3+\mu N^*). \end{aligned} \tag{9.3}$$

It can be readily seen that this system has, say, such solutions:
1. $N_1^* = (\phi - m_1)/\mu$, $N_2^* = N_3^* = 0$.
2. $N_1^* = N_2^* = 0$, $N_3^* = (\phi - m_3)/\mu$.
Interestingly, there is no solution of the form $N_1^* = N_3^* = 0$, $N_2^* \neq 0$. From the biological viewpoint this is quite natural, since no population can consist only of heterozygotes: crossing among any heterozygous couple produces homozygotes in its offspring.

If $\phi > m_1$ and $m_2 > m_1$ then solution 1 is stable, and if $\phi > m_3$ and $m_2 > m_3$ then solution 2 is stable. This implies that when the fecundity coefficient is greater than the coefficient of natural mortality for genotype *AA*, and this coefficient is in turn less than the appropriate coefficient for genotype *Aa*, then only organisms of genotype *AA* remain in the population. A similar statement can be formulated for the *aa* genotype. Curiously enough, in this model the replacement of, say, allele *a*, is determined by inequalities only for ϕ, m_1, m_2. No constraints are imposed on μ and m_3 (except their being positive).

To further our study let us still simplify the problem by assuming $m_1 = m_3 = m$, $m_2 = m - 2s$. Introducing new variables: $x = (N_1 + N_2/2)\mu/m$, $y = (N_3 + N_2/2)\mu/m$, $z = N_2\mu/m$ (x and y are the modified allele numbers), (9.1) can be rewritten in the form:

$$\frac{dx}{d\tau} = x(f - x - y) + \sigma z,$$
$$\frac{dy}{d\tau} = y(f - x - y) + \sigma z, \qquad (9.4)$$
$$\frac{dz}{d\tau} = 2(1+f)\frac{xy}{x+y} - z(1 - 2\sigma + x + y).$$

Here $\tau = mt$, $\sigma = s/m$, $\phi = (1+f)m$. By its biological meaning $\sigma < 1/2$. Since the Equations (9.4) are invariant with respect to the change of variables $x \rightleftarrows y$, their solutions (for symmetric initial conditions) will be symmetric with respect to the plane $x = y$. For the variable $\xi = x - y$ we get the equation

$$\frac{d\xi}{d\tau} = \xi(f - x - y).$$

If $x(\tau) \to x^*$ and $y(\tau) \to y^*$ for $\tau \to \infty$, then in the neighbourhood of these steady-state values $\xi(\tau) \to 0$, when $x^* + y^* > f$ and $\tau \to \infty$. Consequently, if the condition $x^* + y^* > f$ holds, then the plane $x = y$ is an attracting manifold for all the trajectories lying in the vicinity of this plane. Therefore in this vicinity instead of the basic system (9.1) we can study the truncated one with $x(t) = y(t)$:

$$\frac{dx}{dt} = x(f - 2x) + \sigma z \qquad (9.5)$$
$$\frac{dz}{dt} = (1+f)x - z(1 - 2\sigma + 2x).$$

Let us seek for the steady-state solution to (9.5) such that $z^*(N_2^*) = 0$. Besides the natural constraints $x^* > 0$ and $z^* < 2x^*$ should hold. The latter one implies that the number of heterozygotes should not exceed the total population size. One can prove that when $1+f>0$ and $0<\sigma<1/2$, such a solution exists and has the form

$$x^* = \frac{1}{4}(f+2\sigma-1+\sqrt{(1+f)^2+4\sigma^2}), \quad z^* = \frac{x^*(2x^*-f)}{\sigma}. \tag{9.6}$$

Besides, the attraction condition is to hold: $2x^*>f$. By direct substitution we find out that it holds if $1+f>0$, $0<\sigma<1/2$.

For (9.6) to be stable it is necessary and sufficient that

$$12x^{*2}-4x^*(f+2\sigma-1)+(\sigma+f-\sigma f)>0.$$

Substituting the expression for x^* from (9.6) we get

$$f+\sigma>f\sigma. \tag{9.7}$$

Turning to the original notations, we can see, that all the three genotypes can coexist in the population (that is a stable polymorphism can be attained) if

$$0 < m_2 < m, \quad (\phi-m_2)+m_2\frac{(\phi-m)}{m} > 0. \tag{9.8}$$

In other words, if in this population the mortality of the heterozygote is lower than that of both homozygotes and, besides, if an averaged coefficient of natural growth for the homozygote and the heterozygote,

$$\tilde{\epsilon} = m\epsilon_2+m_2\epsilon, \quad \epsilon = \phi-m, \quad \epsilon_2 = \phi-m_2,$$

is positive, then a stable polymorphism is established.

Interestingly, the existence conditions for polymorphism in this model turn to be more complex than in the classical model of Sections 3.5–3.6. However, this distinction disappears if we suppose that $\phi\sim m$ and $m_2<<m$. Then for stability it is necessary and sufficient, that $\phi>m_2$, providing that there is no extinction of the population, and $m_2<m$, providing the existence of a stable steady-state equilibrium for allele frequencies (polymorphism).

For $\sigma<<1$ it follows from (9.6) that $z^*\simeq x^*$, that is $1/2\cdot N_2^*\simeq N_1^*=N_2^*$. The latter equality implies that for small distinctions between the mortality coefficients ('weak selection') the ratio of genotype numbers (and, accordingly, their frequencies) tends to 1:2:1, which is the ratio, given by the Hardy–Weinberg principle.

(b) Suppose

$$\phi_{ij} = \phi = \text{const},$$

$$m_i = m = \text{const for all } i,\ j=1, 2, 3,$$

$$\mu_{ij} = \mu_i, \quad \phi>m.$$

Thus, genotypes are distinguished only by the different effects of competition on the mortality of organisms. Hence, (8.6) can be rewritten in the form

$$\frac{dN_1}{dt} = \frac{\phi}{N}\left[N_1+\frac{N_2}{2}\right]^2-mN_1-\mu_1N_1N,$$

$$\frac{dN_2}{dt} = \frac{2\phi}{N}\left[N_1+\frac{N_2}{2}\right]\left[\frac{N_2}{2}+N_3\right]-mN_2-\mu_2N_2N \tag{9.9}$$

$$\frac{dN_3}{dt} = \frac{\phi}{N}\left[N_3+\frac{N_2}{2}\right]^2-mN_3-\mu_3N_3N.$$

Assuming that $\mu_1=\mu_3=\mu$, $\mu_2=\mu-2s$, and substituting the variables x, y and z, from (9.9) we get ($\tau=mt$, $k=s/\mu$, $\phi=(1+f)m$)

$$\frac{dx}{d\tau} = x(f-x-y)+kz(x+y),$$

$$\frac{dy}{d\tau} = y(f-x-y)+kz(x+y), \tag{9.10}$$

$$\frac{dz}{d\tau} = \frac{2(1+f)xy}{x+y}-z[1+(1-2k)(x+y)].$$

This system displays the same properties of symmetry as (9.4). Therefore, just like above, we will seek for the solution $x(t)=y(t)$, that satisfies the truncated system

$$\frac{dx}{d\tau} = x(f-2x+2kz), \tag{9.11}$$

$$\frac{dz}{d\tau} = (1+f)x-z[1+2(1-2k)x].$$

The non-trivial steady-state solution to (9.11), corresponding to the state of genetic polymorphism, has the form

$$x^* = \frac{1}{4(1-2k)} \times\{-(1-k)(1-f)+\sqrt{(1-k)^2(1-f)^2+4f(1-2k)}\}, \tag{9.12}$$

$$z^* = \frac{2x^*-f}{2k}.$$

One can prove that for $f>0$ and $0<k<1/2$ this equilibrium complies with the natural constraints $x^*>0$, $2x^*>z^*$ and satisfies the condition of attraction: $2x^*>f$. The state of polymorphism is stable, if the condition

$$[(1+f)k-1]x^*+fx^*-\frac{f^2}{4}>0 \tag{9.13}$$

holds. This inequality always holds for $1+f>4k$. Refined sufficient conditions of stability are associated with cumbersome calculations, and for this reason we omit them here. In terms of our original notations the sufficient condition of polymorphism existence can be written in the form $\phi\mu>4sm$. But from the condition $2s<\mu$, which is always satisfied since $2s=\mu-\mu_2<\mu$, it follows that if $\phi>2m$ then $\phi\mu>4sm$.

And finally, a stable polymorphism exists in a population if heterozygotes have competitive advantages in comparison with homozygotes, and the fecundity of individuals is more than twice as large as their natural mortality. Note that the latter condition is sufficient but not necessary.

3.10. Passage from Genetico-Ecological Models to Models in Frequency Form

Let us look at another special case of the general model (8.6). Suppose $m_i = m = \text{const}$, $\mu_{ij} = \mu = \text{const}$ for all $i, j = 1, 2, 3$. As concerns the fecundity coefficients ϕ_{ij} we will assume the fecundity of any couple to be a function only of the female genotype. Then

$$\phi_{11} = \alpha,\ \phi_{22} = \beta,\ \phi_{33} = \gamma,$$

$$\phi_{12} = \phi_{21} = \frac{(\alpha+\beta)}{2},\ \phi_{13} = \phi_{31} = \frac{(\alpha+\gamma)}{2},\ \phi_{23} = \phi_{32} = \frac{(\beta+\gamma)}{2}.$$

In this case (8.6) can be written in the form

$$\begin{aligned}
\frac{dN_1}{dt} &= \frac{1}{N}\left[N_1+\frac{N_2}{2}\right]\left[\alpha N_1+\frac{\beta N_2}{2}\right]-d(N)N_1,\\
\frac{dN_2}{dt} &= \frac{1}{N}\left[\left[\alpha N_1+\frac{\beta N_2}{2}\right]\left[\frac{N_2}{2}+N_3\right]+\right.\\
&\quad+\left.\left[\frac{\beta N_2}{2}+\gamma N_3\right]\left[N_1+\frac{N_2}{2}\right]\right]-d(N)N_2,\\
\frac{dN_3}{dt} &= \frac{1}{N}\left[\frac{N_2}{2}+N_3\right]\left[\frac{\beta N_2}{2}+\gamma N_3\right]-d(N)N_3.
\end{aligned} \tag{10.1}$$

Here $d(N) = m+\mu N$. Define the frequencies of genotypes AA, Aa and aa as $u = N_1/N$, $2v = N_2/N$ and $w = N_3/N$, respectively. Passing to these frequencies in (10.1) we obtain

$$\begin{aligned}
\frac{du}{dt} &= (u+v)(\alpha u+\beta v)-uW,\\
\frac{dv}{dt} &= \frac{1}{2}[(\alpha u+\beta v)(v+w)+(\beta v+\gamma w)(u+v)]-vW,\\
\frac{dw}{dt} &= (v+w)(\beta v+\gamma w)-wW,
\end{aligned} \tag{10.2}$$

where $W = \alpha u+2\beta v+\gamma w$. The equation for the total population can be written in the form

$$\frac{dN}{dt} = N[W-d(N)]. \tag{10.3}$$

It is easily seen that there is no direct way to carry over to the equations for allele frequencies $p=u+v$ and $q=v+w$. Nevertheless we can pass to the allele frequencies, introducing an additional variable $\xi=uw-v^2$, which is nothing else but the index of the deviation of our system from the Hardian equilibrium $u=p^2$, $v=pq$, $w=q^2$. Then

$$u = p^2+\xi, \quad v = pq-\xi, \quad w = q^2+\xi. \tag{10.4}$$

Passing to the new variables, from (10.2) we get

$$\begin{aligned}
\frac{dp}{dt} &= \frac{1}{2}[p(W_p-W_0)+\xi F], \\
\frac{dq}{dt} &= \frac{1}{2}[q(W_q-W_0)-\xi F], \\
\frac{d\xi}{dt} &= -\xi[W_0+(\alpha+\gamma-2\beta)\xi], \\
W_p &= \alpha p+\beta q, \quad W_q = \beta p+\gamma q, \quad W_0 = \alpha p^2+2\beta pq+\gamma q^2, \\
F &= \alpha-\beta-p(\alpha+\gamma-2\beta), \quad p+q=1.
\end{aligned} \tag{10.5}$$

These equations diverge from the frequency equations usually studied in genetics by the terms containing the variable ξ. Let us accept the wide-spread hypothesis about weak selection, that is,

$$\alpha = K+\epsilon\hat{\alpha}, \quad \beta = K+\epsilon\hat{\beta}, \quad \gamma = K+\epsilon\hat{\gamma},$$

where $0\leqslant\epsilon<<1$. Then (10.5) can be presented in the form

$$\begin{aligned}
\frac{dp}{dt} &= \frac{\epsilon}{2}[p(W_p-W_0)+\xi F], \\
\frac{dq}{dt} &= \frac{\epsilon}{2}[q(W_q-W_0)-\xi F], \\
\frac{d\xi}{dt} &= -K\xi-\epsilon\xi[W_0+(\alpha+\gamma-2\beta)\xi].
\end{aligned} \tag{10.6}$$

Here all expressions marked by ^ contain $\hat{\alpha}$, $\hat{\beta}$ and $\hat{\gamma}$ instead of α, β and γ. In this system the variables p and q are 'slow', and ξ is a 'fast' variable. The system dynamics is such that it quickly comes to the vicinity of the plane $\xi=0$ and then allele frequencies start their slow evolution in this vicinity. Therefore over sufficiently long time periods we can describe evolution by a truncated system, which results from (10.5) with $\xi\equiv 0$:

$$\begin{aligned}
\frac{dp}{dt} &= \frac{1}{2}p(W_p-W_0), \\
\frac{dq}{dt} &= \frac{1}{2}q(W_q-W_0).
\end{aligned} \tag{10.7}$$

Let us note that these equations for frequencies can be solved independently from the equations for the total population size. Furthermore, the evolution of allele frequencies is in no way dependent on the function of competition $d(N)$, which can be now chosen quite freely and need not be restricted to the linear relationship (deriving the equations in the frequency form we fixed no particular form for $d(N)$).

Let us concentrate on the equation for the total population. Under weak selection this equation can be written in the form

$$\frac{dN}{dt} = N[K - d(N)] + \epsilon \hat{W}_0 N. \qquad (10.8)$$

Whence one can immediately see that if the equation $d(N) = K$ has the solution $N^* > 0$ and $d(N^*) > 0$, then for sufficiently small ϵ the total population quickly becomes close to N^* and further on remains in the vicinity of this state.

The coefficient $1/2$ in the right-hand sides of (10.7) makes these equations different from the classical equations of population genetics. Whence it follows that (in comparison with the classical equations) in this model the gene structure evolves two times slower than the total population size – quite an interesting fact by itself. It can be associated with the asymmetry of the contributions made by the two sexes to enhance fecundity.

3.11. Notes and Bibliography

To 3.1, 3.2.

The genetical populational model with age structure was first suggested in the paper by

Haldane, J. B. S.: 1927, 'A Mathematical Theory of Natural and Artificial Selection. Part V.', *Proc. Camb. Phil. Soc.* **223**, 607–615.

Assuming that all model functions are weakly varied within one generation, and that individuals of different types have close demographic parameters, Haldane concludes, that if the period between generations, equal to $\int_0^\infty xK(x)\,dx / \int_0^\infty K(x)\,dx$ ($\int_0^\infty K(x)\,dx \approx 1$), is taken as the time unit, then selection takes place as if there were no overlap of generations.

Another model of a one-locus diallele population was suggested and elaborated by H. T. J. Norton in his paper:

Norton, H. T. J.: 1928, 'Natural Selection and Mendelian Variation', Proc. Lond. Math. Soc., **Ser. 2**, 28, 1, 1–45.

Assuming random mating (the ages of parents being mutually independent) and equality of the fecundity coefficients for females of all three genotypes, the author derived sufficient conditions for the population to attain each of the possible states.

However, models of Haldane and Norton are distinguished by their high complexity, and it is hard to apply them to actual biological processes.

To 3.3.

Results of this section may be also found in the paper:

Charlesworth, B.: 1972, 'Selection in Population with Overlapping Generations. III. Conditions for Genetic Equilibrium', *Theor. Pop. Biol.* **3**, 4, 377–395.

The works:

Smirnov, M. V.: 1978, 'Ob usloviajah sushestvovanija polimorfizma v modeljah populjačionnoi genetiki s ucetom vozrastnoi struktury (On the Existence Conditions of Polymorphism in Models of Population Genetics with Account Taken of the Age Structure. In Russian), Tezisy III Vsesouznoi konferencii po biomedkibernetike (Theses of the Third All-Union Conference in Biomedical Cybernetics), Moscow, 333–336;

Smirnov, M. V.: 1980, 'O polimorfizme v populjacii s učetom vozrastnoi struktury (On Polymorphism in

Populations with Age Structure.' In Russian), Zurnal Obshei Biologii (*Journal of General Biology*) **41**, 1, 31–46
concentrate on the case when mating takes place within each particular age in the population (lack of 'age-crossing'). The only result of this constraint is that the form of the equation for λ^* is altered.

To 3.4.
Some of the results, contained here, have been obtained (though, as it seems to us, employing insufficiently rigorous mathematics) in the paper:
Charlesworth, B.: 1973, 'Selection in Populations with Overlapping Generations. V. Natural Selection and Life Histories', *Amer. Natur.* **107**, 954, 303–311.
In more details the main results and conclusions of this section are presented in the work:
Smirnov, M. V.: 'Ob ustoičivosti predelnyh traektoriy dinamiki populjaciy s učetom vozrastnoi struktury (On Stability of Limiting Trajectories for Population Dynamics with Account Taken of the Age-Structure.' In Russian), Tezisy VII Vsesouznovo soveshanija po problemam upravlenija (Theses of the Seventh All- Union Conference on Problems of Control), Tallin, 716–718,
where Equations (2.1) are studied for arbitrary age dependent functions $F_i(x)$, $i = 1, 2, 3$.

To 3.6.
Currently, one of the most interesting problems of the dynamic theory is how 'chaos' originates in dynamical systems. The so- called 'strange attractors' are widely known; these are the limiting sets of very complicated stuctures, being neither points nor cycles, nor sets on a torus. The problem of 'chaos' in ecological systems is treated in a series of papers by R. May with co-authors:
May, R. M.: 1975, 'Biological Populations Obeying Difference Equations: Stable Points, Stable Cycles and Chaos', *Theor. Biol.* **51**, 2, 522–524;
Levin, S. A., May, R. M.: 1976, 'A Note on Difference-Delay Equations', *Theor. Pop. Biol.* **9**, 2, 178–187.

To 3.7.
Genetic polymorphism, in particular the balanced or heterozygous polymorphism, existing due to the enhanced viability of heterozygotes, undergoes an experimental and theoretical analysis in the works
Svirezhev, Yu. M. and Timofeeff-Ressovsky, N. V.: 1966, 'O ravnovesii genotipov v modelnyh populjacijah Drosophila melanogaster (On the Equilibrium of Genotypes in Model Populations of Drosophila Melanogaster.' In Russian), *Problemy Kibernetiki* (*Problems of Cybernetics*) **16**, 123-136;
Svirezhev, Yu. M. and Timofeeff-Ressovsky, N. W.: 1968, 'Some Types of Polymorphism in Populations', In: *Haldane and Modern Biology*, Hopkins Press, J. Baltimore, 141-168.
It is still one of the most delicate problems in population genetics, how to define and measure fitnesses (or the Malthusian parameters). The question: What is genotype fitness? – has found no unique and unambiguous answer as yet. A most interesting discussion of this problem is contained in the book:
Lewontin, R. C.: 1974, *The Genetic Basis of Evolutionary Change*, Columbia Univ. Press, N.Y., L., 346 p.

To 3.8.
In the late 1930's V. A. Kostitzin called attention to the inadequacies and insufficiencies of the classical Fisher–Wright–Haldane equations for the description of the evolutionary process. Pointing out that natural selection in populations is manifested in ecological processes, he derived the equations of evolution as a generalization of the ecological Volterra equations. Kostitzin's works on this topic (which are hardly available at present) have been put together in the recently published book:
Scudo, F. M. and Ziegler, J. R.: 1978, *The Golden Age of Theoretical Ecology: 1923–1940*, Springer-Verlag, Berlin Heidelberg, N.Y., 413–438.

We also recommend, for instance, Chapter 15 from the book:

Kostitzin, V. A.: 1937, *Biologie Mathématique*, A. Colin, Paris, 204–215,
as well as his papers in Comptes rendus de l'Acad. des Sciences (C.R.)

1. 1938, 'Équations differentialles générales du problème de selection naturelle', *C.R.* **206**, 570–572;
2. 1938, 'Sur les coefficients Mendèliens d'héredité, *C.R.* **206**, 883–885;
3. 1938, 'Sur les points singuliers des équations différentielles du problème de la selection naturelle', *C.R.* **206**, 976–978;
4. 1938, 'Sur les équations differentielles du problème de la sélection naturelle dans le cas de mutation d'un chromosome sexual', *C.R.* **206**, 1273–1275.

The equations turned out to be more complicated, but their dynamic behaviour was also enriched. It would be interesting to elaborate on them – nothing of the kind is done yet.

Chapter 4

Multiple Alleles

4.1. Introduction

In the proceeding chapter we have looked at the case, when a gene, acting on a character, can be only in two states. However, for instance the same *ebony* mutation has about ten different forms, all of them initiated by a mutation in one locus. In this case there exists a whole series of alleles for a given gene, that is, a gene can be in several states. They are known as multiple alleles of a given gene (or of a locus, where the given gene is localized). Note that theoretically the case of multiple alleles is similar to the diallele one, but expanding the dimensionality of the phase space of the system, we get a good chance to obtain more interesting dynamic behavior.

Suppose we have a sufficiently large panmictic population, with inheritance of a character controlled by one n-allele gene: $A_1, A_2, \ldots, A_n$, $n \geqslant 2$. There will be $n(n+1)/2$ genotypes A_iA_j in this population. Both sexes are equivalent with respect to both selection and inheritance, that is, the population is 'sexless'. We choose the demographic functions such that the equations of evolution coincide with the classical ones. In this case the equations for evolution of the genetic structure can be considered apart from the equation for the total population size. Therefore we shall investigate only the dynamics of allele frequencies, represented by the equations

$$\frac{dp_i}{dt} = p_i(w_i - w), \tag{1.1}$$

$$w_i = \sum_j w_{ij}p_j, \quad w = \sum_{i,j} w_{ij}p_ip_j, \quad i, j = \overline{1, n},$$

where p_i are defined on the simplex $\overline{\sum}$: $\{\sum_i p_i = 1,\ p_i \geqslant 0\}$. Obviously, $p_i(t) \in \overline{\sum}$ for any $p_i(t_0) \in \overline{\sum}$. In fact, summing up (1.1) over i, we obtain $\sum_i \dot{p}_i = 0$, whence $\sum_i p_i(t) = \sum_i p_i(t_0) = 1$. And since $\dot{p}_i = 0$ on the appropriate faces of the simplex, no trajectory leaves the boundaries of the positive orthant. This proves the statement. Moreover, all trajectories, orginating on a face of the simplex, never leave the boundaries of this face since by (1.1) the appropriate $\dot{p}_i$ are zero.

4.2. State of Genetic Equilibrium. Polymorphism

As it follows from our assumptions, the Malthusian parameters $w_{ij} (w_{ij} \geqslant 0)$ are independent of time. Then the steady-state points of (1.1), found from the equations

$$p_i^*(w_i^* - w^*) = 0, \quad i = \overline{1, n}, \tag{2.1}$$

characterize the state of genetic equilibrium in the population. What are the possible solutions to this system? To answer this question, let us introduce some additional definitions. Let the subsets I_k be made of any k elements of $I (1 \leqslant k < n)$, which is the set of indices I: $\{1, 2, \ldots, n\}$. The number of such subsets is 2^{n-1}. Let $\overline{I}_k$ be the complement of I_k, so that $\overline{I}_k \bigcup I_k = I$, $\overline{I}_k \bigcap I_k = \varnothing$. Obviously, (2.1) can have the following solutions:

(a) $p_i^* = 0, i \in I_k; p_j^* \neq 0, j \in \overline{I}_k, 1 \leqslant k < n$;

(b) $p_i^* \neq 0, i \in I$.

The condition $\sum_i p_i^* = 1$ automatically holds, since $\sum_i p_i^* w_i^* = w^*$. Solutions of type (a) are to satisfy the following system of equations

$$p_i^* = 0, \quad i \in I_k; \quad w_j^* = w, \quad j \in \overline{I}_k, \tag{2.2}$$

those of type (b) should satisfy

$$w_i^* = w^*, \quad i \in I. \tag{2.3}$$

Let $\mathbf{W}^k = \| w_{ij} \|^k$, $i, j \in \overline{I}_k$ be the $(n-k) \times (n-k)$ submatrices of matrix $\mathbf{W} = \| w_{ij} \|$, $i, j \in I$. Suppose $\mathbf{W}^k$ are non-singular, that is $| \mathbf{W}^k | \neq 0$. Let us also introduce matrices $\| v_{ij} \|^k$, where v_{ij} are the cofactors for elements w_{ij}. Then (2.2) can be rewritten in the form

$$p_i^* = 0, \quad i \in I_k; \quad \mathbf{W}^k \mathbf{p}^* = w^* \mathbf{e}, \quad \mathbf{e} = (1, 1, \ldots, 1)^T, \tag{2.4}$$

where $\mathbf{p}^* = \{p_j^*\}$, $j \in I_k$. Since there exists the reciprocal matrix $(\mathbf{W}^k)^{-1}$, we have $(\mathbf{W}^k)^{-1} \mathbf{W}^k \mathbf{p}^* = (\mathbf{W}^k)^{-1} w^* \mathbf{e}$ or $p_j^* = [w^* \sum_s v_{js}] / | \mathbf{W}^k |$. From the normalization condition, $\sum_j p_j^* = 1$, we get

$$w^* = \frac{| \mathbf{W}^k |}{\sum_{j,s} v_{js}}, \quad j, s \in I_k. \tag{2.5}$$

And finally the solutions of type (a) have the form

$$p_i^* = 0, \quad i \in I_k; \quad p_j^* = \frac{\sum_s v_{js}}{\sum_{j,s} v_{js}}, \quad j, s \in \overline{I}_k. \tag{2.6}$$

These solutions are to belong to the $(n-k)$-dimensional faces of the simplex $\sum$. Therefore p_j^* needs to comply with additional conditions

$$\operatorname{sgn}\left[\sum_s v_{js}\right] = +1, \quad \text{or } \operatorname{sgn}\left[\sum_s v_{js}\right] = -1, \tag{2.7}$$

for all $s \in \overline{I}_k$.

Most interesting is the solution for all p_i^* being interior to $\sum$. This state is called the polymorphism state with respect to all alleles of the gene in question. If the state is stable, then all the $n(n+1)/2$ possible genotypes are to be represented in the population in certain concentrations. If matrix $\mathbf{W}$ is non-singular, then

$$p_i^* = \frac{\sum_j v_{ij}}{\sum_{i,j} v_{ij}}, \quad i, j=\overline{1, n}. \tag{2.8}$$

For a non-singular matrix of Malthusian parameters the polymorphism state turns to be unique. The genetic equilibria, corresponding to the steady-state points, located on faces of the $(n-k)$-dimensional simplex, turn to be polymorphism states with respect to a smaller number of alleles. And lastly, the equilibrium for $k=n-1$ corresponds to the genetically homogeneous population, where only one allele took root. The total number of all possible genetic equilibria is 2^n-1.

4.3. Mean Population Fitness. Fisher's Fundamental Theorem

The variable $w=\sum_{i,j} w_{ij}p_ip_j$, which is always present in the evolutionary equations, represents the genotypes' Malthusian parameters, averaged over the genotype frequencies. In fact, by the Hardy–Weinberg principle, $p_ip_j=u_{ij}$ and $w=\sum_{i,j} w_{ij}u_{ij}$. Clearly, w is an average population characteristic, specifying the averaged pressure of selection. This variable is known as the *mean fitness* of the population.

Let us calculate the total derivative of w with respect to time, along the trajectories of (1.1):

$$\frac{dw}{dt} = \frac{\partial w}{\partial t} + \sum_i \frac{\partial w}{\partial p_i}\frac{dp_i}{dt} = \sum_{i,j} \frac{\partial w_{ij}}{\partial t} p_ip_j +$$

$$+ 2\sum_{i,j} w_{ij}\frac{dp_i}{dt}p_j + \sum_{i,j}\frac{\partial w_{ij}}{\partial p_i}p_ip_j\frac{dp_i}{dt}$$

By our assumptions, w_{ij} depends explicitly neither on time, nor on allele frequencies. Then

$$\frac{dw}{dt} = 2\sum_{i,j} w_{ij}p_jp_i\left[\sum_s w_{is}p_s - w\right] = 2\sum_{i,j,s} w_{ij}w_{is}p_ip_jp_s -$$

$$-2w\sum_{i,j} w_{ij}p_ip_j = 2\left[\sum_i p_iw_i^2 - w^2\right].$$

Since $\sum p_i = 1$, the latter expression can be rewritten in the form

$$\frac{dw}{dt} = 2\left[\sum_i p_iw_i^2 - 2w^2 + w^2\right] =$$

$$= 2\left[\sum_i p_iw_i^2 - 2w\sum_i p_iw_i + w^2\sum_i p_i\right] = \tag{3.1}$$

$$= 2\sum_i p_i \left[w_i^2 - 2ww_i + w^2\right] = 2\sum_i p_i(w_i - w)^2.$$

dw/dt is non-negative because $p_i \geqslant 0$, and $w=0$ only at the steady-state points of (1.1). By its definition the quantity $V_g = \sum_i p_i(w_i - w)^2$ is the variance of w_i, whose distribution is characterized by the distribution of allele frequencies p_i. V_g is termed *additive genic variance* of the population.

The result, derived above, can be formulated as a theorem, as follows:

In a sufficiently large panmictic population, with inheritance controlled by one n-allele gene and the pressure of selection, specified by w_{ij}, being constant, the mean population fitness grows, reaching its steady-state value in one of the states of genetic equilibrium. Mean fitness varies at a rate which is in proportion to the additive genic variance, and which is zero at the genetic equilibrium.

This theorem, in a somewhat different formulation, was proved by R. Fisher and became known as the *fundamental theorem of natural selection.*

The function $w(\mathbf{p}) = (\mathbf{p}, \mathbf{W}\mathbf{p})$, $\mathbf{p} = (p_1, p_2, \ldots, p_n)^T$ is continuous and bounded in $\sum$. Hence, either interior to the simplex, or on its boundary it attains a maximum. $w(\mathbf{p})$ is a quadratic form, therefore if this maximum is attained interior to the simplex, then it is unique. If there is no maximum attained interior to the simplex, then local maxima can exist on the simplex faces.

Let us write out the necessary conditions of an extremum of $w(\mathbf{p})$ on $\sum$. Consider the auxiliary function

$$w' = w + \lambda\left[\sum_i p_i - 1\right],$$

where λ is a Lagrange multiplier. Since $\partial w/\partial p_i = 2w_i$, the necessary conditions can be written in the form

$$2w_i(\mathbf{p}^*) + \lambda = 0. \tag{3.2}$$

Whence, multiplying (3.2) by p_i^* and summing up over i, we get $\lambda = -2w(\mathbf{p}^*)$. Then the conditions (3.2) become

$$w_i(\mathbf{p}^*) = w(\mathbf{p}^*), \tag{3.3}$$

which is nothing else, but the equation for the non-trivial equilibrium in (1.1). Likewise we may prove that local extrema of $w(\mathbf{p})$, lying on simplex faces, coincide with the steady-state points of (1.1) which have the appropriate $p_i^* = 0$.

One can prove that if a steady-state point $\mathbf{p}^*$ is asymptotically stable, then $w(\mathbf{p}^*)$ is a local maximum of $w(\mathbf{p})$. In fact, since trajectories of the dynamical system (1.1) are everywhere dense in a certain domain $G \in \sum$, containing $\mathbf{p}^*$, for every point $\mathbf{p}$ from the vicinity of $\mathbf{p}^*$, belonging to G, we can find a trajectory $\mathbf{p}(t)$ passing through $\mathbf{p}$ and tending to $\mathbf{p}^*$. Then, as the function w is continuous and increases strictly along the trajectory $\mathbf{p}(t)$, we have $w(\mathbf{p}^*) > w(\mathbf{p})$. Consequently,

$$w(\mathbf{p}^*) = \max_t w[\mathbf{p}(t)] = \max_{\mathbf{p}\in G} w(\mathbf{p}) = w^*.$$

Thus we proved the necessity of this condition. Sufficiency readily follows from the fact that the function $L(\mathbf{p})=w^*-w$ is a Lyapunov function for (1.1).

4.4. Mean Fitness as a Lyapunov Function

If at some steady-state point $\mathbf{p}^*$ the function $w(\mathbf{p})$ finds its isolated maximum, then the state $\mathbf{p}^*$ is asymptotically stable.

To prove this statement, let us look at the function

$$L(\mathbf{p}) = w(\mathbf{p}^*)-w(\mathbf{p}), \tag{4.1}$$

which is:

(a) continuous together with its first-order partial derivatives in an open domain G, containing the point $\mathbf{p}^*$ and being either a part of the simplex $\sum$, or the whole simplex without its boundary;

(b) non-negative everywhere in G, vanishing only at $\mathbf{p}^*$;

(c) such that $dL/dt=-dw/dt=-2\sum_i p_i(w_i-w)^2\leq 0$ everywhere in G, and $dw/dt=0$ only at p^*. Consequently, $L(\mathbf{p})$ is a Lyapunov function for (1.1) and the state $\mathbf{p}^*$ is asymptotically stable.

If $w(\mathbf{p})$ has an isolated minimum at $\mathbf{p}^*$, then by the definition of a minimum it follows that there are points lying arbitrarily close to $\mathbf{p}^*$ and such that $L(\mathbf{p})=w(\mathbf{p}^*)-w(\mathbf{p})<0$, $\mathbf{p}\in\sum$, and by the first Lyapunov's theorem about instability one can be sure that the state $\mathbf{p}^*$ is unstable.

4.5. Adaptive Topography of a Population

The statements proved above allow us to give a vivid interpretation of the system behavior.

Taking advantage of the relation $p_n=1-\sum_{i=1}^{n-1}p_i$ let us exclude the variable p_n from the expression for $w(\mathbf{p})$:

$$w = \sum_{i,j=1}^{n} w_{ij}p_ip_j = w_{nn}-2\sum_{i=1}^{n-1}A_ip_i-\sum_{i,j=1}^{n-1}B_{ij}p_ip_j, \tag{5.1}$$

where

$$A_i = w_{nn}-w_{in},\quad B_{ij} = w_{in}+w_{nj}-w_{ij}-w_{nn},\quad i,j=\overline{1,n-1}.$$

Obviously, all critical points $w'(p_1,\ldots,p_n)$ and $w(p_1,\ldots,p_{n-1})$ coincide. The necessary extremum conditions have the form:

$$\frac{\partial w}{\partial p_i} = -\sum_j B_{ij}p_j^*-A_i = 0,\quad i,j=\overline{1,n-1}. \tag{5.2}$$

Let us think that this system has a unique solution. The sufficient conditions imply that if the quadratic form with matrix $\| B_{ij} \|$ is positive definite, then $w(\overset{*}{p}_1,\ldots,\overset{*}{p}_{n-1})=\max_{\mathbf{p}} w(p_1,\ldots,p_{n-1})$; if it is negative definite, then $w(\overset{*}{p}_1,\ldots,\overset{*}{p}_{n-1})=\min_{\mathbf{p}} w(p_1,\ldots,p_{n-1})$. The projection of the simplex $\sum$ in the space $\{p_1, \ldots, p_{n-1}\}$ is characterized by the conditions $p_i \geqslant 0$, $\sum_i p_i \leqslant 1$, $i=\overline{1, n-1}$.

Let $\| B_{ij} \|$ be positive definite. Then function $w(p_1, \ldots, p_{n-1})$ is strictly concave (upwards convex). And since the simplex $\sum$ is a convex set, w has a *unique* isolated maximum on this set interior to or on the boundary)*. Consequently, the local maximum of w is also the global one, and (1.1) has a unique stable state of equilibrium. If this maximum lies inside the simplex, then the equilibrium will be a polymorphism with respect to all alleles. Otherwise, some of the alleles are to be eliminated from the population and the equilibrium can be polymorphic only with respect to a part of alleles. The domain of asymptotic stability for both, total and partial, equilibria coincides either with the whole simplex (without boundaries), or also includes the appropriate simplex face, containing the partial polymorphic equilibrium.

Let now $\| B_{ij} \|$ be negative definite. In this case $w(p_1, \ldots, p_{n-1})$ has a unique minimum on the simplex, this statement holding for any simplex face (which is also a simplex of lower dimensionality). Successively carrying on to faces of lower and lower dimension, we come to faces of zero dimension, which are the vertices of the simplex, the minimum of function w being equal to its maximum at these points. Consequently, when $w(p_1, \ldots, p_{n-1})$ has a unique minimum, it also has $n-1$ isolated local maxima at the simplex vertices. This means that the population has $n-1$ stable steady states, each of them characterized by only one fixed allele, all the rest being eliminated. The simplex is split into n domains of asymptotic stability (domains of attraction), one for each of the equilibria, so that the stable state that is reached depends on the choice of initiall conditions.

Even more complex is the case of sign indefinite $\| B_{ij} \|$. Local maxima of the mean fitness function can then be reached on any of the simplex faces.

Consider the surface $w = w_{nn} - 2\sum_i A_i p_i - \sum_{i,j} B_{ij} p_i p_j$, $i,j=\overline{1, n-1}$ in the space $\{w, p_1, \ldots, p_{n-1}\}$. Obviously, its peaks correspond to stable genetic equilibria of the population, and valleys separate their domains of attraction, that is the domains, from each point of which the population comes to its peak. The saddle-points will correspond to unstable states of equilibrium. Since the topography of any quadratic form is such that no closed ring-shaped valleys can occur, it readily follows, that system (1.1) has no steady-state periodic solutions.

Figure 10 displays the topography of the surface $w(p_1)$, $p_1 + p_2 = 1$ for $n=2$ and for various relationships between the Malthusian parameters $w_{11} = \alpha$, $w_{12} = w_{21} = \beta$ and $w_{22} = \gamma$, which is the simplest case. One can see from this Figure that behavior of the population and its limiting state are essentially dependent upon the topography of the mean fitness.

In conclusion let us note that the topography of function $y = w(\mathbf{p})$ is frequently called the *adaptive topography* of a population.

* Cf., for instance, Carr C. R., Howe C. W.: 1964, *Quantitative Decision Procedures in Management and Economics*, McGraw-Hill, New York.

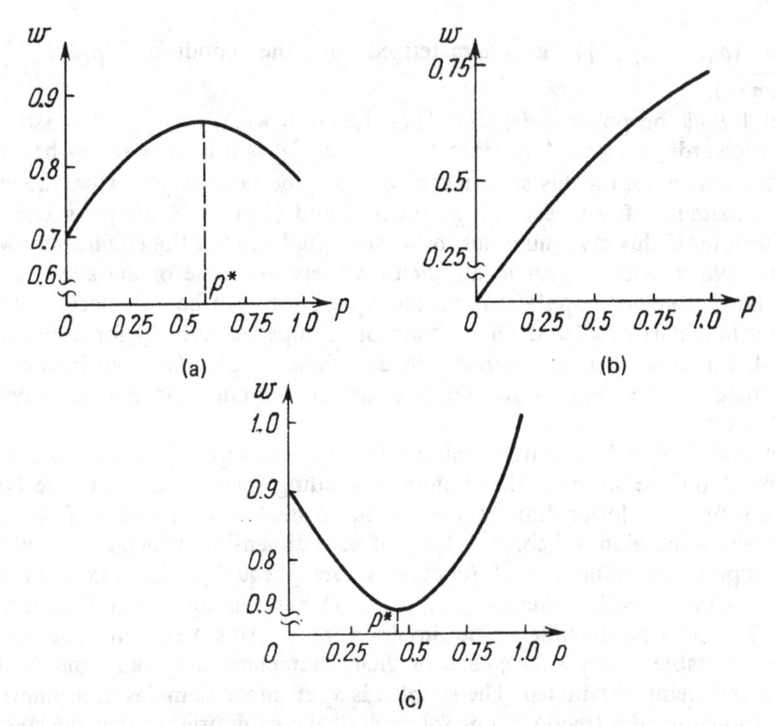

Fig. 10. Graph of the mean fitness function for various relationships between Malthusian parameters. (a) $\alpha=0.8$, $\beta=1$, $\gamma=0.7$; (b) $\alpha=0.75$, $\beta=0.75$, $\gamma=0$; (c) $\alpha=1$, $\beta=0.5$, $\gamma=0.9$.

4.6. The Case of Three Alleles. Search for Domains of Asymptotic Stability

Treating the diallele case we have already come across the example (heterozygote has the minimal viability), when the interval [0, 1] has been split into two domains, each carrying its own asymptotically stable steady-state point. So that one cannot speak about total stability (asymptotic stability on the whole). The problem "How to separate the domains of asymptotic stability?" was easily solved in this case: the domains were separated by a point p^* at which $dw/dt=0$ and $w(p^*)=\min_p w$ (Figure. 10c). The problem becomes considerably more complicated when dimensionality is raised. Nevertheless, analyzing the topography of the mean fitness function, we can separate the domains of asymptotic stability and make some conclusions concerning the system behavior. As an example, let us concentrate on the population with inheritance of a character controlled by a three-allele gene with alleles A_1, A_2, and A_3.

Since $p_3=1-p_1-p_2$, the 3-dimensional simplex can be represented on a plane. Figure 11 presents the phase plane for system (1.1) when $n=3$, and its phase portrait in case there exists a stable state of polymorphism with respect to all three alleles (○ stable point, ◒ semi-stable point, ● unstable point). A semi-stable point

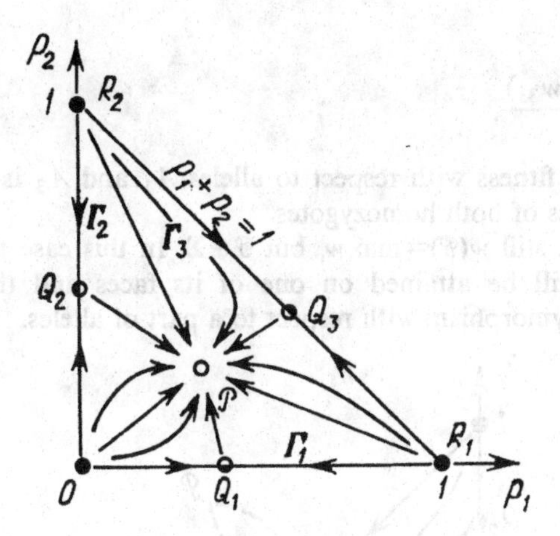

Fig. 11.

is the one which is stable on the boundary Γ and unstable over the whole domain Σ. Thus, only a boundary point can be semi-stable. In the plane (p_1, p_2):

$$\overline{\Sigma} = \Sigma + \Gamma;\ \ \Sigma: p_1, p_2 > 0,\ p_1 + p_2 < 1;$$

$$\Gamma = \Gamma_1 + O + \Gamma_2 + R_2 + \Gamma_2 + R_1.$$

The interior of the simplex will be denoted by $\overline{\Sigma}$, Γ will stand for its boundary. All system trajectories are to belong to the domain $\overline{\Sigma} = \Sigma + \Gamma$. Taking advantage of the relation $p_3 = 1 - p_1 - p_2$, the function of mean fitness can be written in the form of (5.1)

Suppose $w(\mathcal{P}) = \max_{p_1, p_2} w(p_1, p_2)$, where $\mathcal{P}$ is a point with coordinates

$$p_1^* = \frac{(A_2 B_{12} - A_1 B_{22})}{D},\ \ p_2^* = \frac{(A_1 B_{12} - A_2 B_{11})}{D}, \tag{6.1}$$

$$D = B_{11} B_{22} - B_{12}^2,$$

satisfying the necessary conditions for the maximum of w. The sufficient conditions are: $B_{11} > 0$, $D > 0$. If, besides, $\mathcal{P} \in \Sigma$, that is, $p_1^* > 0$, $p_2^* > 0$ (the condition $p_1^* + p_2^* < 1$ automatically holds, see Section 4.2), then the population has a unique stable state of polymorphism (stable polymorphism). The whole domain Σ is attracting with respect to point $\mathcal{P}$, hence from any point inside the simplex the population will come to this state. The phase portrait of such a behavior is displayed in Figure 11. These conditions may be presented in the form

$$B_{11} > 0,\ \ A_2 B_{12} > A_1 B_{22},\ \ A_1 B_{12} > A_2 B_{11},\ \ D > 0. \tag{6.2}$$

Passing on from the variables A_i, B_{ij} to Malthusian parameters we arrive at complicated expressions, and for this reason we omit this passage in its complete form. However, the condition $B_{11} > 0$ yields a simple and clear necessary condition of polymorphism:

$$w_{13} > \frac{(w_{11}+w_{33})}{2}, \tag{6.3}$$

that is heterozygote fitness with respect to alleles A_1 and A_3 is to be higher than the averaged fitnesses of both homozygotes.

Suppose now that still $w(\mathcal{P})=\max w$, but $\mathcal{P}\notin\Sigma$. In this case the maximum of w over the simplex will be attained on one of its faces and the population can develop a stable polymorphism with respect to a part of alleles.

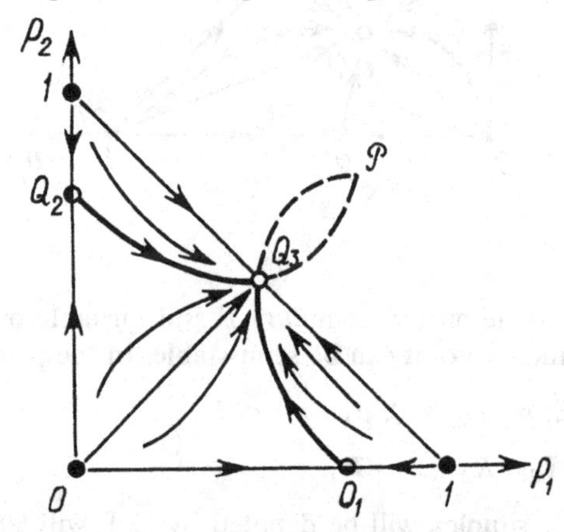

Fig. 12. Phase portrait of system (1.1) for $n=3$, $w(\mathcal{P})=\max w$. Q_3 is the only stable point. Population attains polymorphism with respect to alleles A_1 and A_2.

For instance, if $\mathcal{P}$ lies in the positive quadrant (Figure 12) and, besides, $p_1^*<1$, $p_2^*<1$ but $p_1^*+p_2^*>1$, then polymorphism with respect to alleles A_1 and A_2 will be always attained in such a population.

Consider the situation, when $w(\mathcal{P})=\min w$, that is $B_{11}<0$, $D>0$ (sufficient conditions). In this case the population can have only 'pure' equilibria, i.e. the points $\{0, 0\}$, $\{0, 1\}$ and $\{1, 0\}$ will be stable. What will be the domains of attraction for these points?

If we draw the relief of the function $w(p_1, p_2)$ over the plane $\{p_1, p_2\}$, the surface may be easily shown to be an elleptic paraboloid with its 'apex' at $\mathcal{P}$. Trajectories of the system on the phase plane $\{p_1, p_2\}$ are the projections of the curves onto this surface, those trajectories being proper, which can be associated with curves such that w steadily increases along them. Let us look at the curves, along which:

(1) $\dot{p}_1 = 0, \;\; p_1 \neq 0;$

(2) $\dot{p}_2 = 0, \;\; p_2 \neq 0.$

These are the equations of the valleys, which are either never crossed by trajectories, or trajectories crossing them, abruptly change their directions. Consider a valley with $\dot{p}_1=0$. Its projection on the plane $\{p_1,p_2\}$ passes through the equilibrium points on faces of the simplex (points Q_1, Q_3 in Figure 13 a,b) and separating it into two subdomains ω_1^1 and ω_1^2.

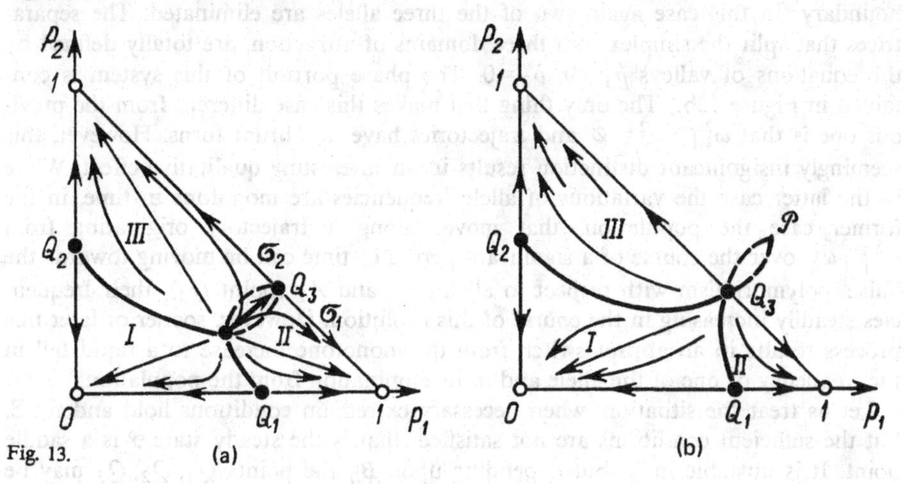

Fig. 13. (a) (b)

Figure 13 shows the phase portrait of system (1.1) for $n=3$, $w(\mathcal{P})=\min w$.

(a) $\mathcal{P}\in\Sigma$, $\omega_1^1 = \text{I}+\text{III}$, $\omega_1^2 = \text{II}+\sigma_1+\sigma_2$, $\omega_2^1 = \text{I}+\text{II}$,

$\omega_2^2=\text{III}+\sigma_1+\sigma_2$. $Q_1\mathcal{P}$ is a separatrix with the equation $\dot{p}_2=0$; $p_2>0$. $Q_2\mathcal{P}$ is another separatrix, its equation being $\dot{p}_1=0$; $p_1>0$. Broken lines indicate those curves, which turn the trajectory that crosses them, changing its direction from one point towards the other. These curves have the same equations as the separatrices.

(b) $\mathcal{P}\in\Sigma$, $\omega_1^1 = \text{I}+\text{III}$, $\omega_1^2 = \text{II}$, $\omega_2^1 = I+\text{II}$, $\omega_2^2 = \text{III}$.

Along the separatrices Q_1Q_3 and Q_2Q_3 we have $\dot{p}_1=0$ and $\dot{p}_2=0$, respectively.

$\dot{p}_1>0$ in ω_1^2 and any trajectory, originating in ω_1^2 tends to the state with $p_1^*=1$. $\dot{p}_1$ is negative in ω_1^1 and for all $\{p_1,p_2\}\in\omega_1^1$ we have $p_1(t)\to0$. The projection of the valley with $\dot{p}_2=0$ passes through the points Q_2, Q_3 and splits the simplex into subdomains ω_2^1 and ω_2^2 where $\dot{p}_2<0$ and $\dot{p}_2>0$, respectively. Evidently, $p_2(t)\to0$ for all $p_1,p_2\in\omega_2^1$ and $p_2(t)\to1$ for $p_1,p_2\in\omega_2^2$.

Suppose $w(\mathcal{P})=\min w$ and $\mathcal{P}\in\Sigma$ (Figure 13a). Then (since both projections are to pass through the point $\mathcal{P}$) there exists a domain such that its points belong to $\omega_1^2\cap\omega_2^2$, that is $\dot{p}_1>0$, $\dot{p}_2>0$ in this domain. But since no trajectory can leave the simplex, for all trajectories originating in this domain either $p_1(t)\to0$ or $p_2(t)\to0$ as $t\to\infty$, and they should necessarily leave this domain. There is only trajectory leading from $\mathcal{P}$ to Q_3, which is the separatrix that divides $\omega_1^2\cap\omega_2^2$ into two subdomains σ_1 and σ_2, pertaining to the domains of attraction for the points $\{1,0\}$

and {0, 1}.

And finally, attracting to the equilibrium {0, 0} will be the domain $\Omega_{00}=\omega_1^1 \bigcup \omega_2^1 \setminus \omega_1^2 \bigcap \omega_2^2$; to the equilibrium {1, 0} – the domain $\Omega_{10}=\omega_1^2 \setminus \sigma_2$, and to the equilibrium {0, 1} – the domain $\Omega_{01}=\omega_2^2 \setminus \sigma_1$.

Let us now $\mathcal{P}\notin\Sigma$, that is the minimum lies outside of the simplex, or on its boundary. In this case again two of the three alleles are eliminated. The separatrices that split the simplex into three domains of attraction, are totally defined by the equations of valleys $\dot{p}_1=0$, $\dot{p}_2=0$. The phase portrait of this system is contained in Figure 13b. The only thing that makes this case different from the previous one is that $\omega_1^2 \bigcap \omega_2^2=\varnothing$ and trajectories have no abrupt turns. However, this seemingly insignificant distinction results in an interesting qualitative effect. While in the latter case the variations of allele frequencies are monotone in time, in the former case the population, that moves along a trajectory originating from $\omega_1^2 \bigcap \omega_2^2$, over the course of a significant period of time can be moving towards the 'false' polymorphism with respect to alleles A_1 and A_2 (point Q_3), their frequencies steadily increasing in the course of this evolution. However, sooner or later this process results in an abrupt switch from the monotone increase to a rapid fall in the frequency of one of the allele and in its elimination from the population.

Let us treat the situation, when necessary extremum conditions hold and $\mathcal{P}\in\Sigma$, but the sufficient conditions are not satisfied, that is the steady state $\mathcal{P}$ is a saddle point. It is unstable in Σ, but depending upon B_{ij} the points Q_1, Q_2, Q_3 may be stable on the boundary. In Figure 14 the phase portraits of system (1.1) are shown for $n=3$:

(a) Depending on the initial conditions either the population develops a polymorphism with respect to alleles A_1 and A_2, or these alleles are eliminated; $\dot{p}_1=0$ on $Q_1\mathcal{P}S_2$ and R_1Q_3, $\dot{p}_2=0$ on $Q_2\mathcal{P}S_1$ and R_2Q_3.

(b) Depending on the initial conditions the population develops a polymorphism either with respect to alleles A_1 and A_2 or with respect to alleles A_1 and A_3; $\dot{p}_1=0$ on $Q_1\mathcal{P}Q_3$, $\dot{p}_2=0$ on $S\mathcal{P}Q_3$ and R_2Q_2. The trajectories $Q_2\mathcal{P}$ and $R_1\mathcal{P}$ are the only ones, that come to the point $\mathcal{P}$, separating the whole simplex into domains of attraction for Q_1 and Q_3, respectively.

(c) The population develops a polymorphism with respect to either the alleles A_1 and A_3, or the alleles A_2 and A_3; $\dot{p}_1=0$ on $Q_1\mathcal{P}S_2$ and R_1Q_3, $\dot{p}_2=0$ on $Q_2\mathcal{P}S_1$ and R_2Q_3. The trajectories $O\mathcal{P}$ and $Q_3\mathcal{P}$ separate the simplex into two domains with either Q_1 or Q_2 being stable in each of them.

$$\text{(a) } D<0,\ B_{11}<0,\ B_{22}<0,\ B_{11}+B_{22}>2B_{12}. \tag{6.4}$$

Then the points Q_1, Q_2 are unstable, Q_3 and 0 are stable (Figure 14a). Besides, the point R_1 is stable in Γ_1 and R_2 is stable in Γ_2. The equations $\dot{p}_1=0$ and $\dot{p}_2=0$ define the curves, which both split into two isolated branches. Parts of these curves, passing through Q_1 and $\mathcal{P}$, Q_2 and $\mathcal{P}$, yield the boundaries for the domains of attraction for the points Q_3 and 0. In such a population, depending on the initial conditions, either a polymorphism is reached with respect to A_1 and A_2, or elimination of these alleles takes place.

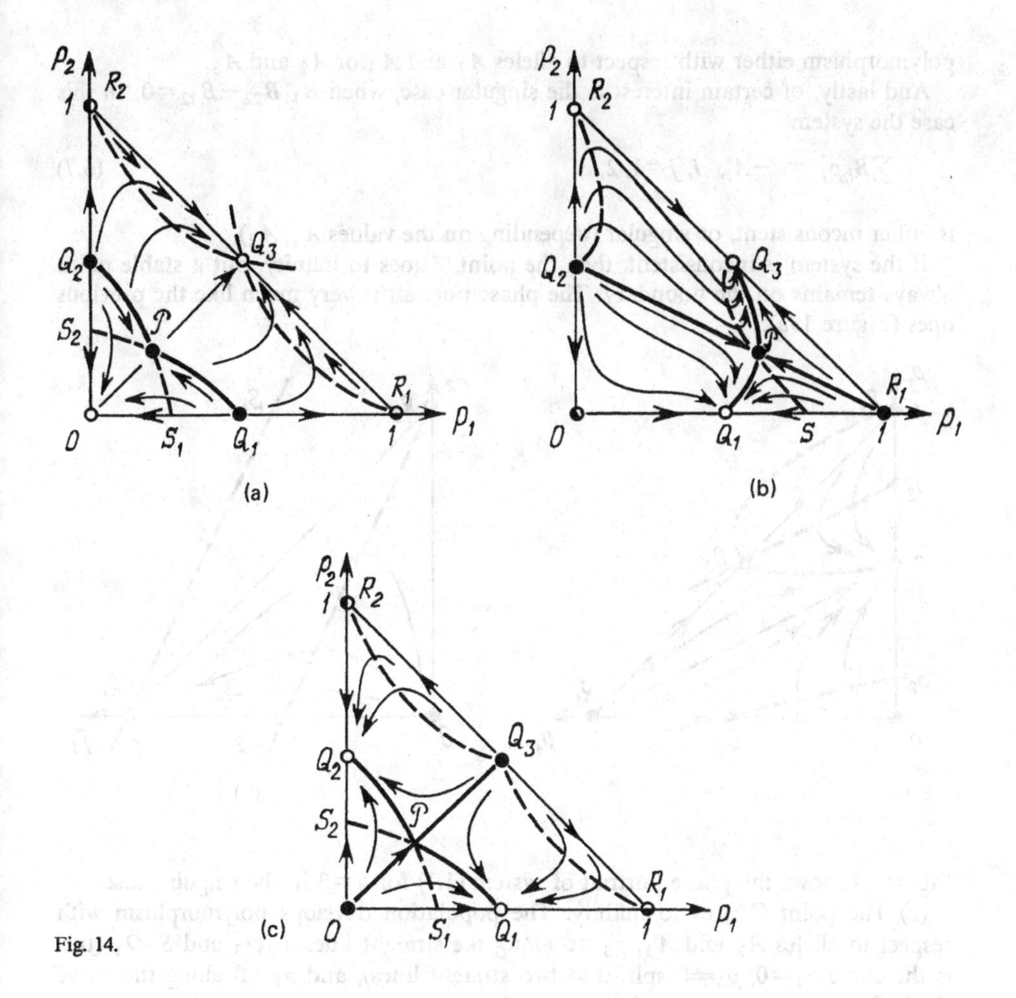

Fig. 14.

(b) $D < 0$, $B_{11} > 0$, $B_{22} < 0$, $B_{11} + B_{12} > 2B_{12}$. (6.5)

Then $Q_1 \in \Gamma_1$ and $Q_3 \in \Gamma_3$ are stable, $Q_2 \in \Gamma_2$ is unstable. Let us again draw the curves $\dot{p} = 0$, $\dot{p} = 0$. As in (a) they split into isolated branches (Figure 14b). The points 0 and R_2 are stable in Γ_2. The separatrices running from Q_2 and R_1 to $\mathcal{P}$ are the boundaries of the attracting domains for Q_1 and Q_3. In this popultion, depending on the initial conditions, polymorphism is attained either with respect to alleles A_1 and A_2, or A_1 and A_3.

(c) $D < 0$, $B_{11} > 0$, $B_{22} > 0$. (6.6)

Let $Q_1, Q_2, Q_3 \in \Gamma$. Then Q_1 and Q_2 are stable, Q_3 is unstable (Figure 14c). The phase portrait of this system resembles those of (a) and (b) and we will not go into details about it. Depending on the initial conditions, such a population reaches polymorphism either with respect to alleles A_1 and A_3 or A_2 and A_3.

And lastly, of certain interest is the singular case, when $B_{11}B_{22}-B_{12}=0$. In this case the system

$$\sum_j B_{ij}p_j^* = -A_i, \quad i, j=1, 2, \tag{6.7}$$

is either inconsistent, or singular (depending on the values A_1, A_2).

If the system is inconsistent, then the point $\mathcal{P}$ goes to infinity, but a stable point always remains on the boundary. The phase portrait is very much like the previous ones (Figure 15a).

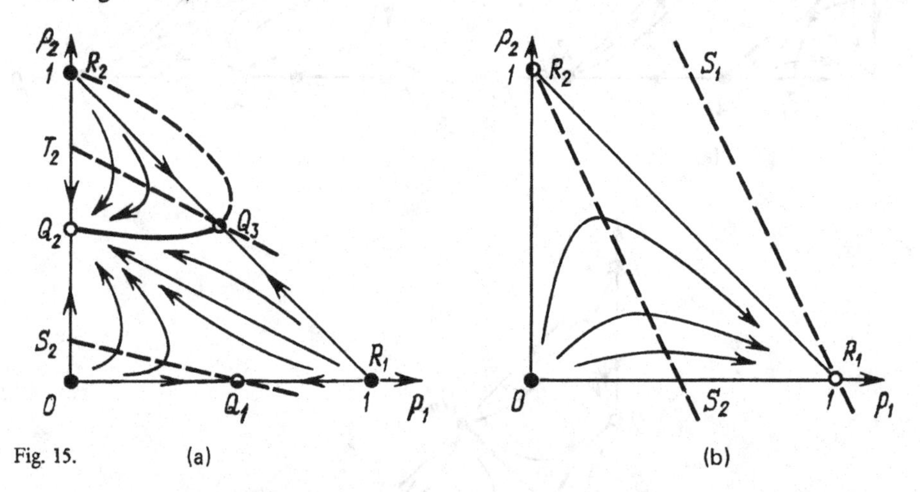

Fig. 15.

Figure 15 shows the phase portrait of system (1.1) for $n=3$ in the singular case.

(a) The point $\mathcal{P}$ goes to infinity. The population develops polymorphism with respect to alleles A_2 and A_3; $\dot{p}_1=0$ along the straight lines T_2Q_3 and S_2Q_1 (this is the curve $\dot{p}_1=0$, $p_1\neq 0$ split into two straight lines), and $\dot{p}_2=0$ along the curve $R_2Q_3Q_2$.

(b) Alleles A_2 and A_3 are eliminated, the population tends to the 'pure' state. $\dot{p}_1=0$ along the straight line R_1S_1, $\dot{p}_2=0$ along the straight line R_2S_2.

If the system is inconsistent, then

$$A_1+\sum_j B_{1j}p_j = k(A_2+\sum_j B_{2j}p_j), \quad j=1, 2,$$

and if $k\neq 1$, then $\dot{p}_1=0$, $p_1\neq 0$, $\dot{p}_2=0$, $p_2\neq 0$ represents two parallel straight lines passing through the points R_1 and R_2. If $k=1$, these two lines merge into one: $p_1+p_2=1$, all points on this line being steady states of the system. Trajectories in this case are straight lines passing through the origin. Depending on the values of the coefficients this line can be either stable or unstable. If it is unstable, then the point 0 will be stable for the whole domain.

Let $k \neq 1$. When $k<1$, the point R_2 is stable; otherwise R_1 is stable (Figure 15b).

The investigation of the three-allele case carried out in this section is far from being complete. But it already shows that even when the population contains only three alleles most various types of dynamic behavior become possible. Naturally, as the number of alleles grows the behavior of the system becomes more and more complicated enriching the set of its various states.

4.7. Necessary and Sufficient Existence Conditions for Polymorphism

Earlier we showed that for a stable polymorphism to exist in a population it is necessary and sufficient that the mean fitness function has a unique isolated maximum interior to Σ. The necessary conditions are:

$$\sum_j B_{ij} p_j^* = -A_i, \quad i,j=\overline{1,n-1}. \tag{7.1}$$

Sufficient conditions require that the quadratic form with matrix $\| B_{ij} \|$ be positive definite. For this all corner minors $|\mathbf{B}_k|$, $k=\overline{1,n-1}$ of matrix $\| B_{ij} \|$ are to be positive.

Let matrix $\| B_{ij} \|$ be non-singular and let system (7.1) has the unique solution

$$p_i^* = \frac{|\mathbf{B}(A_i)|}{|\mathbf{B}|}, \quad i=\overline{1,n-1}, \tag{7.2}$$

where $|\mathbf{B}| = \det \| B_{ij} \|$ and $|\mathbf{B}(A_i)|$ is the determinant of $\| B_{ij} \|$ with the ith column substituted by the column $\| -A_i \|$. From (7.2) it readily follows that for $\mathbf{p}^* \in \Sigma$ it is necessary and sufficient that

$$|\mathbf{B}(A_i)| > 0, \quad \sum_{i=1}^{n-1} |\mathbf{B}(A_i)| < |\mathbf{B}|, \quad i=\overline{1,n-1}, \tag{7.3}$$

since from $\| B_{ij} \|$ being positive definite it follows that $|\mathbf{B}|>0$. Since $|\mathbf{B}(A_i)| \neq 0$ and $|\mathbf{B}| \neq 0$, the solution to (7.2) exists and it is unique.

And finally, for a sufficiently numerous panmictic population, with heredity controlled by one n-allele gene, to have a stable state of polymorphism with respect to all alleles it is necessary and sufficient that:

(a) all corner minors $|\mathbf{B}_k|$ are positive; (7.4)

(b) $|\mathbf{B}(A_i)| > 0, \quad \sum_i |\mathbf{B}(A_i)| < |\mathbf{B}|, \quad i,k=\overline{1,n-1}.$

However, it is hard to check the conditions in this form, since they have no direct relation to the basic characteristics of selection – the Malthusian parameters w_{ij} or some other quantities connected with w_{ij} in a simple manner.

4.8. Theorem About Limited Variations and Another Form of Existence Conditions for Polymorphism

To characterize selection instead of the Malthusian parameters we shall use the variables $a_{ij}=1-w_{ij}$, which can be naturally called the pressures of selection on genotype A_iA_j. Accordingly, instead of the mean fitness function we will consider the function $a=\sum_{i,j} a_{ij}p_ip_j=1-w$ – the mean pressure of selection on the population. Obviously, the function $a(\mathbf{p})$ has an isolated minimum at the point of stable polymorphism.

Let α_{ij} be the cofactors of the elements a_{ij} from matrix $\| a_{ij} \|$. Since $a_{ij}=1-w_{ij}$, applying the well-known relation between a_{ij} and cofactors v_{ij} of w_{ij}

$$\sum_j \alpha_{ij} = (-1)^{n-1}\sum_j v_{ij}, \quad i,j=\overline{1,n}, \tag{8.1}$$

one can derive the expression for coordinates of the steady-state point $\mathbf{p}^*$ in terms of α_{ij} rather than v_{ij}:

$$p_i^* = \frac{\sum_j \alpha_{ij}}{\sum_{i,j} \alpha_{ij}}, \quad i,j=\overline{1,n}. \tag{8.2}$$

Changing the variables: $x_i=p_i-p_i^*$ we yield

$$a = a^* + 2\sum_i x_i \sum_j a_{ij}p_j^* + \sum_{i,j} a_{ij}x_ix_j.$$

Since $\sum_j a_{ij}p_j^*=a_i^*$ and besides $\sum_i x_i=0$ we have

$$2\sum_i x_i \sum_j a_{ij}p_j^* = 2a^*\sum_i x_i = 0,$$

$$a = a^* + \sum_{i,j} a_{ij}x_ix_j = a^* + a_\delta. \tag{8.3}$$

$\mathbf{p}^*$ is the point of an isolated minimum, hence the quadratic form $a_\delta=\sum_{i,j} a_{ij}x_ix_j$ should be positive definite for all x_i, complying with the condition $\sum_i x_i=0$. Let us make use of the result that follows from the Finsler theorem about linked variations. The theorem states that for the quadratic form a_δ to be positive for all nontrivial sets of variables x_i, that satisfy the linear equations $\sum_{j=1}^n b_{ij}x_j=0$, $i=\overline{1,k}$, $k<n$, it is necessary and sufficient, that the quadratic form

$$P = a_\delta + \lambda \sum_{i=1}^{k} \left[\sum_{j=1}^{n} b_{ij}x_j \right]^2 \tag{8.4}$$

be positive definite for all sufficiently large positive λ*. In our case $k=1$ and all $b_{ij}=1$. Then $P=\sum_{i,j}(a_{ij}+\lambda)x_ix_j$, $i,j=\overline{1,n}$ and according to the theorem, the determinant inequalities

$$| a_{ij}+\lambda |_k > 0, \quad i,j=\overline{1,k}, \quad k=\overline{1,n},$$

* Bellman, R.: 1960, *Introduction to Matrix Analysis*, McGraw-Hill, New York.

should hold.

Let us reduce them to a simpler form. Consider the following expression:

$$\begin{vmatrix} a_{11} & \cdots & a_{1k} & \lambda \\ \cdot & \cdots & \cdot & \cdot \\ a_{k1} & \cdots & a_{kk} & \lambda \\ 1 & \cdots & 1 & 0 \end{vmatrix} \cdot \begin{vmatrix} 1 & 0 & \cdots & 0 \\ 0 & 1 & \cdots & 0 \\ \cdot & \cdot & \cdots & \cdot \\ 0 & 0 & \cdots & 0 \\ 1 & 1 & \cdots & 1 \end{vmatrix} = \begin{vmatrix} a_{11} & \cdots & a_{1k}+\lambda & \lambda \\ \cdots & \cdots & \cdots & \cdot \\ a_{k1}+\lambda & \cdots & a_{kk}+\lambda & \lambda \\ 0 & \cdots & 0 & -1 \end{vmatrix}.$$

The second determinant is equal to unity, hence the positiveness of $|a_{ij}+\lambda|_k$ is equivalent to the determinant

$$\begin{vmatrix} a_{11} & \cdots & a_{1k} & \lambda \\ \cdots & \cdots & \cdots & \cdots \\ a_{k1} & \cdots & a_{kk} & \lambda \\ 1 & \cdots & 1 & -1 \end{vmatrix} = \lambda \begin{vmatrix} a_{11} & \cdots & a_{1k} & 1 \\ \cdots & \cdots & \cdots & \cdots \\ a_{k1} & \cdots & a_{kk} & 1 \\ 1 & \cdots & 1 & 0 \end{vmatrix} - \begin{vmatrix} a_{11} & \cdots & a_{1k} \\ \cdots & \cdots & \cdots \\ a_{k1} & \cdots & a_{kk} \end{vmatrix}$$

being negative for large $\lambda>0$. Thus, the sufficient condition for a_δ to be positive under the constraint $\sum_i x_i=0$ is that all bordered determinants

$$\begin{vmatrix} a_{11} & \cdots & a_{1k} & 1 \\ \cdots & \cdots & \cdots & \cdots \\ a_{k1} & \cdots & a_{kk} & \cdots \\ 1 & \cdots & 1 & 0 \end{vmatrix}, \quad k=\overline{1, n} \tag{8.5}$$

are negative. Clearly the conditions

$$\begin{vmatrix} a_{11} & \cdots & a_{1k} & 1 \\ \cdots & \cdots & \cdots & \cdots \\ a_{k1} & \cdots & a_{kk} & \cdots \\ 1 & \cdots & 1 & 0 \end{vmatrix} \leqslant 0, \quad k=\overline{1, n},$$

are necessary. If in this case some lth bordered determinant is zero, then the necessary condition to be positive definite is the inequality

$$\begin{vmatrix} a_{11} & \cdots & a_{1l} \\ \cdots & \cdots & \cdots \\ a_{l1} & \cdots & a_{ll} \end{vmatrix} > 0. \tag{8.6}$$

It is a simple matter to prove that

$$\begin{vmatrix} a_{11} & \cdots & a_{1k} & 1 \\ \cdots & \cdots & \cdots & \cdots \\ a_{k1} & \cdots & a_{kk} & \cdots \\ 1 & \cdots & 1 & 0 \end{vmatrix} = -\sum_{i,j=1}^{k} \alpha_{ij}. \tag{8.7}$$

Then the necessary and sufficient condition of the existence of a minimum for function a is provided by the following inequalities:

$$\sum_{i,j=1}^{k} \alpha_{ij} > 0, \quad k=\overline{1,n}. \tag{8.8}$$

And finally, taking into account the conditions of $\mathbf{p}^*$ being inside the simplex, we can write the necessary and sufficient conditions of polymorphism existence in the form:

$$\text{(a)} \ \sum_j \alpha_{ij} > 0, \quad i,j=\overline{1,n};$$

$$\text{(b)} \ \sum_{i,j=1}^{k} \alpha_{ij} > 0, \quad k=\overline{1,n}, \tag{8.9}$$

or, applying the relations (8.1), we can write them in the form of relationships for cofactors v_{ij}:

$$\text{a}_1) \ (-1)^n \sum_j v_{ij} < 0, \quad i,j=\overline{1,n};$$

$$\text{b}_1) \ (-1)^k \sum_{i,j=1}^{k} v_{ij} < 0, \quad k=\overline{1,n}. \tag{8.10}$$

Since v_{ij} are connected with the entries w^{ij} of matrix W^{-1} by the relationships $w^{ij}=v_{ij} / | W |$, we can give still another form for (8.10):

$$\text{a}_2) \ (-1)^n | W | \sum_j w^{ij} < 0, \quad i,j=\overline{1,n};$$

$$\text{b}_2) \ (-1)^k | W | \sum_{i,j=1}^{k} w^{ij} < 0, \quad k=\overline{1,n}. \tag{8.11}$$

4.9. Elimination of Alleles and Theorem About Dominance

Naturally the question arises: "Is there a chance to judge by the characteristics of selection – the Malthusian parameters and the pressures of seleclion – which of the alleles will be eliminated from the population?" Here we shall use such characteristics as the pressures of selection a_{ij}.

Let us introduce some additional definitions. The row i will be said to be *strictly dominant* over the row j, if $a_{ik}>a_{jk}$, $k=\overline{1,n}$. If $a_{ik}\geqslant a_{jk}$ and $a_{ik}>a_{jk}$ at least for one k, then we shall speak of simply *domination* (similar definitions hold for matrix columns). Both of these relations are transitive. Let us note, that if two rows are different, it does not all imply that one of them dominates over the other. In a symmetric matrix the relationship of dominance between rows results in the same relationship between columns.

Suppose we are given a set of numbers $\{\rho_i \geqslant 0\}$, $\sum_i \rho_i = 1$, $i=\overline{1,s}$. We shall say that x is a convex linear combination of s rows with weights ρ_i if

$$x_j = \sum_{i=1}^{s} a_{ij}\rho_i, \quad j=\overline{1,n}.$$

In case $a_{ij}>x_j$ for all $j=\overline{1,n}$ the ith row will be said to be strictly dominant over those s rows that make up the convex linear combination. If $a_{ij}\geqslant x_j$ with $a_{ik}>x_k$ for at least one k, then the ith row is simply dominant over s rows.

With no loss of generality, let us suppose that matrix $\| a_{ij} \|$ has the last row dominating over the convex linear combination of all other rows.

Deletion of the dominating row and the corresponding column will be called operation of exclusion.

Let I_k be the subset of k indices taken from the set of all indices I, $I_0=\emptyset$. Then the relation of domination for the nth row can be presented in the form

$$a_{nj} = \sum_{i=1}^{n-1} a_{ij}\rho_i,\ j\in I_k,$$
$$a_{ns} > \sum_{i=1}^{n-1} a_{is}\rho_i,\ s\in \overline{I}_k. \tag{9.1}$$

If $j\in I_0$, strict domination takes place.

Let $\mathbf{p}^*$ be a stable steady-state point of system (1.1) such that $p_i^*=0$, $i\in I_k$; $p_j^*>0$, $j\in\overline{I}_k$. In new notations this system can be presented in the form

$$\frac{dp_i}{dt} = p_i(a-a_i),\ a_i=\sum_j a_{ij}p_j,$$
$$a = \sum_i a_ip_i,\ i,j=\overline{1,n}. \tag{9.2}$$

Whence one can see that $a_i^*=a^*$ for $i\in\overline{I}_k$. And since $\mathbf{p}^*$ is stable, $a_i^*\geqslant a^*$ for $i\in I_k$. In fact, in the small vicinity of $p_i^*=0$ we have $\dot p_i\simeq p_i(a^*-a_i^*)$ and $\dot p_i<0$ for $a_i^*>a^*$. If $a_i^*<a^*$ then $\dot p_i>0$, which is in contradiction with our assumption about stability. Consequently, $a_i^*\geqslant a^*$. Let us prove the following auxiliary statement.

LEMMA Let $\overline{I}_k$ *be the set of indices, for which a strict inequality takes place in* (9.1). *Then* $a_n^*>a^*$, *if* $p_s\neq 0$, $s\in\overline{I}_k$; *and* $a_n^*\geqslant a^*$ *if* $p_s^*=0$, $s\in\underline{I_k}$.

Multiplying (9.1) by p_j^* and summing up over $j=1,n$ we get:

(a) if $p_s^*\neq 0$ then

$$a_n^* = \sum_{j=1}^{n} a_{nj}p_j^* > \sum_{j=1}^{n}\sum_{i=1}^{n-1} a_{ij}\rho_ip_j^* = \sum_{i=1}^{n-1} a_i^*\rho_i; \tag{9.3}$$

(b) if $p_s^*=0$ then

$$a_n^* = \sum_{j=1}^{n} a_{nj}p_j^* \geqslant \sum_{j=1}^{n}\sum_{i=1}^{n-1} a_{ij}\rho_ip_j^* = \sum_{i=1}^{n-1} a_i^*\rho_i. \tag{9.4}$$

And since $a_i^*\geqslant a^*$ for all $i=\overline{1,n-1}$ and $\sum_{i=1}^{n-1}\rho_1=1$ we have

(a) $a_n^*>a^*$; (b) $a_n^*\geqslant a^*$.

The lemma is proved.

Let us show, that if the nth row dominates over the rest and if

$$a_{nn} > \sum_{i,j=1}^{n-1} a_{ij}\rho_i\rho_j,$$

then the only stable (asymptotically stable) steady state will be the state with $p_n^*=0$.

(a) Suppose $a_n^* > a^*$. Then the only possible equilibrium will be the state with $p_n^*=0$. Since in a small vicinity of the steady-state point $\dot{p}_n = p_n(a^* - a_n^*)$, we see that for $a_n^* > a^*$ this state will be locally stable, its global stability over the whole simplex following from it being unique.

(b) Suppose $a_n^* = a^*$. The proof will be by contradiction. Let us show that any state with $p_n^* \neq 0$ is unstable. Let us introduce new variables:

$$x_i = p_i - p_i^*, \quad \sum x_i = 0, \quad i = \overline{1, n}.$$

and write out the equation for x_n when $p_n^* \neq 0$ and $a_n^* = a^*$:

$$\begin{aligned}\frac{\mathrm{d}x_n}{\mathrm{d}t} &= p_n^*\left[2\sum_{i=1}^{n-1}\sum_{j=1}^{n} a_{ij}p_i^*x_j - \sum_{j=1}^{n} a_{nj}x_j\right] + 2(p_n^*)^2\sum_{j=1}^{n} a_{nj}x_j + \\ &+ \left\{\left[2\sum_{i=1}^{n-1}\sum_{j=1}^{n} a_{ij}p_i^*x_j - (1-2p_n^*)\sum_{j=1}^{n} a_{nj}x_j\right]x_n + \right. \\ &\left. + p_n^*\sum_{i,j=1}^{n} a_{ij}x_ix_j\right\} + x_n\sum_{i,j=1}^{n} a_{ij}x_ix_j.\end{aligned} \tag{9.5}$$

To reveal instability, it is enough to find at least one trajectory, along which x_n infinitely grows as $t\to\infty$. Let us choose $x_i = -\rho_i x_n$, $i=\overline{1, n-1}$, $x_n \leqslant 0$. This choice is stipulated by the equalities $\sum_{i=1}^{n-1} x_i = -x_n \sum_{i=1}^{n-1}\rho_i = -x_n$. Substituting these values of x_i into (9.5), we get

$$\begin{aligned}\frac{\mathrm{d}x_n}{\mathrm{d}t} &= p_n^* x_n\left[\sum_{j=1}^{n-1} a_{nj}\rho_j - a_{nn}\right] - x_n^2\left[(1-p_n^*)a_{nn} - \right. \\ &\left. -(1-2p_n^*)\sum_{j=1}^{n-1} a_{nj}\rho_j - p_n^*\sum_{i,j=1}^{n-1} a_{ij}\rho_i\rho_j\right] + o(x_n^2).\end{aligned} \tag{9.6}$$

Whence one can see that if $a_{nn} > \sum_{j=1}^{n-1} a_{nj}\rho_j$, then the state with $p_n^* \neq 0$ is unstable, since $\dot{x}_n > 0$ and x_n grows with t.

If $a_{nn} = \sum_{j=1}^{n-1} a_{nj}\rho_j$, we have to look at the following approximation:

$$\frac{\mathrm{d}x_n}{\mathrm{d}t} = -x_n^2 p_n^*\left[a_{nn} - \sum_{i,j=1}^{n-1} a_{ij}\rho_i\rho_j\right] + o(x_n^2).$$

But domination implies that $a_{ns} > \sum_{j=1}^{n-1} a_{sj}\rho_j$ for at least one s. If $\rho_s \neq 0$, then from the condition $a_{nn} = \sum_{j=1}^{n-1} a_{nj}\rho_j$ we immediately get $a_{nn} > \sum_{i,j=1}^{n-1} a_{ij}\rho_i\rho_j$. Then $\dot{x}_n > 0$ and $p_n^* \neq 0$ is again unstable.

One can show that in the most unlikely case, when $a_{nn}=\sum_{i,j=1}^{n-1}a_{ij}\rho_i\rho_j$ then the derivative $\dot{x}_n$ is identically zero and the state with $p_n^*\neq 0$ is the state of neutral equilibrium.

Since instead of the index n we can choose any other index, the derived result can be formulated as a theorem, as follows:

THEOREM ABOUT DOMINATION. *If the matrix of selection pressures* $\| a_{ij} \|$ *has a* jth *row dominating over all the others and* $a_{jj}\neq\sum_{i,j=1}^{n-1}a_{ij}\rho_i\rho_j$, *then the state with* $p_j^*=0$ *will be the steady state of the population, that is the asymptotically stable state.*

When domination is strict, we do not need the inequality for a_{jj}.

This theorem provides a handy method to reduce the dimensionality of the original problem. In fact, suppose we are given a matrix $\| a_{ij} \|$ of a sufficiently high order. Select some dominating row (or column) in this matrix and apply the opertion of exclusion to it. The order of the matrix we get will be less by one. In the new matrix we can again try to select a dominating row or column and again apply the operation of exclusion. We shall go on with this operation till it is possible. As a result we obtain a matrix of a much lower order than the original one, and thus reduce our problem to a problem of lower dimensionality. The operation of exclusion when analyzing polymorphism allows us to neglect the alleles with zero frequencies at steady state, that is the alleles, that are eliminated from the population by the pressure of natural selection.

As an example let us look at the four-allele case with the matrix $\| a_{ij} \|$ of the form

$$\begin{array}{c} \\ A_1 \\ A_2 \\ A_3 \\ A_4 \end{array}\begin{array}{c} \begin{array}{cccc} A_1 & A_2 & A_3 & A_4 \end{array} \\ \left\| \begin{array}{cccc} 0.7 & 0.8 & 0.6 & 0.0 \\ 0.8 & 0.6 & 0.8 & 0.6 \\ 0.6 & 0.8 & 0.6 & 0.0 \\ 0.0 & 0.6 & 0.0 & 0.2 \end{array} \right\| \end{array}.$$

The first row dominates over the others $(\rho_2=\rho_4=0,\ \rho_3=1)$ and $a_{11}>\sum_{i,j=2}^{4}a_{ij}\rho_i\rho_j=a_{33}$, hence, deleting the first row and the first column, we get

$$p_1^*=0;\quad \begin{array}{c} \\ A_2 \\ A_3 \\ A_4 \end{array}\begin{array}{c} \begin{array}{ccc} A_2 & A_3 & A_4 \end{array} \\ \left\| \begin{array}{ccc} 0.6 & 0.8 & 0.6 \\ 0.8 & 0.6 & 0.0 \\ 0.6 & 0.0 & 0.2 \end{array} \right\| \end{array}.$$

In this new matrix again the first row dominates over the rest $(\rho_3=0,\ \rho_4=1)$ and $a_{22}>\sum_{i,j=3}^{4}a_{ij}\rho_i\rho_j=a_{44}$. Deleting the first row and the first column, we get

$$p_2^*=0;\quad \begin{array}{c} \\ A_3 \\ A_4 \end{array}\begin{array}{c} \begin{array}{cc} A_3 & A_4 \end{array} \\ \left\| \begin{array}{cc} 0.6 & 0.0 \\ 0.0 & 0.2 \end{array} \right\| \end{array}.$$

This matrix has no relations of domination, but it is already a 2×2-matrix, while the original one had the order 4×4. The problem is reduced to the diallele case. One can easily see, that there exists a polymorphism with respect to alleles A_3 and

A_4, since

$$a_{34} = 0 < \min\{a_{33}, a_{44}\} = \min\{0.6; 0.2\}.$$

Consequently, in the original 4-allele population polymorphism can also occur only with respect to alleles A_3 and A_4. Alleles A_1 and A_2 will be eliminated from the population by selection.

Interesting corollaries can be easily derived from the theorem proved above.

COROLLARY 1. *If the diagonal elements of matrix* $\| a_{ij} \|$ *are strictly less than the non-diagonal elements of the appropriate rows (columns), then no stable steady state of polymorphism can exist in the population.*

Suppose we have a steady state $\overset{*}{p}_k = 1$, $\overset{*}{p}_i = 0$, $i = \overline{1, n}$, $i \neq k$. Then $\overset{*}{a}_i = a_{ik}$ for all $i \neq k$, and $a_{kk} = \overset{*}{a}_k = a^*$ for $i = k$. $\overset{*}{a}_i > a^*$ for $i \neq k$, since we assumed that $a_{kk} < a_{ik}$, and it immediately follows from the equations that the state with $\overset{*}{p}_k = 1$ is stable by the first-order approximation. If this condition holds for all diagonal elements, then this is the only type of steady-state points, that can exist, and this proves our statement. The biological meaning of this statement is that homozygotes are more viable than the appropriate heterozygotes. Polymorphism becomes impossible in such a population, since heterozygotes, producing different alleles at gamete genesis, loose in competition with homozygotes, which produce gametes of only one type. Sooner or later the population becomes made of only one allele.

COROLLARY 2. *If all rows (columns) strictly dominate over an ith row (column) in matrix* $\| a_{ij} \|$, *then all alleles but the ith one are eliminated from the population.*

4.10. Simple Necessary Conditions of Existence for Polymorphic and 'Pure' Equilibrium

The condition that the mean fitness function be extremal at the points of equilibrium, gives us a whole spectrum of necessary conditions of existence for polymorphic and 'pure' genetic equilibria. As it was shown above, if the population develops a polymorphism, then $\| B_{ij} \|$ is positive definite, and when $\| B_{ij} \|$ is negative definite, the population attains only 'pure' equilibria, when all alleles but one are eliminated.

The necessary condition of being positive definite, $B_{ii} > 0$, implies that

$$2w_{in} > w_{ii} + w_{nn}, \quad i = \overline{1, n-1}. \tag{10.1}$$

And since index n can be replaceld by any other index $k \neq i$, we have

$$w_{ik} > \frac{(w_{ii} + w_{kk})}{2}, \quad i \neq k, \quad i, k = \overline{1, n}. \tag{10.2}$$

This condition has a clear genetic interpretation: in a population with polymorphism with respect to all alleles, the fitness of any heterozygote is always greater than the arithmetic mean of homozygote fitnesses with respect to the alleles contained in the heterozygote.

If $\| B_{ij} \|$ is negative definite, then $B_{ii}<0$ and

$$w_{ik} < \frac{(w_{ii}+w_{kk})}{2}, \quad i\neq k, \quad i, k=\overline{1, n}, \tag{10.3}$$

that is, if all alleles but one are eliminated from the popultion, then heterozygote fitnesses are to be less than the arithmetic mean of the appropriate homozygotes.

If the quadratic form with matrix $\| B_{ij} \|$ is positive definite then

$$\sum_{i,j=1}^{n-1} B_{ij}p_ip_j > 0 \tag{10.4}$$

(at least one of p_i, $i=\overline{1, n-1}$, is non- zero), or

$$2\sum_{i=1}^{n-1} p_i \sum_{j=1}^{n-1} w_{nj}p_j > w_{nn}\left[\sum_{i=1}^{n-1} p_i\right]^2 + \sum_{i,j=1}^{n-1} w_{ij}.$$

Taking into account that the choice of index n is arbitrary to a certain extent, and that $p_n=1-\sum_{i=1}^{n-1}p_i$, simple transformations yield

$$w_k > \frac{(w_{kk}+w)}{2}, \quad k=\overline{1, n}, \tag{10.5}$$

$$w_k - w_{kk} > w - w_k, \quad k=\overline{1, n}. \tag{10.6}$$

By analogy with the mean population fitness w, the quantity $w_k=\sum_{j=1}^{n} w_{kj}p_j$ will be called mean fitness of kth allele. Then from (10.6) it readily follows that in a popultion with polymorphism with respect to all alleles, the difference between the mean fitness of any allele and the homozygote fitness with respect to this allele is always greater than the difference between the mean fitness of the population and that of this allele. In other words, in a polymorphic population the distinction in fitnesses between genotypes should be more pronounced, that than between alleles.

If the population at equilibrium can have only a 'pure' genetic structure, then $\| B_{ij} \|<0$ and

$$w_k - w_{kk} < w - w_k, \tag{10.7}$$

that is, all the aforesaid is correct just the other way round.

4.11. Population Trajectory as a Trajectory of Steepest Ascent

4.11.1. *Introduction of a New Metric Space*

Fisher's theorem only states that mean fitness grows along the population trajectories. It would be fine if these trajectories manifested some extremal properties, say, if they were trajectories of the vector field of the mean fitness gradient, i.e. if out of all the possible directions the population selected the one along which the increment of the mean fitness was maximal. However, as one can easily see, after writing (1.1) in the form

$$\frac{dp_i}{dt} = p_i\left[\frac{1}{2}\frac{\partial w}{\partial p_i} - w\right], \quad i=\overline{1, n}, \tag{11.1}$$

this is not the case, and in the Euclidean space the trajectories of population equations do not provide the steepest ascent for w. However, this does not imply, that there can be no other space with another metric, where trajectories manifest this extremal property.

Let us introduce the metric Riemannian space with the base form $(ds)^2 = g_{ij}\,dx^i\,dx^j$. (Here and further on, if necessary, we shall apply the summation rules adopted in tensor analysis, that is, summation is taken over similar indices, if one of them is a superscript and the other – a subscript. For instance, $(ds)^2 = g_{ij}\,dx^i\,dx^j = \sum_{ij} g_{ij}\,dx^i\,dx^j$.) g_{ij} is a metric tensor of the space R_s, and is defined as follows

$$g_{ij} = \frac{1}{2}\left[\frac{\delta_i^j}{x^j} + \frac{\delta_j^i}{x^i}\right] = \frac{x^i\delta_i^j + x^i\delta_j^i}{2x^i x^j}, \quad i, j=\overline{1, n}. \tag{11.2}$$

Here

$$\delta_i^j = \begin{cases} 1 \text{ for } i=j, \\ 0 \text{ for } i\neq j, \end{cases}$$

$\{x^i\}$ is the contravariant vector in R_s, with components equal to allele frequencies, so that $x^i = p_i$, $i=\overline{1, n}$; $\{x_i\}$ is the associated covariant vector, which can be easily shown to be a vector with constant unit components in R_s, so that $x_i = 1$, $i=\overline{1, n}$. In fact

$$x_i = g_{ij}x^j = \frac{1}{2}\left[\delta_i^j + \frac{\delta_j^i x^j}{x^i}\right] = 1.$$

The squared length of vector x^i in R_s is $x^2 = g_{ij}x^i x^j = 1/2(x^i\delta_i^j + x^j\delta_j^i) = \sum_{i=1}^n x^i$. And since $x^i = p_i$ and p_i complies with the normalization condition $\sum_{i=1}^n p_i = 1$, it follows that

$$x^2 = \sum_{i=1}^{n} x^i = 1,$$

i.e. trajectories, characterizing the variations in the gene structure of the population, are to lie on a unit sphere S in this space.

4.11.2. *Equations of Evolution and Local Extremal Principle*

In R_s the mean fitness function has the form $w = w_{ij}x^i x^j$. It turns out that in R_s the population trajectories are the trajectories of the vector field ∇w. Let us prove this statement.

Write out the equations of gradient ascent for w in R_s under the condition that the trajectories of the vectorial gradient field are to lie on S. In doing this we can invoke the Lagrangian multiplier method.

Define the new, expanded as against R_s, metric space R_s', with the base form

$$(ds')^2 = g_{ij}\,dx^i\,dx^j - \frac{(d\lambda)^2}{\lambda}, \quad i, j=\overline{1, n}, \tag{11.3}$$

and consider the function

$$w' = w + \lambda(g_{ij}x^i x^j - 1) \tag{11.4}$$

in R_s'. The equations of gradient ascent in R_s' for w' have the form

$$\frac{dx^i}{dt} = kg^{li}\frac{\partial w'}{\partial x^l}, \quad k>0, \tag{11.5}$$
$$\frac{d\lambda}{dt} = -k\lambda\frac{\partial w'}{\partial \lambda}.$$

We regard movement along the gradient as a continuous process, so that the parameter t can be identified with time. Equations (11.5) define the movement along the gradient with velocity V', which is in proportion to the norm of the gradient (k is the proportionality coefficient). In fact, multiplying the first n equations in (11.5) by $g_{ij}\,dx^i/dt$, and the last one by $\lambda^{-1}\,d\lambda/dt$, then summing up the first n equations and subtracting the last one, we get

$$g_{ij}\frac{dx^i}{dt}\frac{dx^j}{dt} - \frac{1}{\lambda}\left[\frac{d\lambda}{dt}\right]^2 = kg_{ij}g^{li}\frac{\partial w'}{\partial x^l}\frac{dx^j}{dt} + k\frac{\partial w'}{\partial \lambda}\frac{d\lambda}{dt}. \tag{11.6}$$

And since $g_{ij}x^{li} = \delta^l_j$, it follows from (11.6) that

$$\left[\frac{d}{dt}s'\right]^2 = (V')^2 = k\left[\frac{\partial w'}{\partial x^l}\frac{dx^l}{dt} + \frac{\partial w'}{\partial \lambda}\frac{d\lambda}{dt}\right]. \tag{11.7}$$

The gradient of function w' in R_s' is the contravariant vector, with the squared length equal to

$$|\nabla w'|^2 = g^{kl}\frac{\partial w'}{\partial x^k}\frac{\partial w'}{\partial x^l} - \lambda\left[\frac{\partial w'}{\partial \lambda}\right]^2. \tag{11.8}$$

On the other hand, substituting for dx^l/dt and $d\lambda/dt$ in (11.7) their values from (11.5), we get

$$(V')^2 = k^2\left[g^{kl}\frac{\partial w'}{\partial x^k}\frac{\partial w'}{\partial x^l} - \lambda\left[\frac{\partial w'}{\partial \lambda}\right]^2\right].$$

Comparing this expression with (11.8) we can write

$$|V'| = k\,|\nabla w'|, \tag{11.9}$$

Q.E.D.

Since

$$\frac{\partial w'}{\partial x^l}\frac{dx^l}{dt} + \frac{\partial w'}{\partial \lambda}\frac{d\lambda}{dt} = \frac{dw'}{dt},$$

it follows that

$$|V'| = \sqrt{\frac{k\,dw'}{dt}}. \tag{11.10}$$

Going gack to Equations (11.5) we get

$$\frac{dx^i}{dt} = kx^i(2w^{ij}x^j + \lambda), \tag{11.11}$$
$$\frac{d\lambda}{dt} = -k\lambda(g_{ij}x^ix^j - 1).$$

Here we took into account that $g^{ij} = 1/2(x^i\delta_i^j + x^j\delta_j^i)$. Summing up the first n equations in (11.11) under the condition $\sum_{i=1}^n \dot{x}^i = 0$, we obtain $\lambda = -2w_{ij}x^ix^j = -2w$, whence it readily follows that

$$\frac{dx^i}{dt} = 2kx^i(w_{ij}x^j - w_{ij}x^ix^j), \tag{11.12}$$
$$\sum_i x^i = 1, \quad i, j = \overline{1, n}.$$

But setting $k = 1/2$ in (11.12), we make this system coincide (except for notations) with system (1.1), presenting the dynamics of the population genic composition. Thus we proved that the population trajectories in R_s' are the trajectories of the vector field $\nabla w'$. Since trajectories (11.12) always satisfy the constraint $\sum_{i=1}^n x^i = 1$, and the equations themselves are independent of λ, we can carry on from the space R_s' to R_s and from the function w' to w. Consequently, trajectories of the vector field ∇w, lying on the unit sphere $S \in R_s$, are also the population trajectories.

Let us calculate, what will be the velocity V for the movement of the representing point along the gradient in R_s (here and in what follows by velocity we mean its absolute value). From (11.10), setting $k = 1/2$ and $dw'/dt = dw/dt$ (since all trajectories comply with the condition $\sum_i x^i = 1$), we get

$$V = \sqrt{\frac{1}{2}\frac{dw}{dt}}. \tag{11.13}$$

But $dw/dt = 2V_g = \sum_{i=1}^n p_i(w_i - w)^2$ and

$$V = \sqrt{V_g}. \tag{11.14}$$

We have derived the result, which can be formulated as a local principle of optimality.

If we consider the population dynamics in a Riemannian space with the base form $g_{ij} = (p_i\delta_{ij} + p_j\delta_{ji})/2p_ip_j$, *then all the trajectories of the population in this space belong to the unit sphere. At any other time out of all the possible directions on this sphere the population picks the one that provides the maximal increase to its mean fitness, and moves along this direction with a velocity, which is in proportion to a certain measure of the population genetic diversity*

$$V = \sqrt{\sum_{i=1}^{n} p_i(w_i - w)^2}$$

In other words, along the proper trajectory we have $\delta w^* = \max(\partial w)$ under the condition that

$$\text{(a)} \sum_{i=1}^{n} \delta p_i = 0;$$

$$\text{(b)} \sum_{i=1}^{n} \left[\frac{\delta p_i}{\delta t}\right]^2 \frac{\delta t}{p_i} = \frac{1}{2}\frac{\delta w}{\delta t}.$$

Condition (a) is obvious; condition (b) implies that $(\delta s/\delta t)^2 = 1/2\delta w/\delta t$, that is, the velocity of the movement along the gradient complies with the constraint (11.13).

4.12. Another Form for Equations of Evolution

Invoking the relation $p_n = 1 - \sum_{i=1}^{n-1} p_i$, one can pass over from the n-dimensional space to the space $\{p_1, \ldots, p_{n-1}\}$ which is $n-1$-dimensional. In this case the equations of movement can be written in the form

$$\frac{dp_i}{dt} = \frac{1}{2}\sum_j \sigma^{ij}\frac{\partial \tilde{w}}{\partial p_j}, \quad i, j = \overline{1, n-1},$$

$$\sigma^{ij} = p_i(\delta_{ij} - p_j)$$

$$\tilde{w} = w_{nn} - 2\sum_{i=1}^{n-1} \mathcal{A}_i p_i - \sum_{i,j-1}^{n-1} \mathcal{B}_{ij} p_i p_j, \tag{12.1}$$

where $\mathcal{A}_i = w_{nn} - w_{in}$, $\mathcal{B}_{ij} = w_{in} + w_{jn} - w_{ij} - w_{nn}$.

The form of (12.1) suggests that the population trajectory will be the trajectory of steepest ascent in the metric Riemannian space $\tilde{R}$ with the base form $(d\tilde{s})^2 = \sigma_{ij}\, dx^i\, dx^j$, where σ_{ij} are the elements of the matrix reciprocal to σ^{ij}. Calculating σ_{ij} we get

$$\sigma_{ij} = \frac{\delta_i^j}{x^i} + \frac{1}{1 - \sum_{i=1}^{n-1} x^i}, \quad i, j = \overline{1, n-1}. \tag{12.2}$$

Here $\{x^i\} = \{p_i\}$ is the contravariant vector in $\tilde{R}$; $\{x_i\}$ is the corresponding covariant vector. Calculating its components we get

$$x_i = \sigma_{ij} x^j = \frac{1}{(1-P)}, \tag{12.3}$$

where $P=\sum_{i=1}^{n-1}x^i$, that is, all components of vector $\{x_i\}$ are identic. The squared length of vector $\{x^i\}$ in $\tilde{R}$ is

$$x^2 = \sigma_{ij}x^i x^j = \frac{P}{(1-P)}. \tag{12.4}$$

It follows from (12.3) and (12.4) that as the trajectory approaches the plane $P=1$ (which is one of the simplex faces), the lengths of vectors $\{x^i\}$ and $\{x_i\}$ tend to infinity. This implies, that all trajectories, orginating inside the simplex, never cross this boundary. Since all other boundaries are absorbing, the trajectory can never go beyond the other boundaries as well. Consequently, any trajectory, originating inside the simplex, remains there.

Equations (12.1) in $\tilde{R}$ can be represented in the form

$$\frac{dx^i}{dt} = \frac{1}{2}\sigma^{ij}\frac{\partial \tilde{w}}{\partial x^j}, \quad i,j=\overline{1,n-1}, \tag{12.5}$$

whence it follows, that any population trajectory in $\tilde{R}$ is the trajectory of steepest ascent. At any one time, out of all possible directions in $\tilde{R}$ the population selects the one that provides the maximal increase to its mean fitness, and moves along it with velocity

$$\tilde{V} = \frac{1}{2}\sqrt{\sigma^{ij}\left[\frac{\partial \tilde{w}}{\partial x^i}\right]\left[\frac{\partial \tilde{w}}{dx^j}\right]}. \tag{12.6}$$

Applying the expressions for σ^{ij} and $\tilde{w}$ one can present the velocity $\tilde{V}$ in the form

$$\tilde{V} = \sqrt{\sum_{i,j=1}^{n-1} p_i(\delta_{ij}-p_j)\left[\mathcal{A}_i+\sum_{k=1}^{n-1}\mathcal{B}_{ik}p_k\right]\left[\mathcal{A}_j+\sum_{l=1}^{n-1}\mathcal{B}_{jl}p_l\right]}. \tag{12.7}$$

Since

$$\tilde{V}^2 = \frac{1}{4}\sigma^{ij}\frac{\partial \tilde{w}}{\partial x^i}\frac{\partial \tilde{w}}{\partial x^j} = \frac{1}{2}\frac{\partial \tilde{w}}{\partial x^i}\frac{dx^i}{dt} = \frac{1}{2}\frac{d\tilde{w}}{dt},$$

we obtain another expression for velocity, which is similar to the one derived in Section 4.11.2 ($\tilde{V}=\sqrt{(1/2)d\tilde{w}/dt}$).

Unlike Section 4.11.2, where a restriction was imposed on the movement in the n-dimensional space, no such restriction is needed now, all phase variables are independent and they may be regarded as some generalized coordinates (as it is done in mechanics).

In Chapter 12 one can find an elementary account of the problems touched upon in Sections 4.11–4.12, generalized for the case of the joint actions of selection, mutations and migrations. There we also elaborate on the relationship between the optimized functions and the nature of the steady-state density in the diffusion models of population genetics. It turns out that the optimized functions define the form of the steady-state density, which takes on the greatest values approximately at the points of their maxima. In Section 12.12 we prove that one-locus genetic processes are gradient-wise not only for selection with constant fitnesses w_{ij}, but also under the combined action of other forms of selection (the frequency dependent one can also be among them) together with some forms of migrations and mutations. In terms of the coordinates $\tilde{x}_i = \sqrt{p_i}$ the dynamic equations (being once again differentiated with respect to time) coincide with the equations of mechanical motion in a field of force. Therefore the non-local extremal principle, the least action principle of Hamilton, operates in the analyzed genetic processes, the functional of action being not only stationary along the proper trajectories, but also minimal for sufficiently small intervals of integration.

4.13. Notes and Bibliography

To 4.1.

Models of populations with heredity controlled by one gene with multiple alleles are one of the most elaborated objects in mathematical genetics. Apparently, the reason is that matrix techniques are most natural to describe populations of this kind.

Though equations like (1.1) have been used already by R. Fisher and S. Wright, they were first derived more or less rigorously (with no account of the population age structure) by M. Kimura in his work:

Kimura, M.: 1958, 'On the Change of Population Fitness by Natural Selelction', *Heredity* **12**, 2, 145–167.

To 4.2.

The classification of different types of genetic polymorphism and the appropriate case-studies can be found in:

Timofeeff-Ressovsky N. V. and Svirezhev Yu. M.: 1967, 'O geneticeskom polimorfizme v populjacijah. Experimentalno- teoreticeskoje issledovanije (On Genetic Polymorphism in Populations. Experimental and Theoretical Study. In Russian)', *Genetika* **10**, 152–166.

To 4.3

For the first time this theorem has been formulated (in a somewhat different form) by R. Fisher in his book 'The Genetical Theory of Natural Selection' (1930, Oxford, Clarendon Press). Unfortunately, as a result of the obscurities in the original formulation and some slips in the proof the theorem was considered to be universal (especially among biologists) and its main conclusion was applied to all natural situations.

Later on Fisher himself repeatedly revised this theorem supplementing and correcting its formulation; cf. for instance,

Fisher, R. A.: 1941, 'Average Excess and Average Effect of a Gene Substitution', *Ann. Eugenics* **11**, 1, 53–63.

Some difficulties arise when formulating the discrete analogy of this theorem, which is quite natural, since Fisher's theorem, proving that the total derivative of mean fitness with respect to time is non-negative, bears a local character. The finite increment, however, can be negative as well. In the work:

Kingman, J. F. C.: 1961, 'A Mathematical Problem in Population Genetics', *Proc. Camb. Phil. Soc.* **57**, 3, 574–582,

Fisher's theorem found its rigorous proof for the discrete case. However, difficulties arise when interpreting the result. For more details see:

Li, C. C.: 1967, 'Fundamental Theorem of Natural Selection', *Nature* **214**, 5087, 505–506.

To 4.4.

A. Hasofer suggested to use the direct Lyapunov method to evaluate the stability of the polymorphic state:

Hasofer, A. M.: 1966, 'A Continuous-time Model in Population Genetics', *J. Theoret. Biol.* **11**, 1, 150–163.

Stability in one-locus genetic models was also studied by this method in the paper:

Pyh, Ju. A.: 'Issledovanije ustoičivosti v dinamičeskyh modeljah populjacionnoi genetiki (Stability Analysis in Dynamic Models of Population Genetics. In Russian)' in *Problemy evolucii* (*Problems of Evolution*), Vol. 3, Nauka, Novosibirsk, pp. 214–221.

To 4.5.

The notion of adaptive topography of a population was introduced by S. Wright:

Wright, S.: 1949, 'Adaptation and Selection', in Jenson, G., Simpson, G., and Mary, E. (eds.), *Genetics, Paleontology and Evolution*, Princeton Univ. Press, Princeton.

However, later on with no justification the notion was carried over to models of other types, which could hardly yield the same result. Therefore it was only natural that papers appeared, proving the non-existence of adaptive topography in, say, models with two loci, Cf.:

Moran, P. A. P.: 1964, 'On the Non-Existence of Adaptive Topographies', *Ann. Hum. Genetics* **27**, 383--393.

To 4.7.

Quite a lot of works deal with the search of necessary and sufficient conditions for stability in polymorphic (and not necessarily polymorphic) states in a one-locus model. See, for instance, the work:

Kimura, M.: 1956, 'Rules for Testing Stability of Selective Polymorphism', *Proc. Natl. Acad. Sci.* **42**, 6, 336–340.

Almost simultaneously there appeared a similar work:

Penrose, L. S., Smith, S. M., and Sprott, D. A.: 1956, 'On the Stability of Allelic Systems', *Ann. Hum. Genet.* **21**, 90–93.

General principles to approach the problem of polymorphism were formulated in the paper:

Lewontin, R. G.: 1958, 'A General Method for Investigating the Equilibrium of a Gene Frequency in a Population', *Genetics* **43**, 4, 419–434.

The sufficient conditions in the form of relations for bordered determinants may be found in the paper:

Mandel, S. P.: 1959, 'The Stability of a Multiple Allelic System', *Heredity* **13**, 3, 289–302.

In a way we managed to strengthen the results, derived in this work.

Various steady states in a one-locus model with multiple alleles and their stability criteria are most intensively treated in the above-cited work by Hasofer and in the paper:

Tallis, G. M.: 1966, 'Equlibria Under Selection for *k* Alleles', *Biometrics* **22**, 1, 121–127.

To 4.8.

In the paper

Svirezhev, Yu. M.: 1976, 'Neobhodimyje i dostatocynje uslvoija polimorfizma i teorema dominirovanija (Necessary and Sufficient Conditions of Polymorphism and the Domination Theorem. In Russian)', *Zurnal Obshei Biologii* (*Journal of General Biology*), **37**, 2, 175–183,

it was first suggested to use the theorem about linked variations in order to obtain necessary and sufficient polymorphism conditions.

To 4.9.

In this same work the theorem about domination was proved.

To 4.11–4.12.

The material is presented according to the work:

Svirezhev, Yu. M.: 1972, 'Principy optimalnosti v populjacionnoi genetike (Optimality Principles in Population Genetics. In Russian)', in: *Issledovanija po teoreticeskoi genetike* (*Studies in Theoretical Genetics*), Inst. of Cytology and Genetics, Novisibirsk, pp. 86–102.

An elementary approach is contained in the paper:

Timofeeff-Ressovsky, N. V., and Svirezhev, Yu. M.: 1970, 'Populjacionnaja genetika i optimalnyi processy (Population Genetics and Optimal Processes. In Russian)', *Genetika* **6**, 10, 155–166.

In the former of these papers the considered properties of trajectories are also proved to hold in a Euclidean space, namely on the surface of a unit hypersphere, obtained by the change of coordinates $x_i = \sqrt{p_i}$, $i = \overline{1, n}$. Besides, along the population trajectory under the effect of selection Euler equations turn out to be satisfied for the Lagrange function

$$\sum_i \left[\frac{1}{2p_i} \left[\frac{dp_i}{dt} \right]^2 + \frac{1}{8} p_i (w_i - w)^2 \right].$$

The changes in frequencies of multiple alleles under the effect of selection are analyzed and gradient properties of trajectories are derived in the paper

Shahshahani, S.: 1979, 'A New Mathematical Framework for the Study of Linkage and Selection', *Memoirs of the American Mathematical Society* **17**, 211, 1–34.

In this paper Riemannian metric is applied to the analysis of selection (for the most part, the additive one) in the polylocus case, corresponding to the loci, located in one chromosome with no multiple crossingovers.

Chapter 5

Sex-Limited and Sex-Linked Characters. Models Taking Account of Sex Distinctions

5.1. Introduction

Up till now we treated models of populations with both sexes being equivalent as regards heredity and selection. It was tacitly assumed that characters are controlled by genes pertaining to both sexes (*autosomal genes*) and equally manifested both in males and in females. However these conditions may not hold. They can be violated in two ways.

(a) It often happens, that some characters (for instance beards that men grow) are manifested exclusively by individuals of one sex, though genes, affecting this character, are contained in both sexes. The hereditary transmission of a character has no connection with the sex, however, the way it is manifested, and, consequently, the selection with respect to this character are essentially linked with the sex of an individual. Such characters are said to be *sex-limited.*

(b) The determination of sex is in most cases controlled by the genotype; some or even all sex-controlling genes being located in special sexual chromosomes (for example, human X and Y chromosomes; men have the XY pair, women have the XX pair). But these chromosomes can also contain other genes, having nothing to do with sex determination. Naturally, the transmission of these genes into the offspring depends on the sex of the parent that carries them. Therefore, these genes are said to be *sex-linked*, and the characters they control are called *sex-linked characters.*

5.2. Model Taking Account of Sex Distinctions

5.2.1. *Autosomal Gene. Continuous Model*

Let us look at a sufficiently large bisexual population under panmixia, with male and female genotypes $\{ij\}$, $i, j=\overline{1, n}$ and inheritance of a character controlled by one autosomal gene with multiple alleles. We shall neglect the population age structure and apply the method of Section 2.15 to derive the model equations.

Let N_{ij} and n_{ij} be the numbers of genotypes ♂$\{ij\}$ and ♀$\{ij\}$, respectively, $N=\sum_{i,j} N_{ij}$, $n=\sum_{i,j} n_{ij}$.

Let us concentrate on the mating process in a bisexual population. Under random mating the couple ♂$\{A_iA_j\}$, ♀$\{A_kA_l\}$ appears with probability $(N_{ij}/N)(n_{kl}/n)$. If the numbers of males and females are equal ($N=n$), then the number of such reproductive couples is $[(N_{ij}n_{kl})/(Nn)]N$ or $[(N_{ij}n_{kl})/(Nn)]n$, which is the same. But if $N \neq n$, then the number of couples is determined either by the number of females, or by the number of males. For most animals, even if females are more numerous, males usually manage to fertilize all females. In this case the number of the reproductive couples is determined by the number of females and is equal to $[(N_{ij}n_{kl})/(Nn)]n$. However there are animals whose males can only once perform fertilization. Then the number of the reproductive couples is limited by the number of males: $[(N_{ij}n_{kl})/(Nn)]N$.

In our model we treat only the first case, when the number of reproductive pairs is determined by the total number of females in the population.

Suppose now that each couple produces F male and f female offspring. (Certainly, when sex is genetically determined, that is if sex is controlled by an appropriate chromosome set, the 1:1 relationship always holds under the normal Mendelian segregation. Speaking about different numbers of male and female offspring we imply that their mortality is different at the earliest stages of embryogenesis.) The genotypes of the mating couples define the genotypes of the offspring (cf. Section 2.6). The probabilities for organisms of this generation to live till the reproductive age and to take part in reproduction, are W_{ij} for males and w_{ij} for females. The non-differential mortality, which can depend on the total population size, we denote by D (for males) and d (for females). Then the equations for genotype numbers can be written in the form

$$\frac{dN_{ij}}{dt} = \frac{FW_{ij}}{N}\sum_s N_{is}\sum_k n_{kj} - DN_{ij}, \tag{2.1}$$

$$\frac{dn_{ij}}{dt} = \frac{fw_{ij}}{N}\sum_s N_{is}\sum_k n_{kj} - dn_{ij}, \quad i, j, k, s = \overline{1, n}.$$

Keeping the old notations, define genotype fitnesses according to the scheme $FW_{ij} \Rightarrow W_{ij}$, $fw_{ij} \Rightarrow w_{ij}$. Rewriting (2.1) in terms of allele frequencies,

$$P_i = \sum_j \frac{N_{ij}}{N}, \quad p_i = \sum_j \frac{n_{ij}}{n},$$

and introducing the new variable $\mu = n/N$, which is the ratio between sexes in the population, we get

$$\left(\frac{1}{\mu}\right)\frac{dP_i}{dt} = P_i[W_i(\mathbf{p}) - W] + \frac{1}{2}[p_i W_i(\mathbf{P}) - P_i W_i(\mathbf{p})],$$

$$\frac{dp_i}{dt} = p_i[w_i(\mathbf{p}) - w] - \frac{1}{2}[p_i w_i(\mathbf{P}) - P_i w_i(\mathbf{p})], \tag{2.2}$$

$$i = \overline{1, n},$$

$$\frac{d\mu}{dt} = \mu[(D-d) + w - \mu W]. \tag{2.3}$$

Here

$$W_i(\mathbf{P}) = \sum_j W_{ij}P_j,\quad W_i(\mathbf{p}) = \sum_j W_{ij}p_j,\quad w_i(\mathbf{P}) = \sum_j w_{ij}P_j,$$
$$w_i(\mathbf{p}) = \sum_j w_{ij}p_j,\quad w = \sum_{i,j} w_{ij}p_iP_j,\quad W = \sum_{i,j} W_{ij}p_iP_j,$$

Accepting the hypothesis of weak selection: $W_{ij}=K+\epsilon\hat{W}_{ij}$, $w_{ij}=k+\epsilon\hat{w}_{ij}$, $|\epsilon|<<1$ and assuming that $D=d$, we yield $\dot{P}_i, \dot{p}_j \sim \epsilon$ and $\dot{\mu}=\mu(k-\mu K)$. Whence it follows that under weak selection the population rapidly equilibrates to the ratio between sexes equal to $\mu^*=k/K$, and further on the population genetic structure slowly evolves, retaining this ratio between sexes. Therefore analyzing (2.2) one can put $\mu=\mu^*$ and study its dynamics independently of (2.3). This conclusion holds even if we reject the weak selection hypothesis, but assume that $p_i \to p_i^*$ and $P_i \to P_i^*$ as $t\to\infty$. Then $\mu\to\mu^*=w^*/W^*$ for any initial values of p_i, P_i, μ and the complete system (2.2), (2.3) can be truncated to (2.2) with $\mu=\mu^*$. It becomes immediately clear that this statement is correct, if we look at the matrix of the equations of the linear approximation for (2.2), (2.3) in the vicinity of a steady state $\{P_i^*, p_i^*, \mu^*\}$, $i=\overline{1,n}$, $\mu^*>0$. This matrix has the form

$$A_{2n+1} = \begin{Vmatrix} \mu^*\dfrac{\partial F_i}{\partial P_j} & \mu^*\dfrac{\partial F_i}{\partial p_j} & 0 \\ \dfrac{\partial f_i}{\partial P_j} & \dfrac{\partial f_i}{\partial p_j} & 0 \\ \dfrac{\partial M}{\partial P_j} & \dfrac{\partial M}{\partial p_j} & -\mu^* W^* \end{Vmatrix},$$

where $\partial F_i/\partial P_j$, $\partial F_i/\partial p_j$, $\partial f_i/\partial P_j$, $\partial f_i/\partial p_j$ are partial derivatives of the right-hand sides in (2.2), calculated at the steady-state point; $\partial M/\partial P_j$, $\partial M/\partial p_j$ are the partial derivatives of the right-hand side in (2.3). Whence one can see, that stability of this steady-state point is defined merely by the eigenvalues λ_i, $i=\overline{1,2n}$ of submatrix A_{2n}, obtained from matrix A_{2n+1} by deleting the last row and column, because the eigenvalue $\lambda_{2n+1}=-\mu^*W^*=-w^*$ is negative and the system is always stable with respect to μ. Therefore, in what follows we shall study only the system for allele frequencies, thinking that the evolution of the sex ratio by no means affects the stability of genetic structures at equilibrium.

Like before, we obtain more vivid results, that can be better interpreted, if we consider the special case of $n=2$, that is the two-allele gene. Let us introduce new notations for allele frequencies and Malthusian parameters: $p_i=p$, $P_1=P$, $w_{11}=\alpha$, $w_{12}=w_{21}=\beta$, $w_{22}=\gamma$, $W_{11}=A$, $W_{12}=W_{21}=B$, $W_{22}=\Gamma$. Then from (2.2) we get the following system of equations:

$$\frac{dP}{dt} = \mu^*[P(W_p-W)+\frac{1}{2}B\delta],$$
$$\frac{dp}{dt} = p(w_p-w)-\frac{1}{2}\beta\delta. \tag{2.4}$$

Here

$$w_p = \alpha P+\beta Q,\ W_p = Ap+Bq,\ Q = 1-P,\ q = 1-p,$$
$$w = \alpha pP+\beta(pQ+qP)+\gamma qQ,$$
$$W = ApP+B(pQ+qP)+\Gamma qQ,$$
$$\delta = p-P,\ \mu^* = \frac{w^*}{W^*}.$$

5.3. New Types of Polymorphism and Their Stability

From (2.4) for $\mu\neq 0$ we immediately obtain the equation for steady states (equilibria):

$$(A-B)P^*p^* + \frac{1}{2}B(p^*+P^*) = P^*W^*,$$
$$(\alpha-\beta)P^*p^* + \frac{1}{2}\beta(p^*+P^*) = p^*w^*. \quad (3.1)$$

Obviously, system (3.1) has solutions of the form

1. $p^* = P^* = 0.$ 2. $p^* = P^* = 1,$

that is the population genic structure for sex-limited characters always has trivial states of equilibrium. On the other hand, (3.1) has no solutions of the form $p^*=0$, $p^*=1$, that is the population has no equilibria such that the male subpopulation consists only of individuals *AA*, while all females are *aa* individuals, and vice versa.

Elaborating on the general case we result in very cumbersome calculations, therefore we somewhat simplify the problem, concentrating on some special (but quite typical) cases.

(a) The effect of selection is different only for heterozygotes, so that $A=\alpha$, $\Gamma=\gamma$, $B\neq\beta>0$. Without losing generality, we can set $A=\alpha=\Gamma=\gamma=1$. Then (3.1) yields

$$2(\beta-1)p^*q^*(1-2P^*) = \beta(p^*-P^*), \quad (3.2)$$
$$2(B-1)P^*Q^*(1-2p^*) = B(P^*-p^*).$$

This system has the following solutions

$$1.\ p^* = P^* = 0.\ 2.\ p^* = P^* = 1.\ 3.\ p^* = P^* = \frac{1}{2}. \quad (3.3)$$

$$4,5.\ p^* = \frac{1}{2}\left[1\mp\frac{\Delta}{1-\beta}\right] P^* = \frac{1}{2}\left[\pm\frac{\Delta}{1-B}\right],$$

where $\Delta=\sqrt{1-B\beta}$.

Steady-state points $p^*_{4,5}$, $P^*_{4,5}$ stand for the new type of polymorphism, resulting from sexual dimorphism of the population. Quite natural constraints for the values B, β spring from the fact that $p^*_{4,5}, P^*_{4,5}\in[0, 1]$. For polymorphism $p^*_4=1/2[1+\Delta/(1-\beta)]<1$, $P^*_4=1/2[1-\Delta/(1-B)]$ to exist, the parameters B, β are to satisfy the inequalities

$$1<\frac{\Delta}{1-\beta}<1,\ -1<\frac{\Delta}{1-B}<1,\ B\beta<1,$$

whence it readily follows that

$$B\beta<1,\ B+\beta>2. \tag{3.4}$$

The same inequalities provide the existence of polymorphism $p_5^*=1/2[1-\Delta/(1-\beta)]$, $P_5^*=1/2[1+\Delta/(1-B)]$. This implies that if equilibria of this type appear in a population, then they spring up in conjugated pairs, symmetrical with respect to the point $\{1/2, 1/2\}$. Let us turn to the stability analysis of these equilibria.

1. Let $p^*=P^*=0$. Then the matrix for the linearized system takes the form

$$\left\|\begin{matrix}\frac{\beta}{2}-1 & \frac{\beta}{2}\\ \frac{\beta}{2} & \frac{\beta}{2}-1\end{matrix}\right\|.$$

It is easily seen that for $B+\beta<2$ the equilibrium $p^*=P^*=0$ is stable (a knot). In this state $\mu^*=1$, that is the ratio between sexes in the population at equilibrium is 1:1.

2. Let $p^*=P^*=1$. This equilibrium will also be a stable knot, if $B+\beta<2$. The ratio between sexes at equilibrium is again 1:1.

3. Let $p^*=P^*=1/2$, that is polymorphism exists in the population, and it is stable if $B\beta>1$ (stable knot). Interestingly, in this case the equilibrium ratio between sexes is not 1:1, but equal to $\mu_3^*=(1+\beta)/(1+B)$.

4,5. Let now $p^*=1/2[1+\Delta/(1-\beta)]$, $P^*=1/2[1-\Delta/(1-B)]$. This state is stable (knot) if $B+\beta>2$, $B\beta<1$. Likewise are the conditions for the point $p^*=1/2[1-\Delta/(1-\beta)]$, $P^*=[1+\Delta/(1-B)]$. Comparing these inequalities with (3.4), we see that if only polymorphism 4.5 exists, then it is always stable, the ratio between sexes being $\mu^*=-(1-\beta)/(1-B)$, which is different from unity.

Figure 16 presents the stability domains in the plane of parameters B and β for various equilibria (autosomal gene, $\alpha=A=\gamma=\Gamma=1$).

In domain I the points $p^*=P^*=0$ and $p^*=P^*=1$ are stable, and the point $p^*=P^*=1/2$ is unstable.

In domain II the polymorphisms presented by $p^*=1/2(1+k)$, $P^*=1/2(1-K)$ and $p^*=1/2(1-k)$, $P^*=1/2(1+K)$, $k=\sqrt{1-B\beta}/(1-\beta)$, $K=\sqrt{1-B\beta}/(1-B)$ are stable. Other points are unstable.

In domain III the polymorphism with $p^*=P^*=1/2$ is unstable, no other polymorphism can exist. 'Pure' states are unstable.

One can see that the specific polymorphism, as presented by points 4 and 5, appears due to the sexual dimorphism of the population, and can exist in a quite narrow range of fitnesses which are to be explicitly different for males and females. In Figure 17a, b, c the phase portraits of (2.4) are demonstrated for $A=\alpha=\Gamma=\gamma=1$ under various relationships between B and β taken from: (a) doman I; (b) domain II (its lower part); (c) domain III (see Figure 16).

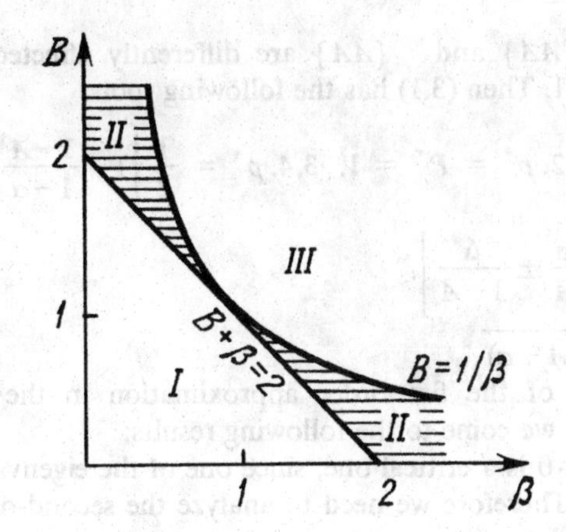

Fig. 16.

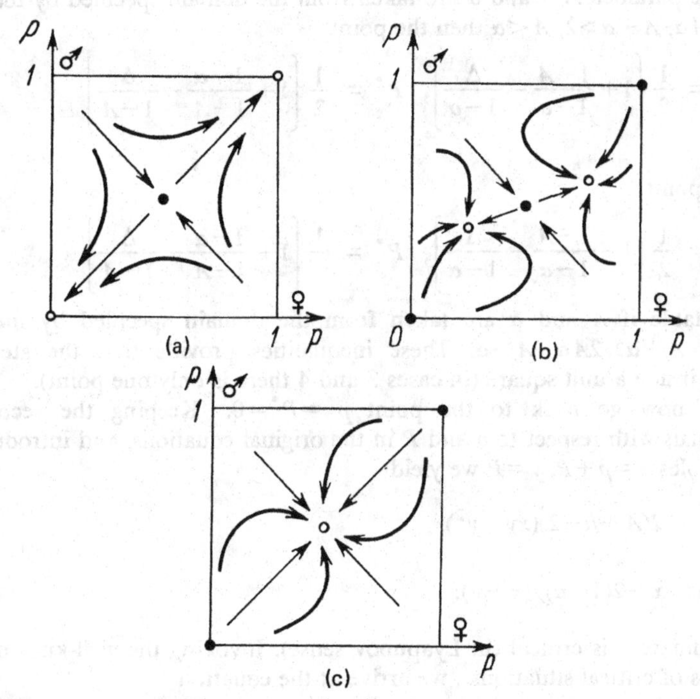

Fig. 17. Phase portrait of system (2.4) for $A=\alpha=\Gamma=\gamma=1$ (○ - stable point, ● - unstable point).

(b) Homozygotes $\{AA\}$ and $\{AA\}$ are differently affected so that $A \neq \alpha$. Suppose $\beta = B = \gamma = \Gamma = 1$. Then (3.1) has the following roots:

$$1.\, p^* = P^* = 0. \quad 2.\, p^* = P^* = 1. \quad 3{,}4.\, p^* = \frac{1}{2}\left[1 + \frac{1-A}{1-\alpha} \mp \frac{\Delta}{1-\alpha}\right],$$

$$P^* = \frac{1}{2}\left[1 + \frac{1-\alpha}{1-A} \pm \frac{\Delta}{1-A}\right].$$

Here $\Delta = \sqrt{(A+\alpha)^2 - 2(A+\alpha)}$.

Studying the system of the first-order approximation in the vicinity of the steady-state points (3.5), we come to the following results:

1. The point $p^* = P^* = 0$ is a critical one, since one of the eigenvalues is zero (the other one is negative). Therefore we need to analyze the second-order approximation, which will be done later on.

2. If $A + \alpha < 2A\alpha$, the point $p^* = P^* = 1$ is stable.

3. If the parameters A and α are taken from the domain specified by inequalities $A + \alpha > 2A\alpha$, $A + \alpha > 2$, $A < \alpha$ then the point

$$p^* = \frac{1}{2}\left[1 + \frac{1-A}{1-\alpha} - \frac{\Delta}{1-\alpha}\right], \quad P^* = \frac{1}{2}\left[1 + \frac{1-\alpha}{1-A} - \frac{\Delta}{1-A}\right]$$

is stable.

4. The point

$$p^* = \frac{1}{2}\left[1 + \frac{1-A}{1-\alpha} + \frac{\Delta}{1-\alpha}\right], \quad P^* = \frac{1}{2}\left[1 + \frac{1-\alpha}{1-A} - \frac{\Delta}{1-A}\right]$$

will be stable if A and α are taken from the domain specified by inequalities $A + \alpha > 2$, $A + \alpha > 2A\alpha$, $A > \alpha$. These inequalities provide that the steady-state points lie inside a unit square (in cases 3 and 4 there is only one point).

Let us now go back to the point $p^* = P^* = 0$. Keeping the second-order infinitesimals with respect to p and P in the original equations, and introducing the new variables $x = p + P$, $y = P$ we yield

$$\frac{dx}{dt} = 2(A + \alpha - 2)(xy - y^2),$$

$$\frac{dy}{dt} = x - 2(1-\alpha)y(x - y). \tag{3.6}$$

The coordinate x is critical (in Lyapunov sense). Invoking the well-known method of analysis of critical situations*, we arrive at the equation

$$\frac{dx}{dt} = \frac{1}{2}(A + \alpha - 2)x^2.$$

* Malkin, I. G.: 1966, *Teoriya ustoichivosti dvizheniya* (*Stability Theory of Motion*), Nauka, Moscow.

We have a typical case of instability in Lyapunov sense.

But since the point $p^*=P^*=0$ belongs to the boundary of admissible values for p and P, it makes sense to concentrate only on those perturbations which deflect the system towards the interior of the square $p, P \in [0, 1]$, that is $x_0 > 0$. Then for $A+\alpha<2$, $\dot{x}<0$, $x_0>0$ the system 'corrects' any sufficiently small positive initial perturbation x_0, tending to the state $p^*=P^*=0$, which is absorbing as if follows from the equations. Thus, if a steady-state point lies on the boundary of the domain admissible for frequencies (usually it is a unit cube of appropriate dimensionality, or a simplex, if we take into account the normalizationm, or even a combination of simplices), then, being unstable in Lyapunov sense, it may present an absorbing state, that is be stable in some other sense. Geometrically it means, that the eigenvector, corresponding to the positive eigenvalue of the linearized operator at the given boundary point, is directed towards the exterior of the admissible domain. Therefore all unstable trajectories take us out of this domain, leaving only stable trajectories inside.

The foregoing reasoning shows that in critical cases, when investigating the stability of boundary points, one cannot apply standard criteria. We have come across a similar problem in Chapter 4, proving the theorem about dominance.

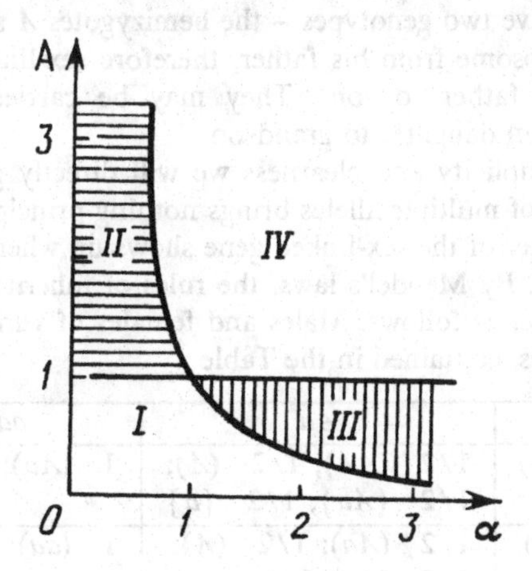

Fig. 18

Figure 18 displays the stability domains in the plane of parameters $\{A, \alpha\}$ for various steady states of (2.4) when $B=\beta=\Gamma=\gamma=1$.

In domain I the point $p^*=P^*=0$ is stable.

In domain II the point $p^*=P^*=1$ is stable and $p^*=P^*=0$ is unstable.

In domain III the point $p^*=1/2(1+(1-A)/(1-\alpha)+k)$, $P^*=1/2(1+(1-\alpha)/(1-A)-K)$, $k=\sqrt{(A+\alpha)^2-2(A+\alpha)\,/(1-\alpha)}$, $K=\sqrt{(A+\alpha)^2-2(A+\alpha)\,/(1-A)}$ is stable, while all other points are unstable.

In domain IV the point $p^* = 1/2(1+(1-A)/(1-\alpha)+k)$, $P^* = 1/2(1+(1-\alpha)/(1-A)-K)$ is stable, all other points are unstable.

If A and α belong to domains III or IV, the population develops the polymorphism, which is totally due to the sexual dimorphism of the population. In Figure 18 one can see that this kind of polymorphism appears only when pressures of selection on males and females are explicitly asymmetric.

We do not display the phase portraits of the system, since in this case they are practically indentical to the previous ones.

5.4. Model Taking Account of Sex Distinctions

5.4.1. *Sex-Linked Gene. Continuous Model*

Sex is determined by a pair of chromosomes, hence, females will have a double set of genes localized in the X-chromosome, while males will have a single one. (Such genes are said to be sex-linked. Typical genes of this type are those that cause hemophilia and daltonism.)

If inheritance in a population is determined by one diallele sex-linked gene, then females will be of three genotypes: AA, Aa and aa, and males, since they carry only one gene, will have two genotypes – the hemizygotes A and a. The son always receives his Y chromosome from his father, therefore sex-linked characters cannot be transmitted from father to son. They may be carried on from father to daughter and then from daughter to grandson.

For the sake of simplicity and clearness we will directly go to the case of two alleles, since the case of multiple alleles brings nothing principally new.

The specific character of the sex-linked gene shows up when we look at the genotypes of the offspring. By Mendel's laws, the rules of inheritance can be presented in the form of a Table, as follows. Males and females of various genotypes can be born with probabilities, contained in the Table

	AA	Aa	aa
A	1 (AA); 1 (A)	1/2 (AA); 1/2 (A); 1/2 $\{Aa\}$; 1/2 $\{a\}$	1 (Aa); 1 (a)
a	1 (Aa); 1 (A)	1/2 (Aa); 1/2 (A); 1/2 (aa); 1/2 (a);	1 (aa); 1 (a)

at the intersections of rows, corresponding to male genotypes and columns, corresponding to female genotypes. These probabilities are conditional, presenting the genotype of the offspring, if we know its sex.

As regards all the rest, the model is formulated exactly as in Section 5.2. Setting $d=D$ and denoting the fitnesses of genotypes $\{AA\}$, $\{Aa\}$, $\{aa\}$, $\{A\}$ and $\{a\}$ by α, β, γ, A and Γ, respectively, we obtain the following equations for allele frequencies P and p, and for the ratio between sexes $\mu = n/N$:

$$\frac{dP}{dt} = \mu(Ap - PW),$$

$$\frac{dp}{dt} = p(w_P - w) - (\frac{\beta}{2})(p - P), \tag{4.1}$$

$$\frac{d\mu}{dt} = \mu(w - \mu W).$$

Here

$$W = Ap + \Gamma q, \ w_P = \alpha P + \beta Q,$$

$$w = \alpha pP + \beta(pQ + qP) + \gamma qQ, \ Q = 1 - P, \ q = 1 - p.$$

Let us treat the behavior of this system under no pressure of selection, that is for $A = \Gamma = \alpha = \beta = \gamma = 1$. Then (4.1) becomes

$$\frac{dP}{dt} = \mu(p - P)$$

$$\frac{dp}{dt} = -\frac{1}{2}(p - P) \tag{4.2}$$

$$\frac{d\mu}{dt} = \mu(1 - \mu).$$

Whence we see that $\mu(t) \to 1$ as $t \to \infty$, and

$$P(t) + 2\mu(t)p(t) = 2\int_{\mu_0}^{\mu(t)} p \, d\mu + P_0 + 2\mu_0 p_0,$$

that is the evolution of the genetic structure in the absence of selection essentially depends on the ratio between sexes in the population. If we select μ_0 equal to 1, then the integral in this expression vanishes and $P(t) + 2p(t) = P_0 + 2p_0 = C$. As $t \to \infty$ we see that $p(t) \to p^*$, $P(t) \to P^*$ with $p^* = P^* = 1/3(P_0 + 2p_0)$.

Just like in Section 5.2 it can be readily shown that if $p(t) \to p^*$ and $P(t) \to P^*$ as $t \to \infty$, then $\mu(t) \to \mu^* = w^* / W^*$. Consequently, to analyze stability of possible equilibria it will suffice to study the first two equations in (4.1) putting $\mu = \mu^*$ in them.

In this system the following states of equilibrium (steady-state points) can exist:

$$1. \ p^* = P^* = 0. \quad 2. \ p^* = P^* = 1. \tag{4.3}$$

$$3. \ p^* = \frac{1}{2}\left[\frac{2\gamma\Gamma - \beta(A + \Gamma)}{\alpha A + \gamma\Gamma - \beta(A + \Gamma)}\right], \quad P^* = \frac{Ap^*}{(A - \Gamma)p^* + \Gamma}.$$

Obviously, while the first two states stand for 'pure' equilibria, the third one is the polymorphism state. Interestingly, if $A = \Gamma$ then $p^* = P^* = (\beta - \gamma)/(2\beta - \alpha - \gamma)$ and we arrive at the polymorphism state, similar to the one obtained for the population which was not subdivided into two sexes (see Section 3.5).

Let us now turn to the stability analysis of the steady-state points (4.3). The matrix of the linearized subsystem (4.1) for p, P has the form

$$\left\|\begin{matrix} -w^* & \dfrac{w^*(AQ^* + \Gamma P^*)}{W^*} \\ \varphi p^* q^* + \dfrac{\beta}{2} & w_P - w^* - p^*[(\alpha - \beta)P^* + (\beta - \gamma)Q^*] - \dfrac{\beta}{2} \end{matrix}\right\|,$$

where $\epsilon=\alpha+\gamma-2\beta$. Whence it readily follows that:

1. Point $p^*=P^*=0$ is stable, if

$$\beta < 4\gamma, \quad \beta(A+\Gamma) < 2\gamma\Gamma, \quad \gamma\Gamma\neq 0. \tag{4.4}$$

It is a simple matter to show that the first inequality in (4.4) results from the second one and, consequently, for the point to be stable it is sufficient that $\beta(A+\Gamma)<2\gamma\Gamma$.

2. Point $p^*=P^*=1$ is stable, if

$$\beta < 4\alpha, \quad \beta(A+\Gamma) < 2\alpha A, \quad \alpha A\neq 0. \tag{4.5}$$

Just like before, the first inequality in (4.5) follows from the second one.

3. Let us give more consideration to the polymorphism case. If fitnesses comply with the inequalities:

$$(a)\ \beta(A+\Gamma) < \{2\alpha A, 2\gamma\Gamma\} \quad \text{or} \quad (b)\ \beta(A+\Gamma) > \{2\alpha A, 2\gamma\Gamma\} \tag{4.6}$$

then always $0<\{p^*, P^*\}<1$ and the third steady-state point is really a polymorphism. Introducing the notations $\hat{\alpha}=\alpha A$, $\hat{\gamma}=\gamma\Gamma$, $\hat{\beta}=\beta/2(A+\Gamma)$ we can present p^* in the form

$$p^* = \frac{(\hat{\beta}-\hat{\gamma})}{(2\hat{\beta}-\hat{\alpha}-\hat{\gamma})},$$

that is, the polymorphic frequency among females can be presented in the same form as in the 'sexless' population.

Polymorphism is stable if

$$\frac{(\hat{\beta}-\hat{\gamma})(\hat{\beta}-\hat{\alpha})}{\hat{\alpha}\hat{\gamma}-\hat{\beta}^2} < 0, \quad \hat{\alpha}\hat{\gamma}+\frac{\beta(\hat{\alpha}A+\hat{\gamma}\Gamma)}{2} < 2\hat{\beta}^2. \tag{4.7}$$

The first inequality immediately implies that if fitnesses comply with (4.6a), then polymorphism is unstable. If inequality (4.6b) holds, then the first of the inequalities in (4.7) always takes place. When $\hat{\beta}>\hat{\alpha}, \hat{\gamma}$, for the second inequality we get the following chain:

$$\hat{\alpha}\hat{\gamma}+\frac{\beta(\hat{\alpha}A+\hat{\gamma}\Gamma)}{2} < \hat{\beta}^2+\frac{\beta(\hat{\beta}A+\hat{\beta}\Gamma)}{2} = 2\hat{\beta}^2,$$

i.e. the condition $\hat{\beta}>\hat{\alpha}, \hat{\gamma}$ ensures that this inequality also holds. Hence, for polymorphism to be stable it is necessary and sufficient that $\hat{\beta}>\hat{\alpha}, \hat{\gamma}$ or

$$\beta(A+\Gamma) > \{2\alpha A, 2\gamma\Gamma\}. \tag{4.8}$$

Let us now compare the existence conditions for polymorphism in a 'sexless' population (see Section 3.5) with those in a population with a sex-linked gene. One can see that they coincide if the values $\hat{\alpha}=\alpha A$, $\hat{\gamma}=\gamma\Gamma$, $\hat{\beta}=\beta(A+\Gamma)/2$ are taken for the Malthusian parameters (fitnesses). Furthermore, the levels of polymorphism coincide as well (in the latter case, the level of polymorphism in the subpopulation of females).

Consider one special case. Let $\beta=\gamma=\Gamma=1$, that is selection differently affects the homozygotes $\{AA\}$ and hemizygotes $\{A\}$. Figure 19 shows the plane $\{A, \alpha\}$ with stability domains for different steady-states. I – stable point $p^*=P^*=0$, II – stable state of polymorphism, III – the state of polymorphism is unstable; depending on the initial conditions the population approaches either the state $p^*=P^*=0$ or the state $p^*=P^*=1$, IV – stable point $p^*=P^*=1$. It can be seen from the Figure that in this case polymorphism is provided only when the pressure of selection has the opposite effect upon the hemizygous male and homozygous female. Moreover, as one can see in Figure 19, the fitness of males should be higher than that of females, that is the selection pressure on males is to be positive ($A>1$), and it should be negative as regards females ($\alpha<1$). And only under these conditions can the population develop a polymorphism.

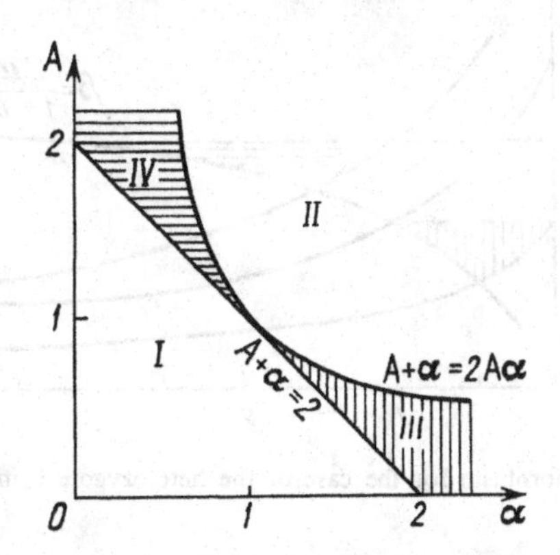

Fig. 19.

If we compare the picture obtained in this example with the pattern of stability domains for the sex-limited gene (see Section 5.3, Figure 18), it leaps to the eye that symmetry is now markedly violated. For a sex-limited gene we can have two states of polymorphism, lying in symmetry with respect to the straight line $A=\alpha$; the stability domains for these states are symmetrical with respect to this line. For the sex-linked gene symmetry is violated, we can have only one state of polymorphism; this state and its domain of stability have no symmetric analogy, as against the case of the sex-limited gene.

Let us note that it is the sexual dimorphism and different selection pressure upon males and females, that develop and fix this distinction. Here we no longer need (as it was in the 'sexless' population) that heterozygotes have advantages for polymorphism to exist: the heterozygote can be worse fit than one of the homozygotes. However, symmetry of selection should be markedly violated among both males and females, the more pronounced the lack of symmetry, the greater the domain of polymorphism existence in the space of parameters. This becomes most obvious from the following example.

Without loss of generality, let us set $\alpha=1$ and accept the following relations to ensure the loss of symmetry: $\mu=A/\Gamma$ and $k=\gamma/\alpha=\gamma$. Evidently, selection is symmetric when $\mu = k = 1$. Then the domain of polymorphism existence is defined by the following inequalities:

$$\beta > \frac{2\mu}{(1+\mu)}, \quad \beta > \frac{2k}{(1+\mu)}.$$

Representing them in Figure 20 on the plane $\{\beta, \mu\}$ for different values of k, we see that when $\mu < 1$ and $k < 1$ there appears a domain of polymorphism existence for $\gamma < \beta < \alpha$, the size of this domain being maximal for m, $k \ll 1$, that is when $A \ll \Gamma$ and $\gamma \ll \alpha$. If $\mu > 1$ and $k > 1$ then polymorphism exists for $\alpha < \beta < \gamma$. Increasing assymetry, we also enhance the domain of polymorphism existence, having no advantages in heterozygotes.

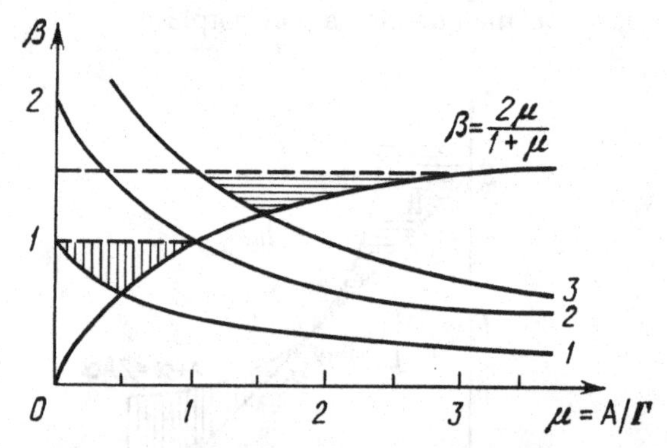

Fig. 20. Domains of polymorphism for the case of the heterozygote being worse fit, than one of the homozygotes.

In Figure 20 the curves 1, 2, 3 stand for the values of $\beta = 2k/(1+\mu)$ with $k = 0.5$; 1.0; 1.5. |||| – marks the domain of polymorphism existence for $\gamma < \beta < \alpha$, $\equiv$ – marks the domain of polymorphism existence for $\alpha < \beta < \gamma$.

5.5. Sex-Linked Gene. Discrete Model

In a 'sexless' population we found no essential difference between the continuous and discrete models when presenting the dynamics of allele frequencies. Will this difference appear when sexuall dimorphism is taken into account?

Invoking the method set forth in Section 2.16 and the hereditary principles of the preceeding section, one can derive the equations of the discrete model for the sex-linked gene as follows:

$$P' = \frac{Ap}{W}, \quad p' = \frac{pw_P}{w} - \frac{\beta(p-P)}{2w}, \quad \mu' = \frac{w}{W},$$

$$W = Ap + \Gamma q, \quad w_P = \alpha P + \beta Q, \tag{5.1}$$

$$w = \alpha pP + \beta(pQ + qP) + \gamma qQ.$$

Here we make use the same notations as in the preceeding section.

From (5.1) we see that while the evolution of the genic structure in the continuous model was essentially dependent on the ratio between sexes μ, in the discrete one the dynamics of μ by no means affects the dynamics of allele frequencies. Therefore we need only the first two equations in (5.1) to study the genetic evolution.

Let us first treat the situation when there is no pressure of selection, that is $\alpha=\beta=\gamma=A=\Gamma=1$. From (5.1) we readily get

$$P' = p,\ p' = \frac{1}{2}(p+P),\ \mu' = 1,$$

that is the 1:1 ratio between sexes is attained already at the next generation. However, unlike the 'sexless' population, where in the discrete model the gene frequency continuously went from one generation into the other, here this variable has a discontinuity, which, say, for the frequency of allele A among females is equal to $[p]=1/2(P-p)$. Thus one new dynamic effect has already showed up. The expressions for allele frequencies in the nth generation have the form

$$P_n = P^* + (-\frac{1}{2})^n (P_0 - P^*),\ p_n = p^* + (-\frac{1}{2})^n (p_0 - P^*),$$

where $p^* = P^* = (P_0 + 2p_0)/3$; P_0 and p_0 are the initial frequencies. Obviously $P_n \to P^*$ and $p_n \to p^*$ as $n \to \infty$. Note that these solutions oscillate and the approach of frequencies to their equilibria is non-monotone.

We now turn to the case with selection. Clearly, the equilibria for (5.1), which satisfy the condition $P'=P$, $p'=p$ coincide with the steady-state points for the system of differential equations (4.1). Let us find the constraints we are to impose on fitnesses in order to make these equilibria stable, that is to ensure that $p_n \to p^*$, $P_n \to P^*$ as $n \to \infty$ (here we denoted $p=p_n$, $p'=p_{n+1}$, $P=P_n$, $P'=P_{n+1}$). P^* and p^* can take on values:

1. $p^* = P^* = 0.$

2. $p^* = P^* = 1.$

3. $p^* = \dfrac{\hat{\beta}-\hat{\gamma}}{2\hat{\beta}-\hat{\alpha}-\hat{\gamma}},\quad P^* = \dfrac{Ap^*}{(A-\Gamma)p^*+\Gamma}.$

It suits us better to replace the first two equations in (5.1) by one equation for p, which will be as follows

$$p_{n+1} = \frac{1}{2}\,\frac{\beta(Ap_{n-1}+\Gamma p_n)+2(\hat{\alpha}-\hat{\beta})p_n p_{n-1}}{\hat{\gamma}+\beta(Ap_{n-1}+\Gamma p_n)-\hat{\gamma}(p_{n-1}+p_n)+(\hat{\alpha}+\hat{\gamma}-2\hat{\beta})p_n p_{n-1}}; \tag{5.2}$$

and to concentrate on this equation. P_{n+1} is related to p_n in a simple manner

$$P_{n+1} = \frac{Ap_n}{((A-\Gamma)p_n+\Gamma)}.$$

Introducing the new variable $x_n = p_n - p^*$, we can represent (5.2) in the form

$$x_{n+1} = (1+b)x_n + ax_{n-1} + R(x_n, x_{n-1}). \tag{5.3}$$

Here

$$a = \frac{\beta A + 2(\hat{\alpha}+\hat{\gamma}-2\hat{\beta}-\beta A)p^* - 2dp^{*2}}{2w^*},$$

$$b = \frac{\beta\Gamma - 2\hat{\gamma} + 2(\hat{\alpha}+3\hat{\gamma}-3\hat{\beta}-\beta\Gamma)p^* - 4dp^{*2}}{2w^*},$$

$$d = \hat{\alpha}+\hat{\gamma}-2\hat{\beta}, \quad w^* = dp^{*2} + 2(\hat{\beta}-\hat{\gamma})p^* + \hat{\gamma}.$$

R is the function of x_n, x_{n-1} raised to powers higher than one, and such that

$$\frac{R(x_n, x_{n-1})}{|x_n| + |x_{n-1}|} \to 0 \text{ as } |x_0| + |x_{n-1}| \to 0.$$

Then the solution $x^* = 0$ is stable (asymptotically), that is $p_n \to p^*$ as $n \to \infty$, if roots of the equation $\lambda^2 - \lambda(1+b) - a = 0$ are less than one in magnitude. This is provided by the following inequalities

$$1.\ a > -1 \quad 2.\ a+b < 0 \quad 3.\ a-b < 2. \tag{5.4}$$

If we write out the stability conditions for steady-state points of the differential equations (4.1), then in terms of these same parameters they will be

$$1.\ b < 1 \quad 2.\ a+b < 0. \tag{5.5}$$

Directly comparing (5.4) with (5.5) we can conclude that the stability domain in the space of these parameters is wider for the continuous model than for the discrete one. However, this is only a seeming effect. Let us compare these inequalities for concrete values of p^*.

1. Let p^* be zero in the discrete model (5.2). The stability conditions immediately follow from (5.4) when concrete values of a and b are substituted:

$$a = \frac{\beta A}{2\hat{\gamma}} > -1, \quad a+b = \frac{\beta A}{2\hat{\gamma}} + \frac{\beta\Gamma}{2\hat{\gamma}} - 1 < 0, \quad \frac{\beta A - \beta\Gamma}{2\hat{\gamma}} < 1. \tag{5.6}$$

The first inequality always holds; the second one implies that $\hat{\beta} < \hat{\gamma}$; the third one always holds, providéd that the second one is satisfied. Consequently, the stability conditions for the 'pure' equilibrium with $p^* = P^* = 0$ are the same in discrete and continuous models. A similar result comes out for the other 'pure' state with $p^* = P^* = 1$.

2. Suppose now that in the discrete model we have the polymorphism state $p^* = (\hat{\beta}-\hat{\gamma})/(2\hat{\beta}-\hat{\alpha}-\hat{\gamma})$. The stability conditions, found from (5.4), have the form

$$a = \frac{\dfrac{\hat{\alpha}\hat{\gamma} - \beta(\hat{\alpha}\Gamma + \hat{\gamma}A)}{2}}{\hat{\alpha}\hat{\gamma} - \hat{\beta}^2} > -1, \quad \frac{(\hat{\beta}-\hat{\gamma})(\hat{\beta}-\hat{\alpha})}{\hat{\alpha}\hat{\gamma}-\hat{\beta}^2} < 0, \tag{5.7}$$

$$\frac{\beta(\hat{\alpha}-\hat{\gamma})(A-\Gamma)}{\hat{\alpha}\hat{\gamma}-\hat{\beta}^2}<2.$$

The necessary polymorphism conditions are $\hat{\beta}<\{\hat{\alpha},\hat{\gamma}\}$ or $\hat{\beta}>\{\hat{\alpha},\hat{\gamma}\}$. Obviously, the second inequality in (5.7) takes place only when $\hat{\beta}>\{\hat{\alpha},\hat{\gamma}\}$. Then it follows from the first inequality that

$$\hat{\beta}^2+\frac{\beta(\hat{\alpha}\Gamma+\hat{\gamma}A)}{2}>2\hat{\alpha}\hat{\gamma}. \tag{5.8}$$

Enhancing this inequality and substituting $\beta=2\hat{\beta}/(A+\Gamma)$, we yield $\hat{\beta}(\hat{\alpha}\Gamma+\hat{\gamma}A)/(A+\Gamma)>\hat{\alpha}\hat{\gamma}$. Since $\hat{\beta}>\hat{\alpha}$ or $\hat{\beta}>\hat{\gamma}$, further enhancing the inequality we get

$$\frac{(\hat{\alpha}\Gamma+\hat{\gamma}A)}{(A+\Gamma)}>\hat{\alpha}\quad\text{or}\quad\frac{(\hat{\alpha}\Gamma+\hat{\gamma}A)}{(A+\Gamma)}>\hat{\gamma}.$$

It readily follows that the first inequality holds if $\hat{\alpha}<\hat{\gamma}$, and the second one holds if $\hat{\alpha}>\hat{\gamma}$ (for $\hat{\alpha}=\hat{\gamma}$ (5.8) always takes place). Hence, if $\hat{\beta}>\{\hat{\alpha},\hat{\gamma}\}$, the first inequality in (5.7) always holds.

The third inequality in (5.7) can be presented in the form

$$\hat{\beta}(\hat{\alpha}-\hat{\gamma})\mu/(\hat{\beta}^2-\hat{\alpha}\hat{\gamma})<1, \mu=(\Gamma-A)/(\Gamma+A), |\mu|<1. \tag{5.9}$$

Setting $\mu=1$ we only intensify (5.9) and obtain $\hat{\alpha}\hat{\beta}-\hat{\beta}\hat{\gamma}<\hat{\beta}^2-\hat{\alpha}\hat{\gamma}$, whence it follows that $-\hat{\gamma}<\hat{\beta}$. Thus we conclude that the third inequality in (5.7) also holds for $\hat{\beta}>\{\hat{\alpha},\hat{\gamma}\}$.

Consequently, the stability conditions of polymorphism in continuous and discrete models are the same. Furthermore, if we introduce new fitnesses $\hat{\alpha}$, $\hat{\beta}$ and $\hat{\gamma}$ in the sex-linked-gene model, then formally both the states of equilibrium and the conditions of their stability are identic in the 'sexless' and sex-linked models.

In the space of parameters the stability conditions for equilibria in the discrete model are such that only one of the following situations can take place at a time: 1. Polymorphism is stable, 'pure' states are unstable. 2. Polymorphism is unstable, 'pure' states are stable. 3. No polymorphism exists, the state with $p^*=P^*=0$ is stable, the state with $p^*=P^*=1$ is unstable. 4. No polymorphism exists, the state with $p^*=P^*=1$ is stable, the state with $p^*=P^*=0$ is unstable. Whence it follows that neither cycles nor 'chaos' can appear in this model. Being intuitively clear, this statement can also find a rigorous proof, based on theorems from the general theory of dynamical systems*.

5.6. Sex-Linked Gene. Multiple Alleles

Concluding this chapter, we shall present the generalization of the diallele continuous model for the case of multiple alleles. The formulation of the model will

* Birkhoff, G. O.: 1927, *Dynamical Systems*, AMS Colloquim Publ., N. Y.

follow exactly the same lines as in the case for two alleles.

Let P_i be the frequency of allele A_i among males, p_i be the frequency of the same allele among females. Denote by w_i and w_{ij} the fitnesses of genotypes $\{i\}$ and $\{ij\}$, respectively. Then the equations for allele frequencies can be written in the form

$$\frac{dP_i}{dt} = \mu\left[W_i p_i - P_i \sum_i W_i p_i\right],$$

$$\frac{dp_i}{dt} = p_i[w_i(\mathbf{P}) - w] - \frac{1}{2}[p_i w_i(\mathbf{P}) - P_i w_i(\mathbf{p})], \quad i=\overline{1,n}. \tag{6.1}$$

Here

$$w_i(\mathbf{p}) = \sum_j w_{ij} p_j, \quad w_i(\mathbf{P}) = \sum_j w_{ij} P_j, \quad w = \sum_{i,j} w_{ij} p_i P_j, \quad i,j=\overline{1,n}.$$

Comparing (6.1) with (2.2) we see, that the equations for female allele frequencies coincide in the models for the sex-linked and sex-limited characters, controlled by the given gene. This is quite natural, since the female genotype-forming mechanism is similar in both cases. In their structure the equations for males stand in marked contrast. However, with no selection the equations for males also coincide. Consequently, the difference between sex-linked and sex-limited characters tells only under the pressure of selection. The equation for the sex ratio $\mu=n/N$ has the form

$$\frac{d\mu}{dt} = \mu[(D-d)+w-\mu W], \quad W = \sum W_i p_i. \tag{6.2}$$

Here D and d are the non-differentiated mortality among males and females, which can be a function of the total population size.

5.7. Minimax Properties of the Mean Fitness Function in a Model of an Sex-Structured Population

Let us give an interesting example, when Fisher's theorem does not hold, but nevertheless the mean fitness function gains peculiar minimax properties. Assume the model of a panmictic population with inheritance of a sex-limited character controlled by one diallele gene (see Section 5.2). Suppose that Malthusian parameters (fitnesses) of genotypes are independent of the organism's sex, that is $A=\alpha$, $B=\beta$, $\Gamma=\gamma$. Then from (2.4) we get

$$\frac{dp}{dt} = p(w_P - w) - \frac{1}{2}\beta\delta,$$

$$\frac{dP}{dt} = \mu^*[P(W_p - w)] + \frac{1}{2}\beta\delta. \tag{7.1}$$

Here

$$w_P = \alpha P + \beta Q, \quad W_p = \alpha p + \beta q,$$

$$w=\alpha pP+\beta(pQ+qP)+\gamma qQ,\quad \delta=p-P.$$

P and p are frequencies of allele A among males and females, respectively.

In contrast to the case, when genotypes of different sexes have different fitnesses, here we have only three steady states

$$p_1^*=P_1^*=0,\ p_2^*=P_2^*=1,$$

$$p_3^*=P_3^*=\frac{(\beta-\gamma)}{(2\beta-\alpha-\gamma)},$$

just like in the model with no consideration given to sex structure. Likewise, the non-trivial state $p_3^*=P_3^*$ is stable when $\beta>\max\{\alpha,\gamma\}$.

It is natural to regard the function $w=\alpha pP+\beta(pQ+qP)+\gamma qQ$ as the mean population fitness. Since genotype fitnesses are independent of sex, the mean fitness of the population coincides with the mean fitness of either the male or of the female population, the fitnesses of these subpopulations being equal, in turn. One can easily show that the point $p_3^*=P_3^*$ is stationary for function w, but if $p_3^*=P_3^*$ is stable, then it will be a saddle-point of function w, regarded as a function of two variables, P and p. This means that unlike the models treated above, where we had to maximize the mean fitness function to find the stable steady states, here this is done by solving a minimax problem. The form of the mean fitness function for $\beta>\max\{\alpha,\gamma\}$ is shown in Figure 21.

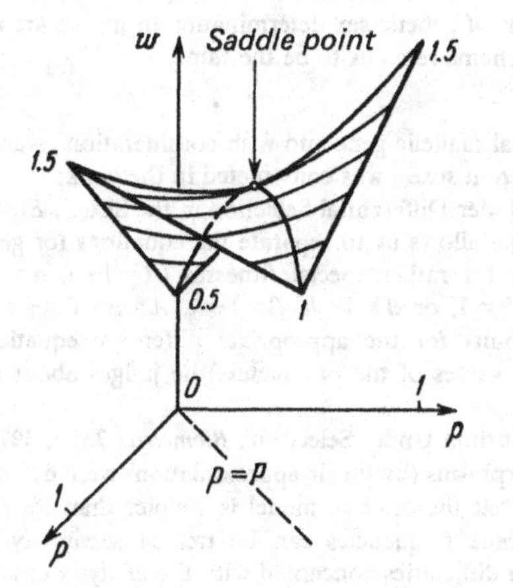

Fig. 21. Function of mean fitness for the model taking account of the population sex structure ($\alpha=1.0$; $\beta=1.5$; $\gamma=0.5$).

An interesting analogy with games theory results from the minimax properties of function w: if subpopulations of males and females are regarded as 'players', and the matrix of coefficients of relative fitness is taken as the pay-off matrix, then frequencies of the optimal strategies in this game are the polymorphic frequencies of alleles A and a, while the value of the game is the mean value of the fitness function at the point of polymorphism. Thus formulated optimal strategies are called minimax or protective. These strategies are optimal only for both 'players' at once and always provide the mean gain (loss) for each 'player', no matter which strategy the opponent employs. Protective strategies are strategies of minimal risk. Thus, a bisexual population with a 1:1 sex ratio is optimal on the average, any random fluctuation in genic content being accompanied by the minimal possible variation in the mean fitness of the population. Since optimal strategies are similar for both subpopulations, we can say that 'players' in this case are not total antagonists, but make up a kind of coalition with no exchange of information.

In conclusion we remark, that the reasoning set forth above is based on a formal analogy. Therefore we should be extremely cautious when giving a concrete interprettaion of a population model in terms of games theory. And generally speaking, any teleological formulation of problems of microevolution is nothing else but a convenient formal instrument; it is hardly possible that real populations in natural conditions are so teleological as we assume they are in our formal models.

5.8. Notes and Bibliography

To 5.1.

Any book in genetics will provide you with quite a lot of examples of sex-limited and sex-linked characters. Generally speaking, here we have assumed a scheme which is rather simple (though generally accepted). Actually, mechanisms of genetic sex determination in nature are more diverse and more complex. However, the principal scheme remains to be the same.

To 5.2.

A discrete model with autosomal diallelic gene and with consideration given to the different pressures of selection on individuals of different sexes, was constructed in the work:

Li, C. C.: 1963, 'Equilibrium Under Differential Selection in the Sexes', *Evolution* **17**, 4, 493–496.

The discreteness of the model allows us to separate the equations for gene frequencies from the one for the sex ratio. Further on, for rather special fitnesses ($A=1-t$, $\alpha=1-s$, $B=\beta=1$, $\Gamma=\gamma=0$, or $A=1-t$, $\gamma=1-s$, $B=\beta=\alpha=\Gamma=1$, or $B=1+h$, $\beta=1-k$, $A=\alpha=\Gamma=\gamma=1$, $k, h>0$) the author finds the non-trivial steady-state points for the appropriate difference equations and by phase portraits (drawn for concrete numerical values of the parameters) he judges about their stability. In the subsequent paper:

Li, C. C.: 1967, 'Genetic Equilibrium Under Selection', *Biometrics* **23**, 3, 397–484,

stability conditions for polymorphisms (by linear approximation) were derived in some special cases.

At first sight it may seem that the discrete model is simpler than the continuous one, since in the former model equations for gene frequencies can be treated separately. However, we pay for this simplification by the additional difficulties concerned with the analysis of solutions to difference instead of differential equations. Note that both cycles and 'chaos' can exist in the discrete model.

To 5.3.

Here we have first come across the situations when a steady-state point lying on the boundary can be unstable by the standard criterion, being stable as an absorbing state. This effect results from the restrictions imposed on the allowed variations, and this is always the case when equilibria lie on the boundary of the admissible domain – the unit simplex.

To 5.4.

The first work that assumed a discrete model for diallelic sex- linked gene (assuming weak selection), was one of the classical papers by J. B. S. Haldane in the *Proceedings of Cambridge Philosophical Society* (1926, **23**, 363–372).

Among more recent works, presenting sufficient stability conditions of polymorphic states for a sex-linked gene, the following ones are worth mentioning:

Bennett, J. H.: 1958, 'The Existence and Stability of Selectively Balanced Polymorphism at Sex-Linked Locus', *Austr. J. Biol. Sci.* **11**, 7, 598–602;

Mandel, S. P. H.: 1959, 'Stable Equilibrium at a Sex-Linked Locus', *Nature* **183**, 467, 1347–1348.

The latter work is more rigorous from the mathematical viewpoint.

An interesting paper by

Haldane, J. B. S. and Jayaker, S. D.: 1964, 'Equilibria Under Natural Selection at a Sex-Linked Locus', *J. Genet.* **59**, 1, 29–36.

though being based on less general assumptions (skew-symmetry of the pressure of selection upon homozygotes), gives very meaningful biological interpretations of the results obtained. An intensive analysis of many special cases for the discrete model is contained in the above mentioned paper by Li.

In the work by

Bennett, J. H., Oertel, C. R.: 1964, 'The Approach to a Random Asociation of Genotypes with Random Mating', *J. Theoret. Biol.* **9**, 2, 67-76,

the autosomal inheritance is compared with the sex-linked one for populations with no pressure of selection.

To 5.5.

The paper

Svirezhev, Yu. M., Timofeeff-Ressovsky, N. V.: 1967, 'O dostatocnyh uslovijah sushestvovanija polimorfizma dlja mutacii sceplennoi s polom (On Sufficient Existence Conditions of Polymorphism for a Sex-Linked Mutation. In Russian), in: *Problems of Cybernetics*, Nauka, Moscow, Vol. 18, 171–174,

proposes a new type of model for a sex-linked gene, which stands in between the continuous and discrete models. Formally, the problem is reduced to the fact that when in Equation (5.2), which has the form $p_{n+1}=f(p_n, p_{n-1})$, we want to change over to the continuous formulation, we are to assume the alteration of gene frequency over two generations to be infinitesimal, which is too restricting. If we require that this alteration be infinitesimal over one generation, then the correct approximation will be

$$\frac{dp(t)}{dt} \simeq p_{n+1}-p_n, \quad p(t)=p_n, \quad p(t-1)=p_{n-1},$$

(here time is measured in generations). Thus we directly arrive at a model characterized by a differential-difference equation, which produces new dynamic effects (as against the purely continuous model formulated in terms of differential equations).

Theoretically it was shown that for certain relations between fitnesses of genotypes a population can attain polymorphism with respect to the sex-linked gene. But the question still remains: "Can relations of this kind occur in real-life populations?". The work:

Svirezhev, Yu. M., Timofeeff-Ressovsky, N. V.: 1967, 'O protivopolo□nyh davlenijah otbora na genotip i na priznak u mutacii sceplennoi s polom (On the Opposite Pressures of Selection on the Genotype and the Sex-Linked Mutation Character. In Russian)', in: *Problems of Cybernetics*, Nauka, Moscow, Vol. 18, pp. 155–170,

gives the positive answer to this question. In a series of experiments on the sex-linked mutation *eversae* of *Drosophila funebris* it was shown that at moderate temperatures (23°*C*) and in moderately congested model popultions (in which approximately half of the larvae die off) this mutation manifests a noticeable increase (about 8%) in its relative viability; viability in underpopulated cultures and under low tempertures is equal to that of the normal form; at high temperatures and under extreme overpopulation it noticeably falls. Polymorphism can exist only in underpopulated cultures at 23°*C*; in this case heterozygotes and hemizygotes of eversae have maximal viability, with $\hat{\alpha}=0.09$, $\hat{\beta}=0.996$, and $\hat{\gamma}=0.986, \hat{\beta}>\hat{\alpha}, \hat{\gamma}$, that is the necessary and sufficient conditions of polymorphism are satisfied. The polymorphic level is $P^*=0.383$; $p^*=0.384$, that is it turns out to be practically equal for males and females.

Chapter 6

Populations with Deviations from Panmixia

6.1. Introduction

Up till now we have examined populations, which mating system was panmixia. Though panmixia is wide-spread in natural populations, just as often various deviations from panmixia occur. For instance, they may be caused by different kinds of preference in mating, when individuals are more likely to form mating pairs by the principle of the greater kinship. It is well known the among birds that particular marriage ritual plays a great role in pair formation, and these behavior reactions are inherited controlled only by the genotype. In a word, everything the suits the saying 'Gentlemen prefer blondes' results in deviations from panmixia.

Another wide-spread type of deviations from panmixia is caused by all sorts of isolating barriers – geographical, physiological, ethnographical and other ones. The opinion of most biologist – evolutionists is that it is the isolation by distance which serves as one of the most important trigger mechanisms in the process of new species formation.

And lastly, we have the artificially evoked deviation from panmixia – inbreeding or incest crossing, which is one of the basic methods of breeding new varieties and stocks.

6.2. Preference in Crossing and Preference Matrix

In Section 2.5 when discussing the notion of 'panmixia', we have introduced the so-called 'preference functions', which characterized the deviation of the mating system from panmixia, when counting the reproductive pairs. Naturally, the preference coefficients we are to introduce now, are the special case of preference functions when age and sexual structure of the population is neglected.

Suppose we are given a population of N individuals; with the 1:1 sex ratio being fixed in the process of the evolution of its genic content. The numbers of genotypes $\{ij\}$ in the population are N_{ij}, so that $\sum_{i,j} N_{ij} = N$, $i, j = \overline{1, n}$. If panmixia or random mating takes place in the population, then a pair $\{ik\}$, $\{lj\}$ is formed with probability $N_{ik}N_{lj}/N^2$ and the number of pairs of this type is $m_{ik}^{lj} = N_{ik}N_{lj}/(2N)$. Let now panmixia be disturbed, and suppose the number of $\{ik\}$, $\{lj\}$ pairs, which is $\hat{m}_{ik}^{lj}$, can be represented as $\hat{m}_{ik}^{lj} = \theta_{ik}^{lj} m_{ik}^{lj}$. The $n^2 \times n^2$-matrix $\| \theta_{ik}^{lj} \|$, $i, k, l, j = \overline{1, n}$ will be called the *preference matrix*, and its elements are the *preference coefficients*. Naturally, if $\theta_{ik}^{lj} = 1$, we have panmixia, when $\theta_{ik}^{lj} < 1$ organisms $\{ik\}$ and $\{lj\}$ avoid crossing, and when $\theta_{ik}^{lj} > 1$ they prefer to mate. Since genotypes $\{ij\}$ and $\{ji\}$ are indistinguishable, we have

$$\theta_{ik}^{lj} = \theta_{ki}^{lj} = \theta_{ki}^{jl} = \theta_{ik}^{jl}, \quad i, k, l, j = \overline{1, n}. \tag{2.1}$$

In the general case preferences are asymmetric and $\theta_{ik}^{lj} \neq \theta_{lj}^{ik}$, that is the attraction of organism $\{ik\}$ to $\{lj\}$ can be stronger than that of organism $\{lj\}$ to $\{ik\}$. However for ease of presentation we assume that preferences are symmetric, that is $\theta_{ik}^{lj} = \theta_{lj}^{ik}$.

If we assume that all males and females in the population make up pairs and that there are no organisms out of reproductive relations, then the total number of pairs is $N/2$, that is

$$\sum_{i,k,l,j} \theta_{ik}^{lj} N_{ik} N_{lj} = N^2. \tag{2.2}$$

Introducing the notation $h_{ik}^{lj} = \theta_{ik}^{lj} - 1$, one can rewrite (2.2) in the form

$$(\mathbf{N}, \mathbf{HN}) = 0, \quad \mathbf{N} = \{N_{ij}; i, j = \overline{1, n}\}, \quad \mathbf{H} = \| h_{ik}^{lj} \|. \tag{2.3}$$

For $\mathbf{N} \neq 0$ this condition holds if $\mathbf{HN} = 0$ or if $\mathbf{N}$ and $\mathbf{HN}$ are orthogonal. The equality $\mathbf{HN} = 0$ can be interpreted as the existence of bilateral monogamy in the population, when each male pairs with only one female and vice versa. In terms of coordinates this condition has the form

$$\sum_{l,j} h_{ik}^{lj} N_{ij} = 0, \quad i, k, l, j = \overline{1, n}. \tag{2.4}$$

In order that (2.4) take place at non-zero numbers, it is necessary that the condition $\det \mathbf{H} = 0$ be satisfied, i.e. under bilateral monogamy the preference coefficients cannot be arbitrary: they are to comply with the condition $\det \mathbf{H} = 0$. Whence it also follows, that numbers cannot be arbitrary as well – at least one of then will always be a linear function of all the rest (with coefficients dependent on θ_{il}^{lj} or h_{ik}^{lj}).

When $\mathbf{N}$ and $\mathbf{HN}$ are orthogonal, we need not require that $\det \mathbf{H} = 0$, however eigenvalues of matrix $\mathbf{H}$ are to have different signs, that is again the preference coefficients cannot be arbitrary. The same with numbers: at least one of them is to be expressed in terms of all the others in keeping with the equation $(\mathbf{N}, \mathbf{HN}) = 0$ (which is non- linear).

For coefficients θ_{ik}^{lj} there is a natural estimate from below: $\theta_{ik}^{lj} \geqslant 0$ $(h_{ik}^{lj} \geqslant -1)$. The estimate from above for these variables will be given later on.

6.3. Model of Population with Deviations from Panmixia Caused by Preference in Crossing

Assume the population with inheritance of a character controlled by one gene with multiple alleles. We shall construct a continuous model, neglecting the sexual and age structure of the population (see Section 2.13).

Let N_{ij} be the number of genotype $\{ij\}$; $N = \sum_{i,j} N_{ij}$, $i, j = \overline{1, n}$ is the total population number. Deviations from panmixia will be characterized by the matrix of preference coefficients $\| \theta^{lj}_{ik} \|$, $i, j, k, l = \overline{1, n}$. Then the number of $\{ik\}$, $\{lj\}$ pairs will be $\hat{\pi}^{lj}_{ik} = \theta^{lj}_{ik} N_{ik} N_{lj} / (2N)$. Suppose that each such pair produces $2F$ offsprings, among which organisms with genotype $\{ij\}$ live till the reproductive age and engage in crossing with probability w_{ij}. The non-differential mortality D can depend on the total population size N. Then the equation for genotype numbers can be written in the form

$$\frac{dN_{ij}}{dt} = \frac{Fw_{ij}}{N} \sum_{k,l} \theta^{lj}_{ik} N_{ik} N_{lj} - DN_{ij}, \quad i, j, k, l = \overline{1, n}. \tag{3.1}$$

If we denote $Fw_{ij} \theta^{lj}_{ik} = \phi^{lj}_{ik}$ then (3.1) will coincide (for $n = 2$) with the Kostitzin-type model (see Section 3.8), presenting a panmictic population, but with fecundity of each $\{ik\}$, $\{lj\}$ pair being $2\phi^{lj}_{ik}$, that is being dependent on genotypes that make up the pair. Consequently, the population with panmixia disturbed by preference in crossing, can be formally regarded as a panmictic population, but with fecundity coefficients depending on genotypes of both individuals tied up in a reproductive pair.

Define the genotype fitnesses as Fw_{ij}, keeping the original notations w_{ij}. Passing two genotype frequencies $u_{ij} = N_{ij} / N$ from (3.1) we get

$$\frac{du_{ij}}{dt} = w_{ij} \sum_{k,l} \theta^{lj}_{ik} u_{ik} u_{lj} - u_{ij} w,$$

$$w = \sum_{i,j,k,l} w_{ij} \theta^{lj}_{ik} u_{ik} u_{lj}, \quad i, j, k, l = \overline{1, n}, \tag{3.2}$$

and the equation for the total population size will be:

$$dN / dt = N(w - D).$$

Just like before, for clearness of presentation, let us look at the diallele case. Suppose $i = j = 1$. Then

$$\sum_{k,l} \theta^{l1}_{1k} u_{1k} u_{l1} = \theta^{21}_{11} u_{11} u_{21} + \theta^{11}_{12} u_{12} u_{11} + \theta^{12}_{12}, u^2_{12} \tag{3.4}$$

$$k, l = 1, 2.$$

Besides, we assume that bilateral monogamy takes place, that is (2.4) holds, or in terms of frequencies:

$$\sum_{l,j} h^{lj}_{ik} u_{lj} = 0 \text{ or } \sum_{l,j} \theta^{lj}_{ik} u_{lj} = 1, \quad i, k, l, j = 1, 2.$$

Adding and subtracting the term $\theta^{22}_{11} u_{11} u_{22}$ in (3.4), and taking into account that $\sum_{l,j} \theta^{lj}_{1k} u_{lj} = 1$, we can rewrite (3.4) as follows:

$$\sum_{k,l} \theta^{l1}_{1k} u_{1k} u_{l1} = u_{11} - (\theta^{22}_{11} u_{11} u_{22} - \theta^{12}_{12} u^2_{12}), \; k, l, = 1, 2. \tag{3.5}$$

Here we took advantage of symmetry ($u_{ij} = u_{ji}$ and, by the first assumption, $\theta^{12}_{11} = \theta^{11}_{12}$), as well as of the properties of θ^{lj}_{ik} (see (2.1)).

Manipulating in a similar manner with the sums $\sum_{k,l}\theta_{ik}^{lj}u_{ik}u_{lj}$

$$\sum_{k,l}\theta_{1k}^{l2}u_{1k}u_{l2} = u_{12}+(\theta_{11}^{22}u_{11}u_{22}-\theta_{12}^{12}u_{12}^2),$$

$$\sum_{k,l}\theta_{2k}^{l2}u_{2k}u_{l2} = u_{22}-(\theta_{11}^{22}u_{11}-\theta_{12}^{12}u_{12}^2). \tag{3.6}$$

Making use of (3.5) and (3.6), we can represent (3.1) in the form

$$\begin{aligned} du_{ij}/dt &= u_{ij}(w_{ij}-w)-(-1)^{i+j}w_{ij}R, \\ R &= \theta_{11}^{22}u_{11}u_{22}-\theta_{12}^{12}u_{12}^2, \\ w &= \sum_{i,j}w_{ij}u_{ij}-(w_{11}+w_{22}-2w_{12})R, \quad i,j = 1,2. \end{aligned} \tag{3.7}$$

Obviously, the trajectory (3.7) never leaves the simplex $\sum_{i,j}u_{ij}=1$, however nothing indicates that it will never leave the manifold $\sum_{l,j}h_{ik}^{lj}u_{lj}=0$, $i, k, l, j=1, 2$, which specifies the bilateral monogamy. Multiplying (3.7) on both sides by h_{ij}^{kl} and summing up over $i, j=1, 2$, we get

$$\sum_{i,j}h_{ij}^{kl}\frac{d}{dt}u_{ij} = \sum_{l,j}w_{ij}h_{ij}^{kl}u_{ij}-R\sum_{i,j}(-1)^{i+j}w_{ij}h_{ij}^{kl} = 0, \quad i,j,k,l = 1,2. \tag{3.8}$$

Thus, for bilateral monogamy to hold under combined action of selection and preference in crossing, it is necessary that the condition (3.8) be satisfied, imposing additional restrictions on genotype frequencies u_{ij}. Apparently, these equations cannot hold for all h_{ij}^{kl}, so besides the condition $\det \mathbf{H}=0$ other conditions will appear, limiting the choice of the preference coefficients.

The complete analysis of (3.8) is rather cumbersome and complicated; therefore we make the simplifying assumptions about weak selection and weak deviations from panmixia, that is we think that $w_{ij}=1+\hat{w}_{ij}$, $|\hat{w}_{ij}|\ll 1$, $|h_{ij}^{kl}|\ll 1$. Then for (3.8) to hold to within $o(\epsilon)$ ($\hat{w}_{ij}, h_{ij}^{kl}\sim\epsilon$) it is necessary and sufficient that

a) $\quad u_{11}u_{22} = u_{12}^2$ or

b) $$\sum_{i,j}(-1)^{i+j}h_{ij}^{kl} = 0, \quad i,j,k,l = 1,2. \tag{3.9}$$

Under weak selection and weak deviations from panmixia to an accuracy of $o(\epsilon)$ we can replace (3.7) by

$$\begin{aligned} du_{ij}/dt &= u_{ij}(w_{ij}-w)+(-1)^{i+j}(\pi-w_{ij}\xi), \\ w &= \sum_{i,j}w_{ij}u_{ij}-(w_{11}+w_{22}-2w_{12})\xi, \quad i,j = 1,2. \end{aligned} \tag{3.10}$$

Here $\pi=-(h_{11}^{12}u_{11}u_{12}-h_{12}^{12}u_{12}^2)$, $\xi=u_{11}u_{22}-u_{12}^2$.

It is only natural to call π the index of deviations from panmixia, since under panmixia $\pi\equiv 0$; the quantity ξ is nothing else but the deviation from Hardian equilibrium. Note that the deviation from panmixia itself is characterized only by two parameters $h_{11}^{22}=h$ and $h_{12}^{12}=H$, which meaning is fairly clear: when $h>0$

homozygotes prefer to mate with other homozygotes, and when $H>0$, heterozygotes prefer heterozygotes. For $h<0$ and $H>0$ organisms prefer to mate with those alike.

Let us now return to conditions (3.9). If we demand that (3.9a) be satisfied that is the Hardy–Weinberg principle holds, then no other additional conditions, but the constraint $\det \| h_{ij}^{kl} \| = 0$, are imposed on the preference coefficients, and consequently, we have five free parameters to specify preference, among which only two affect the genetic evolution of the population. If we require that (3.9b) holds, then the population need not be Hardian, however there remains only two free parameters to specify preference (six preference coefficients are restricted by three conditions (3.9b) and by the constraint imposed on the determinant of the preference matrix). These two parameters can be considered to be h and H.

Turning to allele frequencies $p = u_{11} + u_{12}$ and $q = u_{21} + u_{22}, p + q = 1$, from (3.10) we get ($u_{11} = p^2 + \xi, u_{12} = u_{21} = pq - \xi, u_{22} = q^2 + \xi$)

$$dp/dt = p(w_p - w_0), \quad w_p = \alpha p + \beta q, \qquad (3.11)$$
$$w_0 = \alpha p^2 + 2\beta pq + \gamma q^2,$$

where $\alpha = w_{11}, \beta = w_{12} = w_{21}, \gamma = w_{22}$. Equation (3.11) totally coincides with the equation for allele frequency in the panmictic population. Consequently, if there is a bilateral monogamy in the population, while selection and deviations from panmixia are weak, then preference in mating by no means affects the evolution of the population genic content. However, if $\xi \neq 0$, the population will no longer be Hardian and the evolution of its genotypical frequencies will differ from their evolution in a panmictic population. This difference can be naturally described by ξ, which is deviation from Hardy equilibrium. Taking into account that $u_{11} = p^2 + \xi, u_{12} = u_{21} = pq - \xi, u_{22} = q^2 + \xi$,

$$d\xi/dt = p^2q^2(a-b) - d\xi - b\xi^2, \qquad (3.12)$$

where

$$a = \alpha + \gamma - 2\beta, \quad b = h - H,$$
$$d = (\alpha + h)p^2 + 2(\beta + H)pq + (\gamma + h)q^2.$$

Obviously, under panmixia $\dot{\xi} = ap^2q^2 - w_0\xi$ and if $p(t) \to p^*$ as $t \to \infty$ then $\xi(t)$ goes to zero.

6.4. Evolution and Stability of Deviations from Hardian Equilibrium. Inbreeding

Let us elaborate on the behavior of solutions to (3.12). But first let us find the domain of definition for variable ξ. Since $u_{11}, 2u_{12}$ and u_{22} are to be positive and bounded above by unity (with $u_{12} = u_{12} = 0$ for $u_{11} = 1$, etc.), it immediately follows from the definition of ξ that

$$1.\ \xi \geq -p^2. \quad 2.\ \xi \leq pq. \quad 3.\ \xi \geq -q^2. \qquad (4.1)$$

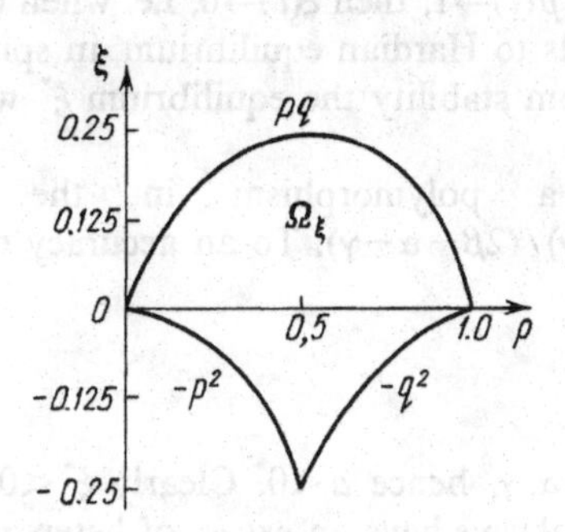

Fig. 22. Domain of definition for the ξ-deviation from Hardian equilibrium.

These inequalities define the domain Ω_ξ, presented in a Figure 22. For any $p \in [0, 1]$ the value of deviation from Hardian equilibrium can never leave the boundaries of this domain ($\xi \in [-0{\cdot}25, +0{\cdot}25]$ for $p=0{\cdot}5$, say).

If in (3.12) the variable p is regarded as a parameter, then this equation will have two states of equilibrium:

$$\xi^*_{1,2} = \frac{1}{2b}[-d \mp \sqrt{d^2+4b(a-b)p^2q^2}\,], \tag{4.2}$$

one of which (the one with the minus) lies beyond the limits of the admissible domain Ω_ξ, being always unstable; the other one (with the plus) lies inside of Ω_ξ, being always stable. In order to prove this statement suffice it to check that $\dot{\xi}>0$ on the lower bound and that $\dot{\xi}<0$ on the upper bound. Substitute the boundary values of ξ into (3.12) to yield

$$\begin{aligned} &1. \quad \xi = -p^2 \Rightarrow \dot{\xi} = p^2(d-b+aq^2). \\ &2. \quad \xi = -q^2 \Rightarrow \dot{\xi} = q^2(d-b+ap^2). \\ &3. \quad \xi = pq \Rightarrow \dot{\xi} = pq[(a-2b)pq-d]. \end{aligned} \tag{4.3}$$

One can show that if $h, H \in [-1, +1]$, then $\dot{\xi}_1>0$ for $0<p<1/2, \dot{\xi}_2>0$ for $1/2<p<1$ and $\dot{\xi}_3<0$ for any $p, q \in (0, 1)$, that is our statement proves to be true. And since $\xi(t)$ can never leave the limits of the admissible domain, this results in the following natural constraints for h and H from above: $h, H \leqslant 1$.

Under weak selection and deviations from panmixia the following estimations hold: $d \sim 1$, $a, b \sim \epsilon$. Furthermore, $\dot{p} \sim \epsilon, \dot{\xi} = -w_o\xi + o(1)$. Whence it follows that allele frequency evolves slowly, while the deviation from panmixia is a fast variable. Over the specific time period there are practically no variations in $p(t)$ and $\xi(t) \to 0$, where $\xi(t) \sim \exp\{-w_o t\}$. However, in the vicinity of the point $\xi=0$, in (3.12) the terms $0(\epsilon)$ come into play, and the system slowly evolves towards the state $\{p^*, \xi^*(p^*)\}$, where $\xi^* \sim \epsilon$. If the state $\xi^*(p)$ is stable for all p and if $p(t) \to p^*$ as $t \to \infty$ then $\xi(t) \to \xi^*(p^*)$.

Obviously, if $p(t)\to 0$ or $p(t)\to 1$, then $\xi(t)\to 0$, i.e. when one of the alleles is eliminated the population tends to Hardian equilibrium, in spite of the deviations from panmixia. This follows from stability the equilibrium ξ^* which is zero for $p=0$ or $p=1$.

Suppose there is a polymorphism in the population, that is $p(t)\to p^*\in(0, 1), p^*=(\beta-\gamma)/(2\beta-\alpha-\gamma)$. To an accuracy of $o(\epsilon)$ the expression for $\xi^*(p)$ will have the form

$$\xi^*(p) \simeq \frac{a-b}{w_0}p^2q^2. \tag{4.4}$$

Under polymorphism $\beta>\alpha, \gamma$, hence $a<0$. Clearly $\xi^*<0$ for $b>0$, that is when $h>H$ the population will always have an excess of heterozygotes (comparing to the Hardian ratio). More accurately, $\xi^*<0$ for $a<b$ and $\xi^*>0$ for $a>b$. Consequently, if $2\beta-(\alpha+\gamma)+(h-H)>0$, that is if heterozygotes have evident advantages in selection and if genotypically different forms prefer to mate, then the population evolves towards a state with an excess of heterozygotes. If $2\beta-(\alpha+\gamma)+(h-H)<0$, that is if advantages of heterozygotes in selections are not so pronounced and genotypically similar individuals prefer to mate, then homozygotes are in excess.

Let us look at the situation when organisms prefer to mate with those alike (incest crossing or inbreeding) and suppose that the extent of this preference is the same for all the three genotypical groups. Then $H=-h=F\geqslant 0$ and $F\leqslant 1$. Suppose also that $\alpha=\gamma=1$, that is the pressure of selections is symmetrical. Then from (4.2) we get (for $p=p^*=1/2$)

$$\xi^* = \frac{1}{4F}(1+\frac{s}{2}-\sqrt{(1+s/2)^2-F(F-s)}), \quad s = 1-\beta, \tag{4.5}$$

whence it is seen that if $F>s$, homozygotes prevail in the population, in spite of the advantages in selection of heterozygotes. In case $F<s$, the advantageous selection of heterozygotes results in increases of their fraction in the population (as against the Hardian equilibrium).

Increased pressure of selection (under fixed inbreeding coefficients F) always raises the fraction of heterozygotes. If we step up the inbreeding coefficients F, the result will not be unambigous. However for small s and F

$$\xi^* \simeq \frac{1}{32}(4F-4s-s^2/F)$$

and $\partial\xi^*/\partial F>0$, that is the increased extent of inbreeding promotes the prevalence of homozygotes in the populations.

Summing up all the aforesaid, we can conclude, that inbreeding results in an excess of homozygotes only under sufficiently weak selection and under a sufficiently strong trend towards incest crossing.

In conclusion, let us look at the situation when there is no selection. If $\alpha=\beta=\gamma$ then $p=\text{const}$, and the stable deviation from panmixia is

$$\xi_0^* = \frac{1}{4F}(d_0-\sqrt{d_0-16F^2p^2q^2}), \quad d_0=1-F(p-q)^2, \tag{4.6}$$

for all $F>0, \xi_0^*>0$, that is without selection inbreeding always raises the fraction of homozygotes in the population. The extent of their prevalence ξ_0^* is essentially dependent on p.

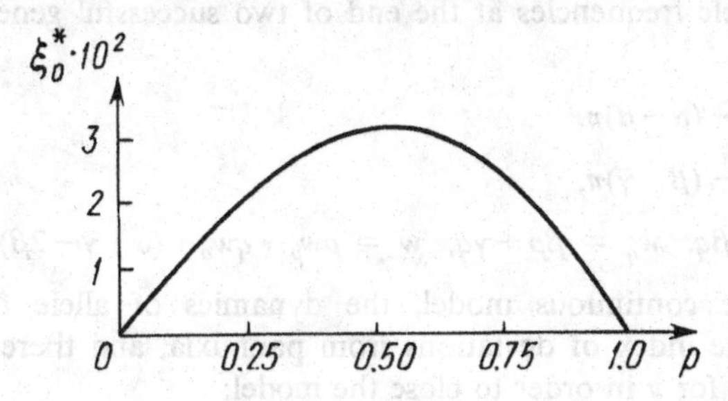

Fig. 23. Extent of prevalence of homozygotes at equilibrium $\xi_0=u_{11}u_{22}-u_{12}^2$ in the absence of selection as a function of the frequency of allele A.

In Figure 23 we graph the function (4.6); whence one can see, that the prevalence of homozygotes is maximal at $p=q=1/2$. Note that speaking about the prevalence of homozygotes, we imply that presence of both homozygotes in the population, that is $p\neq 0, 1$. Evidently, the pure population, that is the population made only of alleles A or a, is always homozygous.

6.5. Preference in Crossing. Discrete Model

In the previous sections quite essential was the assumption about weak selection and weak deviations from panmixia. Rejecting this assumption we faced rather complicated and cumbersome relationships. It turns out that in the discrete model these relationships are simpler and clearer than in the continuous one, and we can do without the hypotheses about weakness. The discrete model is constructed according to the same principles as before (see Section 2.14).

Again we consider the diallele gene and assume bilateral monogamy. Carrying on from one generation to another we get

$$\begin{aligned}(u_{11})_n^+ &= (p^2+\pi)_{n-1}^-, \quad p = u_{11}+u_{12},\\ (u_{12})_n^+ &= (pq-\pi)_{n-1}^-, \quad q = u_{21}+u_{22},\\ (u_{22})_n^+ &= (q^2+\pi)_{n-1}^-, \quad p+q = 1,\end{aligned} \tag{5.1}$$

where $\pi=-(hu_{11}u_{22}-Hu_{12}^2)$ is the index of deviations from panmixia. In our case (just like π in Section 6.3) π also characterizes the extent of the deviation from Hardian equilibrium, but while $\xi=u_{11}u_{22}-u_{12}^2$ was independent of preference coefficients, in π this dependence is obvious. The domain of definition for π coincide with Ω_ξ (see Figure 22). The deviation from panmixia is specified by two free parameters $h=\theta_{11}^{22}-1$ and $H=\theta_{12}^{12}-1$, and the conditions of bilateral monogamy $\sum_{i,j}h_{ij}^{kl}u_{ij}^-=0$ at the end of the generation have been applied to derive (5.1). We can make sure that they hold, if we choose the remaining h_{ij}^{kl} in a special manner.

The pressure of selection can be introduced in a standard way by means of fitnesses $w_{11}=\alpha$, $w_{12}=w_{21}=\beta$, $w_{22}=\gamma$. Then the difference equations for the relation between allele frequencies at the end of two successful generations, will have the form

$$wp' = pw_p+(\alpha-\beta)\pi, \tag{5.2}$$
$$wq' = qw_q-(\beta-\gamma)\pi,$$
$$w_p = \alpha p+\beta q, \; w_q = \beta p+\gamma q, \; w = pw_p+qw_q+(\alpha+\gamma-2\beta)\pi.$$

Here, unlike the continuous model, the dynamics of allele frequency already depends upon the index of deviations from panmixia, and therefore we need still another equation for π in order to close the model:

$$w^2\pi' = -(Ap^2q^2+B\pi+A\pi^2), \tag{5.3}$$
$$A = h\alpha\gamma-H\beta^2, \; B = h\alpha\gamma(p^2+q^2)+2H\beta^2pq.$$

Without the pressure of selection ($\alpha=\beta=\gamma=1$) from (5.2) and (5.3) we get

$$p' = p, \; \pi' = -\{(h-H)(p^2q^2+\pi^2)+\pi[h(p^2+q^2)+2Hpq]\}. \tag{5.4}$$

Whence it is seen that the deviation from panmixia by itself does not change allele frequencies and they remain continuous when carrying on from one generation to another, so that $p_n^+=p_{n-1}^-$, $q_n^+=q_{n-1}^-$, which is quite a natural result. However the index of deviations from panmixia varies even when there is no selection.

Suppose now $\pi=-p^2$, that is the system reached the lower bound of the admissible domain. Then setting $\pi=-p^2$ in (5.4), we obtain $\pi'-\pi=(1+H)p^2$. Likewise, $\pi'-\pi=(1+H)q^2$ when $\pi=-q^2$ and $\pi'-\pi=-(1+h)pq$ when $\pi=pq$. Whence it follows, that once reaching the boundaries of the admissible domain, on the next step the system can move only towards the interior of this domain.

Suppose the system, being inside of Ω_ξ, leaves Ω_ξ on the next step, that is $\pi\in\Omega_\xi$ but $\pi'\notin\Omega_\xi$. Let $\pi'>pq$; then

$$pq < -(h-H)(p^2q^2+\pi^2)-\pi[h(p^2+q^2)+2Hpq],$$
$$\max\{-p^2, -q^2\} < \pi < pq$$

or

$$f(p, h, H) = pq+(h-H)(p^2q^2+\pi^2)+\pi[h(p^2+q^2)+2Hpq] < 0. \tag{5.5}$$

Function f, regarded as the function of h and H takes on the minimal value at one of the corners of the rectangle $\{-1\leqslant h\leqslant h_{\max}; -1\leqslant H\leqslant H_{\max}\}$ (f is linear with respect to h and H). Substituting the appropriate values of h and H in (5.5), we find out that this inequality can hold only if $h_{\max}>1$ and $H_{\max}>1$. In a similar way we can prove that the system cannot leave Ω_ξ if $h, H\in[-1, +1]$. Thus we yield the restriction from above for the preference coefficients h and H. Let us note that these restrictions are similar to those derived for the continuous model.

Equation (5.3) has two steady state points, one of them being unstable and lying outside of Ω_ξ, and the other one lying inside of the admissible domain and being stable when

$$(1+h)^2(p-q)^2+4(1+h)(1+H)pq<16.$$

This inequality always holds, if $h, H\in[-1,+1]$. Consequently, $\pi_n\to\pi^*\in\Omega_\xi$ as $n\to\infty$, i.e. the population always equilibrates with respect to the index of deviations from panmixia, and the ratio of genotype frequencies at equilibrium will be different from the Hardian.

6.6. Evolution of Genetic Structure of Population Under Inbreeding. Discrete Model

Consider the special case of model (5.2), (5.3) where $\alpha=\gamma=1$, $\beta=1+s$, $-h=H=f$, $F\in[0, 1]$. Then

$$\begin{aligned} wp' &= p+s(pq-\pi),\\ w^2\pi' &= F\{[1+(1+s)^2][p^2q^2+\pi^2]+[(p^2+q^2)-2(1+s)^2pq]\pi\}, \\ w &= 1+2s(pq-\pi), q = 1-p. \end{aligned} \tag{6.1}$$

It is more convenient to treat this system in terms of variables p and $y=pq-\pi$. Their domain of definition

$$\Omega = \{0\leqslant p\leqslant 1;\ 0\leqslant y\leqslant p,\ p\in[0, 1/2];\ 0\leqslant y\leqslant q,\ q\in[0, 1/2]\}$$

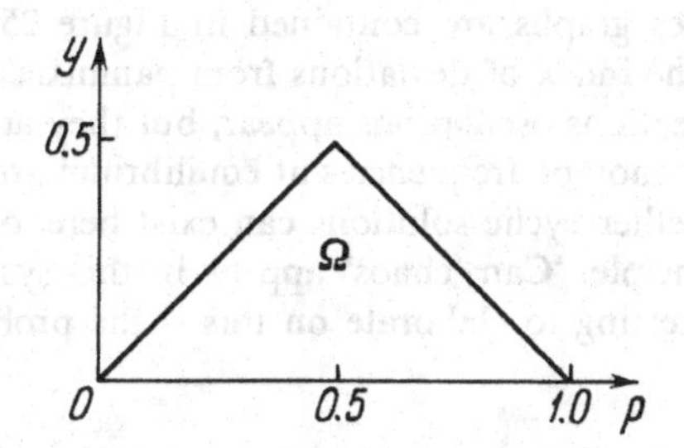

Fig. 24. Domain of definition Ω for the variables y and p in (6.2.)

is shown in Figure 24. Then in place of (6.1) we will have

$$\begin{aligned} wp' &= p+sy,\\ w^2y' &= (1-F)pq+(s+F)y+\{s^2-F\{1+(1+s)^2]\}y^2, \\ w &= 1+2sy. \end{aligned} \tag{6.2}$$

Let us study the character and location of the steady-state points of system (6.2). Evidently, there are the two points $p^*=y^*=0$ and $p^*=1, y^*=0$ which correspond to the "pure" Hardian states with $\pi^*=0$. It can be easily shown that they are stable when $s<0$ and $F<1$, and unstable if $s>0$.

And finally, there is the point $p^*=q^*=1/2$, which stands for the state of polymorphism. The values of y^* are found from the equation

$$4s^2y^{*3}+Ay^{*2}+(1-s-F)y^*-(1-F)/4 = 0, \tag{6.3}$$

where $A=4s-(1-F)s^2+2F(1+s)$, and provided that the condition $y^*\in\Omega$ is satisfied. It follows from the stability analysis of this steady-state point, that if $|1+2sy^*|>1$ and if p_0 is sufficiently close to $1/2$, then $p_n \to 1/2$ as $n\to\infty$. Obviously, the necessary and sufficient condition for this is $s>0, y^*>0$.

For $s>0$ and for any $y^*\neq 0$ the population develops polymorphism with respect to gene frequencies, therefore in order to get a qualitative dynamic picture of π, the index of deviations from panmixia (or of y, which is analogous), it suffices to study the second equation in (6.2), inserting $pq=1/4$. Rewrite this equation in the form

$$y' = \frac{1-F}{4}+\frac{F(1+s)y(1-2y)}{(1+2sy)^2} = f(y). \tag{6.4}$$

Certainly, applying the standard methods of stability analysis of steady-state points, based on the linear approximation, one can define the stability domains of y^* in the space of parameters s and F and accordingly interpret these results. However, we leave this task to the reader. Here we shall illustrate the dynamic behavior of the system by representing the solutions to equation (6.4) for $F=0.96$ (strong inbreeding) and for two values of $s: s_1=1/4$ (weak selection) and $s_2=50$ (strong selection). The solution is obtained by the graphical method ('staircase of Lamerey'). The appropriates graphs are contained in Figure 25a,b. One can see that under weak selection the index of deviations from panmixia equilibrates monotonically; under strong selections oscillations appear, but they are damped. Let us note that in both cases the genotype frequencies at equilibrium are not Hardian.

It is not known, whether cyclic solutions can exist here, or if there is no chance for them to be in principle. 'Can 'chaos' appear in this system?' is another question. It would be interesting to elaborate on this – the problem has not found its overall solution yet.

6.7. Isolation by Distance and Deviations from Panmixia

In Section 2.14 we already shown, that if we assume the existence of panmixia, we thus accept the concept of 'gamete pool', that is the gametes that make up the new zygote, are independently selected out of the set of all gametes of the parental population. But as soon as panmixia is disturbed, this concept no longer works, and we are to treat the relationships at the genotype level, making the model markedly more complex. However there is a kind of intermediate way to describe populations with disturbed panmixia. We can still adopt the concept of 'gamete pool', but think that a zygote is formed with probability, depending upon some new variable, which is the 'distance' between parental gametes.

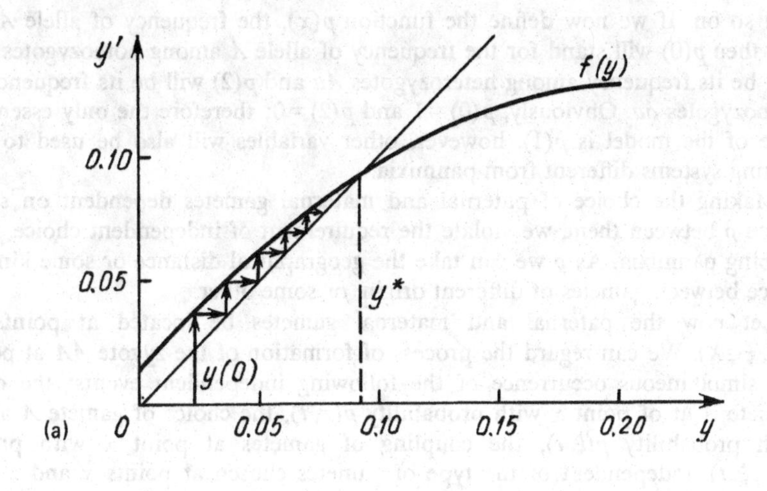

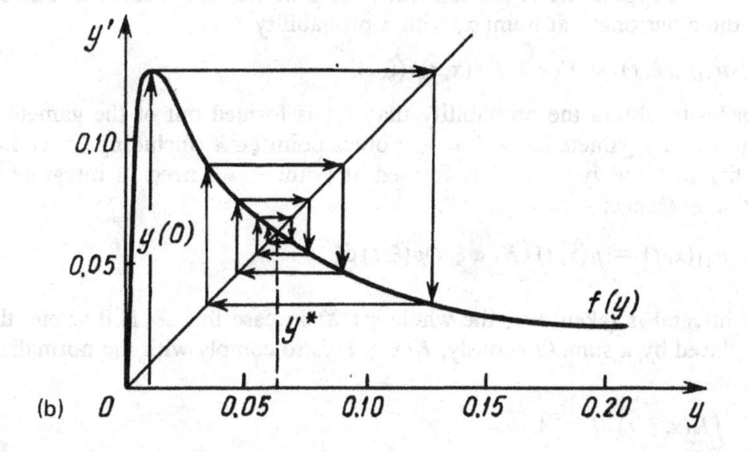

Fig. 25. Graphic solution of Equation (6.4)

Consider a sufficiently large population, with inheritance specified by one diallele gene with alleles A and a. Suppose a set X (discrete or continuous) is given, with elements x and the distance function ρ, and let the frequency of allele A be defined on this set and be a function of time or the generation number, acting as a parameter, so that $p=p(x, t)$. For instance, the set of genotype can be regarded as X, and the metric ρ can be introduced as follows. Enumerate the genotypes: $N\{AA\}=0$, $N\{Aa\}=1$, $N\{aa\}=2$; then

$$\rho(AA, Aa) = |N\{AA\}-N\{Aa\}| = 1,$$

$$\rho(AA, aa) = |N\{AA\}-N\{aa\}| = 2$$

and so on. If we now define the function $p(x)$, the frequency of allele A, on this set, then $p(0)$ will stand for the frequency of allele A among homozygotes $AA, p(1)$ will be its frequency among heterozygotes Aa and $p(2)$ will be its frequency among homozygotes aa. Obviously, $p(0)=1$ and $p(2)=0$; therefore the only essential variable of the model is $p(1)$, however, other variables will also be used to describe mating systems different from panmixia.

Making the choice of paternal and maternal gametes dependent on some distance ρ between them, we violate the requirement of independent choice, thus disturbing panmixia. As ρ we can take the geographical distance or some kind of distance between gametes of different origin, or some other.

Let now the paternal and maternal gametes be located at points x and $\xi\,(x, \xi \in X)$. We can regard the process of formation of the zygote AA at point x as the simultaneous occurrence of the following independent events: the choice of gamete A at of point x with probability $p(x, t)$, the choice of gamete A at point ξ with probability $p(\xi, t)$, the coupling of gametes at point x with probability $K(x, \xi, t)$, independent of the type of gametes chosen at points x and ξ. Then at point x the zygote AA is formed from the gametes, one located at this same point and the other one – at point x, with a probability

$$u_{11}(x, \xi, t) = K(x, \xi, t)p(x, t)p(\xi, t).$$

In order to obtain the probability that AA is formed out of the gamete located at point x and a gamete located at any other point $\xi \in X$ (including $\xi = x$), i.e. the probability that the zygote AA is formed at point x, we need to integrate $u_{11}(x, \xi, t)$ over all ξ. Hence:

$$u_{11}(x, t) = p(x, t)\int_X K(x, \xi, t)p(\xi, t)\,d\xi. \tag{7.1}$$

This integral is taken over the whole set X: in case this set is discrete, the integral is replaced by a sum. Obviously, $K(x, \xi, t)$ is to comply with the normalization condition:

$$\int_X K(x, \xi, t)\,d\xi = 1. \tag{7.2}$$

Similar reasoning can be employed for the formation of zygotes Aa and aa. And eventually

$$\begin{aligned} u_{11}(x, t) &= p(x, t)\int_X K(x, \xi, t)p(\xi, t)\,d\xi, \\ u_{21}(x, t) = u_{12}(x, t) &= \frac{1}{2}\{p(x, t)\int_X K(x, \xi, t)q(\xi, t)\,d\xi + \\ &\quad + q(x, t)\int_X (x, \xi, t)p(\xi, t)d\xi\}. \\ u_{22}(x, t) &= q(x, t)\int_X K(x, \xi, t)q(\xi, t)\,d\xi, \end{aligned} \tag{7.3}$$

where $q(x, t)=1-p(x, t)$. Thus, if the assumption about panmixia fails to hold and if a law is prescribed to limit the random and independent choice of the paternal and maternal gametes, then the frequencies of genotypes AA, Aa and aa in the offspring are defined by (7.3) in terms of the frequencies of parental gametes. These formulae present the principles of inheritance for the case, when the rather restricting requirement of panmixia is relieved, and they can serve as a kind of analogy for the Hardian relations for non-panmictic populations.

If we now apply the Malthusian coefficients α, β and γ and introduce the pressure of selection, then taking into account the obvious relations $p(x, t)=u_{11}(x, t)+u_{12}(x, t), q(x, t)=u_{21}(x, t)+u_{22}(x, t)$, we can write the equation of the continuous model for the gene frequency $p(x, t)$ as follows:

$$\partial p / \partial t = p(w_p - w) - \beta\delta/2, \tag{7.4}$$

where

$$w_p = \alpha\phi + \beta\psi, \quad \phi = \int_X Kp(\xi, t)\,\mathrm{d}\xi,$$

$$\psi = \int_X Kq(\xi, t)\,\mathrm{d}\xi, \quad w = \alpha p\phi + \beta(p\psi + q\phi) + \gamma q\psi,$$

$$\delta = p - \phi$$

Obviously, $\phi+\psi=1$.

Note that the form of this equation resembles that of the equation, derived for the bisexual population in the previous Chapter (see Section 5.2). As a matter of fact, we could also take into account two sexes within the framework of our model: for this it suffices to think that X is a set made of two elements, so that $p(x_1)$ defines the frequency of allele A among males, and $p(x_2)$ – among females. Besides, the function of deviations from panmixia $K(x, \xi)$ should be specially chosen:

$$K(x, \xi) = \begin{cases} 0 & \text{for } x = x_1, \ \xi = x_1; \ x = x_2, \ \xi = x_2, \\ 1 & \text{for } x = x_1, \ \xi = x_2; \ x = x_2, \ \xi = x_1. \end{cases}$$

This implies that the probability that gametes x_1 and x_1 couple and make a zygote is null (quite naturally, since these are male gametes). The same for the female gametes x_2 and x_2. On the other hand there is a unitary probability that gametes x_1 and x_2 couple to form a zygote. Then, if we set $p(x_1)=P$ and $p(x_2)=p$, then $\phi=P, \psi=Q$ and from (7.4) we readily get the Equations (5.2.4), where $\mu^*=1$, that is the ratio of sexes at equilibrium is equal to 1:1.

6.8. Models with Particular Functions of Deviations from Panmixia

a) Let the population be distributed over a uniform area, the straight line $x\,(-\infty \leqslant x \leqslant +\infty)$. All the points of this line can be regarded as the set X, so that $x \in X$. Naturally, the probability, that the individuals, located at points x and $\xi\,(x, \xi \in X)$, couple, is a function of the distance $\rho = |\,\xi - x\,|$ between these individuals, this probability being maximal when $x = \xi$ and falling rapidly with increases in ρ. As such a function satisfying the normalization conditions (7.2), one can take the density function of the normal distribution with some $\sigma \ll 1$, characterizing how rapidly the probability of coupling falls with increases in $|\xi - x|$, hence:

$$K(x, \xi) = \frac{1}{\sqrt{2\pi}\sigma} \exp\{-\frac{(\xi-x)^2}{2\sigma^2}\}, \int_{-\infty}^{\infty} K(x, \xi) = 1.$$

Then the function $\phi(x, t)$ can be represented in the form

$$\phi(x, t) = \int_{-\infty}^{\infty} K(x, \xi) p(\xi, t)\, d\xi =$$

$$= \int_{-\infty}^{\infty} K(x, \xi)[p(x) + (\xi - x)\frac{\partial p}{\partial x} + \frac{1}{2}(\xi - x)^2 \frac{\partial^2 p}{\partial x^2} + \cdots]\, d\xi =$$

$$= p(x) + \frac{1}{2}\frac{\partial^2 p}{\partial x^2} \int_{-\infty}^{\infty} (\xi - x)^2 K(x, \xi)\, d\xi + \cdots = p(x) + \frac{\sigma^2}{2}\frac{\partial^2 p}{\partial x^2} + O(\sigma^4).$$

Since $\sigma \ll 1$, we can neglect the terms $O(\sigma^4)$ and think that

$$\phi(x, t) \simeq p(x) + \frac{\sigma^2}{2}\frac{\partial^2 p}{\partial x^2}. \tag{8.1}$$

Let us also suppose that the pressure of selection is low, i.e. $\alpha = 1 + s_1, \beta = 1 + s_2, \gamma = 1 + s_3$ where $s_1, s_2, s_3 \sim \sigma^2 \ll 1$. Then substituting (8.1) into (7.4) and neglecting the terms of the order of $o(\sigma^2)$ we obtain

$$\frac{\partial p}{\partial t} = \frac{\sigma^2}{4}\frac{\partial^2 p}{\partial x^2} + f(p), \tag{8.2}$$

$$f(p) = p(\hat{w}_p - \hat{w}),\ \hat{w}_p = \alpha p + \beta q,\ \hat{w} = \alpha p^2 + 2\beta pq + \gamma q^2.$$

Thus, we come to the model of the genetic evolution of a spatially distributed population, where the spatial factor results in deviations from panmixia. We shall elaborate on this model in the next Chapter.

b) Let our population be split somehow into r groups, possibly with different gene frequencies. Let us renumber these groups from 1 to r. Suppose, the probability, that a genotype from group i couples with a genotype from group j and forms the appropriate zygote in group i, is a function only of the group numbers and of nothing else. Then our set X is a finite discrete set with r elements, and the function $K(x, \xi)$ can be presented as an $r \times r$-matrix with elements k_{ij}. The normalization condition (7.2) is the condition of matrix stochasticity, i.e.

$$\sum_{j=1}^{r} k_{ij} = 1,\ i = \overline{1, r},$$

and k_{ij} is nothing else, but the probability that a selected gamete from the ith group couples with a jth group gamete (provided that the gamete in this group is already chosen) within the limits of the ith group. In this case integrals in (7.3) are substituted by finite sums, and the dynamic equations of gene frequencies p are written as follows

$$dp^i/dt = p^i(w_p^i - w^i) - \beta\delta^i/2, \quad i = \overline{1, r},$$

$$w_p^i = \sum_{j=1}^{r} k_{ij}(\alpha p^j + \beta q^j),$$

$$w^i = \sum_{j=1}^{r} k_{ij}[\alpha p^i p^j + \beta(p^i q^j + q^i p^j) + \gamma q^i q^j], \tag{8.3}$$

$$\delta^i = p^i - \sum_{j=1}^{r} k_{ij} p^{\alpha}.$$

Actually the derived model is not a model of a single population, but is rather a system of r populations linked together with migration, which has no effect on their numbers, changing only the patterns of mating, that is disturbing panmixia in the united population. Since we already deal with migration, the detailed study of this model is contained in the next Chapter.

c) The situation turns to be more complicated, when the probability that genotypes couple, function K, besides x and ξ also depends upon $p(\xi, t)$ – the concentration of gene frequencies or the concentration of genotypes at the appropriate points of our space. As a result, $K = K(x, \xi, p, t)$ and the unknown function enters non-linearly under the integral sign. This usually makes the solution of the problem markedly more complicated.

6.9. Notes and Bibliography

To 6.1.

The notion of 'systems of mating' was first introduced in the work:

Wright, S.: 1921, 'Systems of Mating', *Genetics* **6**, 1,2, 111–178.

These ideas (especially in application to 'isolation by distance') were furthered in his works:

Wright, S.: 1943, 'Isolation by Distance', *Genetics* **28**, 2, 114–138;
Wright, S.: 1946, 'Isolation by Distance Under Diverse Systems of Mating', *Genetics* **31**, 1, 39–59.

To 6.2.

The idea that deviations from panmixia on the genotype rather than gamete level (i.e. rejecting the concept of 'gamete pool') can be characterized by preference coefficients, has been first stated in the work:

Haldane, J.B.S.: 1939, 'Inbreeding in Mendelian Populations with Special Reference to Human Cousin Marriage;, *Ann. Eugenics* **9**, 321–340.

A similar method was also suggested in the paper:

Bennett, J.H. and Binet, F.E.: 1956, 'Association Between Mendelian Factors with Mixed Selfing and Random Mating', *Heredity* **10**, 1, 51–55.

A short historical digression. Practically in all the first models by Fisher, Haldane, Wright and their successors the concept of 'gamete pool', has been accepted either implicitly or explicitly. The progress of mathematical genetics during the 1920-1930's entirely justified this approach. However towards the end of the 1930's criticism started to be voiced more and more often. Most serious was the criticism by V.A. Kostitzin (see details in the book:

Scudo, F. and J. Ziegier: 1978, *The Golden Age of Theoretical Ecology*, 1923–1940, Springer, Berlin, p. 410–412),

however, the alternative models of Volterra type, that he suggested, have not been widely accepted at that time, apparently due to the purely technical complications in their analysis.

More and more works appear lately, where authors give up the concept of 'gamete' carrying on from the gamete level of description to the level of zygotes. Most systematically this is performed in the works:

Svirezhev, Yu.M.: 1972, 'Mathematical Models in Population Genetics' (Matematicheskye modeli v populyatsionnoi genetike), Review by the author of the doctor's thesis, Institute of Biophysics, Acad. of Sci., U.S.S.R., Pushino. (In Russian);

Kaganova, O.Z. and Korzukhin, M.D.: 1977, *Attempt to Reformulate the Equations of Mathematical Genetics in Terms of 'Zygote Numbers' (for Bisexual Populations) (Opyt pereformulirovki uravneniy matematicheskoy genetiki v peremennykh 'chisla zygot' (dlya dvupolykh populyatsiy))*, Scientific Computer Center, Acad. of Sci., U.S.S.R., Pushino (In Russian).

To 6.3-6.6.

Currently there exist several modeling methods for non- panmictic systems of mating. One of them is represented by the so-called 'coefficients of deviations from panmixia'. They are introduced as follows. While under panmixia the connection between zygote frequencies in the generation and gamete frequencies in the one before is specified by Hardy's formulae, under disturbed panmixia this connection is represented in the form fo $(u_{11})_n^+ = (v_{11}p^2)_{n-1}^-$, $(u_{12})_n^+ = (v_{12}pq)_{n-1}^-$, $(u_{22})_n^+ = (v_{22}q^2)_{n-1}^-$, where the coefficients v_{11}, v_{12} and v_{22} are known as the "coefficients of deviations from panmixia". Assuming that gene frequencies remain continuous when carrying over from one generation to another, we arrive at a restriction imposed on these coefficients: $v_{11}p + v_{12}q = v_{12}p + v_{22}q = 1$, $v_{11}, v_{12}, v_{22} \geq 0$. Obviously, for $v_{11} = v_{12} = v_{22}$ we have panmixia. This description was first suggested by

Bernstein, F.: 1930, 'Forgesetzte Untersuchungen aus der Theorie der Blutgruppen', *Z. Induct. Abst. Vererb.* **56**, 4, 233–273.

Further on the coefficients of deviations from panmixia were widely used in the works of M. Kimura and his co-workers.

In 1922 S. Wright in his paper

Wright, S.: 1922, 'Coefficients of Inbreeding and Relationship', *Amer. Nat.* **56**, 330–338,

introduced the notion of the inbreeding coefficient, which is nothing else, but the coefficient of correlation between two similar gametes that make a zygote. Obviously, if there is a correlation between gametes, then the connection between the frequencies of new zygotes and the gamete frequencies in the previous generation can be given by (5.1), where π may be interpreted as the value of covariance between gametes. On the other hand sampling of gametes out of the 'gamete pool' can be considered as a series of sequential independent trials with the probability of success being equal to the frequency of gamete A. Each sampling is one such trial, therefore the variance is equal to pq. And since by definition the correlation coefficient $F_w = \text{covariation}/\text{variation} = \pi/pq$, we have $\pi = F_W pq$, $|F_w| \leq 1$, and F_w is known as the Wright's coefficient of inbreeding, which may coincide with the probability that two alleles, originating from a common ancestor, come across in one individual. Comparing the coefficients of deviation from panmixia with the inbreeding coefficient, one can easily see that

$$v_{12} = 1 - F_w, \quad v_{11} = 1 + F_w(q/p), \quad v_{22} = 1 + F_w(p/q).$$

Besides the Wright's coefficient of inbreeding, quite widely used is the coefficient of kinship (coefficient de parenté), C_{XY}, suggested by Malecot. This coefficient seems to be more appropriate for the description of deviations from panmixia, than the Wright's coefficient F_W. The coefficient CV_{XY} is defined as follows: let the individuals X and Y have genotypes A_1A_2 and A_3A_4. By $p\{A_1 = A_2\}$ let us denote the probability of the event: "the genes A_1 and A_2 are the same" (say, they originate from one and the same parent). Likewise for other pairs of genes. Then

$$C_{XY} = \frac{1}{4}[p\{A_1 = A_3\} + p\{A_1A_4\} + p\{A_2 = A_3\} + p\{A_2 = A_4\}].$$

For more details about the coefficient C_{XY} see the book:

Malecot, G.: 1948, Les Mathematiques de l'Heredite, Hermann et Cie, Paris. (English translation: 1969, The Mathematics of Heredity, Freeman, San Francisco, XVII, 88, p..

From this viewpoint F_w is defined for one individual X with genotype A_1A_2 and it is equal to $p\{A_1 = A_2\}$. The paper

Malecot, G.: 1969, 'Consanguinite Panmictique et Consanguinite Systematique. (Coefficients de Wright et Malecot)', *Ann. Genet. et Select. Anim.* **1**, 3, 237-242,

deals with the comparison of these two coefficients and elucidate the question: "When C_{XY} should be used when F_w:".

The book:

Fisher, P.A. 1949, *The theory of inbreeding*, Oliver and Boyd, Edingburg, 120 p., attends to a wide range of problems concerned with mathematical models of various schemes of incest crossing and inbreeding.

Many schemes of inbreeding, regarded in Wright's sense, can be represented in terms of linear relations (unlike panmixia, where the relations between genotype frequencies of parents and those of the offspring are essentially non-linear). Therefore the theory of linear transformations can be applied, which is widely performed by Fisher, who managed to obtain a number of fine results.

What makes both the preference coefficients v_{ij} and the Wright's inbreeding coefficient F_w essentially different from the quantities θ_{ij} and F, which we have introduced (chosing the same name for them), is actually the acceptance or non-acceptance of the 'gamete pool' concept. This concept implies that relationships in the genotype level are transformed into the relationships in the gamete level, so that correlation between genotypes is substituted by correlation between gametes. While the statement that correlation between genotypes entirely defines the correlation between gametes is correct, the reverse statement, generally speaking, is not true. We failed to present the model of interest in terms of gene frequencies; we either had to formulate the model in terms of genotype frequencies, or the phase space of gene frequencies needed to be expanded by the addition of one more variable – the index of deviations from panmixia. But accepting the 'gamete pool' concept, we can save the situation to a certain extent and formulate the model only in terms of gene frequencies. However in order to do that, we have to suppose that either v_{ij}=const, or F_w – const. To say nothing about these assumptions being mutually contradictory, we cannot even assume that, says, F_w=const. In fact, $F_w = \pi/(pq)$, but as its results from Section 6.6, this quantity does not stay constant in the evolutionary process of the population. One can try to save the situation, thinking that F_w is explicitly dependent on time, however this is also a palliative solution. From our viewpoint the only way out is to apply the approach suggested in this Chapter, where preference coefficients have a very clear meaning and they can be really considered constant.

To 6.7.

The model, where the probability of reproductive pairing depended upon which of two populations the selected individuals belonged to, was suggested in the above mentioned work of Wright (1943), who implicitly assumed that migration between two populations only redistributes the probabilities of reproductive pairing, without changing the numbers of separate subpopulations. Generally speaking, this is not quite right, since migration essentially alters the numbers of populations linked by flows of migrants. Therefore it is more correct to speak about disturbed panmixia in this case. However, due to S. Wright there appeared a great number of "migration" models, which are actually models of populations with disturbed panmixia.

Let us mention the following ones:

Hanson, W.D.: 1966, 'Effects of Partial Isolation (Distance), Migration and Different Fitness Requirement Among Enviromental Pockets Upon Steady State Gene Frequencies', *Biometrics* **22**, 3, 453-468;

Tallis, G.M.: 1966, 'A Migration Model', *Biometrics* **22**, 1, 17-25.

Models and results of the analysis of the combined action of mutations and migrations are surveyed in Chapter 6 of the book

Nagylaki, T.: 1977, *Selection in One- and Two-Locus Systems*, Springer, Berlin, 208 p.,

Unfortunately, in the above cited works this distinction is not always traced explicitly. More details, concerning these problems, are contained in the following Chapter.

Various cases of disturbed panmixia in populations (in particular, when the originally single population is split into two subpopulations) are studied in the paper:

Svirezhev, Yu.M.: 1968, 'Disturbed Panmixia in Populations (Narusheniye panmixia v populyatsiyakh)', *Genetika* **4**, 12, 120-129 (In Russian).

To 6.8.

In the paper:

Fisher, R.A.: 1937, 'The Wave of Advance of Advantageous Genes', *Ann. Eugen.* **7**, 355-369,

the Equation (8.2) was suggested to describe the evolution of a population with individuals of low mobility distributed along a linear area.

Model (8.3) was suggested and elaborated on in the work:

Svirezhev, Yu.M.: 1968, 'The Systems of Weakly Connected Populations', *Studia Biophysica* **10**, 1, 25-30.

Chapter 7

Systems of Linked Populations. Migration

7.1. Introduction

Up till now we have been looking at the evolution of populations, occupying a fixed uniform area, within which some kind of panmixia was realized. However in real life it is more common, when populations of one and the same species occupy different areas, so that the spatial distribution of the species is represented by a patchy pattern. The areas themselves are not absolutely isolated from each other: there are always some flows of migrants between them, that alter both the sizes of separate populations and their genetic structure. Migration flows connect the originally isolated populations into a single system – the system of linked populations, which evolution can be essentially different from the evolution of an isolated population.

7.2. Migration Between Populations of Different Sizes

Consider two panmictic populations with numbers N_1 and N_2, linked together by flows of migrants. The simplest assumption about the character of migration is that the migration flow (the number of organisms, migrating from one population to the other in unit time) is in proportion to the difference in numbers:

$$M = m(N_1 - N_2). \tag{2.1}$$

Here m is the relative intensity of migration.

Let the evolution of sizes of the genotypic groups in each of the populations be governed by the equations

$$dN_j^i / dt = f_j(N_j^1, \ldots, N_j^n), \quad i = \overline{1, n}; \quad j = 1, 2. \tag{2.2}$$

Then the evolution of a system of two linked populations can be characterized by the following system:

$$dN_j^i / dt = f_j(N_j^1, \ldots, N_j^n) + (-1)^j (N_1^i - N_2^i), \quad i = \overline{1, n}; \quad j = 1, 2. \tag{2.3}$$

Consider the case, when inheritance in each of the populations is determined by one and the same diallele gene with frequencies of allele A being equal to p_1 and p_2 in the first and second populations, respectively. The pressure of selection, being different in different areas, is specified by the finesses $\{\alpha_j, \beta_j, \gamma_j\}, j = 1, 2$. It is assumed that migrants do not affect directly the structure of mating couples (both populations remain panmictic) but just alter the concentration of certain genotypes and the total sizes of the populations. Then instead of the sizes of genotypic groups one can take the numbers of allele A and rewrite (2.3) in the form (see section 2.15)

$$\begin{aligned}
\frac{dx_1}{dt} &= \frac{x_1}{N_1}(\alpha_1 x_1+\beta_1 y_1)-d_1(N_1)x_1-m(x_1-x_2),\\
\frac{dx_2}{dt} &= \frac{x_2}{N_2}(\alpha_2 x_2+\beta_2 y_2)-d_2(N_2)x_2-m(x_1-x_2),\\
\frac{dN_1}{dt} &= \frac{1}{N_1}(\alpha_1 x_1^2+2\beta_1 x_1 y_1+\gamma_1 y_1^2)-d_1(N_1)N_1-m(N_1-N_2),\\
\frac{dN_2}{dt} &= \frac{1}{N_2}(\alpha_2 x_2^2+2\beta_2 x_2 y_2+\gamma_2 y_2^2)-d_2(N_2)N_2-m(N_1-N_2),
\end{aligned} \tag{2.4}$$

Here x_1, y_1, x_2, y_2 are the numbers of alleles A and a in the first and second populations, respectively, $x_1+y_1=N_1$, $x_2+y_2=N_2$. The functions $d_j(N_j)$, $j=1,2$ stand for the effect of the intraspecific non-differential competition on the total mortality in each population. It is only natural to assume that mortality increases with the total population size, that is $d_j'(N_j)>0$. Making use of these functions we take into account the ecological factors, which are not geared to genetics.

Passing to frequencies in (2.4), we get

$$\begin{aligned}
\frac{dp_1}{dt} &= p_1(w_1^p-w_1)-\frac{mN_2}{N_1}(p_1-p_2),\\
\frac{dp_2}{dt} &= p_2(w_2^p-w_2)+\frac{mN_1}{N_2}(p_1-p_2),\\
\frac{dN_1}{dt} &= N_1[w_1-d_1(N_1)]-m(N_1-N_2),\\
\frac{dN_2}{dt} &= N_2[w_2-d_2(N_2)]+m(N_1-N_2),
\end{aligned} \tag{2.5}$$

where $w_j^p=\alpha_j p_j+\beta_j q_j$, $w_j=\alpha_j p_j^2+2\beta_j p_j q_j+\gamma_j q_j^2$, $q_j=1-p_j$, $j=1,2$. Introduce the new variable $\mu=N_1/N_2$ which is the ratio of population sizes. Then instead of (2.5) we will have

$$\begin{aligned}
\frac{dp_1}{dt} &= p_1(w_1^p-w_1)-\frac{m}{\mu}(p_1-p_2),\\
\frac{dp_2}{dt} &= p_2(w_2^p-w_2)-\mu m(p_1-p_2),\\
\frac{d\mu}{dt} &= \mu[w_1-w_2-d_1(N_1)+d_2(\frac{N_1}{\mu})]+m(1-\mu^2),\\
\frac{dN_1}{dt} &= N_1[w_1-d_1(N_1)-m+\frac{m}{\mu}].
\end{aligned} \tag{2.6}$$

Let us concentrate on several special cases of model (2.6)

a) Suppose the size of the second population by far exceeds that of the first, so that μ is small. Then instead of (2.6) for the terms of the order of $O(1/\mu)$ we can write:

$$\frac{dp_1}{dt} \approx -\frac{m}{\mu}(p_1-p_2),\quad \frac{dp_2}{dt} \approx 0,\quad \frac{d\mu}{dt} \approx m,\quad \frac{dN_1}{dt} \approx N_1\frac{m}{\mu}. \tag{2.7}$$

Suppose the second population is of alleles a only, that is $p_2 \approx 0$. Integrating these equations for the initial conditions $p_1(0)=1$, $\mu(0)$, $N_1(0)$ we yield

$$p_1(t) \approx \frac{\mu(0)}{\mu(0)+mt},$$

$$\mu(t) \approx \mu(0)+mt,\quad N_1(t) \approx N_1(0)\left[1+\frac{mt}{\mu(0)}\right].$$

Whence it is seen that migration levels up the genic population contents over the course of time. At first the sizes of populations also tend to level up (μ and N_1 grow), but the further growth of μ and N_1 violates our assumption about them being small, so that the model itself becomes inadequate.

b) Let now the intensity of migration can be low ($m \ll 1$). Besides, suppose that $d_1(N_1)=d_2(N_2)=d=\text{const}$, that is the mortality is the same in both populations, being independent of their sizes. Let us seek for the solution to (2.6) of the form

$$p_1 \approx p_1^0+mp_1^1,\quad p_2 \approx p_2^0+mp_2^1, \tag{2.8}$$

$$\mu \approx \mu^0+m\mu^1,\quad N_1 \approx N_1^0+mN_1^1.$$

Inserting (2.8) into (2.6), equating the terms at common powers of m and neglecting the terms of order $o(m)$, we get

$$\frac{dp_j^0}{dt} = f_j(p_j^0),\quad \frac{d\mu^0}{dt} = \mu^0(w_1^0-w_2^0), \tag{2.9}$$

$$\frac{dN_1}{dt} = N_1(w_1^0-d),\quad \frac{dp_j^1}{dt} = \left(\frac{\partial f_j}{\partial p_j}\right)\bigg|_{p_j^0} p_j^1+\phi_j^0,\quad j = 1, 2,$$

$$\frac{d\mu^1}{dt} = \mu^0\left[\left(\frac{\partial w_1}{\partial p_1}\right)\bigg|_{p_1^0} p_1^1-\left(\frac{\partial w_2}{\partial p_2}\right)\bigg|_{p_2^0} p_2^1\right]+ \tag{2.10}$$

$$+[1-(\mu^0)^2]+\mu^1(w_1^0-w_2^0),$$

$$\frac{dN_1^1}{dt} = N_1^0\left(\frac{\partial w_1}{\partial p_1}\right)\bigg|_{p_0^1} p_1^1+(w_1^0-d)N_1^1-\frac{1-\mu^0}{\mu^0}N_1.$$

Here

$$f_j = p_j(w_j^p - w_j),\ j = 1, 2;\ \phi_1^0 = -\frac{1}{\mu^0}(p_1^0 - p_2^0),$$
$$\phi_2^0 = \mu^0(p_1^0 - p_2^0),\ w_j^0 = \alpha_j(p_j^0)^2 + 2\beta_j p_j^0 q_j^0 + \gamma_j(q_j^0)^2.$$

The equations for p_j^0, p_j^1, μ_0 do not include the variables N_1^0, N_1^1; hence they can be treated separately.

The equations of the zero-order approximation represent the dynamics of two isolated populations. Let each of them have a stable state of equilibrium: $\hat{p}_1^0$ and $\hat{p}_2^0(\hat{p}_1^0 \neq \hat{p}_2^0)$. Then if $w_1(\hat{p}_1^0) > w_2(\hat{p}_1^0)$ then $\mu_0(t) \to \infty$ as $t \to \infty$; otherwise $\mu_0(t) \to 0$. Let these populations be linked by a weak flow of migrants. As it follows from the equations of the first-order approximation (2.9), these relations cannot be preserved, and the genetic structure of the system of linked populations tends to one of the states, typical for the "dominating" population. In fact, let $w_1(\hat{p}_1^0) > w_2(\hat{p}_1^0)$ and $\hat{p}_1^0 > \hat{p}_2^0$. Then $\mu_0(t) \to \infty$ and for sufficiently large t we have $\dot{p}_1^1 \approx (\partial f_1 / \partial p_1)|_{p_1^0} p_1^1$, $\dot{p}_2^1 \approx -C\mu_0(t) \to \infty (C > 0)$. For $\hat{p}_1^0 < \hat{p}_2^0$ we have $\dot{p}_2 \approx -C\mu_0(t) \to -\infty$. And this implies, that as $p_1^1 \to 0$ (it follows from the stability of $\hat{p}_1^0$ that $(\partial f_1 / \partial p_1)|_{p_1^0} < 0$), p_2^1 rapidly grows (or declines), so that the difference between $\hat{p}_1^0$ and p_2 decreases. It can be proved that $p_2 \to \hat{p}_1^0$. Likewise, if $w_1(\hat{p}_1^0) < w_2(\hat{p}_2^0)$ then $p_1 \to p_2$.

It follows from the aforesaid, that in a system of linked populations the population with a higher mean fitness (the 'dominating' one) 'imposes' its genic structure upon the whole system.

Consider the singular case, when $w_1(\hat{p}_1^0) = w_2(\hat{p}_2^0)$, that is fitnesses of isolated populations at stable equilibrium are the same. Then

$$\frac{d\mu_0}{dt} = 0,\ \frac{d\mu_1}{dt} = \mu^0\left[\left.\left(\frac{\partial w_1}{\partial p_1}\right)\right|_{\hat{p}_1} p_1^1 - \left.\left(\frac{\partial w_2}{\partial p_2}\right)\right|_{\hat{p}_2} p_2^1\right] + (1 - \mu_2^0). \tag{2.11}$$

The behavior of the solutions to the system of the first- order approximation is essentially dependent on the choice of the initial value μ^0, which is the classical case for the singular problem. Furthermore, the small parameter m itself is a bifurcational parameter in this case. All this proves that this kind of problem needs to be analysed more carefully.

7.3. Migration Between Populations, Occupying two Similar Ecological Niches

Suppose that both populations, linked by a flow of migrants, are under the same pressure of selection, so that $\alpha_1 = \alpha_2$, $\beta_1 = \beta_2$, $\gamma_1 = \gamma_2$, $d_1 = d_2$. In other words, they occupy two similar ecological niches. Let us further simplify the problem, setting $\alpha_j = \gamma_j = 1$, $\beta_j = 1 + s$, that is the pressures of selection upon homozygotes is the same. Though mortalities $d_j(N_j)$ can depend on the appropriate numbers, the nature of this dependence is the same for both populations ($d_j(N) = d(N)$).

If populations are isolated ($m=0$), they can be in one of the three states:

$$\{p_j^* = 0, N_j^*(0)\},\ \{p_j^* = 1, N_j^*(1)\},\ \{p_j^* = 1/2, N_j^*(1/2)\},\ j = 1, 2.$$

Steady-state numbers N_j^* are the positive solutions to the following equations:

$$d(N_j^*) = 1 \text{ for } N_j^*(0) \text{ and } N_j^*(1);$$

$$d(N_j^*) = 1+s/2 \text{ for } N_j^*(1/2).$$

Suppose now $m \neq 0$. Taking into account all our assumptions, we can rewrite (2.6) in the form

$$\begin{aligned}
\frac{dp_1}{dt} &= sp_1q_1(1-2p_1) - \frac{m}{\mu}(p_1-p_2),\\
\frac{dp_2}{dt} &= sp_2q_2(1-2p_2) - \mu m(p_1-p_2),\\
\frac{d\mu}{dt} &= \mu\left\{\left[\left[\frac{N_1}{\mu}\right] - d(N_1)\right] + 2s(p_1q_1-p_2q_2)\right\} + m(1-\mu^2),\\
\frac{dN_1}{dt} &= N_1\{1-m+\frac{m}{\mu}+2sp_1q_1-d(N_1)\}.
\end{aligned} \tag{3.1}$$

Let us seek for those steady-state points of system (3.1), that comply with the condition $p_1^*q_1^* = p_2^*q_2^*$. Since $w_j = 1+2sp_jq_j$, $j=1, 2$, this condition is equivalent to the equality $w_1(p_1^*) = w_2(p_2^*)$. In other words, we assume that at equilibrium fitnesses of linked populations are equal. Besides, let us think that the effect of ecological factors at equilibrium is the same, that is $d(N_1^*/\mu^*) = d(N_1^*)$. Whence it readily follows that $\mu^*=1$, that is at equilibrium the sizes of linked populations are the same. Since the pressure of selection in both niches is the same, and migration is in proportion to the difference between population sizes, it seems quite plausible to assume that this kind of points exhaust all the set of steady-state points. However, we failed to obtain a rigorous proof of this statement. Calculating these points, we get:

$$\begin{aligned}
&1.\quad p_1^* = p_2^* = 0,\ \mu^* = 1,\ N_1^* = N_1^*(0).\\
&2.\quad p_1^* = p_2^* = 1,\ \mu^* = 1,\ N_1^* = N_1^*(1).\\
&3.\quad p_1^* = p_2^* = 1/2,\ \mu^* = 1,\ N_1^* = N_1^*(1/2).\\
&4.\quad p_1^* = \frac{1}{2}(1+\sqrt{1+4\sigma}),\ p_2^* = \frac{1}{2}(1-\sqrt{1+4\sigma}),\\
&\qquad m^* = 1,\ N_1^* = N_1^*(\sigma).\\
&5.\quad p_1^* = \frac{1}{2}(1-\sqrt{1+4\sigma}),\ p_2^* = \frac{1}{2}(1+\sqrt{1+4\sigma}),\\
&\qquad m^* = 1,\ N_1^* = N_1^*(\sigma).
\end{aligned} \tag{3.2}$$

Here $\sigma = m/s$, and $N_1^*(\sigma)$ is the positive root of the equation

$$d(N_1^*) = 1-2m. \tag{3.3}$$

It is seen that migration results in the arrival of two new steady-states (points 4 and 5), which the isolated population did not have. Since $p_1, p_2 \in [0, 1]$, these states appear only when $\sigma<0\,(s<0)$, that is when unstable polymorphism takes place in isolated populations (the so-called "disruptive selection"). On the other hand, since the subradicand expression is to be positive, there is the lower bound for $\sigma: \sigma>-1/4$, or $s<4m$. There is a natural constraint for $|s|: |s| \leqslant 1\,(\beta \geqslant 0)$, whence immediately follows the necessary existence condition for these equilibria: $m<1/4$. Interestingly, the steady-state sizes of both populations, determined by (3.3), in contrast to the case of isolated populations, are independent of s, being governed only by the intensity of migration. From (3.3) there follows still another constraint for m:

$$m < (1-d(0))/2. \tag{3.4}$$

Thus we can say that under sufficiently low connectedness between populations (weak intensity of migration) in conditions of disruptive selection in each of the niches the system of linked population almost necessarily develops two new (as against the case if isolated populations) types of equilibria.

Let us analyze the stability of equilibria from (3.2). The matrix of linearized system has the form

$$\left\| \begin{matrix} sA_1-m & m & a_{13} & 0 \\ m & sA_2-m & a_{13} & 0 \\ a_{31} & a_{32} & -2_m-b & 0 \\ a_{41} & a_{42} & a_{43} & -b \end{matrix} \right\|, \tag{3.5}$$

where

$$A_i = [1-6p_i^* + 6(p_i^*)^2],$$

$$a_{13} = m(p_1^* - p_2^*), \quad a_{3i} = 2s(1-2p_i^*), \quad i = 1, 2,$$

$$b = d'(N_1^*)N_1^*.$$

One of the eigenvalues of this matrix, $\lambda_4 = d'(N_1^*)N_1^*$, is always negative, since $d'(N)>0$. The stability of steady states 1,2 and 3 is defined by the eigenvalues of matrices

$$\left\| \begin{matrix} s-m & m \\ m & s-m \end{matrix} \right\| \text{ and } \left\| \begin{matrix} -s/2-m & m \\ m & -s/2-m \end{matrix} \right\|,$$

since $\lambda_3 = [2m + d'(N_1^*)N_1^*]<0$. Obviously, when $s>0$ points 3 is stable and points 1 and 2 are unstable. For $s<0$ we get the converse situation: points 1 and 2 are stable, points 3 is unstable.

The eigenvalues of (3.5) for points 4 and 5 are as follows:

$$\lambda_1 = s+4m, \tag{3.6}$$

$$\lambda_{2,3} = \frac{1}{2}[(s-b)+4m \pm \sqrt{(s+b)^2+16mb}\,],$$

$\lambda_4 = -b, b = d'(N_1^*)N_1^*.$

And finally, points 4 and 5 are stable if

$$a)s < -4m, \quad b)(s+6m)b < 2(s+2m)m. \tag{3.7}$$

Since $s+2m<0$ (due to condition a), for b) to hold it is necessary that $s<-6m$, that is the existence domain for stable polymorphism in the space of parameters $\{s, m\}$ is still more constricted.

Since $s<-6m$, we have $|\sigma|=|m/s|<1/6$. Under weak migration and sufficiently strong selection $|\sigma|\ll 1$. Therefore, condition b) from (3.7) can be approximately replaced by

$$b > 2(1+4|\sigma|). \tag{3.8}$$

On the other hand

$$d'(N_1)N_1 \approx \frac{\Delta d}{\Delta N_1/N_1},$$

whence it readily follows that besides the condition $|s|>6m$ (which always holds under weak migration and strong selection) for the population to develop stable divergence we need that

$$\Delta d > (\Delta N_1/N_1)2(1+4|\sigma|) \tag{3.9}$$

at equilibrium. If we still strengthen the inequality (3.9), setting $|\sigma|=1/6$, then

$$\Delta d > 3.4\Delta N_1/N_1. \tag{3.10}$$

In other words, one of the sufficient conditions for the existence of stable divergence between populations is the strong regulation of populations with respect to their sizes, when competitive mortality grows at a rate, by far exceeding the relative growth rate of the population.

As a concrete example consider the so-called "hyperbolic" type of regulation, when $d(N_1)=\gamma N_1^{\nu}$, $\gamma, \nu>0$. For $\nu=1$ we get the logistic rule of the variations of the population numbers, widely used in models of population growth in environments with limited resources.

Calculating $d'(N_1^*)$ and N_1^*, we obtain $b=\nu(1-2m)$. Substituting in (3.7b) we immediately get the lower bound for ν:

$$\nu > 2(s+2m)/[(1-2m)(s+6m)], \tag{3.11}$$

or for small m:

$$\nu > 2(1+2m+4|\sigma|). \tag{3.12}$$

For instance, for $m=0.1$ and $s=-0.7$ it follows from (3.11) that $\nu>25$, and for $m=0.01$ and $s=-0.7$ we get $\nu>2.17$. Even for every small m for a stable genetic divergence we need that $\nu>2$. The logistic rule of regulation ($\nu=1$) cannot ensure stability of migrational polymorphism. Consequently not every ecological mechanism, controlling the size of the population, can ensure the divergent evolution in a system of two linked populations – this mechanism needs to be sufficiently strong.

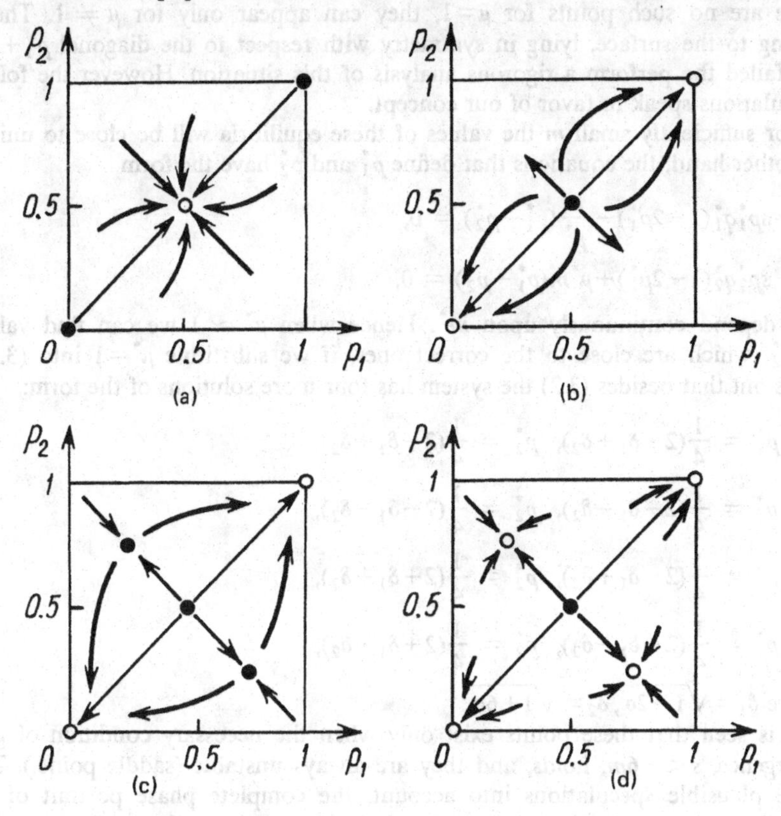

Fig. 26. Projection of the phase portraits of system (3.1) onto the plane $\mu=1$.

Figure 26 a,b,c displays the projections of phase trajectories of system (3.1) onto the plane $\mu=1$, considered in the vicinity of the steady states (3.2) for various relations between s and m. For $s>0$ (Figure 26a) there is only one stable point $p_1^*=p_2^*=1/2$ in the square $p_1, p_2 \in [0, 1]$ and all trajectories are to converge to this point. In other words, under stabilizing selection the system of linked populations can have only one state of polymorphism. For $-4m<s<0$ only the 'pure' genetic states with $p_1^*=p_2^*=0$ and $p_1^*=p_2^*=1$ will be stable; the point $p_1^*=p_2^*=1/2$ is unstable, and there is no other steady states (Figure 26b). If $s<-4m$, but (3.7b) is not satisfied, then still only the corner points will be stable, however new steady states, which are saddle points, appear inside the square (Figure 26c). And lastly, for $s<-4m$ and when (3.7b) holds points 4 and 5 become stable knots (Figure 26d).

The last phase portrait suggests an idea, that in this case there should exist some other steady states of the saddle type, their 'branches' being the separatrices, bounding the domains of attraction for the stable equilibria of the system. Since there are no such points for $\mu=1$, they can appear only for $\mu \neq 1$. They will belong to the surface, lying in symmetry with respect to the diagonal $p_1+p_2=1$. We failed the perform a rigorous analysis of this situation. However the following speculations speak in favor of our concept.

For sufficiently small m the values of these equilibria will be close to unity. On the other hand, the equations that define p_1^* and p_2^* have the form

$$sp_1^*q_1^*(1-2p_1^*)-\frac{m}{\mu^*}(p_1^*-p_2^*) = 0, \tag{3.13}$$

$$sp_2^*q_2^*(1-2p_2^*)+\mu^*m(p_1^*-p_2^*) = 0,$$

and depend continuously upon m^*. Hence when $\mu^* \approx 1$ we can find values of p_1^*, p_2^*, which are close to the correct ones, if we substitute $\mu^*=1$ into (3.13). It turns out that besides (3.2) the system has four more solutions of the form:

$$1.\quad p_1^* = \frac{1}{4}(2+\delta_1+\delta_2),\ p_2^* = \frac{1}{4}(2-\delta_1+\delta_2), \tag{3.14}$$

$$2.\quad p_1^* = \frac{1}{4}(2+\delta_1-\delta_2),\ p_2^* = \frac{1}{4}(2-\delta_1-\delta_2),$$

$$3.\quad p_1^* = \frac{1}{4}(2-\delta_1+\delta_2),\ p_2^* = \frac{1}{4}(2+\delta_1+\delta_2),$$

$$4.\quad p_1^* = \frac{1}{4}(2-\delta_1-\delta_2),\ p_2^* = \frac{1}{4}(2+\delta_1-\delta_2),$$

where $\delta_1=\sqrt{1-2\sigma}, \delta_2=\sqrt{1+6\sigma}$.

It is seen that these points exist only when the necessary condition of genetic divergence, $s<-6m$, holds, and they are always unstable (saddle points). Taking these plausible speculations into account, the complete phase portrait of stable genetic divergence (projected onto the plane $\mu=1$) apparently can be presented as in Figure 27.

7.4. On 'Fast' and 'Slow' Variables in Systems of Linked Populations

Going back to system (3.1), assume that both s and m are small and $|s| \approx m$. Then (3.1) can be presented in the form

$$\begin{aligned} dp_1/dt &= \epsilon f_1(p_1,p_2,\mu), \\ dp_2/dt &= \epsilon f_2(p_1,p_2,\mu), \\ d\mu/dt &= \mu[d(N_1/\mu)-d(N_1)]+\epsilon f_\mu(p_1,p_2,\mu), \\ dN_1/dt &= N_1[1-d(N_1)]+\epsilon f_N(p_1,\mu), \end{aligned} \tag{4.1}$$

where ϵ is a small parameter and functions f_1, f_2, f_μ and f_N are analytical within domain $p_1,p_2 \in [0, 1]$, $\mu>0$, $N_1>0$. Since $\dot{p}_1, \dot{p}_2 \sim \epsilon$ and $\dot{\mu}, \dot{N}_1 \sim 1$, we can say that in the system of two linked populations under weak selection and migration

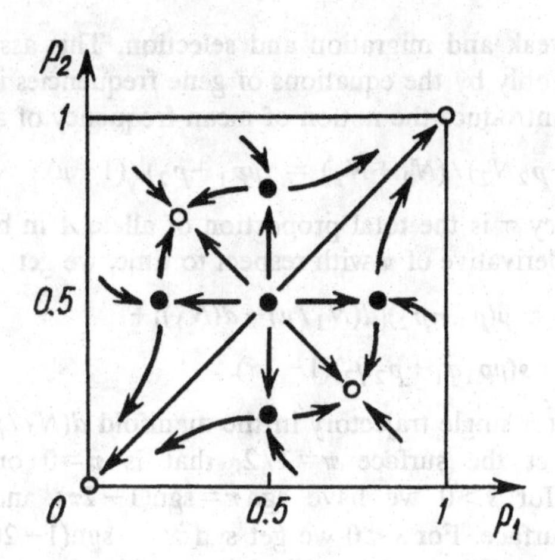

Fig. 27. A phase portrait of system (3.1) (projection onto the plane $\mu=1$) for $s<-6m$.

the variables, defining the genetic structure, are 'slow', while those, defining the sizes of the populations (that is the ecological structure), are 'fast'. Over time intervals $[0, t] \sim 1$ we have $p_1(t) \approx p_1(0), p_2(t) \approx p_2(0)$, and the dynamics of μ and N_1 is governed by the equations, we obtained from (4.1) with $\epsilon \to 0$:

$$d\tilde{\mu}/dt = \tilde{\mu}[d(\tilde{N}_1/\tilde{\mu}) - d(\tilde{N}_1)],$$
$$d\tilde{N}_1/dt = \tilde{N}_1[1-d(\tilde{N}_1)]. \tag{4.2}$$

Since $d(N)>0$ for $N\geq 0$ and $d'(N)>0$, this system has a unique stable equilibrium $\{\tilde{\mu}=1, \overset{*}{N_1}\}$, where $\overset{*}{N_1}$ satisfies the equation $d(\overset{*}{N_1})=1$. Consequently, the trajectories of (4.1) quite rapidly fall into the vicinity of the manifold $\{\tilde{\mu}=1, \overset{*}{N_1}\}$ and further on the system evolves within this vicinity.

Let us assess the rate of system's convergence to the vicinity. For this we linearize (4.2) and write out the solution to the linearized system (C_μ and C_N are constant, depending on the initial conditions)

$$\tilde{\mu} = 1 + C_\mu \exp\{-d'(\tilde{\overset{*}{N_1}})\tilde{\overset{*}{N_1}}t\},$$
$$\tilde{N}_1 = \tilde{\overset{*}{N_1}} + C_N \exp\{-d'(\tilde{\overset{*}{N_1}})\tilde{\overset{*}{N_1}}t\}. \tag{4.3}$$

Whence it is seen that the greater the magnitude of $d'(\tilde{\overset{*}{N_1}})\tilde{\overset{*}{N_1}}$, the quicker the system reaches the vicinity of the manifold. For instance, under the 'hyperbolic' type of regulation, when $d(N)=\gamma N^\nu$, $\gamma, \nu>0$, this index is equal to ν, which is actually the intensity of regulation. Therefore we can think that under strong ecological regulation to the convergence is sufficiently quick.

Since further evolution of the system will mostly results from genetic mechanism, we can describe it using only the first two equations from (3.1), setting $\mu \equiv 1$. Therefore, in what follows we shall often assume (always stipulating it) that sufficiently powerful ecological regulation mechanism operate in systems of linked populations, quickly bringing the system to an ecological equilibrium, which cannot be disturbed by weak and migration and selection. This assumption allows us to describe evolution only by the equations of gene frequencies in each of the populations. Let us now introduce the notion of mean frequency of allele A in the system:

$$\pi = (p_1 N_1 + p_2 N_2)/(N_1 + N_2) = (\mu p_1 + p_2)/(1+\mu). \tag{4.4}$$

The mean frequency π is the total proportion of allele A in both populations. Calculating the total derivative of π with respect to time, we get

$$(1+\mu)d\pi/dt = \mu(p_1 - p_2)[d(N_1/\mu) - d(N_1)] + \\ + s(\mu p_1 q_1 + p_2 q_2)(1-2\pi). \tag{4.5}$$

Hence, there is not a single trajectory in the manifold $d(N_1/\mu) = d(N_1)$, i.e. $\mu = 1$, which can intersect the surface $\pi = 1/2$, that is $\dot{\pi} = 0$ on this surface. Since $\mu p_1 q_1 + p_2 q_2 > 0$, for $s > 0$ we have $\operatorname{sgn} \dot{\pi} = \operatorname{sgn}(1-2\pi)$ and all trajectories are attracted to this surface. For $s < 0$ we get $\operatorname{sgn} \dot{\pi} = -\operatorname{sgn}(1-2\pi)$ and all trajectories are 'repulsed' from it. Whence it readily follows, that the straight line, obtained at the intersection of planes $\mu = 1$ and $p_1 + p_2 = 1$, is a separatrix. When $-4m < s < 0$ it separates the domains of attraction of the stable equilibria $p_1^* = p_2^* = 0$ and $p_1^* = p_2^* = 1$ (see Figure 26,b).

7.5. Genetic Interpretation. Why Stable Divergence is Important in Systems of Linked Populations

In isolated populations disruptive selection (fitness of the heterozygote is lower than those of both homozygotes) always results in the elimination of one of gametes. Consequently, in this case divergence between isolated populations can occur, when diverse forms are fixed in different population. However entirely isolated populations are very scare in nature, therefore, naturally the question arises: "What happens in a system of populations linked by a flow of migrants, even if it is weak?" "Can this system possibly develop a stable polymorphism?"

Why is this problem so important for the evolution theory? The point is that according to the hypothesis of allopatric speciation, in a population with a restricted panmixia (for instance, deviations from panmixia due to certain isolating geographical barriers) even is selection is the same, stable genetic divergence can appear, giving rise to new species.

On the other hand, apparently it is the disruptive selection, which fixes various gametes in different populations, their hybrids being less viable. This process can be regarded as the origin of reproductive isolation. As shown by T. Dobrzhansky, individuals, mating with unlike forms, produce less offspring than the individual mating with those alike. Eventually, the probability of mating is defined by the genotypes of the parental couple, and therefore there appears the factor of selection directed towards the fixation of reproductive isolation. Thus, it still remains to find out: "Can stable divergence occur in a system of populations linked by a two-way flow of migrants?"

Our analysis proved that this divergence can exist, but it cannot be provided by purely genetic mechanisms: the sizes of both populations need to be regulated with respect to density-dependent factors by a strong ecological mechanism. Hence, ecological factors essentially affect the evolutionary processes, and this is another arguments in favor of extending and complementing the classical models of population genetics.

7.6. Systems of Weakly Linked Populations

Consider a natural generalization of the preceding two-population models for the case of r populations. Suppose that migration is weak, and the ecological mechanisms, specific for each population, acting on all genotypes with no differentiation, quickly bringing the population to an equilibrium with respect to numbers. Let us think that the only effect of migration is the violation of local panmixia with each of the populations. The fact that usually organisms prefer not to mate with 'strangers', speaks in favor of this assumption. Then in order to describe the system of r populations we can well use the model of Section 6.7 as presented by (6.8.3). But here we will change it a bit, assuming that each population is characterized by its own pressure of selection, specified by the coefficients α_i, β_i and γ_i, $i=\overline{1,r}$. Taking into account that

$$\sum_{j=1}^{r} k_{ij} = 1,$$

one can rewrite (6.8.3) in the form

$$\frac{dp^i}{dt} = p^i[w_p^i(0)-w^i(0)] - \sum_{\substack{j=1\\ j\neq i}}^{r} k_{ij}\{p^i[\alpha_i(p^i-p^j)+\beta_i(q^i-q^j)-$$

$$-\alpha_i p^i(p^i-p^j)-\beta_i p^i(q^i-q^j)-\beta_i q^i(p^i-p^j)-\gamma_i q^i(q^i-q^j)]+ \qquad (6.1)$$

$$+\frac{\beta_i}{2}(p^i-p^j)\},\quad i=\overline{1,r},$$

$$w_p^i(0) = \alpha_i p^i + \beta_i p^i + \beta^i q^i,\quad w^i(0) = \alpha_i(p^i)^2 + 2\beta_i p^i q^i + \gamma_i(q^i)^2.$$

Obviously, the coefficients of deviations from panmixia k_{ij} are closely related to the characteristics of the migration flows between populations; the less the $k_{ij}(i\neq j)$, the less the intensity of migration, the weaker the links between populations. Suppose the links are weak, that is $k_{ij}(i\neq j)$ is of the order of magnitude of $\epsilon\ll 1$. Besides, suppose that selection is also weak, i.e. $\alpha_i=1+\hat{\alpha}_i$, $\beta_i=1+\hat{\beta}_i$, $\gamma_i=1+\hat{\gamma}_i$, $\hat{\alpha}_i$, $\hat{\beta}_i$, $\hat{\gamma}_i\sim\epsilon\ll 1$. (Let us remark, that weak selection is in no contradiction with the assumption about the existence of strong ecological mechanisms acting without differentiation.) Then from (6.1) to an accuracy of $o(\epsilon)$, we obtain:

$$\frac{dp^i}{dt} = p^i[w_p^i(0) - w^i(0)] - \frac{1}{2}\sum_{\substack{j=1\\ j\neq i}}^{r} k_{ij}(p^i - p^j), \quad i = \overline{1, r}. \tag{6.2}$$

Comparing (6.2) with (2.5), we can say that the quantity $k_{ij}/2$ defines the intensity of migration from the ith population to the jth one; naturally we can denote it by m_{ij}.

Consider two situations: the first one – when all populations are in similar conditions, and the second one is when conditions are different.

If all populations are in similar conditions, then $\alpha_i = \alpha$, $\beta_i = \beta$ and $\gamma_i = \gamma$ for all $i = \overline{1, r}$. Consequently, without the migration the steady-states in all the populations may be the same: $(p_0^i)^* = p_0^*$. Obviously, p_0^* will be equilibria for linked populations, that is $(p^i)^* = p_0^*$ is also the steady-state solution to system (6.2). Certainly, additional solutions can appear (as it was exampled by the system of two populations). Linearizing (6.2) in the vicinity of the steady state, we arrive at a system with matrix $\mathbf{A} = \mathbf{D}_r + \mathbf{M}_r$, where $\mathbf{D}_r$ is a diagonal matrix with equal elements: $\mathbf{D}_r = \mathrm{diag}\{d_i\} = \mathrm{d}I$,

$$d_i = d = \left\{ \frac{\partial}{\partial p^i}[p^i[w_p^i(0) - w^i(0)]] \,|_{p_0^*} \right\}, \quad i = \overline{1, r},$$

and $\mathbf{M}_r$ is the migration matrix with elements

$$M^{ij} = m_{ij} (i \neq j); \quad M^{ii} = -\sum_{\substack{j=1\\ j\neq i}} m_{ij}, \quad i, j = \overline{1, r}.$$

Suppose we know the eigenvalues μ_k, $k = \overline{1, r}$ for matrix $\mathbf{M}_r$. Necessarily there will be one zero value among them, since $\sum_{j=1}^{r} M^{ij} = 0$. On the other hand, since any vector is the eigenvector for the identity matrix I, the eigenvalues of $\mathbf{A}$ are equal to $\lambda_i = \mu_i + d$. Consequently, if the equilibrium $(p_0^i)^* = p_0^*$ for the isolated populations is unstable, then this instability will also remain in the system of linked populations, since one of the λ_i will be equal to $d > 0$. In other words, migration has no stabilizing effect upon the system.

If the isolated equilibrium were stable ($d < 0$), then we need the information about other (non-zero) eigenvalues of matrix $\mathbf{M}_r$ in order to answer the question about stability of the equilibria in the system of linked populations. Let us treat one particular example.Suppose that the areas linked by migration make up a circular pattern (Figure 28), all the intensities being the same and equal to m. Then matrix $\mathbf{M}_r$ is a circulant:

$$M_r = \left\| \begin{matrix} -2m & m & 0 & \cdots & 0 & m \\ m & -2m & m & \cdots & 0 & 0 \\ \cdots & \cdots & \cdots & \cdots & \cdots & \cdots \\ m & 0 & 0 & \cdots & m & -2m \end{matrix} \right\|,$$

which eigenvalues are

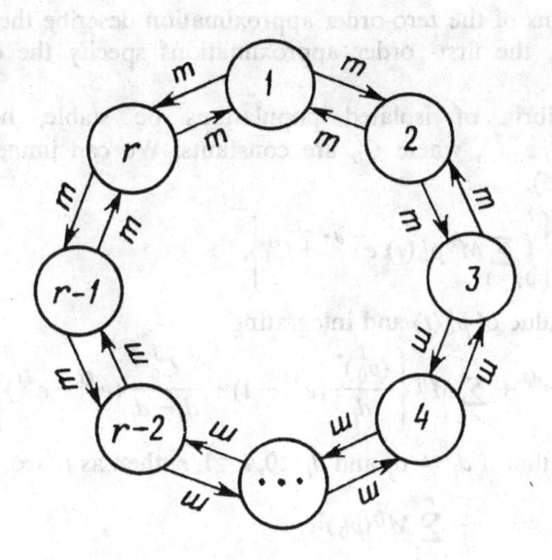

Fig. 28. Circular structure of a system of r populations linked by migration

$$\mu_i = -2m(1-\cos\frac{2\pi(i-1)}{r}), \quad i = \overline{1, r}.$$

All the eigenvalues μ_i are negative, except for μ_1 which is zero. Consequently, stability is not deteriorated when isolated populations are linked into a system in this way, and previously stable equilibria in isolated populations remain to be stable in a system of linked populations.

Let now the isolated populations be in a different conditions, each having its own state of equilibrium $(p_0^i)^*$. These can be either "pure" states with $(p_0^i)^*=0$ or $(p_0^i)^*=1$ or polymorphisms $(p_o^i)^*=(\beta_i-\gamma^i)/(2\beta_i-\gamma_i-\alpha_i)$. Denote $\max_{i,j,i\neq j} m_{ij}=\mu$ and regarding μ as a small parameter, let us seek for the solution to (6.2) in the form of an expansion in powers of μ:

$$p^i = p_0^i + \mu p_1^i + \cdots \tag{6.3}$$

Substituting (6.3) into (6.2) and equating the terms with the same powers of μ, we get

a) $$\frac{dp_0^i}{dt} = p_0^i[\tilde{w}_p^i(0) - \tilde{w}^i(0)], \tag{6.4}$$

$$\tilde{w}_p^i(0) = \alpha_i p_0^i + \beta_i q_0^i, \quad \tilde{w}^i(0) = \alpha_i (p_0^i)^2 + 2\beta_i p_0^i q_0^i + \gamma_i (q_0^i)^2,$$

b) $$\frac{dp_1^i}{dt} = d_i p_1^i + \sum_{j=1}^{r} M^{ij} p_0^i, \quad d_i = \left\{\frac{\partial f^i}{\partial p^i}\,|_{(p_0^i)^*}\right\}, f_i = p^i\{w_p^i(0) - w^i(0)\}.$$

$$i = \overline{1, r}. \tag{6.5}$$

While the equations of the zero-order approximation describe the dynamics of isolated populations, the first- order approximations specify the correction arising from migration.

Let the equilibria of isolated populations be stable, hence $d_i<0$ and $p_0^i(t) \approx (p_0^i)^* + C_0^i e^{-d_i t}$, where C_0^i are constants. We can immediately write out the solution to (6.5):

$$p_1^i(t) = e^{d_i t}\left\{\int_0^t \sum_{j=1}^r M^{ij} p_0^j(\tau)\, e^{-d_i \tau} + C_1^i\right\},$$

or, inserting the value of $p_0^i(t)$ and integrating

$$p_1^i(t) = C_1^i e^{d_i t} + \sum_{j=1}^r M^{ij}\left\{\frac{(p_0^j)^*}{d_i}(e^{d_i t}-1) + \frac{C_0^j}{d_j - d_i}(e^{d_j t} - e^{d_i t})\right\}. \tag{6.6}$$

Whence it is seen that if $d_i \neq d_j$ and $d_i<0$, $i=\overline{1, r}$, then as $t \to \infty$,

$$p_1^i(t) \to (p_1^i)^* = -\frac{1}{d_i}\sum_{j=1}^r M^{ij}(p_0^j)^*. \tag{6.7}$$

Thus the effect of migration displaces the equilibria of isolated populations by the quantity

$$(p_1^i)^* = -\frac{1}{d_i}\sum_{j=1}^r M^{ij}(p_0^j)^* = \frac{1}{d_i}\sum_{\substack{j=1\\ j\neq i}} m_{ij}[(p_0^i)^* - (p_0^j)^*], \tag{6.8}$$

and if the isolated equilibria were stable, then the equilibria in linked populations will be stable as well (for a sufficiently low extend of linkage).

Let the populations be enumerated so that $(p_0^1)^* > (p_0^2)^* > \cdots > (p_0^r)^*$. Then, as it follows from (6.8), $(p_1^1)^* < 0$, $(p_1^r)^* > 0$, i.e. in a system of weakly linked populations the maximal distance between two extreme steady states is less than in the system of isolated populations.

The displacement of steady states in weakly linked populations promotes the appearance of new polymorphic states, even if the isolated populations were 'pure'. For instance, if $(p_0^1)^* = 1$ and $(p_0^r)^* = 0$ then $(p^1)^* < 1$ and $(p^r)^* > 0$, that is populations become polymorphic. Thus in such a system of linked populations the steady states are pulled together towards some average state and and hence the total heterogeneity of the system is reduced. The system of linked populations is more homogeneous, more ordered than the system of that same populations when they are isolated.

One should note that the results obtained can be extended for more general cases with no principal difficulties (for more general rules of inheritance, for multiple alleles, etc.). The appropriate explanations can be found in the Notes to this Section.

7.7. Populations with Continuous Area (Spatially Distributed Populations)

Up till now we have been studying either the isolated populations with common dynamics at all the points of their areas, or systems of populations linked by migration, occupying discrete areas, with the population dynamics being again independent of the locality chosen inside the area. However any organism has its own radius of individual activity and can move in space. If this radius is greater than the distance between discrete areas, then the unified population can be regarded as a system of 'point' populations with migration between 'points'. If the radii of individual activity are small as against the specific dimensions of the area occupied by the population, then we are to assume the model of a spatially distributed population. In nature such a continuous type of inhabitance of vast territories by organisms of one species can be encountered, apparently, as often as the 'local' one.

Suppose that within the time interval between birth and reproduction each organism of the ith type at random moves in some direction (all directions are equiprobable) covering a certain distance. Then if $\phi_i(r)\mathrm{d}r$ is the probability that the size of displacement lies between r and $r+\mathrm{d}r$, we say that

$$\rho_i = \sqrt{\int_0^\infty r^2\phi_i(r)\,\mathrm{d}r}$$

is the mean square displacement, which is usually known in biology as the radius of individual activity. In this way one can calculate it, proceeding from the experimental data.

Let N_i be the density of ith genotype (or gene). If we now characterize the dynamics of N_i at the point by the equations (x and y are the spatial coordinates)

$$\mathrm{d}N_i/\mathrm{d}t = f_i(N_i, \ldots, N_n, x, y),\ i = \overline{1, r}, \tag{7.1}$$

then the increment of the density in the space due to migration and local growth will be equal to

$$\Delta N_i = \int\int_{-\infty}^{+\infty} N_i(x', y')\frac{\phi_i(r)}{2\pi r}\mathrm{d}x'\,\mathrm{d}y' - N_i(x, y) + f_i(N_1, \ldots, N_n, x, y),\quad i = \overline{1, n},$$

$$r = \sqrt{(x-x')^2+(y-y')^2}.$$

Expanding N_i into a Taylor series in powers of $x-x'$ and $y-y'$ and assuming that for the third moments we have

$$\int_0^\infty |\, r^3 \,|\, \phi_i(r)\,\mathrm{d}r \ll \rho_i^2,$$

we can restricts ourselves to the second-order terms in this expansion. Then we can obtain the approximate diffusion type equations in order to describe the evolution of a spatially distributed population:

$$\partial N_i/\partial t = D_i\Delta N_i + f_i(N_1, \ldots, N_n, x, y),\quad i = \overline{1, n}. \tag{7.2}$$

Here

$$\Delta = \partial^2/\partial x^2 + \partial^2/\partial y^2, D_i = \rho_i^2/4.$$

If we assume that there exists a spatially homogeneous steady-state solution to (7.2), then it should comply with the equations $f_i(N_1^*, \ldots, N_n^*)=0, 1=\overline{1,n}$ (there should be no explicit relation between f_i and x, y). Suppose that there is no migration, that is $D_i \equiv 0$. Then the stability of this equilibrium at each point of this space (local stability) is connected with the analysis of the eigenvalues of matrix $\| a_{ij} \| = \| \partial f_i / \partial N_j |_{N^*} \|$. Problems of this kind have been treated up to now. But besides the local temporal perturbations there is a large class of spatial perturbations. Consider perturbations of the form

$$N_i = N_i^* + N_i^0 \cos(k_1 x + k_2 y + \theta) e^{\lambda^D t}. \tag{7.3}$$

In the presence of migration a locally stable solution may turn to be unstable with respect to the perturbations (7.3). In this case the problem is reduced to the eigenvalue analysis for matrix $\| a_{ij} - D_i k^2 \delta_{ij} \|$, where $k = \sqrt{k_1^2 + k_2^2}$ is the wave number of spatial perturbations, δ_{ij} is the Kronecker symbol. And if for a certain value of k^* there appears an eigenvalue with a positive real part, then the amplitudes of all perturbations with the wave number k^* will be growing, i.e. there appears the typical phenomenon of instability, which we shall call *diffusive*. This instability destroys the originally spatially homogeneous distribution. It is quite likely that further development of this process (increases in the amplitude of the perturbations at some points of spatial periodic structure) can result in a collapse of the genetically homogeneous population, of the stable genetic divergence, producing a 'patchy' genetic distribution over a uniform area.

Let all genotypes be characterized by similar mobilities, that is $D_i = D$. Then $\lambda_i^A = \lambda_i^D + Dk^2$, if λ_i^A are the eigenvalues of $\| a_{ij} \|$ and λ_i^D are the eigenvalues of $\| a_{ij} - Dk^2 \delta_{ij} \|$. Whence it is readily seen that if all $\mathrm{Re}\lambda_i^A$ are negative, then $\mathrm{Re}\lambda_i^D$ are negative all the more, that is if equilibrium is locally stable, then migration can only contribute to its stability. Suppose now that there is a positive λ_p^A, that is local equilibrium is unstable. However, this equilibrium will be stable with respect to spatial perturbations with wave numbers $k^2 > (\max_i \mathrm{Re}\lambda_i^A)/D$. Stability of this type will be termed *diffusive stability* or *stabilization by migration*. One can see that migration is most effective in damping short-period spatial perturbations.

From these speculations it already follows that migration results in essentially new effects when we have local instability, say, under disruptive selection. For a more meaningful analysis let us look at a spatially distributed population, with inheritance governed by one diallele gene, with homozygote fitness being equal, and lower fitness of the heterozygote. The numbers are controlled by an ecological mechanism, independent of genetic factors. Then, if there is no dominance, the local equations for numbers of alleles A and a (N_1 and N_2, respectively) can be written in the form

$$\mathrm{d}N_1/\mathrm{d}t = N_1[1 + sN_2/N - d(N)] = f_1(N_1, N_2),$$

$$dN_2/dt = N_2[1+sN_1/N-d(N)] = f_2(N_1, N_2), \qquad (7.4)$$
$$N = N_1+N_2.$$

By our assumptions $\alpha=\gamma=1$, $\beta=1+s$, $s<0$.

For ease of presentation we consider a bounded one- dimensional area of length L, so that $0\leqslant x\leqslant L$. The pressure of selection is the same over the whole area, that is $s=\text{const}$, the radius of individual activity is also the same for all genotype over the whole area. The boundaries of the area will be thought to be absolutely isolating, that is no individual can cross them.

Keeping all this in mind, we can represent the model as the following task: find $N_1(x, t)$ and $N_2(x, t)$, satisfying the equations

$$\partial N_i/\partial t = D\partial^2 N_i/\partial x^2 + f_i(N_1, N_2), i = 1, 2, \qquad (7.5)$$

and boundary conditions

$$\partial N_i/\partial x = 0 \text{ for } x = 0, L, \ i = 1, 2, \qquad (7.6)$$

and some initial conditions, their concrete form being specified below.

It is a simple matter to verify, that the quantity $n^*=N_1^*=N_2^*=\text{const}$, where n^* is the root of the equation $d(2n^*)=1+s/2$, turns out to be the solution to (7.5), satisfying (7.6). If we now calculate the eigenvalues of $\| a_{ij} \|$ for this case ($\lambda_1^A=-s/2, \lambda_2^A=-2b, b=d'(2n^*)n^*$), then obviously the equilibrium is locally unstable ($d'(2n^*)>0$, since the mortality function should grow with increases in number). It is known rather well, that without migration and under lower fitness of heterozygotes polymorphism is unstable.

Let now migration be present. In the vicinity of the equilibrium n^* let us seek for the solution in the form $N_1(x, t)=n^*+N_1^0 \cos kx\, e^{\lambda^D t}$, $N_2(x, t)=n^*+N_2^0 \cos kx\, e^{\lambda^D t}$, where $\lambda_1^D=-s/2-k^2D$, $\lambda_2^D=-2b-k^2D$; N_1^0, N_2^0 are constants defined by the initial conditions. Let us note that choosing such a form for the solution we determine the class of initial conditions (this class is wide enough). The boundary conditions (7.6) imply that $k=m\pi/L$, $m=0, 1, 2, \ldots$

Then for any k greater than $\sqrt{|s|/(2D)}$ we have $N_1(x, t)\to n^*$, $N_2(x, t)\to n^*$ as $t\to\infty$, that is the equilibrium n^* becomes stable with respect to a certain type of spatial perturbations. There appears the effect of migrational stabilization of equilibrium — it becomes diffusively stable.

Since $k=m\pi/L$, the condition of diffusive stability can be written in the form

$$L < m\pi\sqrt{2D/|s|} = m\pi\rho/\sqrt{2|s|}. \qquad (7.7)$$

On the other hand the form of the initial perturbation is characterized by the expressions $N_i(x, 0)=n^*+N_i^0 \cos(m\pi x/L)$. For $m=0$ we obtain a perturbation which is uniform over the whole area. Since L is positive, it follows from (7.7) that for any length of the area, equilibrium n^* is unstable with respect to perturbations of this type. For $m=1, 2, \ldots$ we obtain spatially heterogeneous perturbations. Obviously when $L<\pi\sqrt{2D/|s|}$, all these perturbations are damped. Thus the value $L_{cr}=\pi\sqrt{2D/|s|}=\pi\rho/\sqrt{2|s|}$ defines the maximal size of the area, over which migration damps all spatially heterogeneous perturbations.

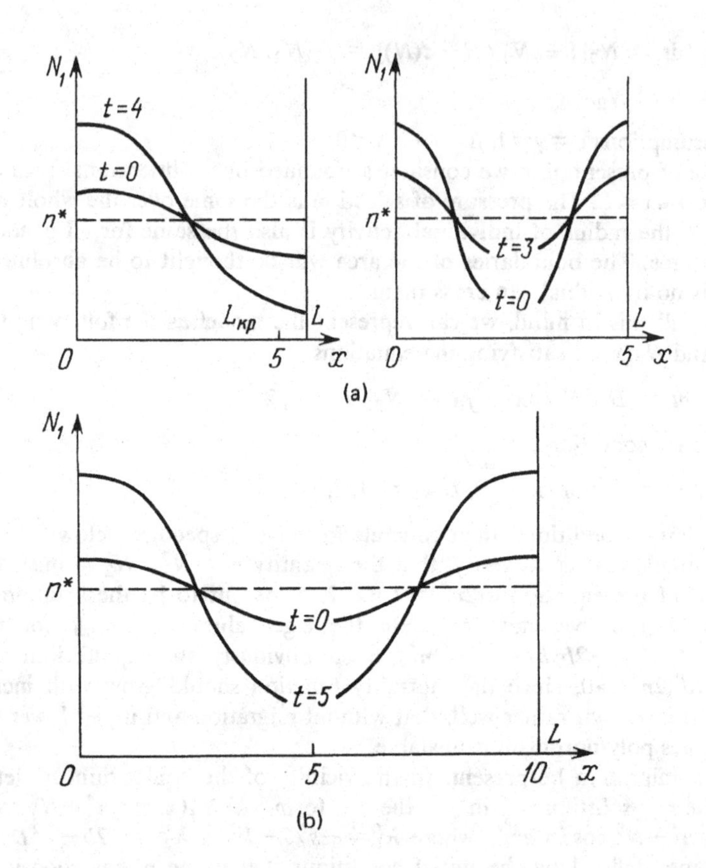

Fig. 29. Initial stage of the arrival of spatially heterogeneous structures for different area sizes and various forms of perturbations when $\rho=1$ and $s=0.25$.

Let us now suppose that $L_{cr}<L<2\pi\sqrt{2D/|s|}$. Here migration can no longer damp the perturbations of the form $N_i(x,0)=n^*+N_i^0\cos(\pi x/L)$, and their amplitude begins to grow exponentially. The effect of diffusive instability springs up, and regions with different genic content and different numbers appear over the homogeneous area. However, smaller-scale perturbations (higher harmonic) are still damped by migration (Figure 29a). Further increases of the area raise the amplitude of higher harmonics, the area becomes 'patchy' (Figure 29b).

Hence, migration acts as a kind of a filter, which transmits and amplifies large-scale spatial perturbations and damps perturbations of lower scales. It is clear that this may produce a 'patchy' structure, characterized by different numbers of organisms and various gene concentration in different localities of the ecologically uniform area. However, it should be noted that the phenomenon of diffusive instability (stability) describes only the initial stage, the starting mechanism for the spatial heterogeneity over a uniform area. As to its fixation and the origination of stable spatial structures, the linear analysis gives no solutions to this problem. Actually in this case we deal with branching of solutions at the bifurcation point $k_{cr} = \sqrt{|s|/(2D)}$ and we are to employ other methods (non- linear ones) in order to analyze this problem. For instance, we can already state that stability of these structures is essentially dependent on the type of ecological regulation, that is on the definite form of the function $d(N)$.

7.8. 'Genic' Waves in Spatially Distributed Populations

Once again, as in Section 6, let us think that migration is weak, that ecological mechanism, independently of genetic factors, maintain the same population size at equilibrium, and that the only effect of migration is the disturbed panmixia. Then for a population distribute over an infinite one-dimensional uniform area $(-\infty < x < +\infty)$ with inheritance controlled by one diallele gene, the genetic evolution can be well described by the model of Section 6.8 (Equation (6.8.2)):

$$\partial p / \partial t = (\sigma^2/4)\partial^2 p / \partial x^2 + p(w_p - w), \tag{8.1}$$

$$w_p = \alpha p + \beta q,\ w = \alpha p^2 + 2\beta pq + \gamma q^2,\ \alpha, \beta, \gamma = \text{const.}$$

Comparing this model with those of the previous Section, we see that the index of deviations from panmixia σ can be identified with the radius of individual activity.ρ.

Therefore let us think that $\sigma = \rho$ and the diffusion coefficient $D = \rho^2/4 = \sigma^2/4$.

In a classical work by A.N. Kolmogorov, I.G. Petrovsky, and N.S. Piskunov* it has been shown that for the equation

$$\partial p / \partial t = D\partial^2 p / \partial x^2 + f(p),$$

where $p \in [0, 1]$; $f(p)$ is a continuous function, which can be differentiated as many times as necessary, and which complies with the conditions

$$f(0) = f(1) = 0; f(p) > 0, 0 < p < 1;$$

$$f'(0) = a > 0; f'(p) < a, 0 < p \leqslant 1, \tag{8.2}$$

there is a solution

$$p(x, t) = p(x + vt),$$

which is a wave that propagates from the right to the left at a rate v. The initial distribution is to have the form of a step function, that is $p(x, 0) = 0$ for $x < x^*$ and $p(x, 0) = 1$ for $x \geqslant x^*$. Furthermore, as $t \to \infty$ the propagation velocity of the front,

* Kolmogorov A.N., Petrovsky, I.G., and Piskunov, N.S.: 1937, 'Issledovanije uravnenija diffuzii, soedinennoi s vozrastaniem veshestva, i jevo primenenije k odnoi biologiceskoi probleme (Analysis of the equation of diffusion, connected with the mounting amount of material, and application of this equation to a biological problem. In Russian)'. *Bjulleten MGU, Seria A. Mathematica i mehanika*, **1**, 6, 1-26

v, approaches (from below) its limit value $v^* = 2\sqrt{aD}$, and its form tends to the limiting form $\hat{p}(x)$, defined by the solution to the equation

$$v^* \mathrm{d}\hat{p} / \mathrm{d}x = D \, \mathrm{d}^2\hat{p} / \mathrm{d}x^2 + f(\hat{p}), \tag{8.3}$$

with boundary conditions $\hat{p}(-\infty)=0$ and $\hat{p}(+\infty)=1$. Such a solution always exists and it is unique up to the transformation $x' = x + c$, which does not change the form of the wave. Let us apply these results to (8.1). First we check for which α, β and γ the function $f(p)=p(w_p - w)$ complies with (8.2). Loosing no generality, we can set $\gamma=1$, and suppose that $\alpha=1+h$, $\beta=1+s$. Then

$$f(p) = p(1-p)[s+(h-2s)p],$$
$$f'(p) = s+2(h-3s)p-3(h-2s)p^2. \tag{8.4}$$

The condition that $f(p)=0$ only at 0 and 1 is then $h \geqslant s$. $f'(0)=s$, consequently, $s>0$. And finally, the condition $f'(p)<s$ for $0<p\leqslant 1$ implies that $h\leqslant 3s$. Therefore, for (8.2) to be satisfied it is necessary and sufficient that $0<s\leqslant h\leqslant 3s$. In this case a 'genic' wave spring up, its propagation velocity being equal to $2\sqrt{sD}$ or $\rho\sqrt{s}$. For this wave to appear it is necessary and sufficient that the fitness of homozygote *aa* be less than the fitness of other genotypes ($0<s\leqslant h$ or $\gamma=1<\min\{\alpha, \beta\}$), while the fitness of homozygote *AA* be greater than *Aa* ($s\leqslant h$ or $\alpha \geqslant \beta$). However the distinction in fitness between *AA* and *Aa* should not be too high ($h\leqslant 3s$ or $\alpha\leqslant 3\beta-2$). In other words the origination of this wave requires a positive selection in favor of allele A, but this selection should not be too strong.

What is this wave? Suppose that initially there exists a vast domain with the concentration of allele A being close to unity. Along the boundaries of this domain there is a transitional zone of intermediate concentrations, the concentration being close to zero beyond this zone. Due to positive selection and migration the domain of $p \approx 1$ will expand, the transitional zone will move towards the territories with $p \approx 0$ at a rate $\rho\sqrt{s}$, the zone itself still being characterized by intermediate concentrations. This picture is what we call the 'genic' wave. Curiously enough, the propagation velocity of this wave is governed only by the fitness of the heterozygote. Thus, even if the fitness of the homozygote *AA* is high as against *Aa* (but not too high, $\alpha\leqslant 3\beta-2$), then for a weakly expressed selective advantage of the heterozygote (as against *aa*) the propagation rate of the wave will be low.

As an example let us look at the case of the dominating allele A. Then $\alpha=\beta>1$ and correspondingly, $h=s>0$. In this case there will always be a 'genic wave', and the width of its intermediate zone can be estimated as follows. From the equation for the form of the wave (8.3), changing the variables for $\xi = \sqrt{s}\,x/\rho$ we get the dimensionless form

$$\mathrm{d}\hat{p} / \mathrm{d}\xi = (1/4)\,\mathrm{d}^2\hat{p} / \mathrm{d}\xi^2 + \hat{p}(1-\hat{p})^2 \tag{8.5}$$

with the same boundary conditions. Whence it is clear that the width of this transitional zone is in proportion to $L=\rho/\sqrt{s}$.

Let us give a concrete example. Observations showed that the radius of individuals activity for the flies *Drosofila funebris* is $\rho=11m$ per one generation, and the selection coefficient for a normal homozygote and a heterozygote with respect to the recessive mutation *scarlet* under moderate temperatures ($\sim 24°C$) is equal to $s=0.064$. Then $v^*=2.78m$ per generation and $L=43.5m$.

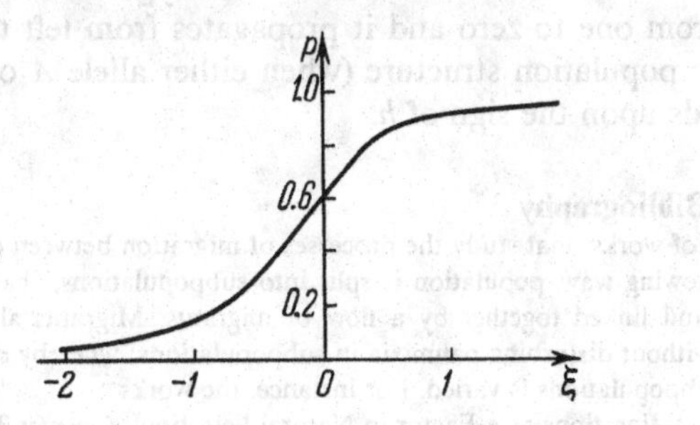

Fig. 30. Graph of the limiting wave for $p(-\infty)=0$ and $p(+\infty)=1$.

Figure 30 contains the graph of the limiting wave,obtained by integration of (8.5) with $p(-\infty)=0$ and $p(+\infty)=1$.

And in conclusion let us briefly go into the following problems. Can waves of this type spring up, if in the local case we have stable or unstable polymorphism? What happens when even under the favorable selection of allele A its pressure is too high ($h \geqslant 3s$)? (the latter implies, that there is a point $0<\tilde{p}<1$, such that $f'(\tilde{p})>f'(0)$). For instance, for $h=3s$ the propagating at a rate $v_0=2\sqrt{s}$ (which is the velocity of the Kolmogorov–Petrovsky–Piskunov wave) will be stable.

For $h \geqslant 4s$ the velocity $v=h/\sqrt{2(h-2s)}$ is the minimal velocity at which the stable wave can propagate. If the selective advantage of homozygote AA as against the heterozygote Aa is markedly pronounced ($h \gg 2s$), then $v \approx \sqrt{h/2}$, and the propagation velocity of the genetic wave will be defined by the selective parameters of homozygotes AA, rather than by the selective advantage of heterozygotes. Note that $v=v_0=2\sqrt{s}$ for $h=4s$ and for $h>4s$ we always have $v>v_0$.

If $s>h\geqslant 0$, that is if the heterozygote Aa is most fit, then there may exist the two so-called 'transfer waves': one from the state $p_0^*=0$ into the polymorphism state with $p_1^*=s/(2s-h)$, and another from the state $p_2^*=1$ into the same polymorphic state. One can show that both these waves will be of the Kolmogorov–Petrovsky–Piskounov type, but while the first one propagates at a rate $v_1=s\sqrt{s}$, the other one has the velocity $v_2=2\sqrt{s-h}$.

And lastly, let $s<0$, $|s|>|h|$, that is the heterozygote Aa is worse fit. In this case there appears a wave that propagates at the only velocity $v=h/\sqrt{2(h+2|s|)}$. Depending upon the sign of the integral $I=\int_0^1 f(p)\,dp$ it will be either the transfer wave from $p_0^*=0$ to $p_2^*=1$, or backwards (for the initial stepwise frequency distribution). Calculating this integral for our particular case, we get

$$I = \int_0^1 \{sp+(h-3s)p^2-(h-2s)p^3\}\,dp = \frac{h}{12}.$$

Whence one can see that if $h>0$, i.e. when the fitness of homozygote AA is higher than that of homozygote aa, then the transfer wave from zero to one appears in the population and its propagates from right to left. Otherwise, if $h<0$, i.e. the fitness of homozygote AA is lower than that of homozygote aa, then there appears the transfer wave from one to zero and it propagates from left to right. Consequently, the final genetic population structure (when either allele A or allele a is present in the area) depends upon the sign of h.

7.9. Notes and Bibliography

There is quite a lot of works, that study the processes of migration between populations. Usually models are built in the following way: population is split into subpopulations, characterized by different pressures of selection and linked together by a flow of migrants. Migrants alter the numbers in various genotypic groups, without disturbing panmixia in subpopulations; whereby due to migration the average fitness of each of subpopulations is varied. For instance, the works

Parsons, P.A.: 1963, 'Migrations as a Factor in Natural Selection', *Genetics* **33**, 3, 184–206;

Edwards, A.W.: 1963, 'Migration Selection', *Heredity* **18**, 1, 101-106,

concentrates on models of migration between two populations with various probabilities of migration between them. Unfortunately, modeling directly in gene frequencies, with no preliminary analysis of models in numbers, results in models being inadequate to their own biological meaning. The stable steady states derived in these works are in fact semi-stable in the entire phase space, including the ration of the two population sizes besides the gene frequencies.

In the paper:

Malecot, G.: 1965, 'Evolution continue des frequences d'ungene mendelien (dans le cas migration homogene entre groupes d'effectife fini constant)', *Ann. Inst. H. Poincare* **2** 2, 137--150,

where the probability of migration is assumed to be the same for all groups, the effect of different numbers in subpopulations is taken into account by weighting them in proportion to their effective sizes.

Starting from the work:

Levene, H.: 1953, 'Genetic Equilibrium When More Than One Ecological Niche is Available', *Amer. Nat.* **87**, 836, 331–333,

consideration is given to models of a population, split into several subpopulations linked by a flow of migrants, each of them occupying its own ecological niche (different pressures of selection correspond to different niches). In the paper:

Deakin, M.A.B.: 1968, 'Genetic polymorphism in a Subdivided Population', *Austr. J. Biol. Sci.* **21**, 1, 165–168,

general conditions for stability of polymorphism in n niches are derived. The different sizes of subpopulations were taken into account by weighting the migration probabilities in proportion to the subpopulation sizes. Unfortunately, the weighting coefficients were considered to be constant, though (as it follows from the made above direct deduction of the equations) they depend on the dynamics of the process itself, which makes them essentially variable. In order that all these models be correct, it is necessary to assume that there is an additional mechanism (in no way appearing in the model), which maintains constant sizes of subpopulations.

There may also be another approach, when effects of migration are assumed to be disturb panmixia only, by no means affecting the total population sizes. This approach was widely used in this Chapter.

To 7.2, 7.3.

Various migration schemes and the appropriate models have been studied in the already cited work:

Svirezehv, Yu.M.: 1972, *Mathematical Models in Population Genetics (Matematicheskye modeli b populyatsionnoi genetike)*, Review by the author of the doctor's thesis, Institute of Biophysics, Acad. of Sci., U.S.S.R., Pushino (In Russian).

The book:

Frisman, E.Ya., and Shapiro, A.P.: 1977, *Selected Models of Divergent Evolution of Populations*

(*Izbranniye mathematicheskiye modeli divergentnoi evolutsyi populyatsiy*), Nauka, Moscow (in Russian), 149,p.,
is concerned with mathematical modeling of the divergent evolution of populations (mostly exampled by two populations).

To 7.5.
Genetic aspects of migration are elaborated on in the book:
Dobzhansky, T.: 1951, *Genetics and the Origin of Species*, Columbia Univ. Press, New York.

To 7.6.
Here we mostly follow the lines of the paper:
Svirezhev, Ju.M.: 1968, 'The Systems of Weakly Connected Populations', *Studia Biophysica* **10**, 1, 25–30.
Generalizations for more complicated cases can be derived, applying the approach formulated in
Svirezhev, Yu.M., Logofet, D.O.: 1983, *Stability of Biological Communities*, Mir, Moscow, (pp. 291–317.
In case the populations are in similar conditions (identical ecological niches), the generalizations are easily derived by applying the techniques of Kronecker products. If the ecological niches are different, then the small parameter method is most effective. This approach (for discrete models) is exampled in the works:
Karlin, S. and McGregor, J.: 1972, 'Application of Method of Small Parameters to Multi-Niche Population Genetic Models', *Theor. Pop. Biol.* **3**, 2, 186–209;
Karlin, S. and McGregor, J.: 1972, 'Polymorphism for Genetic and Ecological Systems With Weak Coupling', *Theor. Pop. Biol.* **3**, 2, 210–238.

To 7.7.
The notion of the radius of individual activity has been introduced in the work:
Timoféeff–Ressovsky, N.V. and Yu.M. Svirezhev: 1967, 'On Opposite Pressures of Selection on the Genotype and on the Character of a Sex-Linked Mutation (0 protivopolozhnykh davleniyakh otbora na genotip i na priznak u mutatsii, stseplennoi s polom)', *Problems of Cybernetics* (*Problemy Kibernetiki*) **18**, 155–170. (in Russian).
When deriving the equations of population dynamics over a continuous area, we followed the method set forth in the above cited work by A.N. Kolmogorov, I.G. Petrovsky and N.S. Piskunov.
As a regards the various aspects of diffusive instability arising in population systems, see the book by Svirezhev and Logofet, pp. 317–328.

To 7.8.
The problem about the dynamics of allele concentrations in space and in time under the impact of selection and migration has been first studied in two papers, which appeared almost simultaneously:
Fisher, R.A.: 1937, 'The Wave of Advance Advantageous Genes', *Ann. of Eugenics* **7**, 355-369,
and the above cited work by Kolmogorov, Petrovsky and Piskunov. It should be noted, that Fisher failed to present the complete solution to the problem, while the paper by Kolmogorov *et al.* contained a complete and mathematically rigorous treatment of this problem. Unfortunately, authors, who know nothing about this publication, still suggests the problems completely solved in this work as topics of investigation. As an example we can mention Chapter 9 of the book, which is quite good in the large:
Moran, P.A.P.: 1962, *The Statistical Processes of Evolutionary Theory*, Clarendon Press, London, 200.p..
More recent works of J. Haldane and R. Fisher:
Haldane, J.B.S.: 1948, 'The Theory of Cline', *J. Genetics* **48**, 277-284;
Fisher, R.A.: 1950, 'Gene Frequencies in a Cline Determined by Selection and Diffusion', *Biometrics* **6**, 3, 353–361,
treated the cases when selection differs at different localities of the one-dimensional area. J. Haldane, for instance, showed that the genetic divergence can take place over an area such that selection favors different alleles at different localities. Both papers elaborate on the conditions, which make the diffusive description valid in populational problems, and elucidate the biological sense of the diffusion coefficient.
These problems are further generalized in the work:
Montroll, E.W.: 1967, 'On Nonlinear Processes Involving Population Growth and Diffusion', *J. Appl. Probab.* **4**, 2, 281–290.

An interesting attempt to derive genetic divergence in a diffusive mode of a population over a continuous uniform area is contained in the work:

Bazykin, A.D.: 1970, 'On the Effect of Disruptive Selection upon a Spatially Extended Population (0 deistvii disruptivnovo otbora na prostranstvenno protyazhennuyu populyatsiyu)', *Problems of Evolution*, **2**, 215–225 (in Russian).

Numerous problems, connected with the applications of the non-linear diffusion equations to biological (mostly ecological topics), can be found in the book:

Fife, P.C.: 1979, *Mathematical Aspects of Reacting and Diffusing Systems*, Springer, Berlin, 185 p.

At present this book can be considered to be the most systematic account of problems on non-linear diffusion.

Interestingly, when we deal with unstable polymorphism, there can exist a stable 'genic' wave. However, unlike the Kolmogorov – Petrovsky – Piskunov wave, where there is a continuous spectrum of wave velocities, bounded from below by $v^* = 2\sqrt{Df'(0)}$ (it is a different matter, that the only stable wave is the one with $v = v^*$), in this case the wave velocity is unique. For more details see:

Kanel, Ya.I." 1960, 'On the Behavior of the Solutions to the Cauchy Problem under Infinite Time Growth for Quasi- Linear Equations Encountered in Combustion Theory (0 povedenii resheniy zadachi Koshi pri neogranichennom vozrastanii vremeni dlya kvazilineinykh uravneniy, vstrechayushikhsya v teorii goreniya)', *Reports of the Academy of Science* **132**, 2, 268–271.

The problem from the combustion theory, studied in this paper, is quite similar to the problem of population genetics. Most different examples of genic waves are treated in detail in the book:

Svirezhev, Yu.M.: 1987, *Nelineinyi volny, dissipativnyi struktury i katastrofy v ecologii* (*Non-Linear Waves, Dissipative Structures and Catastrophes in Ecology*. In Russian), Nauka, Moscow, 366 pp.

Chapter 8

Population Dynamics in Changing Environment

8.1. Introduction

Up till now in all the models considered the environment where the population evolves, was assumed to be invariable. The environmental effects in our models were characterized only by the coefficients of the relative viability, therefore they were considered to be dependent neither on time (the environment is invariable in time), nor on gene frequencies. The latter implies that we do not treat the so-called 'genotypic environment', the pressure of selection being independent of the concentrations of particular genotypes in the population. Otherwise the population in evolution makes up its 'genotypic environment', and since the pressure of selection is a function of gene frequencies, the 'genotypic environment', in turn, determines further population dynamics. The arrival of this feedback can result in most unexpected effects, for instance a stable state may be substituted by a similar but unstable one.

Looking at various types of this dependence, we come to a multitude of interesting problems, which we however leave beyond the framework of this book. We shall mostly bring into focus those cases, when the coefficients of relative viability are either explicit functions of time (for instance, they are periodic functions of time with the period determined by seasonal climatic variations), or depend on the total population size. The latter case has been already encountered in the preceding Chapter; here we shall treat some other versions of this dependence as well.

8.2. Seasonal Oscillations in Coefficients of Relative Viability. Discrete Model

Consider a large enough panmictic population with one diallele gene. Let the genotype fitness be periodic, varying from one generation to another (generations do not overlap) so that, say, for genotype *AA* we have

$$\alpha_0 = \alpha_2 = \alpha_4 = ..., \alpha_1 = \alpha_3 = \alpha_5 = ..., \alpha_0 \neq \alpha_1 \tag{2.1}$$

Similar correlations hold for the other two fitnesses. Thus it is assumed that the durations of seasons coincide with the span of generations, and seasons alternate together with generations.

In this case the equations of populations dynamics can be represented in the form

$$p_n = \frac{p_{n-1} + [(\alpha_{n-1} - \beta_{n-1})p_{n-1} + \beta_{n-1}]}{w_{n-1}} = f_{n-1},$$

$$p_{n+1} = \frac{p_n\,[(\alpha_n - \beta_n)\,p_n + \beta_n]}{w_n} = f_n,\; n = 1, 3, 5, \ldots, \tag{2.2}$$

$$w_k = (\alpha_k - 2\beta_k + \gamma_k)\,p_k^2 + 2\,(\beta_k - \gamma_k)\,p_k + \gamma_k,\; k = 0, 1, 2, \ldots$$

Let us solve these equations graphically, applying the 'Lamerey diagram' (see Section 3.6). Introduce the following notations:

$$\frac{p[(\alpha_0 - \beta_0)p + \beta_0]}{(\alpha_0 - 2\beta_0 + \gamma_0)p^2 + 2(\beta_0 - \gamma_0)p + \gamma_0} = f(p),$$

$$\frac{p[(\alpha_1 - \beta_1)p + \beta_1]}{(\alpha_1 - 2\beta_1 + \gamma_1)p^2 + 2(\beta_1 - \gamma_1)p + \gamma_1} = F(p).$$

The solution will be constructed on coordinates $\{p, p'\}$ corresponding to the gene frequencies in two successive generations. By $\tilde{F}(p)$ denote the function $p = F(p')$ which is in symmetry to $F(p)$ with respect to the straight line $P' = p$.

Consider the following variants of correlations between $f(p)$ and $\tilde{F}(p)$:

a) Let $f(p)$ and $\tilde{F}(p)$ intersect once at point p^* inside the unit square, so that

$$f(p) > \tilde{F}(p) \text{ for } p \in (0, p^*),$$

$$f(p) < \tilde{F}(p) \text{ for } p \in (p^*, 1). \tag{2.3}$$

The solution to (2.2) is constructed the way it is shown in Figure 31a, where the solution is derived for the case when (2.3) is satisfied, and besides $\alpha_0 > \beta_0 > \gamma_0$, $\alpha_1 < \beta_1 < \gamma_1$. It is seen from the Figure that the solution oscillates, and it can be proved that there is a limit cycle ($A_1A_2A_3A_4$) with the half-period being equal to the generation span. If we now draw the graphs of $f(p)$ and $\tilde{F}(p)$ on the plane $\{p, p'\}$, then by the method represented in Figure 31b, one of the envelopes for the total solution can be traced (the sequence $p_0, p_2, p_4, \ldots$ instead of $p_0, p_1, p_2, \ldots$). This is a speedy method to find the limit states for system (2.2), but we are to keep in mind, that in this case non-trivial limit points actually correspond to limit cycles (point Q stands for the cycle $A_1A_2A_3A_4$). The limit cycles appear, firstly, because the direction of selection is different in different seasons: initially selection is advantageous for allele A, in the next season - for allele a, and, secondly, since the action of selection is markedly asymmetric, the curves

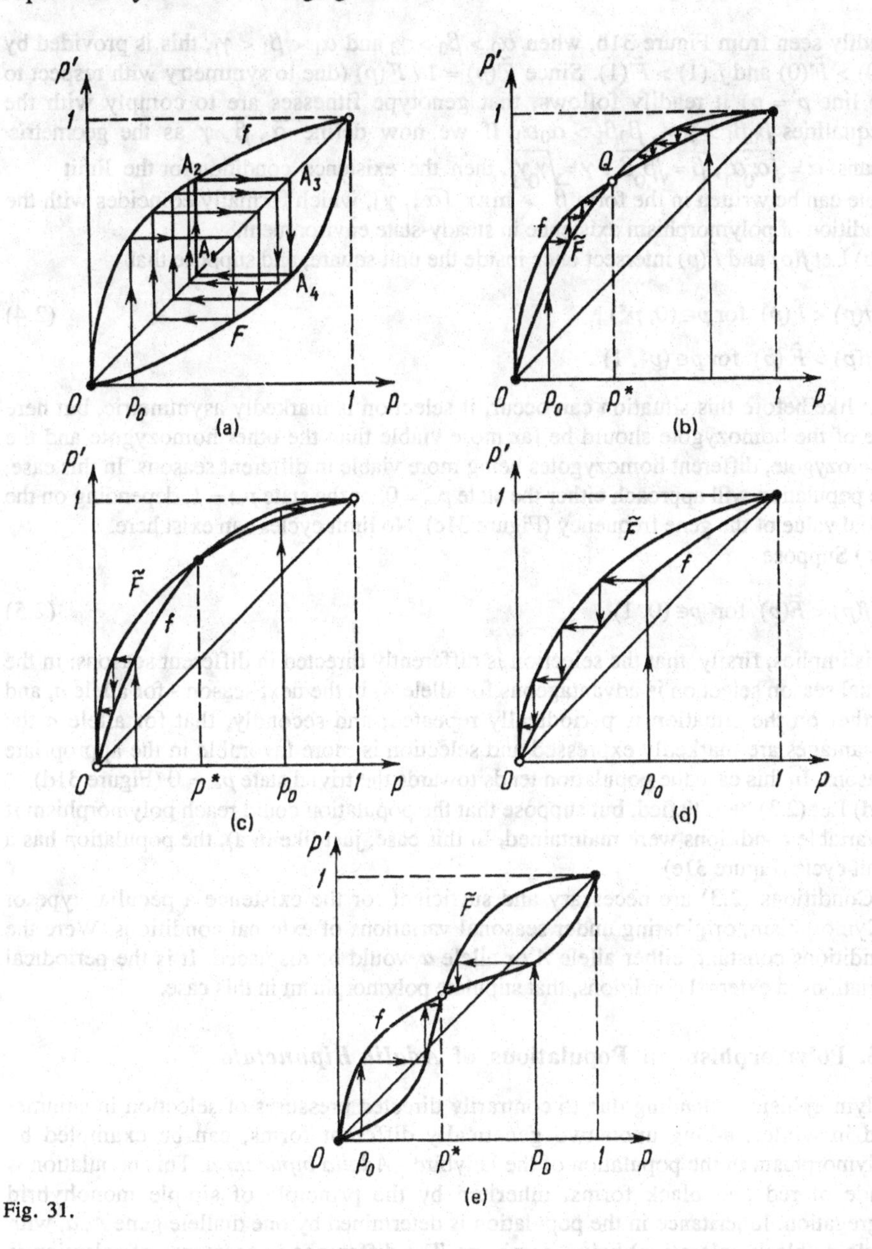

Fig. 31.

$f(p)$ and $\tilde{F}(p)$ intersecting, as a result. Such a situation can take place, when, for instance, one of the homozygotes and the heterozygote are far more viable than the other homozygote, different homozygotes being more viable in different seasons. As it is readily seen from Figure 31b, when $\alpha_0 > \beta_0 > \gamma_0$ and $\alpha_1 < \beta_1 < \gamma_1$, this is provided by $f'(0) > \tilde{F}'(0)$ and $f'(1) > \tilde{F}'(1)$. Since $\tilde{F}'(p) = 1 / F'(p)$ (due to symmetry with respect to the line $p' = p$) it readily follows, that genotype fitnesses are to comply with the inequalities $\beta_0\beta_1 > \gamma_0\gamma_1$, $\beta_0\beta_1 > \alpha_0\alpha_1$. If we now define $\bar{\alpha}$, $\bar{\beta}$, $\bar{\gamma}$ as the geometric means: $\bar{\alpha} = \sqrt{\alpha_0\alpha_1}$, $\bar{\beta} = \sqrt{\beta_0\beta_1}$, $\bar{\gamma} = \sqrt{\gamma_0\gamma_1}$, then the existence condition for the limit cycle can be written in the form $\bar{\beta} > \max\ [\bar{\alpha}, \bar{\gamma}]$, which formally coincides with the condition of polymorphism existence in steady-state environment.

b) Let $f(p)$ and $\tilde{F}(p)$ intersect once inside the unit square, and suppose that

$$f(p) < \tilde{F}(p) \quad \text{for } p \in (0, p^*)\,, \tag{2.4}$$
$$f(p) > \tilde{F}(p) \quad \text{for } p \in (p^*, 1)\,.$$

Just like before this situation can occur, if selection is markedly asymmetric, but here one of the homozygote should be far more viable than the other homozygote and the heterozygote, different homozygotes being more viable in different seasons. In this case, the population will approach either the state $p_\infty = 0$, or the state $p_\infty = 1$, depending on the initial value of the gene frequency (Figure 31c). No limit cycles can exist here.

c) Suppose

$$f(p) < \tilde{F}(p) \quad \text{for } p \in (0, 1)\,. \tag{2.5}$$

This implies, firstly, that the selection is differently directed in different seasons: in the initial season selection is advantageous for allele A, in the next season - for allele a, and further on the situation is periodically repeated; and secondly, that for allele a the advantages are markedly expressed and selection is more favorable in the appropriate seasons. In this case the population tends towards the trivial state $p_\infty = 0$ (Figure 31d).

d) Let (2.3) be satisfied, but suppose that the population could reach polymorphism if invariable conditions were maintained. In this case, just like in a), the population has a limit cycle (Figure 31e).

Conditions (2.3) are necessary and sufficient for the existence a peculiar type of polymorphism, originating under seasonal variations of external conditions. Were the conditions constant, either allele A or allele a would be displaced. It is the periodical variations in external conditions, that stipulate polymorphism in this case.

8.3. Polymorphism in Populations of *Adalia Bipunctata*

Polymorphism, extending due to contrarily directed pressures of selection in summer and in winter, acting upon two genetically different forms, can be exampled by polymorphism in the population of the ladybird - *Adalia bipunctata*. This population is made of red and black forms, inherited by the principle of simple monohybrid segregation. Inheritance in the population is determined by one diallele gene A, a, with allele A (black coloration) being dominant. The difference in pressures of selection is determined by different relative viabilities of the black and red forms in different seasons of the year. Black forms have advantages (apparently, their birth rate is higher) during the summer vegetation period, while the red ones survive winter better.

Periodic time variations in coefficients of relative viability stipulate the origination of a peculiar state of polymorphism (the one predicated theoretically in the previous Section), related to forced oscillations in the system. This type of polymorphism will be termed adaptive.

One and the same natural population of *Adalia bipunctata* has been observed for more than a decade. As a result the coefficients of relative viability could be assessed for various forms in different seasons of the year, and the trajectory of the population could be constructed to describe the variations of its genetic content under the effect of contra-directed pressures of selection. Since allele *A* dominates, we may think that the relative viability of the homozygote *AA* is equal to that of the heterozygote *Aa*. In the vegetation period Adalia usually yields three generations, mostly the third one going into winter. Let us think that one pressure of selection effects the two summer generations, and another one affects the wintering generation; then genotype fitnesses can be regarded as periodic functions with one-year periods. The fitnesses calculated for experimental data are contained in the Table.

Winter	$\alpha=\beta$; $\gamma=1$	Summer	$\alpha=\beta=1$; γ	Winter	$\alpha=\beta$; $\gamma=1$	Summer	$\alpha=\beta=1$; γ
1	0.38	I	0.415	7	0.51	VII	0.66
2	0.32	II	0.78	8	0.605	VIII	0.74
4	0.34	IV	0.47	9	0.545	IX	0.85
5	0.26	V	0.40	10	0.50	X	0.61
6	0.29	VI	0.775	11	0.56	XI	0.55

In order to illustrate the interpopulational polymorphism of Adalia bipunctata, we can make use of the values from the Table to construct the phase trajectory of the dynamical system, characterizing the variations in the frequency of gene *A* for the population effected by contra-directed pressure of selection (Figure 32). Roman numerals stand for the summer seasons, the Arabic ones - for the winter; the dotted line indicates the omitted phase cycle of the winter season III and summer season 3, where experimental data are missing.

It is seen from the phase picture, that the system oscillates with a one-year period around a slowly drifting center, which is shifted apparently due to alterations of the annual average climatic conditions; since the climatic conditions are somewhat periodic, the center can be considered to drift around a certain state of equilibrium, and consequently such a state of polymorphism can be assumed to be stable. On the other hand, in this particular case

$$f(p) = \frac{p}{1 + \lambda q^2}, q = 1 - p, \lambda = \frac{1-\alpha}{\alpha};$$

$$F(p) = \frac{p(1 - \delta q^2)}{(1 - \delta q^2)^2 - \delta q^2 (1 - \delta q^2)^2}, q = 1 - p, \delta = 1 - \gamma$$

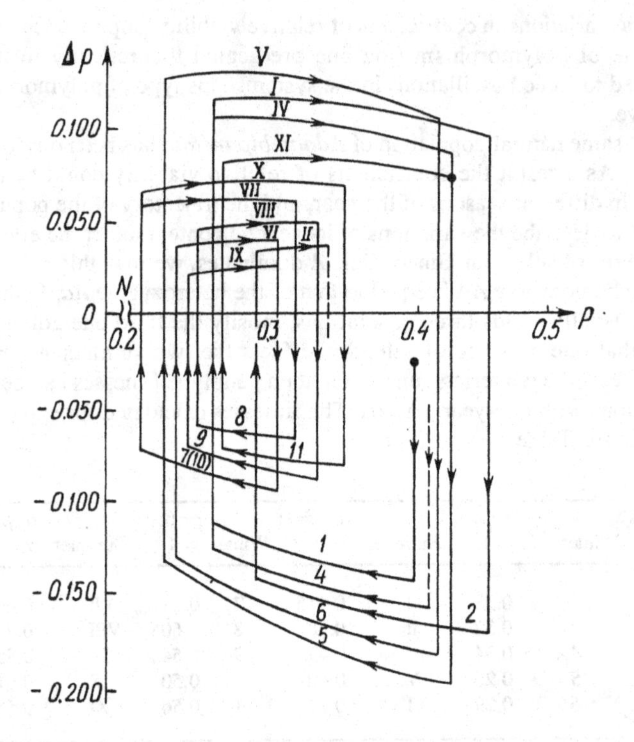

Fig. 32. Phase portrait of *Adalia bipunctata.*

(since two generators elapse during summer). Direct examination proves that (2.3) is almost always satisfied. Whence it follows that our assumption about polymorphism being stable in populations of *Adalia bipunctata* is correct.

While previously polymorphism was related to a stable steady-state point of the system, in this case we connect polymorphism with the existence of a stable limit cycle, and the state of polymorphism is defined by a whole domain. In external environmental conditions were invariable, then the system would be polymorphically unstable (the stable states are $p^* = 0$ and $p^* = 1$). But seasonal environmental variations ensure the existence of a stable polymorphic state. We can say that intrapopulational polymorphism in *Adalia bipunctata* is provided by different fitness of various genotypes to external conditions in winter and in summer seasons, and therefore we can call it 'adaptative polymorphism'.

8.4. Environment Changing with Time. Continuous Model

The simplest model of non-stationary environment is presented by genotype fitness explicitly depending on time. Consider a continuous model for the population with inheritance determined by one gene with multiple alleles (see Section 4.1):

$$dp_i/dt = p_i(w_i - w) \tag{4.1}$$

$$w_i = \sum_j w_{ij}p_j,\ w = \sum_i w_i p_i,\ i, j = \overline{1, n},$$

where the fitnesses $w_{ij} = w_{ij}(t)$. Suppose that $w_{ij}(t) = w^0_{ij} + \omega_{ij}(t)$, where w^0_{ij} are constant. Then (4.1) can be written in the form

$$dp_i/dt = F_i(p_1, ..., p_n) + R_i(p_1, ..., p_n, t), \tag{4.2}$$

where

$$F_i = p_i(\sum_i w^0_{ij} p_j - \sum_{i,j} w^0_{ij} p_i p_j),$$

$$R_i = p_i(\sum_i \omega_{ij}(t) - \sum_{i,j} \omega_j(t) p_i p_j)$$

Let $\omega_{ij}(t) \equiv 0$. In this case the population may have the state of equilibrium $\{p^*_i;\ i = \overline{1, n}\}$, their stability (asymptotic stability) being defined by the form of matrix $\| w_{ij} \|$ (see Section 4.7). Suppose that an equilibrium $\{p^*_i;\ i = \overline{1, n}\}$ is asymptotically stable for $\omega_{ij}(t) \equiv 0$. Then by the theorem about stability under permanent perturbations*, this equilibrium will be also stable for $\omega_{ij}(t) \neq 0$, but only if $| R_i |$ and, consequently, $|w_{ij}(t)|$ are sufficiently small. In other words, for $|w_{ij}(t)| << w^0_{ij}$, once getting into sufficiently small vicinity of the equilibrium, trajectories of (4.1) stay there. And this by no means implies, that if $\omega_j(t) \to 0$ as $t \to \infty$ then $p_i(t) \to p^*_i,\ i = \overline{1, n}$.

However, if $\omega_{ij}(t)$ complies with the additional constraint

$$\int_0^\infty \| \Omega \| \, dt < \infty, \tag{4.3}$$

where $\| \Omega \|$ is the norm of matrix $\| \omega_{ij}(t) \|$, then $p_i(t) \to p^*_i$ as $t \to \infty$. This statement is readily proved, if the appropriate theorems from the book by R. Bellman** are applied to (4.1). Naturally the states of equilibrium $\{p^*_i;\ i = \overline{1, n}\}$ are assumed to be asymptotically stable for $\omega_{ij} \equiv 0$.

And finally, we can always state that if an equilibrium of a population is stable (asymptotically) in steady-state environment, then it will be also stable in varying environment, provided that the perturbations induced by temporal environmental variations are not too large. Of course, here we can no longer speak about asymptotic stability, however if (4.3) is satisfied, then stability will be asymptotic. For instance, if $w_{ij}(t) = w^0_{ij} + c_{ij} \exp\{-\lambda_{ij}t\}$, where w^0_{ij}, c_{ij}, λ_{ij} are constant, and $\lambda_{ij} > 0$, then $p_i(t) \to p^*_i,\ i, j = \overline{1, n}$ as $t \to \infty$, and $\{p^*_i,\ i = \overline{1, n}\}$ is a stable equilibrium for the system $p_i = F_i(p_1, ..., p_n)$, i.e. for the population in steady-state environment.

* Malkin, I.G.: 1966, *Teorija ustoicivisti dvizenija* (*Stability Theory of Motion*. In Russian), Nauka, Moscow, p.301.

** Bellman, R.: 1953, *Stability Theory of Differential Equations*, McGraw-Hill, N.Y., Toronto L., p. 85.

8.5. How Variations in the Total Size of a Population Affect its Genetic Dynamics

In many cases the sizes of the selection pressures, specified by the coefficients of genotype fitness, depend on the total population size, which essentially governs the intensity of competitive interactions under fixed environmental conditions.

Consider the simplest model - the population with inheritance determined by one diallele gene (see Section 3.5):

$$dp/dt = p(1-p)(\lambda - \delta p),$$
$$dN/dt = N[w - d(N)], \tag{5.1}$$

where

$$\delta = 2\beta - \alpha - \gamma,\ \lambda = \beta - \gamma,\ w = \gamma + 2\lambda p - \delta p^2 .$$

It is most ordinary to assume that the function $d(N)$ is linear: $d(N) = \mu N$. In Section 3.5 it was proved that $N(t) \to w(p^*)/\mu = N^*$, as $t \to \infty$, where N^* is the maximal total size of the population at equilibrium. Obviously, μ determines the carrying capacity of the environment for the population, and therefore it is quite natural to suppose that fitnesses are functions of this parameter and, hence, the total population dynamics is to effect the dynamics of the genetic structure. Furthermore, we will assume that there is a direct dependence between fitnesses and total population size.

Let the carrying capacity oscillate periodically about some average state μ^*, so that

$$\mu(t) = \mu^* + m \sin \omega t,\ m \ll \mu^*, \tag{5.2}$$

and suppose that $\alpha(N, \mu)$, $\beta(N, \mu)$ and $\delta(N, \mu)$ can be expanded into a series in the neighborhood of the equilibrium $\{N^*, \mu^*\}$. Taking the first terms of the expansions, we yield

$$\alpha = \alpha^* + K_\alpha(N - N^*) + m_\alpha(\mu - \mu^*),$$
$$\beta = \beta^* + K_\beta(N - N^*) + m_\beta(\mu - \mu^*), \tag{5.3}$$
$$\gamma = \gamma^* + K_\gamma(N - N^*) + m_\gamma(\mu - \mu^*).$$

Linearizing (5.1) in the neighborhood of the equilibrium $\{p^*, N^*, \mu^*\}$ and taking into account (5.2) and (5.3), we obtain a system of two-uniform linear equations. Their treatment implies no principal difficulties, however it is quite cumbersome. Therefore we adopt the following simplifying assumptions. Let $\alpha \equiv 1$, $\beta = \beta^* = \text{const} > 1$, $\delta^* = 1$, $m_\gamma = 0$. This means that there is not a single fitness coefficient explicitly depending on μ and only one coefficient, γ, depends on the total population size. Then

$$\frac{d}{dt}\Delta p + P_p\Delta_p = Q_p, \tag{5.4}$$
$$\frac{d}{dt}\Delta N + P_N\Delta N = R_N \sin \omega t,$$

where

$$\Delta p = p - p^*, \ \Delta N = N - N^*,$$

$$P_p = \tfrac{1}{2}(\beta^* - 1), \ P_N = \frac{\beta^* + 1}{8\mu^*}(4\mu^* - K_\gamma),$$

$$Q_p = -\tfrac{1}{8}K_\gamma \Delta N, \ R_N = -\frac{m(\beta^* + 1)^2}{4(\mu^*)^2}$$

Let us concentrate on the behavior of the solution to (5.4) when $t \to \infty$. For $K_\gamma < 4\mu^*$ we have $P_N > 0$ and $P_p > 0$ (since $\beta^* > 1$). Then after a sufficient period of time t elapses, we get

$$\Delta p \simeq \frac{mK_\gamma(\beta^* + 1)^2}{32\mu^* \sqrt{(P_N^2 + \omega^2)(P_p^2 + \omega^2)}} \sin[\omega t - (\phi_N + \phi_p)], \tag{5.5}$$

$$\Delta N \simeq -\frac{m(\beta^* + 1)^2}{4\mu^* \sqrt{P_N^2 + \omega^2}} \sin(\omega t - \phi_N), \ \mathrm{tg}\, \phi_N = \omega/P_N, \ \mathrm{tg}\, \phi_p = \omega/P_p .$$

Whence it is seen that periodic oscillations of the carrying capacity induce periodic oscillations of both the total populations and the gene frequency. However these oscillations are displaced in phase, and as it is clear from the solution, the displacement in the oscillations of the gene frequency exceeds that of the population size. While the displacement in oscillations of the populations is a function of the viability coefficients at equilibrium and the carrying capacity, as well as of the relationship between the coefficients and the total population size (in this case K_γ), the displacement in oscillations of the gene frequency depend only on the magnitude of the coefficients of relative viability at equilibrium.

If γ varies in a way such that $\delta \leq 1$, then $K_\gamma \leq 0$ and the inequality $K_\gamma < 4\mu^*$ always holds. This implies that if the necessary and sufficient polymorphism condition in steady-state environment, $\beta > \max\{\alpha, \gamma\}$, holds for any N, then the oscillations around this state of polymorphism, caused by small periodic perturbations of the carrying capacity, will always be small. The inequality $\beta(N) > \max\{\alpha(N), \gamma(N)]$ is the sufficient condition of polymorphism stability with respect to periodic perturbations of the environment (certainly, here γ is implicitly assumed to be steadily decreasing, or at least non-increasing with N).

A possible interpretation of the peculiar lag in population oscillations and, to a greater extent, in oscillations of the gene frequency is that the gene structure is a more inertial characteristic of the population, then its size. The population react to environmental perturbations first of all by changing its size and only afterwards its genic content changes.

8.6. How Periodic Variations in Coefficients of Relative Viability Affect the Total Population Size

In this Section we shall study a continuous model, which takes account of the periodic variations in fitness coefficients and considers the effect of these oscillations upon the total population size. Suppose that

$$\begin{aligned} &\alpha = \alpha^* + A \sin \omega t, \ A << \alpha^*, \\ &\beta = \beta^* + B \sin \omega t, \ B << \beta^*, \\ &\gamma = \gamma^* + \Gamma \sin \omega t, \ \Gamma << \gamma^*, \\ &\mu = \text{const}, \ \beta^* > \max\{\alpha^*, \gamma^*\}. \end{aligned} \tag{6.1}$$

Linearizing (5.1) around the steady state $\{p^* = (\beta^* - \gamma^*)/(2\beta^* - \alpha^* - \gamma^*),\ N^* = w^*/\mu\}$ we obtain

$$\begin{aligned} &\frac{d}{dt}\Delta p + P_p \Delta_p = R_p \sin \omega t, \\ &\frac{d}{dt}\Delta N + P_N \Delta N = R_N \sin \omega t, \end{aligned} \tag{6.2}$$

where

$$P_p = \frac{(\beta^* - \alpha^*)(\beta^* - \gamma^*)}{2\beta^* - \alpha^* - \gamma^*}, \quad P_N = \frac{(\beta^*)^2 - \alpha^*\gamma^*}{2\beta^* - \alpha^* - \gamma^*},$$

$$R_p = P_p \frac{A(\beta^* - \gamma^*) + B(\gamma^* - \alpha^*) + \Gamma(\alpha^* - \beta^*)}{(2\beta^* - \alpha^* - \gamma^*)^2},$$

$$R_N = P_N \frac{a(\beta^* - \gamma^*)^2 + 2B(\beta^* - \alpha^*)(\beta^* - \gamma^*) + \Gamma(\beta^* - \alpha^*)^2}{(2\beta^* - \alpha^* - \gamma^*)^2}$$

In this particular case P_p and P_N are always positive, since we assumed that there is always a stable polymorphism in the population in steady-state conditions. Then for $t \to \infty$ we have

$$\begin{aligned} &\Delta p \approx R_p \sin(\omega t - \phi_p) / \sqrt{P_p^2 + \omega^2}, \\ &\Delta N \approx R_N \sin(\omega t - \phi_N) / \sqrt{P_N^2 + \omega^2}, \\ &\operatorname{tg} \phi_p = \omega / P_p, \ \operatorname{tg} \phi_N = \omega / P_N. \end{aligned} \tag{6.3}$$

It is a simple matter to show that $P_p < P_N$ when $\{\alpha^*, \gamma^*\}$, whence it readily follows that $\phi_p > \phi_N$. This implies that even if the environmental variations primarily affect the parameters defined by the genetic structure of individuals (coefficients of fitness), and only through them the total population size is altered, even then the displacement in the oscillations of the gene frequency exceeds that in the oscillations of the population size.

In other words, in this case again the gene structure is a more inertial characteristic of the population, than its total size.

8.7. Changing Environment. Adaptation and Adaptability

In Section 3 of this chapter we have studied adaptational polymorphism in a population of one ladybird species – *Adalia bipunctata,* stipulated by different fitness of the black and red forms of these beetles in different seasons of the year. Basing on experimental data, calculations were made for the coefficients of relative viability for the black and the red forms in winter and in summer. Since frequencies of these forms in the population were also counted in the experiments, we can construct a graph to represent the variations in the average population fitness over the whole period of observations.

In order to be able to compare, we normed the fitness coefficients as follows: the

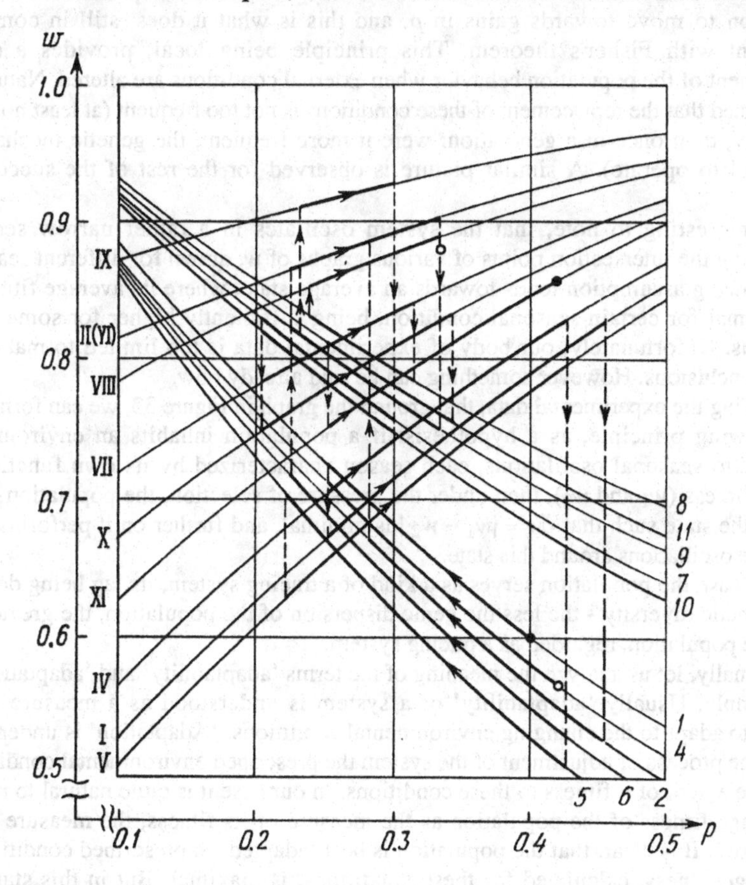

Fig. 33. Seasonal changes in the mean fitness of the population of Adalia bipunctata (1–11 – winter, I–XI – summer).

coefficients, corresponding to the most viable genotype was taken as unity, then fitnesses of other genotypes were less than (or equal to) unity. It is easily seen, that in this case the maximal value of the average population fitness is equal to unity. Figure 33 represents the graph of variations in the average fitness of the *Adalia bipunctata* population, based on the results of observations. It is clear from the Figure, that over the course of one season the average fitness grows while conditions typical for the season are maintained. Consider, say, two successive seasons: the winter season 1 and the summer season I. Starting with $p = 0.40$ the frequency of allele A goes down, since in this situation the magnitude of w, calculated for winter conditions, is increased. Everything proceeds in complete agreement with the fundamental Fisher's theorem. However, by the end of winter season, when $p = 0.254$ external conditions change, the summer season comes. Further reductions of p now results in decreasing average fitness, as calculated for the summer season. It is now more 'profitable' for the population to move towards gains in p, and this is what it does, still in complete agreement with Fisher's theorem. This principle being local, provides a quick readjustment of the population behavior when external conditions are altered. Naturally, it is assumed that the replacement of these conditions is not too frequent (at least no more frequently, then once in a generation: were it more frequent, the genetic mechanism would fail to operate). A similar picture is observed for the rest of the successive seasons.

It is interesting to note, that the system oscillates in a rather narrow section, surrounding the intersection points of various graphs of w, drawn for different seasons. The following assumption tends towards an average state, where its average fitness is not maximal for certain seasonal condition, being sufficiently higher for some other conditions. Unfortunately, our body of experimental data is too limited to make any certain conclusions. However something can be said already now.

Analyzing the experimental data, that ground the graph in Figure 33, we can formulate the following principle, as a hypothesis: if a population inhabits an environment, subjected to seasonal oscillations, each season characterized by its own function of average fitness (w_1 and w_2), then under the pressure of selection, the population tends towards the state such that $\delta w = |w_1 - w_2|$ is minimal, and further on it performs low-amplitude oscillations around this state.

In this case the population serves as a kind of a tracing system, its lag being defined by its genetic diversity - the less the genic dispersion of the population, the greater the lag of the population, regarded as a tracing system.

And finally, let us analyze the meaning of the terms 'adaptability' and 'adaptation' in our example. Usually 'adaptability' of a system is understood as a measure of its abilities to adapt to the changing environmental conditions. 'Adaptation' is understood both as the process of adjustment of the system the prescribed environmental conditions, and as the extent of it fitness to these conditions. In our case it is quite natural to regard the average fitness of the population as the measure of its fitness, the measure of its 'adaptation'. It is clear, that the population is best 'adapted' to prescribed conditions if its average fitness, calculated for these conditions, is maximal. But in this state the genetic diversity of the populations minimal, the population is least of all prepared for alternations in external conditions, and, consequently, its 'adaptability' is minimal.

Therefore it is natural to measure 'adaptability' of a population by its genic dispersion (or by some other, more suitable measure of populational genetic diversity). Whence it is readily seen, that the terms 'adaptability' and 'adaptation' stand for antipodal notions: for maximal values of 'adaptation' the 'adaptability' of the population is minimal. Apparently, in real-life populations there should be some mechanisms, providing the populations with a certain reserve of 'adaptability'. Such mechanisms may be realized in, say, more complicated laws of inheritance (polyhybrid segregation, crossingover), which impose some restrictions on the system (population), preventing it from reaching the state with the maximal degree of 'adaptation' and retaining a certain reserve of 'adaptability', as a result.

8.8. Notes and Bibliography

To 8.1.

An example of interesting and even paradoxical results that may be obtained if coefficients of relative viability are related to gene frequencies, is contained in the work:

Sacks, J.M: 1967, 'A Stable Equilibrium With Minimum Average Fitness', *Genetics* **56**, 4, 705–708.

Among numerous works, the study models with various type of relationships between genotype fitness and gene frequencies, we can mention the following:

Lewontin, R.C.: 1958, 'A General Method for Investigating the Equilibrium of a Gene Frequency in a Population', *Genetics* **43**, 4, 419–439;

Clarke, B., O'Donald, P.: 1964, 'Frequency-Dependent Selection', *Heredity* **19**, 2, 201–206.

Various aspects of population behavior in both spatially and temporally heterogeneous media are treated in the book:

Levins, R.: 1968, *Evolution in Changing Environments*, Princeton Univ. Press, Princeton, 120 pp., which is a collection of numerous papers by this author, that came to light in the period of 1958-1968 in most different journals. Levins suggested the so-called 'adaptive function' (a kind of an analogy for the Fisher's average fitness) for the averaged description of a population in heterogeneous environment. The 'adaptive function' A is to grow steadily with all the w_j (w_j is the average population fitness in j ecological niche) and is to obtain maximum at equilibrium. If π_j^m is the probability that j niche is realized in m generation, p_{ij}^m (α_{ij}) is the frequency (fitness) of genotype $\{i\}$ in j niche, then the adaptive function is chosen in the form

$$A = \exp\left\{\lim_{n\to\infty} \frac{1}{n} \sum_{m=1}^{n} \ln\left(\sum_j \pi_j^m \sum_i \alpha_{ij} p_{ij}^m \right)\right\}.$$

Actually Levins introduced the principle, which states that in heterogeneous environment the population tends to a state where the maximum is attained by the averaged characteristics of its reaction to the environment. In other words, the population constructs an internal averaged model of the environment, and further population behavior is determined just by this averaged model

In spite of its outward elegance and clearness, this concepts calls for some objections. In particular, the observations presented in Section 3 of this chapter indicates that the population traces the seasonal variations of the environment as a system with practically no memory - every time the external conditions are changed the population starts to 'adjust' itself to the new conditions, no matter what were the conditions before that. Such a behavior results in cycles. Nevertheless it is quite plausible that certain averaging mechanisms operates within the population. Special experiments, set forth in the work:

Radchenko, L.A., Svirezhev, Yu.M.: 1972, 'Dinamika populyatsiy v menyayushesya srede. Experimenty s modelnimy populyatsiyami Drosofila melanogaster. (Population Dynamics in Changing Environment. Experiments With Model Populations of *Drosofila melanogaster*.)', *Zhurnal Obshei Biologii* (*Journal Of General Biology*) **33**, 5, 555–561, gave no evidence to decide between the two competing hypotheses: the choice of one or another strategy of behavior depended to a great extent on the external conditions (on the trophic environment).

To 8.2.
Models with coefficients of relative viability periodically varying in time, were treated in the work:
Haldane, J.B.S., Jayakar, S.D.: 1963, 'Polymorphism Due to Selection of Varying Direction', *J. Genet.* **58**, 2, 237–242.
The reasoning set forth is similar to the concept of Levins.
Let us elaborate on this.

Suppose we are given a panmictic population with three genotypes, *AA*, *Aa* and *aa* their fitnesses in two equally common states of the environment being equal to: 1) α, β, γ and 2) γ, β, α. The average population fitness in this case is equal to the mean geometric of fitness w_1 and w_2 defined separately for each of the states. Seeking for the maximum of

$$w = \sqrt{w_1 w_2} = \sqrt{(\alpha p^2 + 2\beta pq + \gamma q^2)(\gamma p^2 + 2\beta pq + \alpha q^2)}$$

we find that it is attained at $p^* = \frac{1}{2}$, if

$$\beta > 2\sqrt{\alpha\gamma} - \tfrac{1}{2}(\alpha + \gamma)\,. \tag{8.1}$$

Whence it is concluded, that if (8.1) holds, then polymorphism can exist in the population.

These speculations have one weak point: it is implicitly assumed that in this case again Fisher's theorem is valid, however, the reasoning employed above does not imply that polymorphism in the population is somewhat unusual, being presented by a cycle, rather than by a steady-state point. Let us note in conclusion, that the existence conditions, which we have derived for such a polymorphism, are more general.

To 8.3.
The paper below contains a full description of the analysis and data used:
Timofeeff-Ressovsky, N.W., Svirezhev, Yu.M.: 1966, 'Ob adaptsionnom polimorphisme v populyatsiyakh Adalia bipunctata (On Adaptational polymorphism in Populations of *Adalia bipunctata*)', *Problyemy kibernetiki (Problems of Cybernetics)* **16**, 137–146,

To 8.4.
An experimental and theoretical treatment of the evolution of populations is non-stationary (non-periodic) medium is contained in the works:
Svirezhev, Yu.M.: 1968, 'Establishment of Heterozygotic Polymorphism in Non-Stationary Population', *D. Inform. Serv.* **49**, 196–197;
Svirezhev, Yu.M., Timofeeff-Ressovsky, N.W.: 1969, 'Ustanovleniye geterozygotmogo polymorfizma v nectatsionarnykh populyatsiyakh (Establishment of Heterozygous Polymorphism in Non-Stationary Populations)', *Genetica (Genetics)* **5**, 1, 154–158.

To 8.5.
In the work:
MacArthur, R.H.: 1962, 'Some Generalized Theorems of Natural Selection', *Proc. Nat. Acad. Sci. USA* **48**, 11, 1893–1898,
Fisher's theorem has been considered with coefficients of relative viability depending on the total population size. It has shown, that in this case the time derivative of the average fitness can be of any sign. However, no special equations for the size have been introduced in this work and variations in the population size were implicitly assumed to be exponential (as it is usually done in frequency models).

To 8.7.
The notions of 'adaptation' and 'adaptability' are intensively discussed in the paper:
Timofeeff-Ressovsk, N.W., Svirezhev, Yu.M.:1972, 'Populationsgenetik und Optimisierungs-prozesses', *Biol. Zbl.* **91**, 1, 3–15.

Chapter 9

Multi-Locus Models

9.1. Discrete Two-Locus Model of Segregation-Recombination and its Continuous Approximation

Let us look at the special features of the genetic content dynamics in a diploid population with respect to several autosomal loci. The state of the population will be presented in terms of frequencies of various types of gametes in the space Σ. The dimensionality of Σ rapidly grows with the number of loci. If distinguish gametes with respect to the genic content of the *i*th locus with n_i alleles, then the dimensionality of Σ is n_i-1. For two loci with n_i and n_j alleles it will be equal to $n_i n_j-1$, if gametes are distinguished with respect to l loci, the dimensionality of Σ will be already $\Pi_{i=1}^{l} n_i-1$, where n_i is the number of alleles at the *i*th locus. Thus for the minimal amount of alleles at each polymorphic locus, which is two, the dimensionality of Σ exceeds 10^3 in case of ten loci. This means it is really hard to study multi-locus systems. Investigations of the system in the level of the whole genome come across practically unmanageable difficulties already due to the dimensionality of the problem.

Variations of gamete frequencies in multi-locus systems are induced by all the factors taken into account in one-locus models, plus by the process of recombination (described in Section 1.6) for *linked* loci (belonging to one chromosome, one *linkage group*) and independent *segregation* in case of several chromosomes. In meiosis elements of different pairs of homologous chromosomes separate independently (segregate) to the daughter cells. As a result, with probability 1/2 the gamete receives any of the two parental alleles at each locus, the events, in which non-homologous chromosomes segregate, being independent. Therefore the probability that a gamete carries, say, k arbitrary genes of parental genotype with no linkage, is equal to $(1/2)^k$.

Let there be no selection, no migrations, no mutations and no other systematic factors. We shall distinguish gametes with respect to their genic content at one (say, *j*th) locus. This means that in the entire *L*-locus system (where *L* is the set of loci $\{1, 2, ..., l\}$) we combine all gametes with one and the same allele of *j*th locus into one gamete. Denote the frequency of the ith *L*-locus gamete by $p_{\mathrm{i}}=p_{i_1 i_2 \ldots i_l}$ (i_j stands for the allele number at *j*th locus in ith gamete), and denote the marginal frequency of the one-locus gamete (carrying the same ith locus allele as the *i*th *L*-locus gamete) by p_{i_j} The quantity p_{i_j} is the concentration of the i_jth allele at jth locus in the population. Index i takes on all possible values when i_j runs from 1 to n_j, $j = \overline{1, l}$. Obviously, the processes of recombination-segregation only reshuffle the combinations of i_jth allele with genes from other loci and by no means affect the concentration of this allele. Whence it follows that without selection concentrations of all alleles at all loci remain constant throughout many generations.

If we assume mating to be random in the population, then even a stronger statement is valid (the already known Hardly-Weinberg principle): with no systematic factors acting in an infinite panmictic diploid population with no overlapping generations the frequencies of alleles at an autosomal locus are constant, and for arbitrary initial values, starting from the following generation, all genotype frequencies are presented by the products of the frequencies of the constituting alleles. This allows us to define the state of a one-locus population by a vector of allele frequencies, which can be easily transferred into genotype frequencies.

When analyzing the genetic content of a diploid population with respect to two autosomal loci, the Hardy-Weinberg relations between allele and genotype frequencies can be generalized to state that combinations of all alleles from all the loci are independent in genotype. Under random mating the fact, that in gametes the combinations of all alleles from different loci are independent, implies that their combinations in genotype are random. Therefore when the Hardy-Weinberg relations hold we can operate in the familiar phase space of gamete frequencies, Σ. In case of two loci the mutual independence of combinations of alleles at each locus does not result in interlocus combinations being random. What turns out to be new, is that the Hardy-Weinberg relations are not attained over the course of one generation (moreover, neither are they attained over a finite number of generations); now they are only limiting.

Denote the concentration of a two-locus gamete by $p_{i_1 i_2}$ assuming, to make it more definite, that we treat alleles of the first and the second loci of the ith L-locus gamete. In the entire L-locus system this concentration is associated with the sum of frequencies of all L-locus gametes, that carry the alleles of interest. Let $r(1|2)$ be the probability of recombination (the exchange of chromosome segments with the first and the second loci as a result of crossing-over) for linked loci, or the probability of segregation, i.e. the probability that chromosomes with the first and second loci are separated between different daughter cells in the process of meiosis. In terms of mathematics both cases are characterized by the parameter $r(1|2)$, which is called the *recombination coefficient*. Though the locations of linked loci are linearly ordered, in our further reasoning the locus numbers have nothing to do with their positions on the chromosomes.

The equations of dynamics in a discrete-time model can be derived as follows. Obviously, if there is no recombination-segregation, the gamete concentrations are constant. The probability of this event is $1-r(1|2)$, the contribution to the concentration of the gamete of interest in the next generation being equal to $[1-r(1|2)]p_{i_1 i_2}$. Recombinations also produce gametes of the type considered, for instance due to crossingover between any two gametes, if one of them carries the i_1st allele, and the other one - the i_2nd. Marginal (total) concentrations of these one-locus gametes were denoted above by p_{i_1} and p_{i_2}, respectively (being invariable in time, as shown above).

The probability of recombination is $r(1|2)$; the probability that under random fusion gametes with i_1st and i_2nd alleles encounter is equal to $2p_{i_1}p_{i_2}$. Therefore the contribution of the recombination-segregation event to the concentration $p_{i_1i_2}$ in the next generation will be $r(1|2)p_{i_1}p_{i_2}$. On the whole, putting a prime over the frequencies in the next generation, we obtain

$$p'_{i_1i_2} = [1 - r(1|2)]\, p_{i_1i_2} + r(1|2)\, p_{i_1}p_{i_2} =$$

$$= p_{i_1i_2} - r(1|2)\,(p_{i_1i_2} - p_{i_1}p_{i_2}, \quad i_1 = \overline{1, n_1}\,; \quad i_2 = \overline{1, n_2} \tag{1.1}$$

Let us note, that equations for the concentrations of various gametes (differing with respect to one allele at least) can be separated, and practically we are to deal with separate equations rather than with a system.

Concentrations p_{i_1} and p_{i_2} have been shown to be constant, hence (1.1) is a linear difference equation. If we expressed p_{i_1} and p_{i_2} in terms of concentrations of two-locus gametes, then the right-hand side in (1.1)(which would be a system already) would be a quadratic function of these concentrations.

The solution to (1.1) is readily obtained. Subtract the constant $p_{i_1}p_{i_2}$ from both sides of the equation:

$$(p_{i_1i_2} - p_{i_1}p_{i_2})' = [1 - r(1|2)]\,(p_{i_1i_2} - p_{i_1}p_{i_2})\,. \tag{1.2}$$

Setting

$$D_{i_1i_2} = p_{i_1i_2} - p_{i_1}p_{i_2}\,. \tag{1.3}$$

we have

$$D_{i_1i_2}(t) = [1 - r(1|2)]^t D_{i_1i_2}(0)\,, \tag{1.4}$$

$$p_{i_1i_2}(t) = p_{i_1}p_{i_2} + [1 - r(1|2)]^t D_{i_1i_2}(0)\,. \tag{1.5}$$

It is seen from (1.5) that if $r(1|2)>0$, then the frequencies of two-locus gametes converge to the equilibria, which are independent of $r(1|2)$, being equal to multiplied frequencies of allele from these gametes, that is equilibria comply with the Hardy-Weinberg relations. According to (1.3) this allows us to regard $D_{i_1i_2}$ as a measure of deviations from the equilibrium state of the population. $D_{i_1i_2}$ vanishes when the limiting state of equilibrium is attained. The index $D_{i_1i_2}$ is quite inadequately termed the *coefficient of linkage disequilibrium*. In fact $D_{i_1i_2}$ specifies the disequilibrium in both linked and non-linked loci, and in both cases its time variations are governed by the same exponential law with $r(1|2)$ in the exponent. The non-linked loci are often called independent (reflecting the independent separation of non-homologous chromosomes in meiosis), however the behavior of $D_{i_1i_2}$ (which can be regarded as the covariance between qualitative presence-absence attributes of alleles of interest in the gamete) indicates, that if the population is not at equilibrium, then in gametes the combinations of alleles from various non-linked loci are correlated just as in the case of linkage.

In the absence of recombination-segregation, when $r(1|2)$ is zero, it follows from (1.1) that gamete frequencies are constant as in the one-locus case. If different gamete types are considered as alleles, we arrive at a situation, which is equivalent to the one-locus case studied above. Therefore, in what follows we assume that there is no such rigid linkage for any pair of loci.

The coefficients of disequilibrium $D_{i_1 i_2}$ are defined by (1.3) for each of the gamete types. However, not all of them are independent (for instance, it is readily seen that summing up $D_{i_1 i_2}$ over the first or the second subscript, we get a zero). In particular, if we look at two diallele loci, then the coefficients of disequilibrium for different gametes can be different only on their signs. In fact, for loci with multiple alleles the concentrations of the latter may be expressed in terms of gamete frequencies as follows: $p_{i_1} = \Sigma p_{i_1 \cdot} = p_{i_1 i_2} + p_{i_1 \bar{i}_2}$ (likewise for p_{i_2}). Here the point stands for the subscript over which summation is being taken, $p_{i_1 \bar{i}_2} = \Sigma_{k,\, k \neq i_2}\, p_{i_1 k}$ is the marginal concentration of the gamete with the i_1st and without the i_2nd allele at the first and second loci, respectively. Then we can rewrite (1.3) as follows

$$D_{i_1 i_2} = p_{i_1 i_2} - (p_{i_1 i_2} + p_{i_1 \bar{i}_2})(p_{i_1 i_2} + p_{\bar{i}_1 i_2}) = \tag{1.6}$$

$$= p_{i_1 i_2}(1 - p_{i_1 i_2} - p_{\bar{i}_1 i_2} - p_{i_1 \bar{i}_2}) - p_{i_1 \bar{i}_2}\, p_{\bar{i}_1 i_2} = p_{i_1 i_2}\, p_{\bar{i}_1 \bar{i}_2} - p_{i_1 \bar{i}_2}\, p_{\bar{i}_1 i_2}$$

It is a simple matter to check that $- D_{\bar{i}_1 \bar{i}_2} = - D_{\bar{i}_1 i_2} = D_{i_1 \bar{i}_2} = D_{i_1 i_2}$. If both loci are diallelic, then i_1 and $\bar{i}_1$ (i_2 and $\bar{i}_2$) are the indices of the two possible alleles of the appropriate loci (and an additional bar over the index, say $\bar{\bar{i}}_1$, makes it equal to i_1). Gametes with arbitrary indices, different from $i_1 i_2$, are obtained from $i_1 i_2$ by the appropriate arrangements of bars, which can only change the sign of $D_{i_1 i_2}$. Therefore, if we write D instead of D_{11}, then (1.1) can be presented in the well-known form

$$p'_{11} = p_{11} - r(1|2)D, \quad p'_{12} = p_{12} + r(1|2)D, \tag{1.7}$$

$$p'_{21} = p_{21} + r(1|2)D, \quad p'_{22} = p_{22} - r(1|2)D, \quad D = p_{11}p_{22} - p_{12}p_{21}.$$

Thus, formally amalgamating alleles of one locus into a diallele system, we get the same equations for combined frequencies as if the locus was really diallelic.

In case of multiple alleles the concentration, say $p_{\bar{i}_1 \bar{i}_2}$, concerns the combination of gametes without the i_1st and the i_2nd alleles at the first and second loci, respectively: $p_{\bar{i}_1 \bar{i}_2} = \Sigma_{m_1 \neq i_1,\, m_2 \neq i_2} p_{m_1 m_2}$. If by analogy with (1.6), we introduce the coefficient of disequilibrium for the pair of gametes $\{i_1 i_2, j_1 j_2\}$ by the formula

$$D_{(i_1 i_2)(j_1 j_2)} = p_{i_1 i_2} p_{j_1 j_2} - p_{i_1 j_2} p_{j_1 i_2} \tag{1.8}$$

which agrees with (1.6) for diallele loci, then for multiple alleles we yield

$$D_{i_1 i_2} = \sum_{j_1, j_2} D_{(i_1 i_2)(j_1 j_2)} = p_{i_1 i_2} - p_{i_1} p_{i_2}. \tag{1.9}$$

In discrete-time models the variations of gamete frequencies are presented by difference equations. The question arises: "When can these equations be approximated by differential ones?" If the span of one generation is taken as the time unit (Δt=1), then (1.1) can be rewritten as follows:

$$\Delta p_{i_1 i_2} = -r(1|2)\,(p_{i_1 i_2} - p_{i_1} p_{i_2})\,\Delta t, \quad i_1 = \overline{1, n_1} \quad i_2 = \overline{1, n_2} \tag{1.10}$$

Introduce a new time scale, assuming that $\tau = r(1|2)t$. For small values of the recombination coefficient $r(1|2)$ the life span of a generation in terms of the new time unit is rather small and the variations in gamete frequencies on this scale can be approximately regarded as continuous, taking on values that correspond to jumps in time $\Delta\tau = r(1|2)\Delta t = r(1|2)$ (since $\Delta t = 1$). For $r(1|2) \to 0$ we have $\Delta\tau \to 0$ and from (1.10) we get

$$\frac{\Delta p_{i_1 i_2}}{\Delta \tau} \underset{r(1|2)\to 0}{\longrightarrow} \frac{\mathrm{d}p_{i_1 i_2}}{\mathrm{d}\tau} = p_{i_1 i_2} - p_{i_1} p_{i_2}. \tag{1.11}$$

If we represent the discrete process by a broken line, connecting the values of $p_{i_1 i_2}$ at points divisible by $\Delta\tau$, then for the integral curve of Equation (1.11) we get an Euler broken line, which is known to be converging towards the curves as $\Delta\tau \to 0$, provided that some weak restrictions are imposed on $\Delta p_{i_1 i_2}$. In this sense the continuous model (1.11) approximates the discrete model (1.1). On the original time scale we have

$$\frac{dp_{i_1 i_2}}{dt} = -r(1|2)\,(p_{i_1 i_2} - p_{i_1} p_{i_2}) = -rD_{i_1 i_2}, \quad i_1 = \overline{1, n_1} \quad i_2 = \overline{1, n_2} \tag{1.12}$$

System (1.10) disintegrates, the solution to each linear (recall that p_{i_1} and p_{i_2} are constant) differential equations has the form

$$p_{i_1 i_2}(t) = p_{i_1 i_2} + \exp\{-r(1|2)\,t\}\, D_{i_1 i_2}(0), \tag{1.13}$$

and the independent combinations of alleles in gametes is only asymptotically attained. For the coefficient of disequilibrium we get

$$D_{i_1 i_2}(t) = \exp\{-r(1|2)\,t\}\, D_{i_1 i_2}(0). \tag{1.14}$$

Thus the solutions to the continuous model are obtained from the solutions to the discrete one by substituting $\exp\{-r(1|2)\,t\}$ for $[1 - r(1|2)]^{t}$.

Let us note that for values of the recombination coefficient being not so small, the differential approximation of difference equations is incorrect. However, close to the states of equilibrium the increments $\Delta p_{i_1 i_2}$ are small and, invoking some reasoning similar to the above, we can prove the solutions to the difference and differential schemes to be close in the vicinity of the equilibrium. Another method to prove that they are close enough has been set forth in Section 2.15. Therefore, generally speaking, the approximation (1.12) is quite good, starting from some time t_0, when $D_{i_1 i_2}$ becomes small. Since $D_{i_1 i_2} = 0$ is an asymptotically stable equilibrium in both (1.1) and (1.12), the approximation (1.12) is valid for any $t > t_0$. The qualitative picture for the discrete-time dynamics of $p_{i_1 i_2}$ and $D_{i_1 i_2}$ is represented by the solution to the differential equation (1.12) over an arbitrary period of time.

9.2. Continuous One- and Two-Locus Models with no Selection. Equations for Numbers and Frequencies, Fast and Slow Variables

Equations like (1.12) can be directly deduced from the continuous model, its simplest version assuming that there is no age or sexual structure and that the natality-mortality processes are continuous, as it is generally accepted in most ecological issues. Such a model has some specific features, which put it in contrast to models with non-overlapping generations (and to their continuous approximations). These features of intrinsically continuous model in question are already distinctly manifested in the one-locus case.

In order to derive the equations let us first look at the dynamics of numbers N_{ij} of the genotypes A_iA_j. For ease of presentation let us distinguish genotypes A_iA_j and A_jA_i. Without selection, mortality m will be the same for all genotypes. The coefficient m can take into account the dependence of mortality on the population size N, the genetic structure $\boldsymbol{p}$ and time, reflecting the regulation of the population size (density) by ecological and other factors. The population can be regulated by different factors: by variations in mortality, or natality, or in both of them together. In what follows we assume that regulation is performed by variable mortality, which is a function of population size, its structure and time, $m(N, \boldsymbol{p}, t)$, while natality b is assumed to be constant. The number of individuals with genotype A_iA_j is Np_{ij}, where p_{ij} is the concentration of the genotype of interest in the population. Mating is assumed to be random. This implies that each of the Np_{ij} individulas of the genotype A_iA_j can mate with the individual of genotype A_kA_l with the probability p_{kl}. Therefore the amount of couples $\{A_iA_j, A_kA_l\}$ is equal to $Np_{ij}p_{kl}$; the fertility of a couple is independent of the genotypes of the mates, being equal to b.

In this ecological-genetical situation the dynamics of genotype numbers is presented by ordinary differential equations of the form:

$$\frac{dN_{ij}}{dt} = bN \sum_{k,\,l} p_{ik}p_{jl} - m(N, \mathbf{p}, t)Np_{ij} . \tag{2.1}$$

Whence for the size of the population we obtain the equation which is dependent on the genetic structure:

$$dN/dt = N\,[b - m\,(N, \mathbf{p}, t)] \tag{2.2}$$

Applying the relation $\dot{p}_{ij} = d(N_{ij}/N)/dt) = \dot{N}_{ij}\,/\,N - p_{ij}\,\dot{N}\,/N$, we arrive at the equations for genotype concentrations:

$$dp_{ij}/dt = bp_{i\cdot}p_{\cdot j} - m(N, \mathbf{p}, t\,)p_{ij} - p_{ij}[b - m\,(N, \mathbf{p}, t)] = b(p_{i\cdot}p_{\cdot j} - p_{ij})\,, \tag{2.3}$$

$$i, j = \overline{1, n}.$$

Equations (2.2), (2.3) characterize the dynamics of the size and the genetic structure of the population, respectively, the latter being separable form the former. Therefore, in the simplest case variations in the genetic structure can be treated separately, apart from the ecological factors (nevertheless this does not mean that the population should infinitely grow or decline, which is specific of models with constant birth-mortality rates, that also result in Equations (2.3)). The population can reach a certain level of saturation, following the s-shaped curve, for example.

In (2.3) we find allele concentrations p_i and p_j: $p_i = \Sigma_j p_{ij}$, $p_j = \Sigma_i p_{ij}$. Summing up (2.3) over j and i we get

$$dp_i/dt = dp_j/dt = 0\,, \quad i, j = \overline{1, n} \tag{2.4}$$

Equations (2.3), (2.4) are known to have the solution

$$p_{ij}(t) = p_i p_j + [p_{ij}(0) - p_i p_j]\, e^{-bt} \tag{2.5}$$

and the time-variations of the disequilibrium measure for combinations of one-locus gametes (alleles) in genotypes, $D^1_{ij} = p_{ij} - p_i p_{ij}$ can be described by a simple equation

$$D^1_{ij}(t) = p_{ij}(t) - p_i p_{ij} = D^1_{ij}(0)\, e^{-bt}. \tag{2.6}$$

Thus, as it was drawn out by P. Moran, already the one-locus case clearly displays one specific feature of the continuous model: the model does not comply with the Hardy-Weinberg principle. Only in equilibrium the genotype concentrations are equal to the product of the constituent gamete frequencies. Deviations from random coupling of gametes is explained by the gradual extinction of organisms: though genotype frequencies of the new-born satisfy the Hardy-Weinberg principle, in the total population (of grown-ups together with the new-born) the principle may not hold.

Let us note, however, that for large b the Hardian relation is attained very soon, and this indicates that there may be a chance to select fast variables (fast time) in more complicated situations. Let us also stress that a large b does not yet imply a rapid population growth, since no restrictions have been imposed on mortality m.

Next consider the two-locus case. Denote the numbers and concentrations of genotypes $A_{i_1}B_{i_2}A_{j_1}B_{j_2}$, made up by the gametes $A_{i_1}B_{i_2}$ and $A_{j_1}B_{j_2}$, by $N_{(i_1i_2)(j_1j_2)}$ and $p_{(i_1i_2)(j_1j_2)}$, respectively, and let $r = r(1|2)$ be the coefficient of recombination between loci. Equations for the dynamics of genotype numbers are derived as follows. Over a period Δt in a population of size N a part of organisms of genotype $A_{i_1}B_{i_2}A_{j_1}B_{j_2}$, equal to $m(N, \mathbf{p}, t)Np_{(i_1i_2)(j_1j_2)}$, dies off. At that same time $N\Delta t$ organisms (to an accuracy of $o(\Delta t)$) take part in reproduction ($Np_{(i_1i_2)(j_1j_2)}\Delta t$ of them have the genotype $A_{i_1}B_{i_2}A_{j_1}B_{j_2}$). In the process of reproduction each organism yields recombinated and non-recombinated gametes in the proportion r:(1−r); fertility of all pairs is b. If Δt goes to zero, we get the following differential equation:

$$\begin{aligned}\frac{dN_{(i_1i_2)(j_1j_2)}}{dt} &= bN[(1-r)^2\Sigma p_{(i_1i_2)(\cdot\cdot)}p_{(j_1j_2)(\cdot\cdot)} + r^2\Sigma p_{(i_1\cdot)(i_2\cdot)}p_{(j_1\cdot)(j_2\cdot)} + \\ &+ r(1-r)\Sigma p_{(i_1i_2)(\cdot\cdot)}p_{(j_1\cdot)(j_2\cdot)} + r(1-r)\Sigma p_{(i_1\cdot)(i_2\cdot)}p_{(j_1j_2)(\cdot\cdot)}] - \\ &- m(N, p, t)\, N_{(i_1i_2)(j_1j_2)} = bN[(1-r)\Sigma p_{(i_1i_2)(\cdot\cdot)} + \\ &+ r\Sigma p_{(i_1\cdot)(i_2\cdot)}]\,[(1-r)\Sigma p_{(j_1j_2)(\cdot\cdot)} + r\Sigma p_{(j_1\cdot)(j_2\cdot)}] - \\ &- m\,(N, \mathbf{p}, t)\, Np_{(i_1i_2)(j_1j_2)}\,.\end{aligned} \tag{2.7}$$

Here points stand for subscript, over which summation is being taken. Just like before, passing to the population size and genotype frequencies, we obtain the system

$$dN/dt = N\,[b-m(N,\mathbf{p},t)], \tag{2.8}$$

$$dp_{(i_1i_2)(j_1j_2)}/dt = b\,[\Sigma p_{(i_1i_2)(\cdot\cdot)} - r\,\Sigma(p_{(i_1i_2)(\cdot\cdot)} - p_{(i_1\cdot)(i_2\cdot)})] \times$$

$$\times[\Sigma p_{(j_1j_2)(\cdot\cdot)} - r\,\Sigma p_{(j_1j_2)(\cdot\cdot)} - p_{(j_1\cdot)}p_{(j_2\cdot)})] - bp_{ij},$$

$$i_1,\ j_1 = \overline{1, n_1};\ i_2,\ j_2 = \overline{1, n_2}$$

Again the equations of the genetic structure dynamics are independent of the equation for the population size, and they can be treated separately. However, they are too cumbersome. Therefore let us change over to new variables: to $p_1 = p_{i_1i_2}$ – the concentrations of gametes $A_{i_1}B_{i_2}$, to $D^1_{(i_1i_2)(j_1j_2)}$ – the measures of randomness for gamete combinations in genotypes (the one–locus analogy is D^1_{ij}), and to $y_{i_1i_2}$- the concentrations of genotypes, carrying allele A_{i_1} in one gamete and B_{i_2} – in another:

$$p_{i_1i_2} = \Sigma p_{(i_1i_2)(\cdot\cdot)},\quad y_{i_1i_2} = \Sigma p_{(i_1\cdot)(\cdot i_2)}, \tag{2.9}$$

$$D^1_{(i_1i_2)(j_1j_2)} = p_{(i_1i_2)(j_1j_2)} - p_{i_1i_2}p_{j_1j_2},\quad i_k, j_k = \overline{1, n_k};\quad k = 1, 2.$$

Next suppose that $b \gg r$ (generally speaking, this does not imply that there is a tight linkage, or that the population grows rapidly). Without loss of generality, to make it simpler we can write $br \sim r \sim \varepsilon \ll 1$. Now if we sum up the equations for $p_{(i_1i_2)(j_1j_2)}$ in (2.8) properly, and isolate a unity and $O(r)$ in the term with $(1-r)^2$ when writing the derivative of $D^1_{(i_1i_2)(j_1j_2)}$, then we arrive at the following system of equations:

$$dp_{i_1i_2}/dt = br(y_{i_1i_2} - p_{i_1i_2}) = O(\varepsilon),$$

$$dD^1_{(i_1i_2)(j_1j_2)}/dt = -bD^1_{(i_1i_2)(j_1j_2)} + O(\varepsilon),$$

$$dy_{i_1i_2}/dt = b\,(p_{i_1}p_{i_2} - y_{i_1i_2}) + O(\varepsilon), \tag{2.10}$$

$$i_1,\ j_1 = \overline{1, n_1};\quad i_2, j_2 = \overline{1, n_2},$$

where p_{i_1} and p_{i_2} are the concentrations of the i_1st allele at the first locus and of the i_2nd allele at the second one, respectively.

From (2.10) one can see, that $p_{i_1i_2}$ are 'slow' variables, while $D^1_{(i_1i_2)(j_1j_2)}$ and $y_{i_1i_2}$ are 'fast', since $b \gg r$. Roughly speaking, the evolution of $p_{i_1i_2}$ proceeds for the equilibrium values of 'fast' variables, their dynamics being described by the equations, derived from (2.10) with $\varepsilon \to 0$:

$$dD^1_{(i_1i_2)(j_1j_2)}/dt = -bD^1_{(i_1i_2)(j_1j_2)},$$

$$dy_{i_1i_2}/dt = -\,b(p_{i_1}p_{i_2} - y_{i_1i_2}), \tag{2.11}$$

$$i_1,\ j_1 = \overline{1, n_1};\quad i_2, j_2 = \overline{1, n_2}.$$

In (2.11) the slow variables $p_{i_1 i_2}$ are 'frozen' and they are regarded as the parameters that determine the equilibrium of the fast variables.

The globally stable equilibria in (2.11) are $D^1_{(i_1 i_2)(j_1 j_2)}=0$ and $y_{i_1 i_2}=p_{i_1}p_{i_2}$. Whence by the Tychonoff theorem, the dynamics of $p_{i_1 i_2}$ over a finite time interval can be approximated by the solution to

$$\mathrm{d}\, p_{i_1 i_2}/\mathrm{d}t = br(p_{i_1}p_{i_2} - p_{i_1 i_2}) = -\, brD_{i_1 i_2}, \quad i_1=\overline{1, n_1}\,;\ i_2=\overline{1, n_2}\,, \tag{2.12}$$

where $D_{i_1 i_2}$ is the coefficient of linkage disequilibrium (1.3).

Formally this equation coincides with (1.12), the only difference is that br substitutes r. Besides, in contrast to (1.12) we derive (2.12) without requiring that the system be close to equilibrium or that r be small (we only need that b>>r).

In what follows we shall repeatedly take advantage of the equations for slow variables (gamete frequencies p_I); unlike (2.12) in more complicated situations (say, if selection is taken into account) these equations may have no explicit solutions. In these cases we shall be concerned with equilibria of p_I and their stability, that is with the limiting behavior of gamete concentrations as $t\to\infty$. Therefore we need to make sure that the approximation (2.12) is correct all over the semi-infinite time interval $0\le t<\infty$. Let us make use of the conventional vector notations: $\mathbf{Z}$ will stand for the fast variables ($\mathbf{D}^1_{ij}$, y_I), the appropriate right-hand side in (2.10) will be $\mathbf{F}$, and $\mathbf{y}$ will stand for the slow variables p_I with the right-hand side $\varepsilon\mathbf{f}$. Then the dynamics of slow variables are correctly approximated by Equation (2.12) if the following condition holds: eigenvalues ρ_i of matrix

$$\| \mathbf{f_y} \| - \| \mathbf{f_z} \| \, \| \mathbf{F_z} \|^{-1} \| \mathbf{F_y} \| \tag{2.13}$$

(for $\mathbf{y}(t)$ defined by (2.12) and $\mathbf{Z}(\mathbf{y}(t))$ defined as the asymptotically stable equilibrium in (2.11)) comply with the inequality $\rho_i \le \kappa < 0$, $t\in[T,\infty)$. Here T is an arbitrarily large but fixed number.

In case of (2.10) the condition imposed on the matrix (2.13) can be rapidly verified, since the appropriate derivatives make up block matrices with zero blocks and diagonal blocks of constants to within negligible additions.

The solution to (2.12) is $p_{i_1 i_2}(t) = p_{i_1}p_{i_2} + \exp\{-\,brt\}D_{i_1 i_2}(0)$, hence, $p_{i_1 i_2}(t)\to p_{i_1}p_{i_2}$, as $t\to\infty$, that is the allele combinations in gametes are asymptotically independent. Thus, in the limit gametes in genotypes and alleles in gametes combine randomly, that is the Hardy-Weinberg principle holds with respect to two loci. The following hierarchy takes place in this case (agreeing with the situation for the discrete-time model).

First (and very quickly), the Hardian relations (or, more accurately, the quasi-equilibrium relations close to the Hardian ones) are attained with respect to each of the loci separately. This is induced by the high fecundity under panmixia, which results in random fusion of gametes in the genotypes of the newborn. Therefore the quickly 'renewed' population becomes quasi-Hardian with respect to gamete combinations. Next, just as in the discrete model, the processes of recombination-segregation in 'slow' time reshuffle the alleles of different loci in gametes to yield a random combination of alleles in them, that is we arrive at the Hardy-Weinberg principle with respect to two loci simultaneously. We can still regard the space of gamete frequencies Σ as the space of the genetic states of the population, since the dynamics of genotype frequencies can be defined by the gamete frequencies. Simplex Σ in its turn is represented as a direct product of allele frequency simplices.

9.3. Formalization of Recombination-Segregation in a Discrete-Time Multi-Locus System. Equations of Dynamics, Equilibria

In the qualitative respect the situation in the multi-locus system is similar to the two-locus one: the equilibria are characterized by independent combinations of alleles in gametes, trajectories converge to them at an exponential rate, all trajectories, originating from the states with equal allele frequencies, have one and the same limit.

The explicit form of the relationships between gamete concentrations and time is specified by the type of recombinations. In the general case they are determined by single, double, triple, etc. crossing-overs and by the number of linkage groups, resulting in fairly complicated gene exchanges between gametes in meiosis. Obviously, for the set of loci $L=\{1, 2,...,l\}$ these exchanges can be described by all kinds of partitions of L into two classes U and V. If the loci are split into U and V, then after the exchange the gametes are made of U-loci from one of the parental gametes and V-loci from another. Over the set of partitions the probabilities of crossing-overs and the linkage groups define the *linkage distribution* - a probability distribution $\{r(U|V)\}$ such that

$$r(U|V)\geq 0,\ \sum_{U|V} r(U|V) = 1\,. \tag{3.1}$$

In $\{r(U|V)\}$ let us distinguish the element $r(\varnothing|L)$, corresponding to the absence of exchange of genes:

$$r(\varnothing|L) = 1 - R(L)\,,$$

where

$$R(L) = \sum_{U|V,\ U\neq\varnothing,L} r(U|V)\,. \tag{3.2}$$

is the 'non-breakage parameter' for the set of loci L.

Obviously, the foregoing recombination probability for the first and second loci $r(1|2)$ is induced by the L-locus linkage distribution, being equal to the sum of $r(U|V)$ over all partitions $U|V$ such that the first locus belongs to U, and the second one - to V. In general, it is readily seen if we distinguish gametes with respect to a subset of L, then the linkage distribution, induced over this subset will also be a probability distribution (and this fact was already applied to treat the two-locus case).

Suppose that the linkage distribution is such that only the $U|V$-exchanges of loci can take place. Then the ith gamete can appear as a result of the $U|V$-exchange between L-locus gametes, one of them carrying the allele of the ith gamete at the U-loci, the other one - at the V-loci, their remaining genetic content being arbitrary. Let us denote the concentrations of these gametes with U- and V-loci (implying all L-locus gametes carrying alleles of the ith gamete at U- and V-loci) by p_{i_U} and p_{i_V}, respectively. Equations of dynamics under random combinations of gametes in genotypes are as follows:

$$p'_i = [1-r(U|V)]p_i + r(U|V)p_{i_U}p_{i_V} =$$
$$= p_i - r(U|V)(p_i - p_{i_U}p_{i_V}) = p_i - r(U|V)D_{i,U|V}.$$

It is clear that these equations coincide with the two-locus ones (see (1.1)), if all kinds of U- and V-locus gametes are regarded as alleles of two loci with the recombination coefficient $r(U|V)$. Therefore in the limit, as $t \to \infty$, the combinations of 'alleles' from U- and V-loci in L-locus gametes are independent, while the coefficient of disequilibrium $D_{i,U|V}$ vanishes exponentially.

In the general case, all types of exchanges are to be taken into account simultaneously. For instance, if we distinguish gametes with respect to three first loci, then invoking the linkage distribution we can present the dynamic equations in the following form:

$$p_{i_1i_2i_3}(t+1) = [1-R(1,2,3)]\,p_{i_1i_2i_3}(t) + r(1|2,3)p_{i_1}(t)\,p_{i_2i_3}(t) + \tag{3.3}$$
$$+ r(2|1,3)p_{i_2}(t)\,p_{i_1i_3}(t) + r(3|1,2)p_{i_3}(t)\,p_{i_1i_2}(t),$$
$$i_1 = \overline{1, n_1};\quad i_2 = \overline{1, n_2};\quad i_3 = \overline{1, n_3}.$$

If we recall that p_{i_j} are constant, and that from (1.5) we know the concentrations of two-locus gametes as functions of time, then it is clear, that (3.3) disintegrates into separate linear non-uniform equations. Substituting (1.5) into (3.3) (here we present the explicit form for one term, say, the one with $p_{i_2i_3}$, all the rest being similar) we get

$$p_{i_1i_2i_3}(t+1) = [1-R(1,2,3)]p_{i_1i_2i_3}(t) +$$
$$+ r(1|2,3)[p_{i_1}p_{i_2}p_{i_3} + p_{i_1}D_{i_2i_3}(0)(1-r(2|3))^t] + \ldots. \tag{3.4}$$

In the complete presentation of (3.4), raised to the power t are the probabilities of non-breakage by crossing-over for various two-locus subsets of the set of all three loci. The solution to a non-uniform difference equation

$$y(t+1) = ay(t) + b + cd^t \tag{3.5}$$

is known to have the following form:

$$y(t) = a^t y(0) + b\frac{1-a^t}{1-a} + c\sum_{n=0}^{t-1} a^{t-1-n}d^n =$$
$$= \frac{b}{1-a} + c\frac{d^t}{d-a} + [y(0) - \frac{b}{1-a} - \frac{c}{d-a}]a^t. \tag{3.6}$$

In our case $a = 1-R(1,2,3)$, $b = [\sum r(\cdot|\cdot\cdot)]p_{i_1}p_{i_2}p_{i_3} = R(1,2,3) \times p_{i_1}p_{i_2}p_{i_3}$, c and d take on one of three values according to the crossing-over type. For instance, if the partition is $1|2,3$, then $c = r(1|2,3)p_{i_1}D_{i_2i_3}(0)$, the probability of non-breakage by crossing-over for two (the second and the third) loci is $d = 1-r\,(2|3) = 1-r\,(2|1, 3) - r(3|1, 2) = 1-R(1, 2, 3) + r\,(1|2, 3)$, whence $d-a = r(1|2, 3)$. Each of the three values of (c,d) in (3.4) is associated with a term similar to those in (3.6), hence

$$p_{i_1 i_2 i_3}(t) = p_{i_1} p_{i_2} p_{i_3} + \sum_{\cdot|\cdot\cdot} p_{\cdot} D_{\cdot\cdot}(0)[1 - R(\cdot\cdot)]^t + \\ + [p_{i_1 i_2 i_3}(0) - p_{i_1} p_{i_2} p_{i_3} - \sum_{\cdot|\cdot\cdot} p_{\cdot} D_{\cdot\cdot}(0)](1-R(1, 2, 3))^t. \tag{3.7}$$

Here and above summation is being taking over all partitions .|.. of the set of three loci into one and two, $p_{\cdot}$ is the concentration of the corresponding allele at one locus (in the partition), $D_{\cdot\cdot}(0)$ is the initial value of the disequilibrium coefficient for the appropriate alleles of the two other loci, $R(..) = r(.|.)$ is the recombination coefficient for these loci (and the non-breakage parameter at the same time), $R(1, 2, 3)$ is the non-breakage parameter for the whole set of three loci, and $1-R(..)$ is the probability of non-breakage by crossing-over for the appropriate set.

From (1.5) and (3.7) one can see, that gametes frequencies as functions of time are represented by the sum of a constant with the linear combination made of the powers of probabilities, that there is no breakage in various subsets of the considered set of loci. The constant is equal to the product of initial frequencies of the alleles that make up the gamete. This results in an exponential tendency of gamete frequencies towards their equilibria, characterized by independent allele combinations with no rigid linkage in any pair of loci.

Let us note that if a subset of loci K belongs to a subset M, then the inequality $R(K) \leq R(M)$ is correct. In fact, in $R(K)$ we sum up the various partitions of the considered set into subsets (with no empty subsets among them), therefore the contribution of each summand to $R(M)$ is the same, but additionally $R(M)$ includes, say, $r(K|M \setminus K) \geq 0$. Consequently, the asymptotic rate of convergence towards equilibrium is equal to the value of the maximal non-breakage probability for different pairs of loci.

When analyzing the behavior of gametes frequencies, we carried on from one locus to two and further on to three loci. This suggests the idea about applying induction, as it was done by Ju.I. Ljubic, who gave a complete explicit description of the dynamics of gamete frequencies in a multi-locus discrete model, invoking the methods of genetic algebras.

Suppose that the frequencies of gametes, classed with respect to an arbitrary subset of loci $K \subset L$, can be represented as functions of time t in the form of a constant (equal to the product of frequencies of the alleles that enter into the K-locus gamete) summed with the linear combination of various products of probabilities, that crossing-over does not break different disjoint subsets of K, raised to the power t. Obviously, the concentration $p_{\mathrm{i}} = p_{i_1 \ldots i_l}$ of the ith L-locus gamete among all gametes, subjected to no exchanges, is constant (this event is associated with the parameter $R(L)$). But if recombination or segregation breaks L into U and V, then the ith gamete can appear due to a $U|V$-exchange between U- and V-locus gametes (containing the subsets of U-and V-genes of the ith gamete, respectively, and being arbitrary at the rest loci as all L-locus gametes), their concentrations denoted above by p_{i_U} and p_{i_V}. If combinations of gametes are random the probability of this event is $r(U|V)p_{i_U}p_{i_V}$. Therefore the equations of dynamics are as follows:

$$p'_{i_1...i_l} = [1 - R(L)]p_{i_1...i_l} + \sum_{U|V,\, U\neq\varnothing,L} r(U|V)p_{i_U}p_{i_V},$$

$$i_1 = \overline{1, n_1};...;i_l = \overline{1, n_l}. \tag{3.8}$$

Taking (3.2) into account, we can rewrite (3.8) in the form:

$$p'_{i_1...i_l} = p_{i_1...i_l} - \sum_{U|V,\, U\neq\varnothing,L} r(U|V)D_{\mathbf{i},U|V},$$

$$i_1 = \overline{1, n_1};...;i_l = \overline{1, n_l}, \tag{3.9}$$

where the coefficient of $U|V$-disequilibrium is

$$D_{\mathbf{i},U|V} = p_{\mathbf{i}} - p_{i_U}p_{i_V}. \tag{3.10}$$

If there can be only one type of the $U|V$-exchanges, then (3.9) stands for the two-locus situation, and the general case is obtained as if the two-locus ones were summed up.

Just as in the two-locus case the $U|V$-disequilibrium (3.10) can be rewritten in terms of the L-locus gamete concentrations, by analogy with (1.6):

$$D_{\mathbf{i},U|V} = p_{\mathbf{i}}p_{\bar{\mathbf{i}}} - p_{\mathbf{i}_U\bar{\mathbf{i}}_V}\, p_{\bar{\mathbf{i}}_U\mathbf{i}_V} \tag{3.11}$$

where the stroked index, say $\bar{\mathbf{i}}_U$, still indicates that it never takes on the values $\mathbf{i}_U$ among the U-loci. Actually this means that the join of gametes is indexed: $p_{\mathbf{i}_U\bar{\mathbf{i}}_V} = \sum_{\mathbf{j}_V,\, \mathbf{j}_V\neq\mathbf{i}_V} p_{\mathbf{i}_U\mathbf{j}_V}$. Extending the analogy with the two-locus case, let us introduce the $U|V$-coefficients of disequilibrium for a couple of gametes $\{\mathbf{i}, \mathbf{j}\}$:

$$D_{\mathbf{i},\mathbf{j},U|V} = p_{\mathbf{i}}p_{\mathbf{j}} - p_{\mathbf{i}_U\mathbf{j}_V}p_{\mathbf{i}_V\mathbf{j}_U}. \tag{3.12}$$

Then

$$D_{\mathbf{i},U|V} = \sum_{\mathbf{j}} D_{\mathbf{i},\mathbf{j},U|V} = p_{\mathbf{i}} = p_{\mathbf{i}_V}p_{\mathbf{i}_U} \tag{3.12a}$$

Let us note that summation of the equations (3.8) over some proper subset of values of the index $i_j, j \in L$ results in equations of the same form with respect to frequencies of gametes with joined alleles. Such a summation corresponds to a formal join of the subset of the jth locus alleles into one allele (j can also be a multi-index denoting the numbers of several loci). The situation was likewise in the two-locus case (see, (1.6), (1.7)). Summing up (3.8) over all indices $i_2...i_l$, we yield $p'_{i_1} = p_{i_1}$; summing up over $i_3 ... i_l$, we arrive at the equations for two-locus gametes, and so on. Thus, we could have first formulated the system for L-locus gametes, and then deduce the equations for the K-locus ($K \subset L$) case.

If we write out $p_{\mathbf{i}_V}$ and $p_{\mathbf{i}_U}$ in terms of the L-locus gamete concentrations, then the right-hand side of (3.8) will be a quadratic function of these frequencies. If the values of

p_{i_V} and p_{i_U} are substituted by the functions of time, which are considered to be known by the assumption of induction, then (3.8) falls into separate linear non-uniform equations.

The solution to these equations can be presented in the form:

$$p_i(t) = [1-R(L)]^t p_i(0) + \sum_{U|V,\, U\neq\varnothing,L} r(U|V) \sum_{n=0}^{t-1} [1-R(L)]^{t-1-n} \times$$

$$\times p_{i_U}(n) p_{i_V}(n) = [1-P(L)]^t \left\{ p_i(0) + \sum_{U|V,\, U\neq\varnothing,L} \frac{r(U|V)}{1-R(L)} \times \right.$$

$$\left. \times \sum_{n=0}^{t-1} p_{i_U}(n) p_{i_V}(n) [1-R(L)]^{-n} \right\}. \qquad (3.13)$$

For any $U|V$-partition the constant in $p_{i_U} p_{i_V}$ is equal to the product of constants from the expansions of p_{i_U} and p_{i_V} which is equal, by the assumption of the induction, to

$$\left(\prod_{i_j \in U} p_{i_j}\right)\left(\prod_{i_k \in V} p_{i_k}\right) = \prod_{j=1}^{l} p_{i_j},$$

that is to the product of concentrations of all alleles contained in the ith L-locus gamete. The coefficient for this term will be $r(U|V)$. Summing up over all $U|V$-partitions, and taking account of (3.2), after summation is being taken also over n, we find the constant in the expansion of $p_i(t)$ to be equal to the product of concentrations of the alleles that make up the gamete.

By the assumption of induction, in addition to the constant, the expansion of $p_{i_U}(n)$ also contains the linear combination of various products of nth powers of the non-breakage probabilities for all kinds of disjoint subsets of U. Multiplying this combination by the expansion of $p_{i_V}(n)$, we again obtain a linear combination of multiplied nth powers of non-breakage probabilities $\{1-R(K_i)\}$ for the disjoint subsets $\{K_i\}$ already of the whole set L:$\lambda^n_{K_1|\ldots|K_s} = \prod_{j=1}^{s}[1-R(K_j)]^n$. The substitution of various $\lambda_{K_1|\ldots|K_s}$ into (3.13) yields summands of the form

$$[1-R(L)]^{t-1} \sum_{n=0}^{t-1} \{\lambda_{K_1|\ldots|K_s}/[1-R(L)]\}^n =$$

$$= [1-R(L)]^t/[\lambda_{K_1|\ldots|K_s} - 1 + R(L)] - \lambda^t_{K_1|\ldots|K_s}/[\lambda_{K_1|\ldots|K_s} - R(L)],$$

where the constants are omitted. Therefore (3.13), which is the concentration of L-locus gametes presented as a function of time, can be rewritten as follows:

$$p_i(t) = \prod_{j=1}^{l} p_{i_j} + \sum_{K_1|\ldots|K_s} C_{K_1|\ldots|K_s} \prod_{j=1}^{s} [1-R(K_j)]^t, \qquad (3.14)$$

where $C_{K_1|\ldots|K_s}$ are constants, depending only on the initial state and the linkage distribution.

The explicit form of $C_{K_1|...|K_s}$ (which is quite cumbersome), derived by Ju.I. Ljubic, can be also deduced by induction. However we shall not dwell on this, confining ourselves to (3.14). Let us only note that there can be such a 'singular' occasion, when $1\text{-}R(\cup_{i=1}^{s} K_i)$ coincides with one of the $\lambda_{K_1|...|K_s}$ (we can by-pass this, if we slightly deviate the parameters of the linkage distribution). Then in the expansion of $p_{\mathrm{i}}(t)$ we will have a term with the product of the form $t[1-R]^t$. If we have also come across such an occasion previously, then we will have $t^2\lambda^t$.

Thus in the non-singular case with non-rigid linkage between loci the gamete frequencies are exponentially converging towards the equilibria, characterized by random allele combinations in gametes. The manifold of equilibrium states is independent of the linkage distribution. Its dimensionality is far less than that of the space of gamete frequencies Σ, being equal to the total number of alleles minus the number of loci.

In order to treat the problem about the approximation of difference equations for multi-locus gamete frequencies by the differential ones, let us rewrite (3.8), regarding the generation span as the time unit ($\Delta t = 1$):

$$\Delta p_{i_1...i_l} = -\Big[\sum_{U|V,\,U\neq\varnothing,L} r(U|V)D_{\mathrm{i},U|V}\Big]\Delta t, \quad i_1 = \overline{1, n_1};...; \quad i_l = \overline{1, n_l}\,. \tag{3.15}$$

Reasoning along the same lines as in the two-locus case, we find that close to the state of equilibrium or for small parameters of the linkage distribution $r(U|V)$, the Equations (3.15) can be approximated by the differential ones, as follows:

$$\frac{dp_{i_1...i_l}}{dt} = -\sum_{U|V,\,U\neq\varnothing,L} r(U|V)D_{\mathrm{i},U|V}, \quad i_1 = \overline{1, n_1}; \quad i_l = \overline{1, n_l}, \tag{3.16}$$

if only time is measured in generations.

The solution to (3.16) is defined by induction, just as in the scheme with difference equations, and it can be obtained from (3.14) by substituting $\exp\{-R(K_i)t\}$ for $[1-R(K_i)]^t$. Like before the gamete frequencies are in equilibrium if and only if they are equal to the product of concentrations of their constituent alleles.

9.4. Recombination-Segregation Model in a Multi-Locus Continuous-Time System

If instead of the continuous approximation of a discrete model, we look at a population with no age structure and with parallel processes of reproduction and mortality, which is usually done in ecological models, then we also arrive at the equations of the (3.16) type. First, let us note, that under panmixia hypothesis the dynamic equations for genotypes numbers (cf. with (2.7)) can be presented as follows:

$$\frac{dN_{\mathbf{ij}}}{dt} = bN\,\Big\{[1 - R(L)]\sum p_{\mathrm{i}\cdot} + \sum_{U|V,\,U\neq\varnothing,L} r(U|V)\sum p_{(\mathrm{i}_U\cdot)(\mathrm{i}_V\cdot)}\Big\} \times$$

$$\times \{[1 - R(L)]\sum p_{\mathbf{j}\cdot} + \sum_{U|V,\, U\neq\varnothing,L} r(U|V)\sum p_{(\mathbf{j}_U\cdot)(\mathbf{j}_V\cdot)}\} - m(N, \mathbf{p}, t)Np_{\mathbf{ij}},$$

$$i_1 j_1 = \overline{1, n_1};\ldots;\ i_l, j_l = \overline{1, n_l}. \qquad (4.1)$$

Here points stand for the multi-indices, over which summation is being taken. Taking account of (3.2), the equations for genotype numbers N and frequencies $p_{\mathbf{ij}}$ have the form

$$\frac{dN}{dt} = N[b - m(N, \mathbf{p}, t)],$$

$$\frac{dp_{\mathbf{ij}}}{dt} = b\left[\sum p_{\mathbf{i}\cdot} - \sum_{U|V,\, U\neq\varnothing,L} r(U|V)\sum (p_{\mathbf{i}\cdot} - p_{(\mathbf{i}_U\cdot)(\mathbf{i}_V\cdot)})\right] \times$$

$$\times\left[\sum p_{\mathbf{j}\cdot} - \sum_{U|V,\, U\neq\varnothing,L} r(U|V)\sum (p_{\mathbf{j}\cdot} - p_{(\mathbf{j}_U\cdot)(\mathbf{j}_V\cdot)})\right] - bp_{\mathbf{ij}},$$

$$\mathbf{i} = \{i_k\},\ \mathbf{j} = \{j_k\},\ i_1 j_1 = \overline{1, n_1};\ldots;\ i_l, j_l = \overline{1, n_l}. \qquad (4.2)$$

Equations for frequencies are independent of numbers, but they are still too complicated. Therefore let us change over to new variables: $p_{\mathbf{i}}$ are the frequencies of the gametes with alleles A_{i_j}, $j = \overline{1, l}$, $D^1_{\mathbf{ij}}$ are the measures of randomness for gametes combinations in genotypes $\{\mathbf{i}, \mathbf{j}\}$, and $y_{\mathbf{i}_U \mathbf{i}_V}$ are the concentrations of genotypes carrying alleles A_{i_j}, $j \in U$ in one gamete and alleles A_{i_k} $k \in V$-in another:

$$p_{\mathbf{i}} = \sum p_{\mathbf{i}\cdot},\ y_{\mathbf{i}_U \mathbf{i}_V} = \sum p_{(\mathbf{i}_U\cdot)(\mathbf{i}_V\cdot)},$$

$$D^1_{\mathbf{ij}} = p_{\mathbf{ij}} - \sum p_{\mathbf{i}\cdot} \sum p_{\mathbf{j}\cdot} = p_{\mathbf{ij}} - p_{\mathbf{i}} p_{\mathbf{j}}, \qquad (4.3)$$

where in the expression for $y_{\mathbf{i}_U \mathbf{i}_V}$ summation is being taken over all kinds of gamete 'tails'. Assuming that

$$b >> \max_{U|V,\, U\neq\varnothing,\, L} r(U|V) = r,$$

without loss of generality, we can write that $r(U|V) = 0\ (\varepsilon)$, $0<\varepsilon<<1$, for all non-trivial $U|V$-partitions. An appropriate summation of (4.2) under the condition $br \sim 0(\varepsilon)$ yields

$$\frac{dp_{\mathbf{i}}}{dt} = b \sum_{U|V,\, U\neq\varnothing,L} r(U|V)(y_{\mathbf{i}_U \mathbf{i}_V} - p_{\mathbf{i}}) = 0(\varepsilon),$$

$$\frac{dy_{\mathbf{i}_U \mathbf{i}_V}}{dt} = b(p_{\mathbf{i}_U} p_{\mathbf{i}_V} - y_{\mathbf{i}_U \mathbf{i}_V}) + 0(\varepsilon),$$

$$\frac{dD^1_{\mathbf{ij}}}{dt} = -b\, D^1_{\mathbf{ij}} + 0(\varepsilon),\quad \mathbf{i} = i_1 \ldots i_l;\ \ \mathbf{j} = j_1 \ldots j_l;\ \ i_k, j_k = \overline{1, n_k};\ \ k = \overline{1, l}, \qquad (4.4)$$

where p_{i_U} and p_{i_V} are the concentrations of U-and V-locus gametes with alleles from the ith gamete.

By (4.4), p_i are 'slow' variables, while the rest ones are 'fast'. When the slow variables are fixed, the globally stable equilibria of the fast ones, as $\varepsilon \to 0$, are $D^1_{ij}=0$ and $y_{i_U i_V} = p_{i_U} p_{i_V}$, which means that gametes and allele subsets in genotypes combine at random in complete agreement with the two-locus case of Section 9.2. By Tychonoff theorem, over a finite time interval the dynamics of p_i can be approximated by the solution of the first equation in (4.4), assuming that $y_{i_U i_V} = p_{i_U} p_{i_V}$:

$$\frac{dp_{i_1 \dots i_l}}{dt} = -b \sum_{U|V,\, U \neq \varnothing, L} r(U|V) D_{i,U|V}\,, \quad i_1 = \overline{1, n_1};\dots;\quad i_l = \overline{1, n_l} \tag{4.5}$$

where $D_{i,U|V} = p_i - p_{i_U} p_{i_V}$ as it was defined in (3.10) when the discrete model was studied.

If we drop the coefficient b, then (4.5) becomes identic to the equation (3.16) for the continuous approximation of the discrete model. But this time we did without the burdensome assumption about the proximity of the state to the equilibrium, or about tight linkage, which excludes the biologically important situations such as, say, the case when some of the loci of interest are not linked.

Summing up (4.5) over $i_2, \dots, i_l$, we find out that $\dot{p}_{i_1} = 0$, that is the allele frequencies are constant. If summation is being taking over all indices but the first two, then we arrive at equation (2.12) for the frequency of two-locus gamete, and this equation is linear for the known (from the preceding step) values of p_{i_1} and p_{i_2}. Let us now suppose that the concentrations of U-and V-locus gametes are equal to a constant (which is the product of allele frequencies for the $U(V)$ loci of the considered gamete) summed with the linear combination of exponentials, their exponents being equal to time multiplied by various sums of the non-breakage parameters for disjoint subsets of the $U(V)$ loci. Then in the robust case a similar expansion holds for L-locus gametes as well.

In fact, substituting p_{i_U} and p_{i_V} as the functions of time, we split (4.5) into separate linear non-uniform equations.

The solution to these equations can be represented as follows

$$p_i(t) = e^{-bR(L)t} \left[\sum_{U|V,\, U \neq \varnothing, L} r(U|V) \int_0^t p_{i_U}(s)\, p_{i_V}(s)\; e^{bR(L)s}\, ds \; + p_i(0) \right].$$

Obviously, the constant in the product $p_{i_U} p_{i_V}$ for any $U|V$-partition is equal to the product of the concentrations of alleles, contained in the ith L-locus gamete. The coefficient for this term will be $r(U|V)$. Summing up over all $U|V$-partitions, and taking account of (3.2), after integration we find the constant in the expansion of p_i to be equal to the product of the concentrations of alleles, carried by the gamete in question, just as it could be expected.

Multiplying the linear combination of exponential in the expansion of p_{i_U} (their exponent being equal to time multiplied by various sums of non-breakage parameters R for all kinds of disjoint subsets of U) by p_{i_V}, we again arrive at a linear combination of exponentials. Therefore, after integration the expansions of the L-locus gametes frequencies will contain exponentials with exponents defined by the sums of the non-breakage parameters for the disjoint subsets already of all the L loci, as it was assumed by the induction. Whence the asymptotic behavior of the continuous-time model breaks with the dynamics in the discrete case by the exchange of the probabilities of non-breakage of subsets K_i of the set L, that is $1\text{-}R(K_i)$, for $\exp\{-bR(K_i)\}$ in the appropriate solution.

For (4.5) one can find some functions steadily changing along the trajectories. The simplest of them is the two-locus coefficient of linkage disequilibrium (1.3), its relative rate of variation being constant. One can construct similar functions depending on the frequencies of three-locus gametes and so on. Their form becomes rather complicated already for a small number of loci. Therefore the dynamics of the population genetic structure is better represented by the entropy, which is simpler and easier to interpret and which also grows steadily with time. Though the rate of its variations is not constant, the fact that this characteristic defines the statistical diversity of the population genetic content, makes it so attractive. In a more general context the monotonicity of entropy has been indicated by L.A. Kun and Ju.I. Ljubic. The entropy of the distribution of gamete frequencies is defined as

$$H = -\sum_{\mathbf{i}} p_{\mathbf{i}} \ln p_{\mathbf{i}} \,. \tag{4.6}$$

Differentiating H with respect to time along trajectories of (4.5) and thinking that all the frequencies $\{p_{\mathbf{i}}\}$ are independent, we obtain

$$\frac{dH}{dt} = \sum_{\mathbf{i}} (1 + \ln p_{\mathbf{i}}) b \sum_{U|V,\, U \neq \emptyset, L} r(U|V)(p_{\mathbf{i}} - p_{\mathbf{i}_U} p_{\mathbf{i}_V}) =$$

$$= b \sum_{U|V,\, U \neq \emptyset, L} r(U|V) \left[\sum_{\mathbf{i}} p_{\mathbf{i}_U} \ln p_{\mathbf{i}} - \sum_{\mathbf{i}} p_{\mathbf{i}_U} p_{\mathbf{i}_V} \ln p_{\mathbf{i}} \right] \geq 0 \,.$$

Here we dropped the unity in $1 - \ln p_{\mathbf{i}}$ (since the sum of the right-hand sides of (4.5) over $\mathbf{i}$ is zero due to the identity $\Sigma_{\mathbf{i}} p_{\mathbf{i}} \equiv 1$), and took into account that for the two distributions $\{p_{\mathbf{i}}\}$, $\{q_{\mathbf{i}} = p_{\mathbf{i}_U} p_{\mathbf{i}_V}\}$ the quantity $\Sigma_{\mathbf{i}} q_{\mathbf{i}} \ln p_{\mathbf{i}}$ is maximal when $p_{\mathbf{i}} = q_{\mathbf{i}}$.

In the limit the combinations of alleles at various loci in gametes are independent and the entropy (the maximal one) of gamete frequencies will be equal to the sum of allele entropies at each of the loci:

$$H = -\sum_{k=1}^{l} \sum_{i_k=1}^{n_k} p_{i_k} \ln p_{i_k},$$

where p_{i_k} is the concentration of the ith allele at the kth locus.

9.5. Additivity of Interaction Between Selection and Recombination-Segregation in Multi-Locus Models Presented by Differential Equations

The processes of selection and recombination-segregation occur at different stages of the life-cycle. Therefore in the model formulated in terms of differential equations, the rate of variations in gamete frequencies due to the combined action of these factors is equal to the sum of the rates corresponding to the individual contributions of each of the factors. For instance, if the continuous version is regarded as the approximation of the discrete one, then the effect of selection and recombination over one generation should be assumed to be small. Let the selection-induced increment in the vector of gamete frequencies be characterized by the function $\Delta_w(\mathbf{p}) = \varepsilon\mathbf{f}_w(\mathbf{p})$ (or $\varepsilon\mathbf{f}_w(\mathbf{p})\Delta t$ if the generation span Δt is regarded as the time unit), and let the recombination-induced increment be $\Delta_R = \varepsilon f_R(p)\Delta t$. Then the difference equation for the dynamics of the gamete frequency vector will be as follows (the prime indicates that the variables belong to the next generation):

$$\mathbf{p}' = \mathbf{p} + \varepsilon\mathbf{f}_w(\mathbf{p})\Delta t + \varepsilon\mathbf{f}_R[\mathbf{p} + \varepsilon f_w(p)\Delta t]\Delta t =$$
$$= \mathbf{p} + \varepsilon\mathbf{f}_w(\mathbf{p})\Delta t + \varepsilon\mathbf{f}_R(\mathbf{p})\Delta t + o(\varepsilon^2\Delta t^2)\,. \tag{5.1}$$

Introducing once again the new time scale $\tau = \varepsilon t$, we derive that the length of one generation in terms of the new time is very small, and the variations in gamete frequencies in terms of this time can be approximately regarded as continuous. Consequently, as $\varepsilon \to 0$, assuming that the functions $\mathbf{f}$ are sufficiently good, from (5.1) we obtain

$$d\mathbf{p}/d\tau = \mathbf{f}_w(\mathbf{p}) + \mathbf{f}_R(\mathbf{p})\,. \tag{5.2}$$

We would have resulted in a similar equation, if recombination preceded selection. Therefore in the continuous-time model the order of the factors' action does not matter, and parameters defining segregation (selection) do not enter into the functions $\mathbf{f}_w(\mathbf{f}_R)$. On the time scale with the generation as the time-unit, (5.2) assumes the conventional form:

$$d\mathbf{p}/dt = \Delta_w(\mathbf{p}) + \Delta_R(\mathbf{p})\,. \tag{5.3}$$

The smallness of $\Delta(\mathbf{p})$ was applied to derive (5.3). The biological meaning of this assumption may be the weakness of selection and tightness of linkage, or the proximity of the states to equilibria.

Equations of the (5.3) type can be derived directly from the continuous model, that implies that there is no age structure (for instance, if a quick-stabilization is assumed) and that the processes of birth and death are simultaneous. Roughly speaking, these assumptions indicate that the process is analyzed on a time-scale such that the length of generation is small and, accordingly, the effect of the age distribution dynamics, of natality and mortality upon the genetic structure over this time period is negligible, making the model close to the discrete version.

Taking no account of the age, we can determine the dynamics of the genetic structure by selection and recombination-segregation. Generally speaking, the processes of recombination-segregation are associated in time with one of the components of selection - with differential fecundity. If the differential fecundity is taken into account, then the analysis of the population genetic structure in the level of one locus already results in equations of dynamics which are more complicated then the classical ones (except for the simplest case of multiplicative effect of the mating individuals upon fecundity of the pair). That is why in what follows we actually confine ourselves to the investigation of only one component of selection, namely, the selection with respect to viability. In formal terms this situation implies that the fecundity of mating pairs is independent of the genetic construction of individuals.

In this case the dynamic equations for genotype numbers have the form

$$dN_{\mathbf{ij}}/dt = -m_{\mathbf{ij}}(N, \mathbf{p}, t)\, N_{\mathbf{ij}} + b\tilde{f}_{\mathbf{ij},R}(N)\,, \tag{5.4}$$

where $\tilde{f}_{\mathbf{ij},R}$ is the function, presenting the rate of variations in the numbers of the {**i**, **j**}th genotype (this function appears in Equation (4.1)) as a result of recombination-segregation, and $m_{\mathbf{ij}}(N, \mathbf{p}, t)$ presents the rate of the variations induced by (differential) mortality. If we carry on to genotype frequencies **p**, in the vector form we get

$$d\mathbf{p}/dt = \mathbf{f}_w + b\,\tilde{\mathbf{f}}_R \tag{5.5}$$

where $\mathbf{f}_w$ reflects the effect of differential mortality (selection), as if the one-locus structure were studied (with no recombination), and $\tilde{\mathbf{f}}_R$ stands for the effect of recombination (with no selection and mortality at all). As a result, just as in the approximation of the discrete model, the derivations of the genotype concentrations are equal to the summed rates of variations in concentrations induced by selection and by the recombination-segregation processes (separately) as functions of one and the same current value of **p**.

The explicit form of the functions contained in the right-hand sides of (5.2), (5.3), can be obtained as follows. First consider the discrete model of population with non-overlapping generations, and write out the functions $\Delta_w(\mathbf{p})$ and $\Delta_R(\mathbf{p})$ for the multi-locus version of this model. Next, assuming selection to be weak (the differences between fitnesses are of the order of ε) and linkage to be tight ($r(U|V)$ is of the order of ε), let us modify Δ_w and Δ_R, rounding them off to the terms of the order of $o(\varepsilon)$. In this way we arrive at the differential equations, approximating the discrete-model dynamics. In case of the originally continuous model, let us carry on from the equations for genotypes to the equations for gametes. Unlike the previous case, gamete combinations in genotypes will no longer be random. However, assuming the effect of systematic factors to be weak, we quickly come to a quasipanmictic situation with gamete fusions being close to random. Actually, the equations for gamete frequencies asymptotically coincide with the continuous approximation of the discrete model.

9.6. Selection of Zygotes and Gametes in a Discrete-Time Model and its Continuous Approximation

Without recombination the multi-locus model can be formally considered within the framework of one-locus equations with multi-locus gametes playing the part of alleles. In the discrete case frequencies of such 'alleles' p_i comply with the difference equation (see Section 2.16)

$$\Delta p_i = p_i \sum_j p_j w_{ij} \Big/ \sum_{i,j} p_i p_j w_{ij} - p_i = p_i \frac{w_i - w}{w}\,, \tag{6.1}$$

where w_i is the fitness of the ith allele, and w is the average fitness of the population.

Equations (6.1) are usually analysed under the assumption that fitnesses w_{ij} are constant and non-negative. In this case the average fitness is equal to the ratio between the population sizes in successive generations, which is an important factor in evolution of the population.

Let us note that (6.1) does not change, if all w_{ij} are multiplied by one and the same function (say, of the population size, allele frequencies and time), which makes fitnesses variable. Therefore from (6.1) w is defined only to within a coefficient (though allele numbers define it uniquely). This coefficient (for instance, when it depends only on the population size, as in one of the formulae contained in the paper by May and Oster) can reflect the non-differential pressure of external factors, which is independent of the genetic structure.

For variable fitnesses of this kind the equations for allele frequencies can be separated from the one for the total population size. The dynamics of the former can be studied separately, abstracting from ecological factors. At the same time for changes in the population size a good agreement with experimental data can be achieved in models without the exponentially infinite or damped growth (which is specific of models with constant fitnesses), as well as in models with exotic, say, chaotic population behavior.

The genetic structure can be still analyzed by means of the relatively simple equations (6.1), where fitnesses can be assumed constant. It appears that this can be the reason why the isolated analysis of the dynamics of genetic structure is so common: in the simplest case the genetic structure can be studied independently of the ecological effects on the population size.

Thus, if Equations (6.1) are regarded as a part of more realistic models, taking account of ecological effects, then the average fitness, defined under the assumption of constant genotype fitness, can no longer be interpreted as the ratio between population sizes in neighboring generations. However it still effects the growth rate of the population: other things being equal, the rate is in proportion to the average fitness.

The coefficient of fitness w_{ij} in (6.1) are assumed to be symmetric. The dynamics and statics of allele frequencies and related populational characteristics are essentially based on this symmetry of fitnesses. One of the conclusions here is as follows: under the effect of selection and random mating the average fitness of the population grows (Fisher's fundamental theorem of natural selection). Applying the expressions for the rate of increases in average fitness, one can show that the population equilibrates for any constant non-negative value of w_{ij}, which is an important conclusion for population genetics.

If in addition to selection of genotypes, we introduce the selection of gametes, employing the coefficients v_i, which present the elimination intensity for the allele of the ith type, then we arrive at relations for allele frequencies of the (6.1) type, but the already generalized fitness coefficients will be non-symmetric in the general case. It turns out that the behavior of a number of populational characteristics will be also altered. For instance, the average fitness no longer needs to grow with the passage of time. Stability conditions for the equilibrium states will be also different, and consequently additional efforts are required in order to analyze this model.

Let us show that by choosing the right moment in the life-span when to treat the gene frequencies of the population, we may reduce the case of gamete selection to the ordinary symmetric case.

If p_i are the allele frequencies at the beginning of the generation, then under random mating the numbers of genotypes $\{ij\}$ at that time are in proportion to $p_i p_j$ (taking into account the order of alleles). As a result of the action of genotypic selection, specified by the fitness coefficients $w_{ij}(w_{ij} = w_{ji})$, at the end of the generation genotype numbers will become in proportion to $p_i p_j w_{ij}$. Next, assuming fecundity to be non-differential, we are to take into account the process of segregation and differential survival of gametes. Suppose that coefficients υ_i specify the intensity of variations in allele frequencies, induced by selection of gametes, the allele numbers being in proportion to these coefficients. Then as it was proved by V.A. Ratner,

$$p_i' = \sum_j p_i p_j w_{ij} \upsilon_i / \sum_{i,j} p_i p_j w_{ij} \upsilon_i = p_i \sum_j p_j G_{ij} / G \,,$$

or

$$\mathbf{p}_{n+1} = \mathbf{D}(\mathbf{p}_n)\, \mathbf{V}\mathbf{W}\mathbf{p}_n / (\mathbf{e}, \mathbf{D}(\mathbf{p}_n)\mathbf{V}\mathbf{W}\mathbf{p}_n)\,. \tag{6.1a}$$

Here the later formula is presented in the vector-matrix form: $G_{ij} = w_{ij}\upsilon_i$, $G = \sum_{i,j} p_i p_j w_{ij} \upsilon_i = (\mathbf{e}, \mathbf{D}(\mathbf{p})\mathbf{V}\mathbf{W}\mathbf{p})$ is termed generalized fitness and plays the part of a normalizing factor in (6.1a), such that the sum of new allele frequencies is equal to unit: $\mathbf{D}(\mathbf{p})$ and $\mathbf{V}$ are diagonal matrices with diagonal entries p_i and υ_i, respectively; $\mathbf{p}$ is the vector of allele frequencies with coordinates p_i; $\mathbf{W}$ is the matrix of fitnesses w_{ij}; $\mathbf{e}$ is the vector with unitary coordinates; index n is the generation number.

Recall that in (6.1a) the basic characteristic of the genetic structure are presented by allele frequencies p_i at the beginning of the generation; that is prior to the action of selection. Allele frequencies (denoted by x_i) after the action of selection can be regarded as the basic characteristics of the genetic structure. The Mendelian process of segregation does not alter the frequencies x_i, when one-locus gametes are formed, and under the action of gamete selection the allele frequencies becomes proportional to $x_i \upsilon_i$. Next goes the process of random mating, which makes the frequencies of genotypes $\{ij\}$ proportional to $x_i \upsilon_i x_j \upsilon_j$ at the beginning of the next generation, and proportional to $x_i \upsilon_i x_j \upsilon_j w_{ij}$- after selection. Therefore

$$x_i' = \sum_j x_i x_j \upsilon_i w_{ij} \upsilon_j / \sum_{i,j} x_i x_j \upsilon_i w_{ij} \upsilon_j \,.$$

Thus, if fitnesses of genotypes are assumed equal to $\upsilon_i w_{ij} \upsilon_j$ and symmetric, then the dynamics of x_i are equivalent to those in the common case without gamete selection.

These conclusions can be supported by a formal deduction, which is based solely on Equation (6.1a), and does not appeal to the genetic mechanisms, invoked in order to prove that equation. This enables us to reduce relationships of this kind to those already studied, regardless of the nature of the considered phenomena and the changes for a sound interpretation of the variables x_i.

Let us change the variables (genetically this implies that we carry on backwards from the allele frequencies at the beginning of each generation to those at the end of the one before, the nth one):

$$\mathbf{x}_n = \mathbf{V}^{-1}\mathbf{p}_{n+1}/(\mathbf{e}, \mathbf{V}^{-1}\mathbf{p}_{n+1}) \,. \tag{6.2}$$

Hence, $\mathbf{p}_{n+1}$ is to comply with the equality

$$\mathbf{p}_{n+1} = (\mathbf{e}, \mathbf{V}^{-1}\mathbf{p}_{n+1})\mathbf{V}\mathbf{x}_n. \tag{6.2a}$$

The inverse transformation has the form

$$\mathbf{p}_{n+1} = \mathbf{V}\mathbf{x}_n/(\mathbf{e}, \mathbf{V}\mathbf{x}_n) \,. \tag{6.2b}$$

Substituting $\mathbf{p}_{n+1}$ from (6.2a) and $\mathbf{p}_n$ calculated by (6.2b), into (6.1a), we get

$$(\mathbf{e}, \mathbf{V}^{-1}\mathbf{p}_{n+1})\mathbf{V}\mathbf{x}_n = \frac{1}{(\mathbf{e}, \mathbf{D}(\mathbf{p}_n)\mathbf{V}\mathbf{W}\mathbf{p}_n)} \frac{\mathbf{D}(\mathbf{V}\mathbf{x}_{n-1})}{(\mathbf{e}, \mathbf{V}\mathbf{x}_{n-1})} \mathbf{V}\mathbf{W} \frac{\mathbf{V}\mathbf{x}_{n-1}}{(\mathbf{e}, \mathbf{V}\mathbf{x}_{n-1})} \tag{6.3}$$

Note that $\mathbf{D}(\mathbf{V}\mathbf{x}) = \mathbf{V}\mathbf{D}(\mathbf{x})$. We can write the scalar product, contained in (6.3) as a factor on the left, substituting $\mathbf{p}_{n+1}$ from (6.1a) and $\mathbf{p}_n$ as in (6.2b):

$$\begin{aligned}(\mathbf{e}, \mathbf{V}^{-1}\mathbf{p}_{n+1}) &= \frac{1}{(\mathbf{e}, \mathbf{D}(\mathbf{p}_n)\mathbf{V}\mathbf{W}\mathbf{p}_n)} \times \left(\mathbf{e}, \mathbf{V}^{-1}\frac{\mathbf{V}\mathbf{D}(\mathbf{x}_{n-1})}{(\mathbf{e}, \mathbf{V}\mathbf{x}_{n-1})} \mathbf{V}\mathbf{W}\frac{\mathbf{V}\mathbf{x}_{n-1}}{(\mathbf{e}, \mathbf{V}\mathbf{x}_{n-1})}\right) = \\ &= \frac{(\mathbf{e}, \mathbf{D}(\mathbf{x}_{n-1})\mathbf{V}\mathbf{W}\mathbf{V}\mathbf{x}_{n-1})}{(\mathbf{e}, \mathbf{V}\mathbf{x}_{n-1})^2(\mathbf{e}, \mathbf{D}(\mathbf{p}_n)\mathbf{V}\mathbf{W}\mathbf{p}_n)} \,.\end{aligned} \tag{6.4}$$

Here the subscript for $\mathbf{p}$ and $\mathbf{x}$ stands for the generation number. All υ_i are supposed to be non-zero, which makes the matrix $\mathbf{V}$ non-singular. Multiplying (6.3) on the left by $\mathbf{V}^{-1}$ and dividing it by (6.4), we get

$$\mathbf{x}_n = \frac{\mathbf{D}(\mathbf{x}_{n-1})\mathbf{V}\mathbf{W}\mathbf{V}\mathbf{x}_{n-1}}{(\mathbf{e}, \mathbf{D}(\mathbf{x}_{n-1})\mathbf{V}\mathbf{W}\mathbf{V}\mathbf{x}_{n-1})} \,. \tag{6.5}$$

Equation (6.5) totally corresponds to the dynamics of gene frequencies $\mathbf{x}$, when the matrix of fitnesses $\mathbf{VWV}$ is symmetric. All the results, known for this case, can be rewritten in terms of $\mathbf{p}$, applying (6.2). In particular, we derive that over the course of time the function $F = (\mathbf{x}, \mathbf{V}\mathbf{W}\mathbf{V}\mathbf{x})$ is non-decreasing along the trajectories. This function has the biological meaning of average population fitness after the action of selection and in terms of $\mathbf{p}$ (applying (6.2)) it has the form

$$F = \frac{(\mathbf{p}, \mathbf{W}\mathbf{p})}{(\mathbf{e}, \mathbf{V}^{-1}\mathbf{p})^2} = \sum_{i,j} p_i p_j w_{ij} \Big/ \left(\sum_i \frac{p_i}{\upsilon_i}\right)^2$$

It defines the adaptive topography of system (6.1a), attaining the maximum (we denote it by F^*) at the asymptotically stable point of the system, and the function $F^*\text{-}F(\mathbf{p})$ can be regarded as the Lyapunov function for the stability analysis.

The proof of monotonicity of F in the discrete case is quite cumbersome. Let us present the simple proof, which is obtained when the difference scheme (6.1a) is approximated by the system of ordinary differential equations. Let

$$w_i = \sum_j p_j w_{ij}, \; w = \sum_{i,j} p_i p_j w_{ij}, \quad G = \sum_i \sum_j p_i p_j \upsilon_i w_{ij}.$$

Then

$$dp_i/dt = (\upsilon_i w_i - G), \; i = 1, 2, \ldots \tag{6.6}$$

Here the subscript i is related to the allele number. Next we get

$$\frac{\partial F}{\partial p_i} = \frac{\partial}{\partial p_i}\left[w \Big/ \left(\sum_j \frac{p_j}{\upsilon_j}\right)^2 \right] = \frac{2w_i}{\left(\sum_j p_j/\upsilon_j\right)^2} - \frac{2w}{\upsilon_i\left(\sum_j p_j/\upsilon_j\right)^3},$$

$$\frac{dF}{dt} = \sum_i \frac{\partial}{\partial p_i} F \frac{d}{dt} p_i = \frac{2}{\left(\sum_j p_j/\upsilon_j\right)^2} \sum_i p_i w_i (\upsilon_i w_i - G$$

$$- \frac{2w}{\left(\sum_j p_j/\upsilon_j\right)^3} \sum_i \frac{p_i}{\upsilon_i}(\upsilon_i w_i - G) = \frac{2}{\left(\sum_j p_j/\upsilon_j\right)^2} \left[\sum_i p_i \upsilon_i w_i^2 - \frac{w^2}{\sum_j p_j/\upsilon_j} \right].$$

Obviously, the sign of dF/dt coincides with the sign of the expression in square brackets. Let us note that by the Cauchy-Schwarz-Buniakowski inequality

$$w^2 = \left(\sum_j p_j w_j\right)^2 = \left[\sum_j \sqrt{p_j/\upsilon_j}\,\sqrt{p_j \upsilon_j} w_j\right]^2 \le \left(\sum_j \frac{p_j}{\upsilon_j}\right)\left(\sum_j p_j \upsilon_j w_j^2\right). \tag{6.7}$$

Therefore $dF/dt \geq 0$. The equality in (6.7) is reached only on proportional vectors, that is when $\sqrt{p_j \upsilon_j}\, w_j = \alpha \sqrt{p_j/\upsilon_j}$, $j = 1, 2, \ldots$. Whence for any j the equality $\upsilon_j w_j = \alpha$ holds.

Then $\alpha = G$. It follows from (6.6) that if $\upsilon_j w_j = G$ then $\dot{p}_j = 0$. Thus, F grows steadily along the trajectories of (6.6), being constant only at the stationary points of this system.

Let us justify the differential approximation of the difference equation, that was used in (6.6). It has been repeatedly mentioned, that this approximation is correct, for instance if the effect of systematic factors (which is the selection of genotypes and gametes in our case) is weak. Therefore, let us present the coefficients of generalized fitnesses in the form $G_{ij} = 1 - \varepsilon g_{ij}$ (recall that all G_{ij} can be written an accuracy of one and the same factor). Then it follows from (6.1a) that

$$\Delta p_i = p_i \frac{1 - \varepsilon \sum_j p_j g_{ij} - 1 + \varepsilon \sum_{i,j} p_i p_j g_{ij}}{1 - \varepsilon \sum_{i,j} p_i p_j g_{ij}} =$$

$$= \varepsilon p_i (g - g_i)(1 + \varepsilon g) + o(\varepsilon) = \varepsilon p_i (g - g_i) + o(\varepsilon)$$

Here g_i and g are the fitnesses of the ith allele and of the whole population, defined by the coefficients of 'fitness' g_{ij}. Since $\varepsilon(g - g_i) = G_i - G = \upsilon_i w_i - G$, neglecting the term $o(\varepsilon)$ we yield, according to (5.3):

$$dp_i/dt = p_i(v_i w_i - G_i),\ i = 1, 2,...$$

that is the Equation (6.6).

If we approximate (6.1), assuming that $w_{ij} = 1 - m_{ij}$, $m_{ij} \sim \varepsilon$, then the appropriate equation will be

$$dp_i/dt = p_i(w_i - w) = p_i(m - m_i)\ ,\ \ w_{ij} = w_{ji}, i,j = 1, 2,... \tag{6.8}$$

Further on we will see that the coefficients m_{ij} are similar to the Malthusian parameters in continuous-time models.

Sometimes when the difference scheme is approximated by the differential one, the expression for Δ_w is treated without passing to the limit with respect to ε to within $o(\varepsilon)$. Then instead of (6.6) we get the equations

$$dp_i/dt = p_i(G_i - G)/G,\ \ i = 1, 2,... \tag{6.9}$$

The right-hand sides in (6.6) and (6.9) are the same, except for the positive coefficient G. Therefore the trajectories of these systems coincide, only the rate of the movement being different.

Let us note, that there is another way to approximate the difference scheme (6.1a). When (6.6) and (6.9) were derived, the difference between generalized fitnesses G_{ij} were assumed to be weak. If the intensities of selection among zygotes and gametes are supposed to be of the same order of smallness, and if we think that in any stage of the life-cycle the differential approximation can be applied, then $w_{ij} = 1 - m_{ij}$, $v_i = 1 - s_i$, where $m_{ij} \sim s_i \sim \varepsilon << 1$. Hence $G_{ij} = v_i w_{ij} = 1 - m_{ij} - s_i + o(\varepsilon)$. Neglecting the term $o(\varepsilon)$ in this expression, we obtain the following system of differential equations as an approximation of the difference scheme (6.1a):

$$dp_i/dt = p_i(m - m_i) + p_i(s - s_i)\ ,\ s = \sum_i p_i s_i\ . \tag{6.10}$$

Such an approach to the presentation of the equations, specifying the variations in gamete frequencies in the succession of life stages, corresponds to the summation of the right-hand sides from the equations of the dynamics in each of the stages separately, presented as functions of one and the same current value of the gamete concentrations.

These examples already demonstrate, that the small increments Δp_i (the necessary condition for the differential approximation) can be formulated in different (though asymptotically close) ways. Analysis of thus derived systems of differential equations results in similar results for the robust cases.

In conclusion we can remark, that applying ordinary differential equations to the approximation of the model with non-overlapping generations, we can confine our study (in case of gamete selection as well) to the case of symmetric fitness coefficients. When analyzing the multi-locus model, the effect of selection on gamete concentrations can be characterized by the function $\Delta_w(\mathbf{p})$ from the difference equations, presented to an accuracy of $o(\varepsilon)$ (where ε is the order of differences between fitnesses) in the following form:

$$(\Delta_w)_i \simeq p_i(w_i - w),\ \ i = 1, 2,... \tag{6.11}$$

As mentioned above, the same function describes the effect of selection in the one-locus case.

9.7. Equations of Dynamics Under the Combined Action of Selection and Recombination-Segregation in Discrete- and Continuous-Time Models

In the L-locus case, when processes of segregation-recombination and selection are taken into account, the differential equations, that approximate the difference ones, due to (3.16) and Section 9.5, have the following form:

$$\frac{dp_{\mathbf{i}}}{dt} = \frac{dp_{i_1 \ldots i_l}}{dt} = p_i(w_i - w) - \sum_{U|V,\, U \neq \emptyset, L} r(U|V) D_{\mathbf{i},\, U|V} = p_i(m - m_i) -$$

$$- \sum_{U|V,\, U \neq \emptyset, L} r(U|V) D_{\mathbf{i}, U|V}, \quad i_1 = \overline{1, n_1}\,; \ldots;\; i_l = \overline{1, n_l}\,. \tag{7.1}$$

Here the selection-induced term is presented according to the Equation (6.8), the coefficients $r(U|V)$ are assumed to be small, and the parameters of fitnesses do not enter into the coefficients of disequilibrium $D_{\mathbf{i}, U|V}$ (as well as into the whole sum over all $U|V$-partitions, representing the effect of recombination-segregation).

In the discrete case the equations turns to be more sophisticated. Since the recombination-segregation processes effect the gamete frequencies, already altered by selection, here we can no longer present the increments in concentrations by separate terms corresponding to selection and recombination of the gamete content in a way such that the parameters, specifying selection, do not enter into the recombination increment:

$$p_i' = p_{i_1 \ldots i_l}' = \frac{1}{w}\Big[\sum_{j} (1 - R) w_{\mathbf{ij}} p_{\mathbf{i}} p_{\mathbf{j}} +$$

$$+ \sum_{U|V,\, U \neq \emptyset, L} r(U|V) \sum_{\mathbf{j}} w_{(\mathbf{i}_U \mathbf{j}_V)(\mathbf{i}_V \mathbf{j}_U)} p_{\mathbf{i}_U \mathbf{j}_V} p_{\mathbf{i}_V \mathbf{j}_U}\Big], \quad i_1 = \overline{1, n_1}\,; \ldots;\; i_l = \overline{1, n_l}\,. \tag{7.2}$$

Here $(\mathbf{i}_U, \mathbf{j}_V)$ is a multi-index, its kth item being i_k if $k \in U$, and j_k if $k \in V$; w is the average fitness, defined as in the one-locus case: $w = \sum_{\mathbf{i},\mathbf{j}} w_{\mathbf{ij}} p_{\mathbf{i}} p_{\mathbf{j}}$. If the fitness of the ith gamete is expressed by the formula

$$w_{\mathbf{i}} = \sum_{j} w_{\mathbf{ij}} p_{\mathbf{j}},$$

and if, like before, R is written out as the sum of coefficients $r(U|V)$, over $U|V$ then (6.14) can be rewritten as

$$\Delta p_{i_1 \ldots i_l} = \Delta p_{\mathbf{i}} = p_{\mathbf{i}} \frac{w_{\mathbf{i}} - w}{w} - \frac{1}{w} \sum_{U|V,\, U \neq \emptyset, L} r(U|V) D^{w}_{\mathbf{i},\, U|V}\,,$$

$$i_1 = \overline{1, n_1}\,; \ldots;\; i_l = \overline{1, n_l}. \tag{7.3}$$

Here the first term in the right-hand side is independent of the linkage distribution and formally corresponds to the one-locus dynamics under the effect of selection. The coefficients $D^w_{\mathbf{i},U|V}$ are more complicated than the coefficients of $U|V$ -linkage disequilibrium, defined in (3.10) and appearing in (4.5) and (7.1):

$$D^w_{\mathbf{i},U|V} = \sum_{\mathbf{j}}(w_{\mathbf{ij}}p_{\mathbf{i}}p_{\mathbf{j}} - w_{(\mathbf{i}_U\mathbf{j}_V)(\mathbf{i}_V\mathbf{j}_U)}p_{\mathbf{i}_U\mathbf{j}_V}p_{\mathbf{i}_V\mathbf{j}_U}). \tag{7.4}$$

If all the fitness coefficients $w_{\mathbf{ij}}$ are equal to one and the same constant, say, unity, then $D^w_{\mathbf{i},U|V}$ coincides with the measure of disequilibrium $D_{\mathbf{i},U|V}$ defined by (3.10) in the absence of selection. Let us treat the relationship between $D^w_{\mathbf{i},U|V}$ and $D_{\mathbf{i},U|V}$ in case of selection. Suppose that the fitnesses of same genotypes, made up be different gametes, are equal, i.e. in (7.4) $w_{\mathbf{ij}} = w_{(\mathbf{i}_U\mathbf{j}_V)(\mathbf{i}_V\mathbf{j}_U)}$ for any $U|V$-partition of the L-loci. Exceptions from this rule are encountered in the molecular level. Taking $w_{\mathbf{ij}}$ outside the parenthesis, we get

$$D^w_{\mathbf{i},U|V} = \sum_{\mathbf{j}} w_{\mathbf{ij}}D_{\mathbf{ij},U|V}, \tag{7.5}$$

where $D_{\mathbf{ij},U|V}$ are defined in (3.12). Comparing (7.5) with (3.12a) we see, that while the $U|V$ disequilibrium $D_{\mathbf{i},U|V}$ is defined by the summation of coefficients of pairwise $U|V$-disequilibriums $D_{\mathbf{ij},U|V}$, in the presence of selection $D^w_{\mathbf{i},U|V}$ is obtained by the summation of pairwise coefficients with weights $w_{\mathbf{ij}}$.

Let us note, that not all of the $D^w_{\mathbf{i},U|V}$ are independent. In the particular case of selection with respect to two diallele loci only one disequilibrium parameter enters into the equations for the dynamics of gamete frequencies. If by $D = D(\mathbf{p})$ we denoted $D_{11} = p_{11}p_{22} - p_{12}p_{21}$ (by (1.6) all the other values of D_{ij} can differ from D_{11} only in their sign), then (7.3) can be written out in the conventional form first suggested by R. Lewontin and R. Kojima:

$$\Delta p_{11} = p_{11}\frac{w_{11} - w}{w} - \frac{r(1|2)}{w}w_{(11)(22)}D,$$

$$\Delta p_{12} = p_{12}\frac{w_{12} - w}{w} + \frac{r(1|2)}{w}w_{(11)(22)}D,$$

$$\Delta p_{21} = p_{21}\frac{w_{21} - w}{w} + \frac{r(1|2)}{w}w_{(11)(22)}D, \tag{7.6}$$

$$\Delta p_{22} = p_{22}\frac{w_{22} - w}{w} - \frac{r(1|2)}{w}w_{(11)(22)}D.$$

Let us now look at the functions, characterizing the action of selection and recombination-segregation in the continuous-time model. Here, even without selection (see Section 9.2), the state of the population in the general case is defined by numbers (concentrations) of genotypes – not gametes, which markedly raises the dimensionality of problems in question. First let us call to mind the question in terms of numbers. Suppose that mortality depends on the genotype of the organism $\{\mathbf{ij}\}$, on the total size of the population N, on the genotypic structure - the vector of genotype frequencies **p** and on the time t according to the formula

$$m_{ij}(N, \mathbf{p}, t) = m_{ij} + \phi(N, \mathbf{p}, t) ,$$

where the coefficients m_{ij} are constant. Fecundity of all couples is assumed to be constant and equal to b. Taking account of the recombination processes in the L-locus case with n_k alleles at the k-th locus (see Section 9.4) the equation for the dynamics of genotype frequencies becomes as follows:

$$\frac{dN_{ij}}{dt} = \{N - [m_{ij} + \phi(N, \mathbf{p}, t)]p_{ij} + b[(1-R)\Sigma p_{i.} + \sum_{U|V,\, U\neq\varnothing, L} r(U|V)\Sigma p_{(i_U.)(i_V.)}]\times$$

$$[(1-R)\Sigma p_{j.} + \sum_{U|V,\, U\neq\varnothing, L} r(U|V)\Sigma p_{(i_U.)(i_V.)}]\} , \qquad (7.7)$$

$$\mathbf{i} = \{i_k\}, \mathbf{j} = \{j_k\},\ i_1, j_1 = \overline{1, n_1} ;\dots;\ i_l, j_l = \overline{1, n_l}$$

Here points stand for the multi-indices, over which summation is being taken, $p_{i.}$ is the concentration of the genotype, made up two gametes, one of which is denoted by the index **i**, and the other one – by the point. The index $(\mathbf{i}_U.)(\mathbf{i}_V.)$ indicates that one gamete of the genotype contains alleles of the U-loci and the other one - of the V-loci of the **i**th gamete, the points are related to the indices of gamete 'tails'.

From equations for genotype numbers we go over to the system for genotype frequencies and the total population size N, as it was done in Section 9.4:

$$\frac{dN}{dt} = N\{b - [m + \phi(N, \mathbf{p}, t)]\} ,$$

$$\frac{dp_{ij}}{dt} = p_{ij}(\overline{m} - m_{ij}) + b\,[\Sigma p_{i.} - \sum_{U|V,\, U\neq\varnothing, L} r(U|V)\Sigma(p_{i.} - p_{(i_U.)(i_V.)})]\times$$

$$\times[\Sigma p_{j.} - \sum_{U|V,\, U\neq\varnothing, L} r(U|V)\Sigma(p_{j.} - p_{(j_U.)(j_V.)})] - bp_{ij},$$

$$\mathbf{i} = \{i_k\}, \mathbf{j} = \{j_k\},\ i_1, j_1 = \overline{1, n_1} ;\dots;\ i_l, j_l = \overline{1, n_l} \qquad (7.8)$$

Here $\overline{m} = \Sigma_{i,j} p_{ij} m_{ij}$. From (7.8) one can see that an adequate description of the population size dynamics can be achieved by the choice of the appropriate function $\phi(N, \mathbf{p}, t)$, reflecting the regulation of the population by means of density – dependent (N), competitive (**p**) and temporal (t), say, seasonal or epochal, factors. The equations for genotype frequencies can be treated apart from the equation for the number, N. However, their study is too cumbersome, therefore let us try to simplify the analysis, changing over to new variables, corresponding to (4.3), As before, suppose that $p_i = \Sigma p_{i.}$, is the **i**th gamete frequency among genotypes of organisms in the population; $y_{i_U j_V}$ is the concentration of the genotype made up by gametes, one of which contains alleles of U-loci, and the other one of the V-loci of **i**th gamete: $D^1_{ij} = p_{ij} - \Sigma p_{i.}\,\Sigma p_{j.}$ is the measure of non-randomness for gamete combinations in genotypes.

Suppose that

$$b >> \max\{r = \max_{U|V,\, V\neq\varnothing, L} r(U|V),\ \max_{\mathbf{i},\mathbf{j},\mathbf{k},\mathbf{l}} \{|m_{\mathbf{ij}} - m_{\mathbf{kl}}|\}\},$$

i.e. the birth processes, resulting in random gamete combinations in genotypes of newborn, proceed at an essentially higher rate, than the processes of recombination and selection, that vary the gamete concentration and, hence, generally speaking, violate the Hardy-Weinberg principle in the total population. Without the loss of generality, we can write $r(U|V) \sim \varepsilon$ for all non-trivial $U|V$-partitions, $|m_{\mathbf{ij}} - m_{\mathbf{kl}}| \sim \varepsilon$. In terms of new variables the dynamics equations will be

$$\frac{dp_{\mathbf{i}}}{dt} = p_{\mathbf{i}}\overline{m} - \sum_{\mathbf{j}} p_{\mathbf{ij}} m_{\mathbf{ij}} + b \sum_{U|V,\, U\neq\varnothing, L} r(U|V)(y_{\mathbf{i}_U \mathbf{j}_V} - p_{\mathbf{i}}),$$

$$\frac{dD^1_{\mathbf{ij}}}{dt} = -bD^1_{\mathbf{ij}} + O(\varepsilon), \tag{7.9}$$

$$\frac{dy_{\mathbf{i}_U \mathbf{i}_V}}{dt} = b(p_{\mathbf{i}_U} p_{\mathbf{i}_V} - y_{\mathbf{i}_U \mathbf{j}_V}) + O(\varepsilon),$$

$$\mathbf{i} = i_1, \ldots, i_l,\ \mathbf{j} = j_1, \ldots, j_l;\ i_k, j_k = \overline{1, n_k};\ k = \overline{1, l},$$

where $p_{\mathbf{i}_U}$ and $p_{\mathbf{i}_V}$ are the concentrations of U- and V-locus gametes, corresponding to $\mathbf{i}$, among genotypes of organisms in the population. Let us call attention to the following distinctions between the first equation in (7.9) and the differential approximation of the discrete model (7.1). First of all, the function of average fitness $\overline{m}$ is defined in terms of frequencies of genotypes – not gametes, and $\Sigma_{\mathbf{j}} p_{\mathbf{ij}} m_{\mathbf{ij}}$ serves as $p_{\mathbf{i}} m_{\mathbf{i}}$. Moreover in place of $D_{\mathbf{i},U|V}$ we have $p_{\mathbf{i}} - y_{\mathbf{i}_U \mathbf{j}_V}$, and equations for gamete frequencies remain non-closed. Note that all distinctions vanish, if gamete combinations in genotypes are random.

Due to the adopted assumptions, we have $p_{\mathbf{i}}\overline{m} - \Sigma_{\mathbf{j}} p_{\mathbf{ij}} m_{\mathbf{ij}} = O(\varepsilon)$, whence (for $br \sim \varepsilon$) $\dot{p}_{\mathbf{i}} = O(\varepsilon)$, that is the gamete frequencies are 'slow' variables. Freezing $\{p_{\mathbf{i}}\}$ and making ε approach zero, as in Section 9.4, we find that for any initial state, $D^1_{\mathbf{ij}}$ and $y_{\mathbf{i}_U \mathbf{j}_V}$ tend to zero and $p_{\mathbf{i}_U} p_{\mathbf{i}_V}$, respectively. Applying Tychonoff's theorem, we can approximate the behavior of $p_{\mathbf{i}}$ over a finite period of time by the equation, which implies that $y_{\mathbf{i}_U \mathbf{j}_V} = p_{\mathbf{i}_U} p_{\mathbf{i}_V}$ and $p_{\mathbf{ij}} = p_{\mathbf{i}} p_{\mathbf{j}}$:

$$\frac{dp_{i_1 \ldots i_l}}{dt} = \frac{dp_{\mathbf{i}}}{dt} = p_{\mathbf{i}}(m - m_{\mathbf{i}}) - b \sum_{U|V,\, U\neq\varnothing, L} r(U|V) D_{\mathbf{i},U|V},$$

$$i_1 = \overline{1, n_1};\ldots;\ i_l = \overline{1, n_l}. \tag{7.10}$$

This equation, to an accuracy of a factor b in the disequilibrium coefficients, coincides with the differential approximation (7.1) of the model with non-overlapping generations. The coefficients $m_{\mathbf{ij}}$ from the continuous model are known as the Malthusian parameters. They correspond to $1 - w_{\mathbf{ij}}$, where $w_{\mathbf{ij}}$ are the genotype fitnesses in the discrete case. In what follows we shall use the most common notations $w_{\mathbf{ij}}$, without specifying which of the models – with overlapping or non-overlapping generations - is implied, and we shall think that fecundity b in (7.10) is equal to unity.

9.8. Comparing the Dynamics in One-Locus and Multi-Locus Systems in the Presence of Selection

Results of Section 9.7 suggest that for analysis of multi-locus systems we need study equations (7.1) (or (7.10), which are practically equivalent). If all recombination coefficients $r(U|V)$ are zero, then (7.1) turn into the dynamics equations for the one-locus case. When all the $w_{\mathbf{ij}}$ are equal to one and the same constant, (7.1) defines the evolution of a multi-locus system when effected by the processes of recombination and segregation. This system can be studied in the levels of one, two or more loci, applying the marginal gamete frequencies $p_{\mathbf{i}_U}$. Marginal frequencies result from summation of concentrations of all L-locus gametes made of one and the same alleles from the considered set of loci U (that is there is no discrimination between the genetic content with respect to the rest of the loci).

Unfortunately, under the combined action of recombination-segregation and selection in the general case, from the very beginning we are to carry out the analysis in the level of all the L loci, since the equations for K-locus gametes ($K \subset L$) turn to be non-closed due to the action of selection, while selection cannot be treated in the one-locus level because of segregation-recombination. These peculiarities make the treatment markedly more complicated as against the case of one locus (where already we had to confine ourselves mostly to the study of the equilibriums and their stability).

Equilibrium of system (7.1) can be derived from the equations:

$$p_{\mathbf{i}}(w_{\mathbf{i}} - w) = \sum_{U|V,\ U \neq \varnothing, L} r(U|V) D_{\mathbf{i},U|V}, \tag{8.1}$$

$$\mathbf{i} = \{i_k\},\ \mathbf{j} = \{j_k\},\ i_1 = \overline{1, n_1};...;\ i_l = \overline{1, n_l}.$$

It is a laborious task to solve these equations, but it becomes much more simple, when the right-hand sides of (8.1) are equal to zero. In this case the only possible state of polymorphic equilibrium (just as for the frequencies of the one-locus multiple alleles) complies with the equality

$$\mathbf{p} = \|w_{\mathbf{ij}}\|^{-1}\mathbf{e}/(\mathbf{e}, \|w_{\mathbf{ij}}\|^{-1}\mathbf{e}),\ \mathbf{e}^T = (1, 1, ..., 1), \tag{8.2}$$

if only the matrix of fitnesses $\| w_{\mathbf{ij}} \|$ is non-singular.

Even if one of the coefficients of equilibrium is non-zero, we are to study equation (8.1) (or (7.3) for the model with non-overlapping generations). There are very few results for this case.

Let us remark, that for zero right-hand sides in (8.1), what makes the equilibria even more attractive, in addition to the simplicity of their explicit representation by (8.2), is the fact that they can be defined by gene frequencies. The equilibrium concentration of the $\mathbf{i}$th gamete in this case is equal to the product of its constituent alleles, since the results of Section 9.3 indicate, that this equality is necessary and sufficient for the right-hand sides of (8.1) to become zero. Such equilibria will be called Hardy-Weinberg equilibria. Obviously, for fitness matrices of general form such kind of equilibria are rather an exclusion, than a rule. In fact, in the space Σ of gamete frequencies, Hardian equilibria are to belong to a hypersurface of considerably lower dimensionality (defined by the number of allele - not gamete - types), where the point $\mathbf{p}$, defined by (8.2), can be found. This markedly restricts the admissible set of genotype frequencies.

Obviously, at polymorphic Hardian equilibria the average fitness of the population w, expressed as a function of independent frequencies, takes on stationary values. However, even these equilibria lack the one-to-one relation, existing in the one-locus case, between Lyapunov stability for system (7.1) and the type of the surface specified by the function of average fitness. R. Lewontin observed that in the general case the maximum of w is attained only under complete linkage (which is equivalent to the one-locus situation). For instance, if the maximum is associated with the equilibrium state of polymorphism $\mathbf{p}^*$, then introducing an arbitrary linkage distribution we cannot enhance the equilibrium average fitness. In fact, if at that same time there appears a new state of equilibrium $\tilde{\mathbf{p}}$, different from $\mathbf{p}^*$, then its average fitness will be lower (since the maximum attained at the interior point of Σ is unique and global); if $\tilde{\mathbf{p}} = \mathbf{p}^*$, the average fitness will not grow. If we look at the boundary equilibrium, we see that it is associated with a local maximum of w in $\overline{\Sigma}$. Introducing sufficiently tight linkage, instead of the arbitrary one, we only weakly alter the state of equilibrium, which means that the corresponding average fitness will be no higher than the original one.

In general, it is hard to find any general regularities in dynamics and statics of multi-locus systems, but the 'negative' ones, that is those that are different from the regularities of the one-locus case. For instance, as a rule, in the multi-locus case not only there is no simple relation between the type of the average fitness function and the features of the equilibrium states, but also there is no monotone growth of the average fitness along the trajectories of system (7.1). Taking $\mathbf{p}^*$, the point of the maximum of w, as the initial polymorphic state and choosing fitness and linkage distribution such that $\mathbf{p}^*$ is not equilibrium, we can make the average fitness fall away over some period of time.

Stability analysis of the equilibria, derived from (8.1), causes some additional difficulties. Even in the most simple two-locus diallele model with overdominance with respect to each of the loci, the dependence of the number of equilibria and their stability on the linkage distribution is fairly complicated. S. Karlin and M. Feldman, applying numeric methods, and A. Hastings analytically showed that in case of multiplicative fitness there exist equilibria with positive and negative coefficients of linkage disequilibrium, as well as the Hardian equilibrium. The latter one is unstable for small recombination coefficients r, while the rest are locally stable. When r grows to reach a value r_0, one of the equilibria merges with the Hardian ones, which becomes locally stable. Further growth of r from r_0 to some r^* is characterized by local stability of two types of equilibria: one with $D = 0$ and the other one with $D \neq 0$. For $r = r^*$ the only globally stable equilibrium will be Hardian. Therefore, in the behavior of multi-locus systems it is hard to find any general regularities, similar to the one-locus case. Thus, already the example of two-locus systems proves, that for constant non-negative fitnesses the genetic content of the population does not necessarily reach equilibrium, as in the one-locus case. Situations are known, when trajectories converge to a limite cycle.

Nevertheless, under certain correlations between fitnesses and linkage parameters the population quite rapidly reaches the state, which M. Kimura called quasi-linkage equilibrium. In this state, in the two-locus diallele case, alleles from different loci combine in gametes in a way, which deviates from the random one approximately by a constant, while the average fitness of the population steadily grows, i.e. Fisher's fundamental theorem and Wright's principle of adaptive topography are valid.

The proof of this statement fails to be absolutely rigorous mathematically, but it is well supported by computer runs. In the haploid case the concept of quasi-linkage equilibrium can be applied if the recombination coefficient r by far exceeds Fisher's coefficients of epistasis, E, which is equal to $w_{11} - w_{12} - w_{21} + w_{22}$, where w_{ij} is the fitness of the $\{ij\}$th two-locus haploid genotype (indexing corresponds to gamete types under diploidy). The diploid case requires that all epistasis coefficients $E_i = w_{i1} - w_{i2} - w_{i3} + w_{i4}$, $i = \overline{1, 4}$ be small. If all these conditions hold, the value of disequilibrium index $z = p_{11}p_{22}/p_{12}p_{21}$ rapidly attains its quasi-stationary value, which is close to unity. Next we need that initially the gene frequencies be not close to equilibrium, so that some space is still available for the dynamics after the quasi-stationary value of z is attained. After this happens, there comes the most interesting period of dynamics. Over this period z remains practically constant, and variations in gene frequencies are such that the population fitness grows, just as in the one-locus case. Besides, there is a connection between the steady-state points of the average fitness surface and the equilibria of the equations of dynamics: these equilibria merge if fitness is treated under the condition that z is equal to the equilibrium value (provided that, as usually, the sum of gamete concentrations is equal to unity). Let us stress, that if the above-mentioned relation between epistasis coefficients and the recombination parameter is not satisfied, then the dynamics can be strikingly different from the described above.

S. Shahshahani elaborated on the more general case, characterized by an arbitrary amount of loci with any number of alleles at each of them, restricted by somewhat artificial parameters of recombination associated with one linkage group in the absence of multiple crossing-overs (that is, in meiosis chromatids can break only in one, but not the same, point). Basing on qualitative analysis and applying Riemannian metrics, the following specific traits of population behavior were demonstrated in the model of random gamete fussion with weak selection. If $r = \min_i \{r_i\} >> \varepsilon > 0$, where r_i is the recombination coefficient associated with the exchange of chromosome segments before the ith locus inclusively, and after it, then the trajectories of a system with selection, regarded as a small perturbation of the system evolving due to recombinations only, converges exponentially towards the surface of quasi-linkage equilibrium. This surface is close to the equilibrium one in the absence of selection. On the equilibrium surface, attached to the perturbed system, the rate of change in disequilibrium coefficients has the order of $o(1/r^2)$. The steady-state points in this case are well approximated by the points with linkage equilibrium.

An increase in the average fitness over a finite time interval was demonstrated by F. Hoppensteadt in a model with two diallelic loci similar to the one considered in the previous section. He selected the fast and slow variables for the recombination parameters r being essentially less than the weak intensity of selection ε, $1 >> \varepsilon >> r > 0$, and then he concentrated on the analysis of the case of loose linkage for $r \in (0, 1/2)$ and $0 \le \varepsilon << 1$. Similar methods were applied by T. Nagylaki to study the effect of weak selection on Hardy-Weinberg relations, linkage disequilibrium and the behavior of average fitness.

9.9. Model of Additive Selection in a Multi-Locus System

Results of the previous section demonstrate how complicated is the behavior of multi-locus systems as against the case of selection with respect to one locus. However, in some particular situations the equilibiria and their stability in a multi-locus system are governed by one-locus characteristics. Such a system is exampled by the case of selection with additive fitness of genotypes. Fitnesses are said to be additive, if for any **i,j** the equality

$$w_{\mathbf{ij}} = \sum_{k=1}^{l} w_{i_k j_k},\ w_{i_k j_k} = w_{j_k i_k} \geq 0,\ k = \overline{1, l} \tag{9.1}$$

is satisfied. Constants $w_{i_k j_k}$ can be called fitnesses of genotypes of the kth locus. This definition is reasonable, since under random gamete coupling the marginal fitnesses of genotypes $\{i_k, j_k\}$, associated with the L-locus genotypes distinguished only with respect to the kth locus, will be equal to

$$\overline{w_{i_k j_k}} = \frac{1}{p_{i_k} p_{j_k}} \sum_{\mathbf{m}:\ m_k = i_k;\ \mathbf{n}:\ n_k = j_k} \left(\sum_{l} w_{m_l n_l}\right) p_{\mathbf{m}} p_{\mathbf{n}} =$$

$$= w_{i_k j_k} + \frac{1}{p_{i_k} p_{j_k}} \sum_{l,\ l \neq k} \left[\sum_{m_l,\ n_l} w_{m_l n_l} p_{i_k m_l} p_{j_k n_l}\right]. \tag{9.2}$$

If w_l is the average population fitness with respect to the lth locus (with fitnesses of one-locus genotypes being $w_{i_l j_l}$), then for independent allele combinations in two-locus gametes (when $p_{i_k m_l} = p_{i_k} p_{m_l}$) (9.2) yields $\overline{w_{i_k j_k}} = w_{i_k j_k} + \Sigma_{l,\ l \neq k}\, w_l$. Thereby, in this case all marginal fitnesses of genotypes of the kth locus differ from $w_{i_k j_k}$ by one and the same function, which is cancelled out in the difference $w_{i_k} - w_k$. Consequently, $w_{i_k j_k}$ can be regarded as the fitnesses of the kth locus genotypes.

Hence, if the population with additive selection is in linkage equilibrium, then the variations in allele frequencies with respect to each of the loci are independent and governed by their fitness matrices. On the other hand, when the population is in equilibrium with respect to concentrations of alleles rather than gametes, the selection induced terms in the dynamics equations vanish, since fitnesses depend only on the equilibrium frequencies of alleles and $w_{\mathbf{I}} = w$. Therefore the dynamics of gametes concentrations coincide with the dynamics under the effect of recombination-segregation processes with no selection, the entropy calculated for the distribution of gamete concentrations grows, until the combinations of alleles from different loci become independent.

In a wider context of disequilibrium in frequencies of both gametes and alleles, the dynamics becomes more complicated and the behavior even of the neutral loci becomes dependent on the behavior of those linked with them. However here again for any kind of additive selection we can find some general regularities in dynamics, for instance, one can show that the average population fitness is non-decreasing over the course of time. In order to prove this, let us note that, as it is readily seen from (9.1), the gamete fitnesses $w_{\mathbf{i}}$ and the average fitness w depend only on frequencies of alleles - not gametes:

$$w_{\mathbf{i}} = \sum_{\mathbf{j}} p_{\mathbf{j}} w_{\mathbf{ij}} = \sum_{k,\mathbf{j}} p_{\mathbf{j}} w_{i_k j_k} = \sum_{k, j_k} p_{j_k} w_{i_k j_k} = \sum_k w_{i_k}\,, \tag{9.3}$$

$$w = \sum_{\mathbf{i},\mathbf{j}} p_{\mathbf{i}} p_{\mathbf{j}} w_{\mathbf{ij}} = \sum_{k,\mathbf{i},\mathbf{j}} p_{\mathbf{i}} p_{\mathbf{j}} w_{i_k j_k} = \sum_k w_k\,.$$

Whence it is clear that summing up the equations in (7.1) over all indices, associated with gametes that carry the k-th locus allele with the number i_k, we arrive at the derivative concentration p_{i_k}, which is independent of the linkage distribution, because the sum of the recombination-segregation induced terms yields a zero, while the selection induced terms are independent of recombination-segregation (note, however, that $\dot{p}_{i_k} \neq p_{i_k}(w_{i_k} - w_k)$ under linkage disequilibrium). Consequently, the derivative of the average fitness is also independent of the linkage distribution. Therefore, formally the distribution can be regarded as rigid, which is in accord with the one-locus case. At that same time the derivative of the average fitness is known to be greater than zero, if the population is in disequilibrium with respect to allele frequencies. This reasoning scheme, first employed by W. Ewens, results in the following conclusion: in case of additive selection for arbitrary linkage distribution the average fitness of a population in disequilibrium is steadily non-decreasing. It is known that the rate of change in the average fitness will be equal to the genetic variance of gamete fitnesses:

$$\frac{dw}{dt} = \sum_{\mathbf{i}} \frac{\partial w}{\partial p_{\mathbf{i}}} \frac{dp_{\mathbf{i}}}{dt} = \sum_{\mathbf{i}} 2\, w_{\mathbf{i}}[p_{\mathbf{i}}(w_{\mathbf{i}} - w) +$$

$$+ \sum_{U|V,\, U \neq \varnothing, L} r(U|V) D_{\mathbf{i},U|V}] = 2 \sum_{\mathbf{i}} p_{\mathbf{i}}(w_{\mathbf{i}} - w)^2, \tag{9.4}$$

which formally coincides with the (4.3.1) in the one-locus case. Here we took into account that $2w$ can be substracted from the coefficient $2w_{\mathbf{i}}$ (since $\sum_{\mathbf{i}} \dot{p}_{\mathbf{i}}$ is identically zero), and that the sum over all $U|V$-partitions can be neglected. To prove the latter it suffices to show that $\sum_{\mathbf{i}} w_{\mathbf{i}} D_{\mathbf{i},U|V}$ be equal to zero for any $U|V$. Due to additivity of fitness, we have $w_{\mathbf{i}} = w_{\mathbf{i}_U} + w_{\mathbf{i}_V}$. Here $w_{\mathbf{i}_U}$ is the average fitness of a U-locus gamete (containing the same allele at the U-loci as the gamete with number $\mathbf{i}$), and defined by fitnesses $w_{i_k j_k}$ its concentration being $p_{\mathbf{i}_U}$. By (3.10) $D_{\mathbf{i},U|V} = p_{\mathbf{i}} - p_{\mathbf{i}_U} p_{\mathbf{i}_V}$, hence the sum of all $D_{\mathbf{i},U|V}$ over all kinds of subscripts $\mathbf{i}_U$ (or $\mathbf{i}_V$) is equal to zero. As a result

$$\sum_{\mathbf{i}} w_{\mathbf{i}} D_{\mathbf{i},U|V} = \sum_{\mathbf{i}_U} w_{\mathbf{i}_U} \sum_{\mathbf{i}_V} D_{\mathbf{i},U|V} + \sum_{\mathbf{i}_V} w_{\mathbf{i}_V} \sum_{\mathbf{i}_U} D_{\mathbf{i},U|V} = 0$$

and therefore (9.4) holds.

Let us now concentrate on the equilibria and their stability. First of all note that if the allele concentrations $p^*_{i_k}$ are in equilibrium with respect to one-locus selection with fitnesses $w_{i_k j_k}$, then the gamete concentrations $p^*_{\mathbf{i}}=\Pi_k p^*_{i_k}$ are in equilibrium in the multi-locus system. Moreover, if $p^*_{i_k}$ are locally (globally) stable with respect to $w_{i_k j_k}$, then the concentrations of multi-locus gametes $p^*_{\mathbf{i}}$ are also locally (globally) stable. The proof of these facts for the state $\{p^*_{\mathbf{i}}\}$ follows from the equalities $p^*_{\mathbf{i}}(w^*_{\mathbf{i}}-w^*)=0$ for all $\mathbf{i}$ (which is due to (9.3) and the relationships $w^*_{i_k}=w^*_k$ for $p^*_{i_k}\neq 0$) and from the Hardian structure of concentrations $p^*_{\mathbf{i}}$, which imply that the recombination-segregation terms are equal to zero. Therefore $\dot{p}^*_{\mathbf{i}}=0$.The stability properties depend on how the allele frequencies at each of the loci approach the values $p^*_{i_k}$ (since, roughly speaking, in equilibrium the average fitness attains its local (global) maximum, and the gamete concentrations start to determine the allele frequencies $p^*_{i_k}$). Under fixed (equilibrium) values $p^*_{i_k}$ the dynamics of gametes frequencies is independent of fitnesses (see Section 9.4), the state of equilibrium is unique and Hardian, that is $p^*_{\mathbf{i}} = \Pi_k p^*_{i_k}$.

Up till now we excluded from our analysis the structurally unstable (non-robust) situations, where the qualitative picture of dynamics is altered by small deviations of parameters. For instance, we assumed that the steady-state point of function w are isolated. The usual reasoning scheme, justifying the exclusion of non-robust cases, is roughly as follows. Since all modeling efforts address real-world phenomena, while the nature of these phenomena is only approximately known, the model parameters can be only estimated, say, in the appropriate experiments. As a rule, the evaluation of a model is eventually based on its forecasting capacity. If parameters are inexactly specified, the non-robust model can forecast a behavior, which would be qualitatively different from the actual one. In this sense the value of such a model is not too high.

The reasoning set forth is too general to take it for granted when all kinds of natural phenomena are analyzed. In connection with the genetic processes we attended to, the formally non-robust phenomena are presented by the widespread occasions of dominance and recessivity of alleles in the level of one locus, recessive epistasis, dominant suppresion, complementarity, etc. in the level of two loci and so on. Therefore a priori the steady-state points of the function of average fitness need not be isolated in case of multiple alleles or in the multi-locus situation.

The monotonicity of average fitness w in unsteady one-locus population with multiple alleles ensures the absence of cycles (since variations of w would have been cyclic on closed trajectories) for all symmetric matrices $\|w_{ij}\|$, $w_{ij}\geq 0$.

In case of a finite number of equilibria each trajectory is converging, that is there exists a limit to $p(t)$ as $t\to\infty$. The phase space Σ can be separated into domains of attraction corresponding to the local maxima of average fitness, which is an implication of the Lyapunov theory. Things are different if there is a continuum of equilibria (for instance, when the matrix of fitnesses is singular): convergence of the trajectory towards a point is not obvious. However in this case, applying the selection-induced monotonicity of the population average fitness w, Ju.I. Ljubic with co-authors proved that a more complicated model with non-overlapping generations also demonstrates a convergence towards an equilibrium.

In case of additive selection in a multi-locus model with non-overlapping generations a similar statement about convergence was proved by L.A. Kun and Ju.I. Ljubic. The authors first invoked the monotonicity of the behavior of w to show that the trajectory of gene frequencies converges, just as in the one-locus case, the average population fitness being constant and equal to gamete fitnesses (for gametes with non-zero concentrations) on the limit set Ω of the trajectory. The convergence of gamete concentrations is proved by the behavior of the trajectory on Ω. It turns out that entropy grows, attaining the only maximum if alleles from different loci are randomly coupled in gametes. The maximum point turns to be the limit of the trajectory.

In the continuous-time model the qualitative dynamic picture is the same and the corresponding results are obtained from the treatment of differential equations.

9.10. Models of Multiplicative and Additively Multiplicative Selection

Let us now assume the model with multiplicative fitnesses, defined by the relation

$$w_{\mathbf{ij}} = \prod_k w_{i_k j_k} . \tag{10.1}$$

Biologically these relations are justified, say, in case if the action of various genes tells at different ages. Then the probability of survival at the time of reproduction is equal to the product of survival probabilities over the appropriate age intervals, into which the whole period before reproduction can be split.

Note, that if the continuous-time model is regarded as the approximation of the one with non-overlapping generations, then under multiplicative fitnesses, $w_{\mathbf{ij}}$ can be presented in various variety of forms. For instance, if we assume that $w_{i_k j_k}$ at each locus differ among themselves by $O(\varepsilon)$, i.e. that we deal with weak selection, its intensity being of the same order of magnitude at all loci, then it seems reasonable to apply the additive scheme $w_{\mathbf{ij}} = \Sigma_k w_{i_k j_k}$, which we studied earlier, since it defines the difference $w_{\mathbf{i}} - w$ to an accuracy of $O(\varepsilon)$. If the intensity of selection has different orders of magnitude with respect to different loci, then fitnesses will be additively multiplicative.

Constants $w_{i_k j_k}$ in (10.1) can be termed fitnesses of kth locus genotypes, since the dynamics of the population state with respect to this locus is determined by fitnesses $w_{i_k j_k}$, when Hardian linkage equilibrium is attained. In this case the gamete concentration $p_{\mathbf{i}}$ equals $\Pi_k p_{i_k}$, while the fitnesses of the gamete and the population are defined as follows:

$$w_{\mathbf{i}} = \sum_{\mathbf{j}} p_{\mathbf{j}} w_{\mathbf{ij}} = \sum_{k,\, j_k} \prod_m p_{j_m} w_{i_m j_m} = \prod_m w_{i_m} ,$$

$$w = \sum_{\mathbf{i}} p_{\mathbf{i}} w_{\mathbf{i}} = \sum_{k,\, i_k} \prod_m p_{i_m} w_{i_m} = \prod_m w_m \tag{10.2}$$

where w_{i_m} and w_m are the fitnesses of allele $\{i_m\}$ and of the one-locus population with the survival coefficients $w_{i_m j_m}$ respectively.

Whence it follows that the derivative of the concentration of, say, the allele at kth locus in $\mathbf{i}$th gamete p_{i_k} (which is obtained by summation of the dynamics equations over gametes, containing this allele) will be

$$\frac{dp_{i_k}}{dt} = \left(\prod_{m,\, m \neq k} w_m \right) p_{i_k} \, (w_{i_k} - w_k) \,. \tag{10.3}$$

Here we take into account that the sum of recombination-segregation induced terms equals zero. Let us note that (10.3) breaks with the one-locus equation of dynamics under the effect of selection with fitnesses $w_{i_k j_k}$ only by the factor $\Pi_{m, m \neq k} w_m$ (one and the same for all kth locus alleles). If at any one time all $w_m > a > 0$, then the trajectories of (10.3) in the phase space coincide with the trajectories of the appropriate one-locus population, justifying the term fitnesses of the kth locus genotypes, which was chosen for the coefficients $w_{i_k j_k}$. In the model with non-overlapping generations the factor $\Pi_{m, m \neq k} w_m$ is cancelled out and the equations for allele frequencies, written for each of the loci, exactly coincide with the dynamics equations for one-locus selection.

Modifying the results of S. Karlin and U. Liberman for the case of the continuous-time model, we can now concentrate on the Hardy-Weinberg equilibria and their stability. Obviously, the population with gamete concentrations $p^*_{\mathbf{i}} = \Pi_k p^*_{i_k}$ is in equilibrium, if allele frequencies $p^*_{i_k}$ are in steady state with respect to selection in a one-locus population with genotype fitnesses $w_{i_k j_k}$. This follows from (10.3) and the equality $w^*_{i_k} = w^*_k$ for $p^*_{i_k} \neq 0$.

As for the stability of the state $\{p^*_{\mathbf{i}}\}$, the analysis becomes more sophisticated than in the case of additive selection. Let us treat the stability by the first-order approximation, linearinzing the dynamics equations in the vicinity of the state $\{p^*_{\mathbf{i}}\}$. Let us bring into focus only the robust cases, when the matrix of the linearized system is non-singular. First we remark, that the matrix of fitnesses $\| w_{\mathbf{ij}} \|$ can be represented as the Kronecker-product of one-locus fitness matrices:

$$\| w_{\mathbf{ij}} \| = \| w_{i_1 j_1} \| \otimes \| w_{i_2 j_2} \| \otimes \ldots \otimes \| w_{i_l j_l} \| \,. \tag{10.4}$$

Recall the definition and properties of the Kronecker-product. For two $n_1 \times n_1$ and $n_2 \times n_2$ square matrices $A_1 = \| a_{ij} \|$ and A_2 the Kronecker-product $A_1 \otimes A_2$ is defined by the formula

$$A_1 \otimes A_2 = \left\| \begin{matrix} a_{11} A_2 & a_{12} A_2 & \cdots & a_{1n_1} A_2 \\ a_{21} A_2 & a_{22} A_2 & \cdots & a_{2n_1} A_2 \\ \ldots & \ldots & \ldots & \ldots \\ a_{n_1 1} A_2 & a_{n_1 2} A_2 & \cdots & a_{n_1 n_1} A_2 \end{matrix} \right\| \tag{10.5}$$

It is a simple matter to check directly, that if λ_{1i} and $\mathbf{e}_{1i}$ are n_1 eigenvalues and eigenvectors of A_1, while λ_{2i} and $\mathbf{e}_{2i}$ are n_2 eigenvalues and eigenvectors of A_2, then the eigenvalues of $A_1 \otimes A_2$ equal $\lambda_{1i_1} \lambda_{2i_2}$ and the eigenvectors equal $\mathbf{e}_{1i_1} \otimes \mathbf{e}_{2i_2}$, $i_1 = \overline{1, n_1}$; $i_2 = \overline{1, n_2}$. The Kronecker-product of several matrices $\{A_k\}$ will be denoted by $\Pi_k \otimes A_k$. For the case of several matrices the eigenvalues and eigenvectors of their Kronecker-product can be represented as follows:

$$\lambda_{\mathrm{i}} = \prod_k \lambda_{ki_k}, \quad \mathbf{e}_{\mathrm{i}} = \prod_k \otimes \mathbf{e}_{ki_k}. \tag{10.6}$$

There is also the equality $(\mathbf{A}_1 \otimes \mathbf{A}_2)(\mathbf{B}_1 \otimes \mathbf{B}_2) = (\mathbf{A}_1\mathbf{B}_1) \otimes (\mathbf{A}_2\mathbf{B}_2)$ which can be generalized for more co-factors in the following way. If the products $\mathbf{A}_k\mathbf{B}_k$ are defined, then

$$\left(\prod_k \otimes \mathbf{A}_k\right)\left(\prod_k \otimes \mathbf{B}_k\right) = \prod_k \otimes \mathbf{A}_k\mathbf{B}_k. \tag{10.7}$$

This formula results from successive applications of the above mentioned property of pairwise product to the left-hand side of (10.7), thereby yielding

$$(\mathbf{A}_1 \otimes \tilde{\mathbf{A}}_2)(\mathbf{B}_1 \otimes \tilde{\mathbf{B}}_2) = \mathbf{A}_1\mathbf{B}_1 \otimes \tilde{\mathbf{A}}_2\tilde{\mathbf{B}}_2,$$

where

$$\tilde{\mathbf{A}}_2 = \prod_{k>1} \otimes \mathbf{A}_k, \quad \tilde{\mathbf{B}}_2 = \prod_{k>1} \mathbf{B}_k.$$

The property (10.7) holds not only for square matrices, if there exist the products $\mathbf{A}_k\mathbf{B}_k$. In particular, when $\mathbf{A}_k^T$ is a vector-row and $\mathbf{B}_k$ is a vector-column, then the products $\mathbf{A}_k^T\mathbf{B}_k$ and $(\Pi_k \otimes \mathbf{A}_k^T)(\Pi_k \otimes \mathbf{B}_k)$ are scalars, and the Kronecker-product of scalars is the ordinary multiplication. Therefore in this case (10.7) becomes

$$\left(\prod_k \otimes \mathbf{A}_k^T, \prod_k \otimes \mathbf{B}_k\right) = \prod_k (\mathbf{A}_k, \mathbf{B}_k). \tag{10.8}$$

If at least one of the pairs of vectors $\mathbf{A}_k, \mathbf{B}_k$ is orthogonal, then both $\Pi_k \otimes \mathbf{A}_k$ and $\Pi_k \otimes \mathbf{B}_k$ are orthogonal, and further on we shall make use of this fact.

Recall that the dynamics equations for the multi-locus system with selection are

$$\frac{\mathrm{d}p_{i_1 \ldots i_l}}{\mathrm{d}t} = \frac{\mathrm{d}p_{\mathrm{i}}}{\mathrm{d}t} = p_{\mathrm{i}}(w_{\mathrm{i}} - w) - \sum_{U|V,\, U \neq \varnothing, L} r(U|V)(p_{\mathrm{i}} - p_{\mathrm{i}_U} p_{\mathrm{i}_V}). \tag{10.9}$$

In order to study the stability of the equilibrium $\mathbf{p}^* = \{p_{\mathrm{i}}^* = \Pi_k p_{i_k}^*\} = \Pi_k \otimes \mathbf{p}_k^*$, suppose that at each of the loci the state of polymorphism $\mathbf{p}_k^* = \{p_{i_k}^*\}$ is asymptotically stable. Linearizing (10.9) in the vicinity of $\mathbf{p}^*$, let us separately treat the components of the linearized system, associated with the selection and recombination-segregation-induced terms in (10.9).

First let us concentrate on selection. In the vector-matrix form, presenting the population state $\mathbf{p}$ as $\mathbf{p}^* + \Delta$, we find that the contribution of selection to $\dot{\Delta}$ equals

$$\mathbf{D}(\mathbf{p}^* + \Delta) \,\|\, w_{\mathrm{ij}} \,\|\, (\mathbf{p}^* + \Delta) - w\,(\mathbf{p}^* + \Delta)(\mathbf{p}^* + \Delta), \tag{10.10}$$

that is the effect of selection is defined by the expression, which agrees with the one-locus case, when L-locus gametes plays the part of alleles. In (10.10) $\mathbf{D}(\mathbf{p})$ is a diagonal matrix with the coordinates of vector $\mathbf{p}$ on the diagonal, $w(\mathbf{p}^* + \Delta) = w^* + 2(\Delta, \|w_{\mathrm{ij}}\|\mathbf{p}^*) + (\Delta, \|w_{\mathrm{ij}}\|\Delta)$, $\mathbf{D}(\mathbf{p}^*)\|w_{\mathrm{ij}}\|\mathbf{p}^* - w^*\mathbf{p}^* = 0$, since $\mathbf{p}^*$ is an equilibrium, $w^* = w(\mathbf{p}^*)$). The increment Δ in gamete concentrations satisfies the relation

$$(\Delta, \mathbf{e}) = 0, \quad \mathbf{e} = (1, 1, \ldots, 1)^T, \tag{10.11}$$

because the sums of coordinates in $\mathbf{p}^* + \Delta$ and $\mathbf{p}^*$ are equal to unity, whence the sum of coordinates of Δ is to be zero. Dropping the terms of the second order with respect to coordinates of Δ, we arrive at the selection-induced component of the linearized system:

$$\mathbf{D}(\mathbf{p}^*)\|w_{ij}\|\Delta + \mathbf{D}(\Delta)\|w_{ij}\|\mathbf{p}^* - w^*\Delta = \mathbf{D}(\mathbf{p}^*)\|w_{ij}\|\Delta . \qquad (10.12)$$

Here we have taken into account that by (10.11), $\mathbf{D}(\Delta)\|w_{ij}\|\mathbf{p}^* = \mathbf{D}(\Delta)w^*\mathbf{e} = w^*\Delta$, $(\Delta, \|w_{ij}\|\mathbf{p}^*) = w^*(\Delta,\mathbf{e}) = 0$.

Due to (10.4) and applying (10.7), the matrix $\mathbf{D}(\mathbf{p}^*)\|w_{ij}\|$, its eigenvalues and eigenvectors can be represented as follows:

$$\left[\prod_k \otimes \mathbf{D}(\overset{*}{p_k})\right]\left[\prod_k \otimes \| \overset{*}{w_{i_kj_k}} \|\right] = \prod_k \otimes \mathbf{D}(\overset{*}{p_k})\| w_{i_kj_k} \|, \qquad (10.13)$$

$$\lambda_{i_1...i_l} = \prod_k \lambda_{i_k}, \quad \mathbf{e}_{i_1...i_l} = \prod_k \otimes \mathbf{e}_{i_k}$$

for i_k=1, $\mathbf{e}_{i_k} = \overset{*}{p_k}$. Next we need to know the properties of the matrices $\mathbf{D}(\overset{*}{\mathbf{p}_k})\|w_{i_kj_k}\|$, which corresponds to the one-locus linearization and follows the assumption about asymptotic stability of one-locus polymorphisms $\overset{*}{\mathbf{p}_k}$. In the general case, eigenvalues of these matrices should have negative real parts. In our case the eigenvalues are known to be real, since matrix $\mathbf{D}(\overset{*}{\mathbf{p}_k})\|w_{i_kj_k}\|$ is similar to the symmetric one $\mathbf{D}(\sqrt{\overset{*}{\mathbf{p}_k}})\|w_{i_kj_k}\|\mathbf{D}(\sqrt{\overset{*}{\mathbf{p}_k}})$ (and hence, to the diagonal one), which is derived by multiplications on the left and on the right by $\mathbf{D}^{-1}(\sqrt{\overset{*}{\mathbf{p}_k}})$ and $\mathbf{D}(\sqrt{\overset{*}{\mathbf{p}_k}})$ respectively, where $(\sqrt{\overset{*}{\mathbf{p}_k}})^T = \{\sqrt{\overset{*}{p}_{i_k}}\}$. However, the requirement that all eigenvalues be negative is too restrictive, since we are considering not all kinds of increments Δ, but rather treat only those, that belong, by (10.11), to the subspace, orthogonal to the vector $\mathbf{e}^T$=(1, 1,...,1). Let us note that $\mathbf{e}^T$ is the eigenvector of $\mathbf{D}(\overset{*}{p_k})\|w_{i_kj_k}\|$ with the eigenvalue $\lambda_{k1} = \overset{*}{w_k} > 0$, since $\mathbf{e}^T\mathbf{D}(\overset{*}{\mathbf{p}_k}) = (\overset{*}{\mathbf{p}_k})^T$, $(\mathbf{p}_k)^T\|w_{i_kj_k}\| = \overset{*}{w_k}\mathbf{e}^T$ where $\overset{*}{w_k}$ is the average fitness with respect to the kth locus in the state of equilibrium $\overset{*}{p_k}$. Therefore, all right eigenvectors with eigenvalues different from $\overset{*}{w_k}$, are orthogonal to $\mathbf{e}$. Any increment Δ, complying with (10.11), can be expanded in these vectors. Consequently, all the rest of the eigenvalues of $\mathbf{D}(\overset{*}{\mathbf{p}_k})\|w_{i_kj_k}\|$ are negative due to model robustness and asymptotic stability of the equilibrium $\overset{*}{\mathbf{p}_k}$. It can be directly verified, that $\overset{*}{\mathbf{p}_k}$ is the right eigenvector, corresponding to $\overset{*}{w_k}$. Obviously, $\overset{*}{\mathbf{p}_k}$ does not satisfy (10.11). As a result, in an asymptotically stable equilibrium the matrix $\mathbf{D}(\overset{*}{\mathbf{p}_k})\|w_{i_kj_k}\|$ should have one positive eigenvalue $\lambda_{k1} = \overset{*}{w_k}$ and n_k-1 negative ones, λ_{ki} (corresponding to eigenvectors $\mathbf{e}_{ki}$, orthogonal to $\mathbf{e}$). Whence it follows that by the properties of Kronecker-products, matrix (10.13) has one positive eigenvalue $w^* = \Pi_k \overset{*}{w_k}$, the rest of eigenvalues are equal to $\Pi_k \lambda_{ki_k}$ (where $i_k = \overline{1, n_k}$, but all i_k cannot be equal to unity simultaneously) and can be both positive and negative. The corresponding eigenvectors are orthogonal to $\mathbf{e}$ - a vector of appropriate dimensionality, which can be represented as a Kronecker-product of l vectors $\mathbf{e}^k$ with unit coordinates, their dimensionality being n_k. Whence, by (10.8) we have $(\Pi_k \otimes \mathbf{e}^k, \Pi_k \otimes \mathbf{e}_{ki_k}) = \Pi_k(\mathbf{e}^k, \mathbf{e}_{ki_k}) = 0$, since there is at least one $i_k \neq 1$, and by the property of one-locus systems, proved above, for this i_kth locus $(\mathbf{e}^k, \mathbf{e}_{ki_k}) = 0$.

Let us now treat the recombination-segregation-induced component in system (10.98), its ith coordinate being equal to the appropriate contribution to $\dot{\Delta}_{\mathbf{i}}$:

$$\sum_{U|V,\, U\neq\varnothing,L} r(U|V)[p_{\mathbf{i}}^* + \Delta_{\mathbf{i}} - (p_{\mathbf{i}_U}^* + \Delta_{\mathbf{i}_U})(p_{\mathbf{i}_V}^* + \Delta_{\mathbf{i}_V})].$$

Due to the Hardian structure of gamete frequencies, $p_{\mathbf{i}}^* - p_{\mathbf{i}_U}^* p_{\mathbf{i}_V}^* = 0$ for all $\mathbf{i}$ and $U|V$, whence the linearized system can be presented as follows

$$\frac{d\Delta_{\mathbf{i}}}{dt} = -\sum_{U|V,\, U\neq\varnothing,L} r(U|V)(\Delta_{\mathbf{i}} - \Delta_{\mathbf{i}_U} p_{\mathbf{i}_V}^* - p_{\mathbf{i}_U}^* \Delta_{\mathbf{i}_V}) \,. \tag{10.14}$$

In this formulation the matrix of the linearized system remains obscure. Let us find out what is the form of $\Delta_{\mathbf{i}_U}$ in terms of Δ. Obviously, $\Delta_{\mathbf{i}_U}$ is equal to the sum of those coordinates of Δ, which corresponds to the gametes, that carry the same alleles $\{i_k, k\in U\}$ at the U-loci as the $\mathbf{i}$th gamete. Therefore $\Delta_{\mathbf{i}_U}$ can be represented as a scalar product of a vector $\mathbf{d}_{\mathbf{i}}(U)$, made of zeros and ones, and the vector Δ. It is convenient to arrange the coordinates of the later in the order, that corresponds to the succession of coordinates of the formal product $\Gamma = \Pi_k \otimes (A_1^k, A_2^k, ..., A_{n_k}^k)^T$, where n_k is the number of kth locus alleles. Clearly, the $\mathbf{i}$th coordinate of vector Γ represents the content of the $\mathbf{i}$th gamete $A_{i_1}^1, A_{i_2}^2, ..., A_{i_l}^k$; $\{A_{i_l}^l\}$ are the allele symbols; i_k equals the number of the kth locus allele, contained in the gamete $\Pi_k A_{i_l}^l$ (carrying the multi-index $\mathbf{i} = (i_1, i_2, ..., i_l)$).

Our task is construct the vector $\mathbf{d}_{\mathbf{i}}(U)$. Obviously, every coordinate of $\mathbf{d}_{\mathbf{i}}(U)$ is to be an indicator, that is it should equal one, if it matches i_k for some $k\in U$, and it is to be zero otherwise. Let us construct $\mathbf{d}_{\mathbf{i}}(U)$ as a Kronecker-product of vectors with zero and unitary coordinates, so that as a result the coordinates of $\mathbf{d}_{\mathbf{i}}(U)$ would induce the product of absence-presence indicators for the appropriate alleles. Let the n_k-vector $\mathbf{d}_{i_k}$, attached to the kth locus, be such that its i_kth coordinate is a one, while all the rest are zeros. Suppose that $\mathbf{d}_{\mathbf{i}}^{k(U)} = \mathbf{d}_{i_k}$ for $k(U) = 0$ and $\mathbf{d}_{\mathbf{i}}^{k(U)} = \mathbf{e}$ (its dimensionality being n_k) for $k(U) = 1$, while $k(U) = 1$ for $k\in U$ and $k(U) = 0$ for $k\notin U$. Then one can directly verify that $\mathbf{d}_{\mathbf{i}}(U)$ is defined by the formula

$$\mathbf{d}_{\mathbf{i}}(U) = \prod_k \otimes \mathbf{d}_{\mathbf{i}}^{1-k(U)} \,. \tag{10.15}$$

In fact, the structure of $\mathbf{d}_{i_k}(U)$ is similar to that of Γ, but the symbols of alleles are equal to zero or one for the set of loci U and they are equal to one for all other loci. Thus, the product of such symbols satisfies the conditions imposed on coordinates of $\mathbf{d}_{\mathbf{i}}(U)$.

If we represent the linearized system, assigned to recombination-segregation, in its matrix form, then for a fixed $U|V$-partition the matrix $\mathbf{L}_U$, that relates Δ_U to Δ, has the rows made of $\mathbf{d}_{\mathbf{i}}(U)$. This implies that if for a $n_k\times n_k$ matrix made of ones, $\mathbf{J}_k = \mathbf{e}\mathbf{e}^T$, we assume that $\mathbf{J}_k^{k(U)} = \mathbf{I}_k$ (unit matrix) for $k(U) = 0$ and that $\mathbf{J}_k^{k(U)} = \mathbf{J}_k$ for $k(U)=1$, then we obtain

$$\Delta_U = \left[\prod_k \otimes \mathbf{J}_k^{1-k(U)}\right]\Delta = \mathbf{L}_U\Delta. \tag{10.16}$$

The correctness of this representation is due to the fact that the $\mathbf{i}$th row of $\mathbf{L}_U$ (which can be associated with the multi-index $(i_1, i_2, ..., i_l)$) can be presented as a Kronecker-product $\Pi_k \otimes \mathbf{e}_{ik}$, where $\mathbf{e}_{ik}$ is the i_kth row of matrix $\mathbf{J}_k^{1-k(U)}$. It remains only to note that $\mathbf{e}_{ik} = \mathbf{d}_{\mathbf{i}}^{1-k(U)}$, that is, by (10.15), the $\mathbf{i}$th row of $\mathbf{L}_U$ is equal to $\mathbf{d}_{\mathbf{i}}(U)$.

Finally we remark, that applying (10.16) and (10.7), the column vector with coordinates $\Delta_{i_U} \overset{*}{p}_{i_V}$ can be written as

$$\mathbf{D}\Big[\prod_k \otimes (\overset{*}{\mathbf{p}}_k)^{1-k(U)}\Big]\Big[\prod_k \otimes \mathbf{J}_k^{1-k(U)}\Big]\Delta = \Big\{\prod_k \otimes \mathbf{D}[(\overset{*}{\mathbf{p}}_k)^{1-k(U)}]\mathbf{J}_k^{1-k(U)}\Big\}\Delta, \tag{10.17}$$

since $\overset{*}{p}_{i_V} = \Pi_k(\overset{*}{p}_{i_k})^{1-k(U)}$, and raising of a vector to a power should be understood as a coordinate-wise operation. The right eigenvectors of $\mathbf{D}(\overset{*}{\mathbf{p}}_k)\mathbf{J}_k$ will be any of the n_k-vectors orthogonal to $\mathbf{e}$ (in particular, eigenvectors of $\mathbf{D}(\overset{*}{\mathbf{p}}_k)\|w_{i_k j_k}\|$), and corresponding to the eigenvalues $\mu_{ki} = 0$, $i>1$. The only non-zero eigenvalue will be $\mu_{ki} = 1$ with the eigenvector $\overset{*}{\mathbf{p}}_k$. Therefore for all U the matrix in (10.17) will have a non-zero eigenvalue, which is equal to one, and its eigenvector $\Pi_k \otimes \overset{*}{\mathbf{p}}_k$ obviously does not comply with the conditions (10.11) imposed on Δ. The rest of the eigenvectors are orthogonal to $\mathbf{e}$ and correspond to the eigenvalues zero or one. The eigenvectors of (10.17) can be considered to be the same as the eigenvectors in (10.13).

So for the linearized system we found the matrix associated with the term $\Delta_{i_U} \overset{*}{p}_{i_V}$ in (10.14) for any fixed $U|V$-partition. The vector of increments in gamete concentrations, Δ, can be expanded in eigenvectors of this matrix, orthogonal to $\mathbf{e}$.

When summation is being taken over all $U|V$, we arrive at the matrix $\mathbf{L}$, which also has the same eigenvectors. It should be noted that the terms $\Delta_{i_U} \overset{*}{p}_{i_V}$ and $\overset{*}{p}_{i_U} \Delta_{i_V}$ are analogous in the representation of the sums over $U|V$- the only difference between them is that the indices U and V are transposed. Therefore the right eigenvectors of matrix (10.13) and those of the appropriate transformation matrices summed up over $U|V$ are the same, while the eigenvalues of the linearization (10.14), affecting the dynamics of Δ, are equal up to a sign to

$$\mu_{i_1 \dots i_l} = \sum_{U|V,\, U \neq \emptyset, L} r(U|V)\Big(1 - \prod_k \mu_{ki_k}^{1-k(U)} - \prod_k \mu_{ki_k}^{1-k(V)}\Big), \tag{10.18}$$

where all i_k cannot be equal to 1 simultaneously. Since in (10.18) the expressions in brackets are non-negative, the eigenvalues of the system that takes into account selection and recombination, are less than the eigenvalues of matrix (10.13) by $\mu_{i_1 \dots i_l}$, that is the recombination-segregation processes contribute to stability of the Hardy-Weinberg equilibrium.

For R=0, that is under complete linkage, the Hardy-Weinberg equilibrium $\Pi_k \otimes \overset{*}{\mathbf{p}}_k$ in a multi-locus system with multiplicative fitnesses is unstable, because among the eigenvalues of (10.13) there are positive ones. Only when the recombination-segregation processes, specified by parameters r, are sufficiently active, the equilibrium $\Pi_k \otimes \overset{*}{\mathbf{p}}_k$ becomes stable. The exact stability criterion has the form

$$\prod_k \lambda_{ki_k} - \mu_{i_1 \dots i_l} < 0, \quad k = \overline{1, l}; \quad i_k = \overline{1, n_k}\,, \tag{10.19}$$

where λ_{ki_k} is the i_kth eigenvalues of the matrix of the linearized system for selection with respect to the kth locus, with not all of the i_k being equal to one.

At the beginning of this section we mentioned that under selection of different intensity with respect to separate loci the additive multiplicative model of fitnesses is reasonable, and it had been also treated by S. Karlin and U. Liberman for the case of non-overlapping generations. For continuous-time models the appropriate results are modified as follows.

First of all, let us note that if a locus is neutral, then the corresponding fitness matrix, appearing in the Kronecker-product (10.4), will be equal to $\mathbf{e}\mathbf{e}^T = \mathbf{J}$. Therefore, if selection with respect to any two loci is additive, then the genotype fitness is equal to the sum of fitnesses, obtained when the first one and then the other locus is assumed to be neutral. Accordingly, we substitute the matrix $\mathbf{J}$ of the appropriate dimensionality first instead of one of the one-locus fitness matrices in the Kronecker-product (10.4), and then instead of the other one, and then we sum them up. The general case of non-epistatic selection is defined by the above mentioned authors as follows. All kinds of vectors η, with dimensionality l and made of zeros and ones (l is the number of loci), are introduced, and the matrix of L-locus fitnesses is assumed to be

$$\| w_{ij} \| = \sum_{\eta} c(\eta) \prod_k \otimes \| w_{i_k j_k} \|^{\eta_k} \tag{10.20}$$

with the condition $\|w_{i_k j_k}\|^0 = \mathbf{J}_k$, $\|w_{i_k j_k}\|^1 = \|w_{i_k j_k}\|$. Here $c(\eta)$ are arbitrary chosen coefficients, complying with the only restriction that the resulting values of w_{ij} be positive. Obviously, for each of the η we obtain a combination of neutrally multiplicative interactions between loci, the additivity being a result of summation over η.

Under the made above assumptions about the type of equilibrium $\mathbf{p}^*$, the matrix of the linearized system, taking account of selection, has the form

$$\sum_{\eta} c(\eta) \prod_k \otimes \mathbf{D}(\mathbf{p}_k^*) \| w_{i_k j_k} \|^{\eta_k}. \tag{10.21}$$

For each of the summands, the eigenvectors that specify stability with respect to perturbations Δ of the state $\mathbf{p}^*$, are the same (orthogonal to $\mathbf{e}$), while their eigenvalues are $\Pi_k[\lambda_{ki_k}^{\eta_k} \mu_{ki_k}^{1-\eta_k}]$, $k=\overline{1, l}$; $i_k = \overline{1, n_k}$, not all of the i_k being equal to one simultaneously. Here μ_{ki_k} stand for the eigenvalues of $\mathbf{D}(\mathbf{p}_k^*)\mathbf{J}_k$, $\mu_{k1}=1$, $\mu_{ki_k}=0$ for $i_k>1$. Consequently, for equilibrium $\mathbf{p}^*$ with coordinates, associated with one-locus equilibria with respect to selection specified by fitness matrices $\|w_{i_k j_k}\|$, the stability criterion will be as follows

$$\sum_{\eta} c(\eta) \prod_k \left[\lambda_{ki_k}^{\eta_k} \mu_{ki_k}^{1-\eta_k} \right] - \mu_{i_1 \ldots i_l} < 0, \; k = \overline{1, l}; \;\; i_k = \overline{1, n_k}, \tag{10.22}$$

where not all of the i_k on the left equal unity simultaneously.

9.11. Notes and Bibliography

To 9.1 and 9.2

The dynamics of genetic content in one- and two-locus models without selection is well known. For instance, a discrete model is set forth in the monograph:

Moran, P.A.P.: 1962, *The Statistical Processes of Evolutionary Theory*. Clarendon Press, London, 200 pp.

The author proves that there is an exponential convergence towards the Hardy-Weinberg equilibrium in the one-locus (frequency) continuous-time model, and also analyze a discrete three-locus model.

Systems for differential equations with fast and slow variables are analyzed over a finite time interval in the book:

Vasilyeva, A.B. and Butuzov, V.F.: 1973, *Asimptoticheskiye* (*Asymptotic Expansions of Solutions to Singularly Perturbed Equations*, Nauka, Moscow, 272 pp.

The applicability conditions for these asymptotic expansions over semi-infinite time intervals are presented in the work:

Butuzov, V.F.: 1963, *Asymptoticheskiye formuly dlya resheniya sistemy differentsialnykh uravneniy s malym parametrom pri proizvodnoi na polubeskonechnom promezhutke* ($0 \le t < \infty$))' (*Asymptotic Formulas for Solutions to Systems of Differential Equations with a Small Parameter at the Derivative over Semi-Infinite Interval* ($0 \le t < \infty$) Vestnik MGU (Bulletin of the Moscow State University), N4, 3-14.

Singular perturbations are analyzed in the works:

Hoppensteadtr, F.: 1966, 'Singular Perturbations on the Infinite Interval', *Trans. Amer. Math. Soc.* **123**, 2, 521–535;

Hoppenstead, F.: 1974, 'Asymptotic Stability in Singular Perturbation Problems. II: Problems Having Matched Asymptotic Expansion Solutions', *J. Dif. Equat.* **15**, 3, 510–521.

To 9.3 and 9.4.

In formalizing recombination-segregation we follow the work of Ju.I. Ljubic, who applied the techniques of genetic algebras to give a complete solution to the problem of explicit determination of the relationships between the state of a multi-locus population and time in a discrete model with arbitrary linkage distribution:

Ljubic, Ju.I.: 1971, 'Osnovniye ponyatiya i teoremy evolutsionnoi genetiki svobodnykh populyatsiy (Basic Notions and Theorems of Evolutionary Genetics of Free Populations)', *UMN(Russian Mathematical Reviews*); **26**, 5(161), 51–116.

In the works:

Kun, L.A. and Ljubic, Ju.I.: 1980, 'H-teorema i skhodimost k ravnovesiyu dlya svobodnykh polilokusnykh populyatsiy 'H-Theorem and Convergence Towards Equilibrium in Free Multi-locus populations)', *Cybernetics* 2, 137–138,

it is proved that entropy of the distribution of gamete frequencies grows in the process of evolution, and this fact is applied to study the type of the equilibrium and the convergence towards it in a multi-locus discrete-time system without selection. The similar behavior of entropy in a more general context with selection, when the trajectory attains the set, on which the average population fitness is constant, was applied to prove the convergence of the trajectory. See the paper:

Kun, L.A. and Ljubic, Ju.I.: 1979, `Convergence to Equilibrium Under the Action of Additive Selection in a Multilocus Mutliallelic Population', *Soviet Math.Dokl.***20**, 6, 1380–1382.

See also the monograph:

Ljubic, Ju.I.: 1983, *Mathematicheskije struktury v populjatsionnoi genetike* (*Mathematical Structures in Populational Genetics*), Naukova Dumka, Kiev, 296 pp.

To 9.5 and 9.6.

Section 9.6 is set forth in keeping with the paper:

Passekov, V.P.: 1979, 'K Analyzu populyatsionno-geneticheskoy modeli otbora s uchotom differentsialnoi vzyhivayemosti gamete (On the analysis of a Populational-Genetic Model of Selection with Differential Viability of Gametes)', *Genetics*, **15**, 1, 77–83.

See also the paper:

Gregorius, H.F.: 1982, 'Selection in Diplo-Haplonts', *Theor. Pop. Biol.* 21, 2, 289–300.

The model of selection among zygotes and gametes with non-symmetric generalized fitnesses is introduced in the work:

Ratner, V.A.: 1971, 'Uravneniya dinamiki mendelevskikh populyatsiy i kontseptsiya obobshennykh prisposoblennostey (Equations of Dynamics in Mendelian Populations and the Concept of Generalized Fitnesses)', in *Sbronik trudov po agronomi cheskoi fizike* (*Transactions on Agronomical Physics*), Vol. 30, Gidrometeoizdat, Moscow, 131–141.

Density-dependent growth rates, that result in chaotic regimes in populations, are represented in the paper:

May, R.M. and Oster, G.F.: 1976, 'Bifurcation and Dynamical Complexity in Simple Ecological Models', *American Naturalist,* **110**, 974, 573–599.

In the work:

Ljubic, Ju.I., Maistrovskiy, G.D. and Olkhovskiy, Yu.G.: 1980, 'Skhodimost k ravnovesiyu pod deistviyem otbora v odnolokusnoi autosomnoi populyatsii (Convergence towards Equilibrium Under the Effect of Selection in One-Locus Autosomal Population)', *Problemy peredachi informatsii (Problems of Information Transmission),* **16**, 1, 93–104,

with no assumptions about non-singularity of the fitness matrix, it is proved that the trajectory of a one-locus population, affected by selection, converges. See also the paper:

Losert, V. and Akin, E.: 1983, 'Dynamics of Gametes and Genes: Discrete versus Continuous Time', *J. Math. Biology* **17**, 2, 241–251.

To 9.7.

Equations for a two-locus diallele model were first derived in the paper:

Lewontin, R.G., Kojima, K.: 1960, 'The Evolutionary Dynamics of Complex Polymorphisms', *Evolution* **14**, 4, 458–472.

The general case is presented, say, in the work:

Crow, J.F. and Kimura, M.: 1970, *An Introduction to Population Genetics Theory,* Harper and Row, New York, 591 pp.,

and in the latter of the above cited papers by Kun and Ljubich.

The equations for gamete frequencies in a continuous-time model are presented in the above mentioned monograph by Crow and Kimura. They assume gamete combinations in genotypes to be random under panmixia and overlapping generations (which is not obvious from biological reasons).

In the work:

Hoppenstead, F.C.: 1976, 'A Slow Selection Analysis of Two Locus, Two Allele Traits', *Theor. Pop. Biol.* **9**, 1, 68–81,

a model, similar to the one we presented for continuous time, is suggested for the special case of a two-locus diallele system. Unlike our treatment, the author assumes that not only the mortality, but also the natality depends upon the genotypes (the natality being determined only by the female genotype). Distinguishing fast and slow variables, he managed to make the model analysis much more simple over a finite time interval.

A similar approach is developed in the paper:

Nagylaki, T.: 1976, 'The Evolution of One- and Two-Locus Systems', *Genetics* **83**, 3, 583–600.

To 9.8.

The fact that average fitness is maximized under complete linkage, is proved in the work:

Lewontin, R.C.: 1971, 'The Effect of Genetic Linkage on the Mean–Fitness of a Population', *Proc. Nat. Acad. Sci. USA* **68**, 5, 984–986.

Numeric methods were applied in the paper:

Karlin, S., Feldman, M.W.: 1978, 'Simultaneous Stability of D=0 and D≠0 for Multiplicative Viabilities at Two Loci', *Genetics* **90**, 3, 813–825,

to show that there is a complex relationship between the extent of linkage and the behavior in the simplest two-locus diallele (with overdominance) model of multiplicative fitnesses.

Analytically this problem was treated by Hastings:

Hastings, A.: 1981, 'Simultaneous Stability of **D**=0 and **D**≠0 for Multiplicative Viabilities at Two Loci: an Analytical Study', *J. Theor. Biol.* **89**, 1, 69–81.

An example of a limit cycle for a model with non-overlapping generations is contained in the above cited work by Kun and Ljubic on additive selection. Problems of cyclic dynamics are also considered in the works:

Hastings, A.: 1981, 'Stable Cycling in Discrete-Time Genetic Models', *Proc. Nat. Acad. Sci. USA* **78**, 11, 7224–7225;

Akin, E.: 1982, 'Cycling in Simple Genetic Systems', *J. Math. Biology* **13**, 3, 305-324;

Akin, E.: 1983, 'Hopf Bifurcation in the Two Locus Genetic Model', *Memoirs of the Amer. Math. Soc.* **44**, 284, V, 190 pp.

The concept of quasi linkage equilibrium was introduced in the work:

Kimura, M.: 1965, 'Attainment of Quasi Linkage Equilibrium when Gene Frequencies are Changing by Natural Selection', *Genetics* **52**, 5, 875–890.

This approach is advanced, generalized and treated from various viewpoints in the works:

Shahshahani, S.: 1979, 'A New Mathematical Framework for the Study of Linkage and Selection', *Memoirs of the American Mathematical Society* **17**, 211, 1–34;

Akin, E.: 1979, *The Geometry of Population Genetics*, Springer, Berlin, Heidelberg, N.Y., 205 pp.

Hoppensteadt, F.C.: 1976, 'A Slow Selection Analysis of Two Locus, Two Allele Traits', *Theor. Pop. Biol.* **9**, 1, 68–81;

Nagylaki, T.: 1976, 'The Evolution of one- and Two-Locus Systems', *Genetics* **83**, 3, 583–600.

The paper

Passekov, V.P.: 1984, 'Asimpoticeskij Analiz otbora v polilokusnoi i poloallelnoi populjatsii (Asymptotic Analysis of Selection in Multi-locus Multi-Allelic Population)', *Reports Acad. Sci. USSR* **277**, 6, 1338–1342 elaborates on the case when recombination coefficients for all kinds of pairs of loci by far exceed the differences between viabilities of multi-locus genotypes. It is shown that in this case the allele frequencies are the slow variables, while the coefficients of linkage disequilibrium are the fast ones. Linkage equilibrium is quickly attained, and afterwards the dynamics of allele frequencies becomes gradientwise.

To 9.9.

The monotonicity of changes in average fitness under additive selection is proved in the paper:

Ewens, W.J.: 1969, 'A Generalized Fundamental Theorem of Natural Selection', *Genetics* **63**, 2, 531-537.

In the above mentioned works of Ju.I. Ljubic *et al.* it is proved that in the discrete model trajectories converge under additive fitnesses in a multi-locus system, if stationary points are non-isolated in case of one locus.

To 9.10.

The results of this section are the modifications of the proves presented in the paper:

Karlin, S. and Liberman, U.: 1979, 'Representation of Nonepistatic Selection Models and Analysis of Multilocus Hardy-Weinberg Equilibrium Configurations', *J. Math. Biol.* **7**, 4, 353–374.

PART 2

STOCHASTIC MODELS OF MATHEMATICAL GENETICS

Chapter 10

Diffusion Models of Population Genetics

10.1. Types of Random Processes Relevant to Models of Population Genetics

Random influences of various factors of evolution, which may be highly important in population life, are not covered by deterministic analysis of population genetics models. Therefore, stochastic (probability) models arise quite naturally in population genetics, reflecting conditions which are not 'exotic'.

The fact is that any natural population has a finite size. When describing dynamics of its genetic structure, one should take into account the random character of survival and reproduction processes, including the Mendelian segregation, inherent in the very nature of changes in the sequence of generations. Random mechanism reflecting this character should therefore be included into any model of a finite-sized population. The same requirement springs up in description of random character of an environment pressure ensuing from e.g., fluctuation in the direction or intensity of selection.

The stochastic models applicable in these cases permit a description of population characteristics to be more complete, accounting for both all deterministic factors and random aspects. These models, moreover, can help in revealing principally new features in the dynamics of a population. Random effects may drastically change a conclusion from a deterministic model, while the idea that the deterministic analysis shows the behavior of average population characteristics is far from being always true.

For example, by the deterministic approach to the conventional problem of the conditions for a genetic polymorphism to exist under selection pressure, the relations among genotype fitness values can be found which guarantee a population to be genetically heterogeneous (see Chapter 4, Part I). The stochastic analysis of the problem results in the conclusion that a finite population comes inevitably to one of the complete homozygous states, i.e. the polymorphism existence time is limited under any fitness pattern (see Section 10.5).

At the same time, a knowledge of the population dynamics in a deterministic model generates useful information on behavior of the trajectories in its stochastic version. In the deterministic case, we suppose the behavior of trajectories in the n-dimensional space to be determined by an autonomous system of ordinary differential equations. A probability generalization can then be obtained if small random, diffusion-type perturbations are introduced into the model. When these perturbations are sufficiently small, it appears that one can infer the behavior of trajectories in the stochastic model from solving a fairly close deterministic model instead of the original one. Within small time intervals, the motion proceeds mainly along a deterministic trajectory, while being specified by Gaussian deviations from it.

Under small perturbations, properties of the equilibrium states in some modified deterministic model determine essential features in the behavior of trajectories of the probability model, the modification arising because the diffusion coefficient matrix differs from the identity matrix (see 12.11.7). In the case where the right-hand side of the modified system represents the gradient of a function (a potential), the behavior of solutions to the system is quite obvious: the motion goes in the direction which is always perpendicular to a level surface of the potential. Local minima of the potential function surface indicate stable equilibrium points, while local maxima correspond to unstable points. A trajectory of the system can be imagined as the trajectory of a small ball rolling along the potential surface under the action of the gravity force (see Section 12.12). It appears that, if there is a *steady-state* (i.e. invariable in time) distribution of probabilities in the stochastic version, then its density function is related to the pattern of the potential surface in a way that is intuitively clear. It looks as if a population state were 'smeared' over stable equilibrium points of the deterministic model, the probability density minima being attained at unstable equilibria. The probability is 'condensed' in asymptotically stable equilibrium states, the deeper a well in the potential surface, the greater is the probability 'concentration' (see Section 12.11).

If a deterministic model has a unique stable equilibrium and the stochastic version proposes a steady-state probability density function, then it can be shown, as the magnitude of random perturbations tends to zero, one can get a picture of how the steady-state distribution 'shrinks up' to the equilibrium point.

In the present book, the stochastic models for changes in the population state are described by means of random processes. It is fairly common in genetics to believe that the dynamics of a population in the condition of its current state does not depend on the way this state has been reached (i.e., under the fixed present, the future does not depend on the past). Such random processes are called *Markov processes*.

Genetic diversity of a limited population, although being certainly finite, is extremely great. It is determined by genotypes of individuals composing the population and changes discretely by birth-death events. Therefore, a corresponding process of changes in the population genetic state is to be a Markov chain with either discrete or continuous time.

The genetic structure of a population can be described in terms of gene, gamete, or genotype frequencies. This structure is discrete due to the discreteness of individuals and discrete nature of the gene. If, however, the size of a population is not too small, then one can regard those frequencies as roughly continuous variables. It is highly probable that their changes in a unit of time (e.g. during the life-span of a generation or in some other time scale) are negligible under the conditions characteristic for evolution. The discrete random process of changes in the genetic structure will thus be approximated by a continuous-time Markov process having continuous trajectories in its space too. Such a process is termed a *diffusion process*.

10.2. Fundamental Problems in the Analysis of Stochastic Models

In a number of fairly regular cases, the state of a population can be sufficiently described by the gene or gamete frequencies, p_i, in whose terms the genotypes frequencies, specifying the genetic structure, can be expressed as well. As the sum of all frequencies is always equal to unity, the state space is represented by the simplex, $\overline{\Sigma}$, where e.g. the last frequency is thought off as being a dependent variable:

$$\overline{\Sigma} = \left\{ p_i \leq 0, \sum_i p_i \leq 1 \right\} , \tag{2.1}$$

with the interior

$$\Sigma = \left\{ p_i > 0, \sum_i p_i < 1 \right\} . \tag{2.2}$$

The points of the simplex will be denoted by letter $\mathbf{p}$ when related to an initial state of the process, and by other letters (most often by $\mathbf{x}$) when standing for a current state. The coordinates of point $\mathbf{p}=(p_1, p_2, ...)$ will be called the *spatial* or *phase variables*. The boundary of simplex is formed by hyperplanes in which one of the coordinates becomes zero. Note that these faces, in turn, are also simplices of type (2.1), though of the dimensionality lesser by one.

A trajectory originating from a point $\mathbf{p} = (p_1, p_2, ...)$ at time moment t_0 (in what follows we assume $t_0=0$ without loss of generality) will have certain probabilities of being in different regions of the space at time moment t.

Let $\mathbf{x}$ designate a current state of the population. A fundamental problem is to determine the density, $f(\mathbf{p}, \mathbf{x}, t)$, of the probability that the population is in state $\mathbf{x}$ at time t if the initial state was $\mathbf{p}$. Knowing the probability density, we are able to solve all the problems described below, the solution often being reached by an extremely tedious way though.

In some models there exists a non-degenerate limit of $f(\mathbf{p}, \mathbf{x}, t)$ as $t \to \infty$, which is called a *steady -state density*. To find a steady-state distribution (which is an analogue to the equilibrium state of the deterministic model) is an essential (and more simple than finding $f(\mathbf{p}, \mathbf{x}, t)$) problem of stochastic model analysis.

If we consider a process with *absorption*, i.e. when a trajectory ceases being under concern once it has reached a boundary point (for instance, having a homozygouse state reached, a population always remains in it provided there is no mutation), then of principal importance are the following characteristics of the process.

First of all, we need to know probabilities of absorption in different parts of the boundary (i.e. the probabilities of a trajectory to come into these parts). If, for example, the population state is described by frequency, x, of an allele in a diallelic locus, then a trajectory coming into the point $x = 0$ corresponds to loss of the allele and into the point $x = 1$ to its fixation.

Then, it is desirable to find a mean absorption time, e.g. the time necessary to attain homozygosity in the above case. To describe the process more thoroughly, it is necessary to learn also the higher moments of the absorption time, namely, its variance and the third and forth moments characterizing asymmetry and excess of the absorption time distribution curve, and finally to learn the entire generating function of the distribution.

Some of these problems are concerned with finding out a mathematical expectation of a functional defined on process trajectories. Let $\tau(\omega)$ designate a random time moment when the trajectory, ω, come out of a certain domain (for instance, the interior of the state space, Σ); let, furthermore, $u(\mathbf{x}_t)$ be a 'penalty' function defined on current states of the process; $h(\mathbf{x}_\tau)$ be 'penalty' depending on a point where the trajectory has reached a boundary of domain. Then the average 'payment' for a trajectory, including its coming out, is the mathematical expectation of the following functional:

$$\int_0^{\tau(\omega)} u[\mathbf{x}_t(\omega)]\,\mathrm{d}t + h[\mathbf{x}_\tau(\omega)]\,. \tag{2.3}$$

It is known that, when selection acts on a locus where one of the alleles has a selective advantage, s, over the other, the function $u(x) = s(1\text{-}x)$ determines the portion of total population size that is rejected by selection (the genetic death-rate) and hence the value of reproductive excess to preserve the population size. If we set $h(x)\equiv 0$, then the expectation of (2.3) with $u(x) = s(1\text{-}x)$ will give us the average value of elimination in the course of reaching homozygosity.

Sometimes, it is not sufficient to know the functional mean alone, but the higher moment are to be found, too.

Note that all these problems may not be necessarily posed over the whole state space Σ. When we are interested in the above-described characteristics before the coming out of a domain D, $D\subset\Sigma$, the corresponding equations must not change (in D the process is the same as in Σ), whereas the boundary conditions can do.

10.3. Forward and Backward Kolmogorov Equations

In the present section, the equations are presented which give solution to a number of problems considered above. A rigorous presentation of these topics would be too cumbersome and require an advanced level of the reader's mathematical background. At the same time, more simple, heuristic arguments can be enough to see why one or another equations are used in those problems.

Let us consider, for example, a simple model for discrete diffusion, $x(t)$. We define the process $x(t)$ by the formula:

$$x(t+\delta) = x(t) + M[x(t)]\delta + \sigma[x(t)]\xi_\delta(t+\delta)\,,\qquad x(0) = p, \tag{3.1}$$

where δ is a rime interval between successive changes of the state, $M(x)$ and $\delta(x)$ are non-random functions, and $\xi_\delta(0)$, $\xi_\delta(\delta)$, $\xi_\delta(2\delta)$,... compose a set of independent random variables with the properties that

$$E\{\xi_\delta(t)\} = 0\,,\ E\{\xi_\delta^2(t)\} = \delta\,,$$
$$E\{\xi_\delta^m(t)\} = o(\delta)\,,\ m>2\,, \tag{3.2}$$

for any $\delta \geq 0$. By $\Delta_t x$ we denote the difference $x(t+\delta)-x(t)$. Defined so, the process is Markov one, the coefficients M and $V = \sigma^2 \geq 0$ having a clear probability meaning:

$$\begin{aligned} &M[x(t)]\delta = E\{\Delta_t x|x(t)\}\,, \\ &V[x(t)]\delta = E\{[\Delta_t x - M(x(t))\delta]^2|x(t)] = \\ &\qquad = E\{(\Delta_t x)^2|x(t)\} + o(\delta)\,, \\ &E\{(\Delta_t x)^m|x(t)\} = o(\delta),\ m>2\,. \end{aligned} \tag{3.3}$$

It is clear that M and $V = \sigma^2$ represent the mean and the variance of the process increment per unit of time. They are called the *drift* and *diffusion coefficients*, respectively. In what follows, we assume functions M and V to be bounded and sufficiently smooth, the function V not vanishing inside Σ.

For a process (3.1) the value of the *generating operator* $\mathfrak{A}_\delta$ on a function $u(x)$ of process states is defined in the following way:

$$(\mathfrak{A}_\delta u)[x(t)] = \frac{1}{\delta}E\{u[x(t+\delta) - x(t)]\}\,. \tag{3.4}$$

Thus a function $u(x)$ is mapped by operator $\mathfrak{A}_\delta$ to the function that equals the expected increment of $u(x)$ over the process trajectories in the unit of time. The domain of operator $\mathfrak{A}$'s definition covers all functions u whose mathematical expectations (3.4) are finite. Let δ tend to zero. In the limit, time proceeds continuously, so that the process itself can be also supposed to converge to the limit one with continuous trajectories. The corresponding limit of the generating operator $\mathfrak{A}_\delta$ will be denoted by $\mathfrak{A}$.

We present now a heuristic proof for passage to the limit in operator $\mathfrak{A}_\delta$. Let us suppose $u(x)$ to be a sufficiently smooth function:

$$\begin{aligned} &E\{u[x(t+\delta)] - u[x(t)]\} = \\ &= E\left\{\Delta_t x\frac{du}{dx} + \frac{1}{2}(\Delta_t x)^2\frac{d^2u}{dx^2} + o(\Delta_t x)^2\right\} = \\ &= \delta\left\{M[x(t)]\frac{du}{dx} + \frac{1}{2}V[x(t)]\frac{d^2u}{dx^2}\right\} + o(\delta)\,. \end{aligned}$$

Dividing the both parts by δ and passing to the limit as $\delta \to 0$, we have:

$$\mathfrak{A}_u = M(x)\frac{du}{dx} + V(x)\frac{d^2u}{dx^2} \tag{3.5}$$

In the deterministic case, the differential equation $du/dx = M(x)$ yields apparently $\mathfrak{A}_u = M(x)\,du\,/\,dx$.

If we define operator T_t on a function u to be the operator of averaging u over the process states,

$$(T_t u)(p) = E\{u(x_t)|x_0 = p\}\,, \tag{3.6}$$

then clearly $T_0 u = u$ i.e. T_0 is the identity operator. By means of T_t, the generating operator $\mathfrak{A}$ can be written in the form

$$\mathfrak{A} = \lim_{\tau \to 0} \frac{1}{\tau}(T_\tau - T_0) = M(p)\frac{d}{dp} + \frac{1}{2}V(p)\frac{d^2}{dp^2}. \tag{3.7}$$

The domain of operator $\mathfrak{A}$'s definition consists of those functions u for which there exists a finite limit

$$\lim_{\tau \to 0} \frac{1}{\tau} E\{u(x_\tau) - u(p)\} .$$

In accordance with the above-stated, any twice continuously differentiable function (with the second derivative meeting the Lipschitz condition) belongs to the operator $\mathfrak{A}$'s domain of definition. In what follows, the $\mathfrak{A}$'s domain of definition is confined to bounded, twice continuously differentiable functions only.

Recall that, due to the Markov property, the density function, $f(p,x,t)$, for the probability of the process being in state x at time t conditioned by initial state p, obeys the Kolmogorov-Chapman equation

$$f(p, x, t + \tau) = \int f(p, y, \tau) f(y, x, t)\, dy. \tag{3.8}$$

The integral here is taken over the entire state space. The equation reflects the mere fact that, to reach a state x at time $t + \tau$, a trajectory can pass through one of the states y at time τ with probability density $f(p, y, \tau)$ and then pass from y to x in time t with the density $f(y, x, t)$ (independently of what is the way the trajectory gets into the state y).

From (3.8) it follows that, given a function $u(x)$ on the process states, then

$$(T_{t+\tau} u)(p) = \int f(p, y, \tau)[\int f(y, x, t) u(x)\, dx] dy = \\ = \int f(p, y, \tau)(T_t u)(y)\, dy = (T_\tau T_t u)(p) .$$

In the similar way, we have

$$(T_{t+\tau} u)(p) = (T_t T_\tau u)(p) ,$$

i.e. the following relation is true for the operators:

$$T_{t+\tau} = T_t T_\tau = T_\tau T_t . \tag{3.9}$$

By (3.9) it is easy to see that

$$\lim_{\tau \to 0} \frac{1}{\tau}(T_{t+\tau} - T_t) = \begin{cases} \lim_{\tau \to 0} \frac{1}{\tau} (T_\tau - T_0) T_t = \mathfrak{A} T_t, \\ \lim_{\tau \to 0} \frac{1}{\tau} T_t (T_\tau - T_0) = T_t \mathfrak{A} . \end{cases} \tag{3.10}$$

This means that, for the mathematical expectations

$$U(t, p) = (T_t u)(p) = E\{u(x_t) | x(0) = p\} ,$$

the following differential equation holds

$$\frac{dU}{dt} = \mathfrak{A}U = [M(p)\frac{\partial}{\partial p} + \frac{1}{2}V(p)\frac{\partial^2}{\partial p^2}]U\,,$$

$$U(0, p) = u(p)\,. \tag{3.11}$$

Since averaging u can only strengthen its smoothness, the function U will be twice continuously differentiable.

Equation (3.11) is called the *backward* (or *second*) *Kolmogorov equation*.

In (3.11) the independent variable is denoted by p to stress that mathematical expectation U is a function of the initial state p. If we choose a function u to be a step of the unit height over the interval $(a, b)\subset(0, 1)$, the step being a limit of smooth 'steps', then its expectation will represent the probability of the process being in (a, b). Thus, a probability of the process being a given interval obeys equation (3.11).

If the probability density $f(p, x, t)$ is treated as a function of time and an initial state, then it also obeys Equation (3.11). In fact, the density $f(p, x, t)$ can be set equal to the expectation of the delta-function: $g(x) = \delta(x-y)$.

A delta-function is defined by the condition that

$$\int \delta(x - y)h(x)\, dx = h(y)\,,$$

where the integration is to be done over any interval containing the point y; $h(x)$ is an arbitrary function continuous in the point y.

It is clear that

$$E\{\delta(x_t - y)|x_0 = p\} = \int \delta(x_t - y)f(p, x, t)\, dy = f(p, y, t)\,,$$

$$f(p, y, 0) = \delta(y - p)\,.$$

If the 'penalty' is $g(x)=\delta(x-y)$ and the process, once having reached a boundary point y, remains in it forever, then Equation (3.11) determines the absorption probability as a function of time and an initial state.

So, to study temporal changes in the mathematical expectation of a function on the process states, the operator $\mathfrak{A}$ can be used as shown above. To study temporal evolution of probability distributions in the state space is another important problem. Let $v(x)$ be a probability density at the initial time moment. Then, at a moment t, it is determined by the relation

$$v(x, t) = \int f(p, x, t)v(p)\, dp\,. \tag{3.12}$$

Let $v(x, t)$ be written down differently, by making use of the Kolomogorov-Chapman Equation (3.8):

$$v(x, t) = \iint f(p, y, s)v(p)f(y, x, t - s)\, dp\, dy =$$
$$= \int v(y, s)f(y, x, t - s)\, dy\,.$$

Differentiating both sides of this equality with respect to s and granting (3.11), we have

$$0 = \int \left[\frac{\partial}{\partial s}v(y, s)f(y, x, t - s) - v(y, s)\mathfrak{A}f(y, x, t - s)\right] dy.$$

Now, we explicate the meaning of $\mathcal{a}$ and integrate the last summand twice by parts, the terms being assumed vanishing which arise as values of the functions on the boundary of the entire state space. This results in

$$\int\left[\frac{\partial}{\partial s}v(y, s) - \mathcal{a}^*v(y, s)\right]f(y, x, t-s)\, dy = 0\,, \tag{3.13}$$

where

$$\mathcal{a}^*v = -\frac{\partial}{\partial y}[M(y)v(y, s)] + \frac{1}{2}\frac{\partial^2}{\partial y^2}[V(y)v(y, s)]\,. \tag{3.14}$$

Hence,

$$\partial v(y, s)/\partial s = (\mathcal{a}^*v)(y, s) \tag{3.15}$$

almost everywhere in y. If, in particular, $v(x)$ is chosen to be $\delta(x\text{-}p)$, then Equation (3.15) (which is called the *forward Kolmogorov equation*) is satisfied with the density $f(p, x, t)$, the *fundamental solution* to (3.15). This fundamental solution was shown above to satisfy the backward Kolmogorov Equation (3.11) too.

Note that the forward Kolmogorov equation for $f(p, x, t)$ can be written in another form. Let $P(p, x, t)$ be defined by the formula

$$P(p, x, t) = M(x)f(p, x, t) - \frac{1}{2}\frac{\partial}{\partial x}[V(x)f(p, x, t)]\,. \tag{3.16}$$

Then, by means of (3.14), the Equation (3.15) takes on the form

$$\partial f(p, x, t)/\partial t = -\partial P(p, x, t)/\partial x\,. \tag{3.17}$$

Let $I = (a, b)\subset(0, 1)$ be an interval and $F(p, I, t)$ be the probability that a state of the process originated from p belongs to the interval I at time t. Then

$$\begin{aligned}\frac{\partial}{\partial t}F(p, I, t) &= \int_a^b \frac{\partial}{\partial t}f(p, x, t)\, dx = -\int_a^b \frac{\partial}{\partial x}P(p, x, t) = \\ &= P(p, a, t) - P(p, b, t)\end{aligned} \tag{3.18}$$

and $P(p, x, t)$ can be interpreted as the *flow of probability*. The difference between the values of the flow through the left and right bounds of the interval I determines the rate of variation in the probability of process being in I.

If the process under study is one with absorbing boundaries $a= 0$ and $b= 1$, then the flow directed to them will result in all the probability 'mass' eventually 'flowing out' through the boundaries. The probabilities, $U_0(p, t)$ and $U_1(p, t)$, that a trajectory comes out via the left and the right bounds respectively, are related with the flow by the following differential equations:

$$dU_0(p, t)/dt = -P(p, 0, t)\,, \tag{3.19}$$

$$dU_1(p, t)/dt = P(p, 1, t)\,. \tag{3.20}$$

10.4. Diffusion Approximation of the Fisher-Wright and the Moran Models

The passage, heuristically reasoned above, from discrete diffusion (3.1) to the diffusion process, can be associated with the Fisher-Wright nonoverlapping generation model widely applicable in population genetics.

In this model, the changes in gamete frequencies that are caused by evolutionary factors during one generation life-span are assumed to permit a deterministic description. Genetic composition of a new generation is determined by the reproduction process that is assumed to a be a random sampling with replacement from the set of gametes produced by individuals of the previous generation. The number of gametes sampled corresponds to the population size, N. The assumption of the gamete sampling with replacement is justified by the fact that the number of sexual cells which are produced, actually or potentially, by the individuals during their life-span is extremely large, so that the gamete 'expenditures' per each offspring do not affect the probabilities of subsequent gamete 'choices'.

In the simplest case, i.e. that of a haploid population of constant size N treated with respect to one locus with two alleles, A and a, the genetic composition of the population can be described by the frequency, for instance, of allele A alone. Let this frequency be p at the start of generation. By the end of the generation it will be equal to some other value, $\tilde{p}$, due to action deterministic factors. Let the increment, $M(p)=\tilde{p}-p$, be written down in the form of $m_N(p)/N$. Reproduction then takes place and, at the start of the next generation, the number of A-alleles is to be determined by the N Bernoulli trials, the probability of A's appearance to be equal to $\tilde{p}$. Hence, the variance in the number of A-alleles in the next generation equals $N\tilde{p}(1-\tilde{p})$. If we consider the share of A-alleles among N members of the population, rather than their absolute number, then the previous expression must be divided by N^2 and the variance of the A-allele frequency will be equal to $\tilde{p}(1-\tilde{p})/N$.

The process of changes in the gene frequency can be, furthermore, described by the discrete diffusion model, by setting the new time-scale unit equal to N generations. Note also, that $\tilde{p}-p = O(1/N)$ whereby $\tilde{p}(1-\tilde{p})/N = p(1-p)/N + O(1/N^2)$. During one generation, the time increases by the amount $\delta = 1/N$ of the new time unit and, therefore,

$$x\left(t+\frac{1}{N}\right) = x(t) + m_N[x(t)]\,\frac{1}{N} + \\ + \sqrt{x(t)[1-x(t)]+O(1/N)}\;\frac{\xi_N(t+1/N)}{\sqrt{N}}. \tag{4.1}$$

Here, $\xi_N(t+1/N)$ represents a random variable having zero mean and unit variance that appears as a result of normalizing the binomial random variable with parameters N and $\tilde{x}(t)$. The higher than the second-order moments of ξ_N will be equal to $o(1/N)$. For different values of t, those of ξ_N are not correlated. By tending t to infinity, we have ξ_N to be distributed normally in the asymptotics and be independent (due to their being uncorrelated). Suppose then $m_N(x)$ to converge to a function, $m(x)$, the term $O(1/N)$ not affecting the limiting behavior of the process (4.1) and $m_N(x)$ permitting replacement by $m(x)$. In the limit, therefore, the diffusion process appears which has the drift and diffusion coefficients equal to $m(x)$ and $p(1-p)$. If N is sufficiently large, the discrete process (4.1) can be approximated by the diffusion one. With the time unit equal to only one generation, the drift and diffusion coefficients of the approximation will be equal to $m_N(x)/N = M(x)$ and $x(1-x)/N$, respectively.

Similarly, the passage to a diffusion process can be also grounded for the Moran model of overlapping generations. In its simplest version, considered is a constant-size population of N haploid individuals sharing two alleles, A and a. Only *one* birth-death event occurs in the unit of time. The probability that an allele, A or a, dies is proportional to its concentration in the population. The birth event can be interpreted as a result of sampling one gamete from the gamete pool that has been formed up to the time moment prior to death.

The gamete concentrations in the gamete pool reflect the population processes (of selection, mutation, etc.) shifting the state of the population (that is described, for instance, by concentration, x, of allele A) from the point x to point $\tilde{x}$, the x characterizing the population at the previous birth moment. Let the resulting increment be written in the form of $M(x)=\tilde{x}-x=m_N(x)/N^2$. Sampling a gamete corresponds to one Bernoulli trial with the probability that borned is allele A being equal to $\tilde{x}$. As a result of birth, the population state can alter by no more than $\pm 1/N$, i.e. quite insignificantly for a large N. The variance of the random increment equals $\tilde{x}(1-\tilde{x})/N^2$.

By passing to the new time unit that corresponds to N^2 birth-death event and by tending N to infinity, we have a diffusion process in the limit (by the reasons similar to those presented above). Its drift coefficient equals $m(x)$ while the diffusion one is equal to $x(1-x)$.

Thus, the diffusion approximations to the Fisher-Wright and the Moran models are the same (in the proper time scale), once the same are the factors considered that change the genetic structure. In a similar way, the passage to diffusion can be done also for the continuous-time Moran model where the probability of a birth-death event in any time interval $(t, t+\Delta t)$ is assumed equal to $N\lambda\, dt + o(dt)$. In the limit as $N\to\infty$ we obtain the same diffusion process as above whereas the time is measured in the units each consisting of N^2 events of birth-death rather then in those of a continuous process.

In what follows, when interpreting outcomes of the diffusion approach, we shall mean the approximation of the Fisher-Wright model, while, in the proper time scale, the outcomes will be also true for the Moran model with overlapping generations.

If one consider a population of diploids, rather than that of haploids, then, under the random mating hypothesis, the generation change in the Fisher-Wright model will be equivalent to sampling $2N$, rather than N, gametes from the parent generation. In the diffusion approximation, therefore, the diffusion coefficient will be equal to $x(1-x)/(2N)$. The model premises resulting in the random gamete sampling scheme can often be violated. If, nevertheless, the variance of gene frequencies in a time interval can be represented as $x(1-x)/(2N_e)$ and if the higher moments have orders of $o(1/N_e)$, where N_e may differ from the actual population size N, then the N_e must be substituted for N in the diffusion coefficient formula. The quantity N_e is called the *variance effective size* of the population.

For example, as known from observations on natural populations, some of them undergo fairly regular and significant oscillations in size. If k denotes the period of oscillations, it is reasonable to choose k generations as a new time unit. In this time interval, the gene frequency variance will approximately equal

$$\sum_{i=1}^{k} \frac{1}{2N_i} x(1-x) = \frac{kx(1-x)}{2N_e},$$

where N_i is a population size at the i-th stage of the period. The effective size will, therefore, be equal to the harmonic mean of the population sizes which vary deterministically over the period. When the population size, the direction and intensity of regular factors to change the genetic structure do vary randomly, one should take into account both some patterns in their variability and the auto-correlation in the sequence of generations. If the higher than second-order moments of the process increment in a chosen unit of time are negligibly small, then the limiting diffusion process can have both the drift and the diffusion coefficients depending on the auto-correlation and the mean shift in gene frequencies (due to, for instance, variations in the intensity of selection).

In what follows, we make no distinction in the notation of the actual and the effective population size, implying the necessary correction to have been done and the N symbol to refer to the variance effective size.

Note also that convergence to a one-dimensional diffusion process takes place for a population with two sexes too, the state of the population being determined in general by the subpopulation sizes and the allele frequencies defined separately for the male and female subpopulations, i.e. the behavior of average gene concentrations being no longer Markov.

10.5. Classification of Boundaries in Diffusion Models

It is typical for genetic models that the diffusion coefficient vanishes at the bounds of interval (0, 1) (*singularity*). The boundary point can be *accessible* from the interval (with a non-zero probability of being attained in a finite time), any point inside (0, 1) can be accessible from that bound, but the bound itself is impassable to outside. Such a point will be called a *reflecting boundary* . An accessible boundary point can be such that, once a trajectory has gotten into this point, it remains here forever. Getting inside (0, 1) is impossible from this point, so that it is called a *capturing boundary*. If, however, a boundary is not accessible from the inside, but inside points themselves can be reached from it, the boundary is called a *releasing* one.

As to an *inaccessible* (with a positive probability in a finite time) boundary, x_B, it may be an *attracting* one if, for any $\varepsilon > 0$, there exists $\delta > 0$ such that

$$P\left\{ \lim_{t \to \infty} x_t = x_B \right\} = 1 - \varepsilon$$

for any initial point p within (0, 1) that is apart from x_B by no more than δ. An inaccessible boundary x_B is called a *repelling* one if a trajectory starting at any interval within [0, 1] that includes x_B, comes out of the interval through its bound opposite to x_B with the unit probability.

Behavior of the process in boundary points is determined by its coefficients. To investigate the boundaries the following functions can be used:

$$R_1(x) = \exp\left\{ -\int_p^x \frac{2M(y)}{V(y)} dy \right\}, \quad R_2(x) = \frac{1}{V(x)R_1(x)},$$

$$R_3(x) = R_1(x) \int_p^x R_2(y)\, dy. \tag{5.1}$$

If the integral of R_1 over a vicinity of the boundary point under concern equals $+\infty$, then the point is a repelling boundary. Otherwise, the behavior of R_3 is to be considered: if the integral of R_3 over a vicinity of the boundary turns into $+\infty$, the boundary is an attracting one.

If R_1 and R_3 are integrable and the integral of R_2 over a vicinity of the boundary equals $+\infty$, the boundary is a capturing one. Otherwise, it will be a releasing boundary.

Integrability of R_2 is a sufficient condition for a steady-state distribution to exist.

In genetic models, the diffusion coefficient $V(x) = x(1-x)/(2N)$ is positive in the interval (0, 1) and vanishes in its boundary point, the derivative $V'(x)$ being positive in the left bound and negative in the right one. The drift may change its sign in (0, 1), but it is non-negative in the left bound and non-positive in the right one. Due to these properties, the investigation of the boundary types becomes essentially easier.

Let, for example, the drift be zero in the boundary $x_B = 0$. Then the boundary is capturing. This can be shown by approximation of the drift and diffusion coefficients near the point $y = 0$:

$$V(y) \sim V(0) + V'(0)y = V'(0)y,$$

$$M(y) \sim M(0) + M'(0)y = M'(0)y.$$

The following expressions then approximate the functions $R_i(x)$ for a small x accurately to $o(x)$:

$$R_1(x) \sim \exp\left\{ -\frac{2M'(0)}{V'(0)}x \right\} \sim 1 - \frac{2M'(0)}{V'(0)}x,$$

$$R_2(x) \sim \left[1 + \frac{2M'(0)}{V'(0)}x \right] / [V'(0)x],$$

$$R_3(x) \sim \left[1 - \frac{2M'(0)}{V'(0)}x \right] \left[\frac{\ln x}{V'(0)} + \frac{2M'(0)}{(V'(0))^2}x \right].$$

Thus, the functions R_1 and R_3 are integrable in the vicinity of the boundary $x_B = 0$, while the R_2 is not. The boundary is hence a capturing one. The boundary $x_B = 1$ is of the same type if $M(1) = 0$. To prove, we may approximate the functions R_i near $x_B = 1$, but it would be more easy if we reduce the case to the previous one by the change of variables $z = 1 - x$ transferring the bound into the origin of coordinates.

This result shows that genetic homogeneity is to be reached in a population under any form of selection with constant values of genotype fitness. In fact, the selection does render influence on the genetic structure if there are options to select; in a homozygous population (i.e. in the boundary states) the drift coefficient, therefore, equals zero.

Another important case is represented by genetic conditions where drift values at the boundaries are directed inside the interval (0, 1). For example, the drift is directed inside if migrants bring the different-type alleles into the population, or if the missing allele appears as a result of mutation. A steady-state probability distribution of the gene frequencies then exists there in the population, the integrability of function R_2 being an analytical condition for the existence. Let us verify the integrability in the vicinity of the boundary $x_B = 0$ (the integrability at $x_B = 1$ being verifiable similarly). Since $M(0)>0$, we have for a small x:

$$R_1(x) \sim \exp\left\{ -\frac{2M'(0)}{V'(0)} \ln x \right\} = x^{-2M(0)/V'(0)},$$

$$R_2(x) \sim x^{2M(0)/V'(0)}/[V'(0)x] .$$

As the sign of $V'(0)$ coincides with that of $M(0)$, we have $M(0)/V'(0)>0$ and R_2 is integrable near zero.

Due to the singularity of boundary points, the boundary conditions are not arbitrary in the Kolmogorov equations. If, in a finite time, the process does not reach a boundary with a non-zero probability, then the boundary does not affect anyhow the behavior of the process. That is why there is no need to specify the boundary conditions when we are searching for the fundamental solution. Since jump-wise passages are impossible in the genetic case, there must be only absorption at a capturing bound. In this case, the boundary conditions can also remain unspecified.

The Kolmogorov equation should not be necessarily considered over the entire state space. When we study the process on an interval $(a, b) \subset (0, 1)$, the boundaries will no longer be singular, requiring the proper boundary conditions to be ascribed to the equation. One may investigate, for instance, the problem of the first passage time for a point $a \in (0, p)$ attainable by a trajectory originating from p. To do this, one should consider the process in the interval $(a, 1)$ where the boundary a should be an absorbing one: then the distribution of the time to come out through the bound a is identical to that of the a's first passage time. Having point a reached, the trajectory is unable to come back inside $(a, 1)$, so that the boundary condition takes the form of $f(a, x, t) = 0$. If we have to study the conditional probability of the first passage through a under the condition of not passage through a point $b>p$, we should consider then the probability to come out through a for the process in (a, b) where both boundaries are absorbing ones.

10.6. Multidimensional Diffusion Models

When studying models with many alleles, or in other cases where the state of a population is a vector variable, we have the random variation of this vector to be approximated now by a multidimensional diffusion process. In this case, the components of the drift vector $\mathbf{M}^T(\mathbf{x}) = (M_1(\mathbf{x}), M_2(\mathbf{x}), \ldots)$ determine the expected increments of the coordinates per unit of time, while the entries in the diffusion matrix $\|V_{ij}(\mathbf{x})\|$ corresponding to the average pair products (or the covariances) of increments in various coordinates. Thus, the vector, $\Delta\mathbf{x}$, of the coordinate increments $(\Delta x_1, \Delta x_2, \ldots)$ in a small time interval δt satisfies the following relations:

$$E\{\Delta x_i\} = M_i(\mathbf{x})\delta t + o(\delta t)\,,$$
$$E\{\Delta x_i \Delta x_j\} = V_{ij}(\mathbf{x})\delta t + o(\delta t)\,, \qquad (6.1)$$
$$E\{\Delta x_i^n \Delta x_j^m\} = o(\delta t)\,,\ n+m \geq 3$$

In genetic applications, $M_i(\mathbf{x})$ corresponds to the increment in the ith coordinate per unit of time due to the action of deterministic forces, while $V_{ij}(\mathbf{x})$ shows the covariance of random increments in the ith and jth coordinates per unit of time (the passage to the limit is indifferent to whether the covariances or the mixed product moments are chosen).

Coefficients $V_{ij}(x)$ make up the diffusion matrix $\| V_{ij} \|$. While the diffusion coefficient is non-negative in the one-dimensional case, the multi-dimensional counterpart of this property is the non-negative definiteness of the diffusion matrix $\| V_{ij} \|$. In the Fisher-Wright model (where the state of a diploid population is specified by the gamete frequencies, $\{x_i\}$), the gamete sampling at the change of generations is of the polynomial nature, so that, in the diffusion approximation, the diffusion matrix entries have the following form:

$$V_{ij}(\mathbf{x}) = x_i(\delta_{ij} - x_j)/(2N)\,, \qquad (6.2)$$

where N stands for the variance effective size of the population and δ_{ij} for the Kronecker delta.

If the population state is described by concentrations of all the gametes excepting one, the diffusion process will be singular, as it was in the one-dimensional case, since the matrix with entries (6.2) degenerates in boundaries (where some of the coordinate turns into zero).

The operators $\mathfrak{A}$ and $\mathfrak{A}^*$ that correspond to the backward and forward Kolmogorov equations, have the following forms:

$$\mathfrak{A} = \frac{1}{2}\sum_{i,j} V_{ij}(\mathbf{p})\frac{\partial^2}{\partial p_i \partial p_j} + \sum_i M_i(\mathbf{p})\frac{\partial}{\partial p_i}\,, \qquad (6.3)$$

$$\mathfrak{A}^* = \frac{1}{2}\sum_{i,j}\frac{\partial^2}{\partial x_i\, \partial x_j}[V_{ij}(\mathbf{x})\ldots] - \sum_i \frac{\partial}{\partial x_i}[M_i(\mathbf{x})\ldots] \qquad (6.4)$$

while the density function $f(\mathbf{p}, \mathbf{x}, t)$ obeys the forward and the backward Kolmogorov equations:

$$\frac{\partial}{\partial t} f(\mathbf{p}, \mathbf{x}, t) = \mathfrak{A}^* f(\mathbf{p}, \mathbf{x}, t)\,, \qquad (6.5)$$

$$\frac{\partial}{\partial t} f(\mathbf{p}, \mathbf{x}, t) = \mathcal{Q} f(\mathbf{p}, \mathbf{x}, t) .$$

The forward equation $\partial f/\partial t = \mathcal{Q}^* f$ can be rewritten in the form

$$\frac{\partial}{\partial t} f(\mathbf{p}, \mathbf{x}, t) = -\sum_i \frac{\partial}{\partial x_i} P_i(\mathbf{p}, \mathbf{x}, t) , \tag{6.6}$$

where

$$P_i(\mathbf{p}, \mathbf{x}, t) = M_i(\mathbf{x}) f(\mathbf{p}, \mathbf{x}, t) - \frac{1}{2} \sum_j \frac{\partial}{\partial x_j} [V_{ij}(\mathbf{x}) f(\mathbf{p}, \mathbf{x}, t)]. \tag{6.7}$$

Let D be a domain within Σ, with the boundary being denoted by $B(D)$; let also $F(\mathbf{p}, D, t)$ be the probability that the process (starting from a point $\mathbf{p}$) is being in D at time moment t. Then it is clear that

$$\frac{\partial}{\partial t} F(\mathbf{p}, \mathbf{x}, t) = -\int_D \sum_i \frac{\partial}{\partial x_i} P_i(\mathbf{p}, \mathbf{x}, t) \, d\mathbf{x} . \tag{6.8}$$

By the Gauss-Ostrogradskii formula,

$$\int_D \sum_i \frac{\partial}{\partial x_i} P_i(\mathbf{p}, \mathbf{x}, t) \, d\mathbf{x} = \int_{B(D)} (\mathbf{P}, \mathbf{n}) \, d\mathbf{S} , \tag{6.9}$$

where the vector $\mathbf{P}$ is composed by $(P_1, P_2, \ldots)$, $\mathbf{n}$ is a vector of the outward normal to the boundary of D, and $(\mathbf{P}, \mathbf{n})$ stands for their inner product; the right-hand side of (6.9) represents a surface integral of the first kind.

Vector $\mathbf{P}$ is well-known to have quite a definite interpretation: in this particular case it is the flow of probability. Its ith component, $P_i(\mathbf{p}, \mathbf{x}, t)$, is equal to the flow of probability through point $\mathbf{x}$ in the direction of the ith coordinate axis. The equalities (6.8) and (6.9) thus show that a variation in the probability of being in a domain is determined by the flow through the boundary of the domain. In the one-dimensional case the equations (6.8) and (6.9) reduce to (3.18).

In case of inhomogeneous diffusion process, the drift and diffusion coefficients depend non-randomly upon both the spatial coordinates and the temporal ones. The density, $f(s, \mathbf{p}, \mathbf{x}, t)$, of the transition probability that, from state $\mathbf{p}$ at time moment s, the process comes to state $\mathbf{x}$ at time t, obeys the Kolmogorov equations

$$-\partial f/\partial s = \mathcal{Q} f; \quad \partial f/\partial t = \mathcal{Q}^* f,$$

where the operators $\mathcal{Q}$ and $\mathcal{Q}^*$ have the same form as those in the homogeneous case (6.3) - (6.4) but with the coefficients depending additionally on time.

10.7. Solutions to the Kolmogorov Equations by the Fourier Method. Transformations of Diffusion Processes. The Steady-State Density

The forward and the backward Kolmogorov equations are partial differential equations of the parabolic type. To solve them one can use a standard method of separation of variables, namely, the Fourier method. In the one-dimensional case, for example, the forward Equation (3.15) is supposed to be complied with a function that can be represented as a product $X(x)T(t)$. If we substitute it into (3.15), group the terms containing the function T and its derivatives in the left-hand side while those containing X with its derivative in the right-hand side, and divide both sides by $X(x)T(t)$, we then obtain an equality whose one side depends solely on x, while the other depending exclusively on t. It is possible only when the left and right expressions are both equal to the same constant value, λ, termed an *eigenvalue* .

The equation for T has a fairly simple form,

$$(1/T)\, dT/dt = \lambda\,, \tag{7.1}$$

from which $T(t) = e^{\lambda t}$. To find the function X we have an ordinary differential equation which has a solution (commonly termed an *eigenfunction* or a *characteristic function*) under certain values of λ, normally in discrete points $\lambda_n(\lambda_n \leq 0)$ making up a monotone decreasing sequence termed the *spectrum* (sometimes, the spectrum can be continuous). The solution for the probability distribution density $f(p, x, t)$ can be written down as the series (or the integral in the continuous-spectrum case)

$$f(p, x, t) = \sum_{n=1}^{\infty} X(x, A_n, B_n, \lambda_n) e^{\lambda_n t}, \tag{7.2}$$

where A_n, B_n, and λ_n are to be specified by the initial and boundary conditions.

If all the values $\lambda_n<0$, then $f(p, x, t)$ converges exponentially to zero as $t \to \infty$ (the case of an absorption process, for instance), of most importance being the main term in expansion (7.2) having the maximum eigenvalue, λ_{max}. For a sufficiently great t the form of the probability distribution density $f(p, x, t)$ is determined by the characteristic function that corresponds to the greatest eigenvalue. In the asymptotics as $t \to \infty$, the distribution form is invariable, while the density decreases at a constant rate λ_{max}.

To find λ_{max} and the corresponding eigenfunction is a critical problem, whose solution yields a picture of the asymptotic behavior of the probability distribution density. For example, under the combined action of selection and fluctuation in sample gene frequencies that is known (see Section 10.5) to lead the population eventually to genetic homogeneity, the λ_{max} shows the asymptotic rate at which the homozygosity is attained, while the corresponding eigenfunction shows the asymptotic density of the allele frequency distribution in still segregating polymorphic populations.

If the maximum eigenvalue is equal to zero, then, as $t \to \infty$ the probability distribution density converges to the characteristic function associated with λ_{max} (for instance, the case where a steady-state distribution exists). The difference between the function and the density $f(p, x, t)$ converges exponentially to zero. The convergence rate is asymptotically equal to the second-magnitude eigenvalue, while the corresponding eigenfunction specifies the asymptotic form of the difference.

The most comprehensive characteristic of a diffusion process is represented by the transition probability density that can be obtained from the fundamental solution of (3.15) corresponding to the initial condition in the form of the delta-function. This solution, however, is difficult to find in explicit form. Yet sometimes, by transforming the diffusion process, one can have a more simple one, e.g. a Wiener process. An explicit form of the fundamental solution for the Wiener process either in the entire real axis or in some of its intervals is known, which greatly facilitates the solution.

In the case where an inhomogeneous process has the smooth drift and diffusion coefficients, the necessary and sufficient conditions for a process to admit the transformation into a Wiener one, were obtained by I.D. Cherkasov. He has also described the explicit, though fairly tedious, form of the change of variables in terms of the process coefficients, their derivatives up to the second order, and some determinants composed of them. No conditions of this kind are known for a multidimensional process.

In the case of one-dimensional homogeneous diffusion process, a one-to-one transformation, $\tilde{p} = \phi(p)$, of the state space generates the diffusion process whose drift and diffusion coefficients have the following forms (as functions of the original variable):

$$\tilde{M}(p) = \phi'(p)M(p) + \frac{1}{2}\phi''(p)V(p)\,, \tag{7.3}$$

$$\tilde{V}(p) = [\phi'(p)]^2 V(p)\,.$$

In the multidimensional case, a one-to-one change of variables, $\tilde{p}_i = \phi_i(\mathbf{p})$, results in the following transformation:

$$\tilde{M}_i(\mathbf{p}) = \sum_j \left[\frac{\partial}{\partial p_j}\phi_i(\mathbf{p})\right] M_j(\mathbf{p}) + \frac{1}{2}\sum_{k,l}\left[\frac{\partial^2}{\partial p_k\,\partial p_l}\phi_i(\mathbf{p})\right] V_{kl}(\mathbf{p})\,,$$

$$\tilde{V}_{ij}(\mathbf{p}) = \sum_{k,l}\left[\frac{\partial}{\partial p_k}\phi_i(\mathbf{p})\right]\left[\frac{\partial}{\partial p_l}\phi_j(\mathbf{p})\right] V_{kl}(p)\,. \tag{7.4}$$

These formulae are easy to remember: since $\tilde{M}\delta t$ and $\tilde{V}_{ij}\delta t$ represent the expected values of infinitely small increments in ϕ_i and $\phi_i\phi_j$ in the δ-increment of time, to find them one can expand the functions $\{\phi_i\}$ into the power series of $\{p_i\}$ and make use of the fact that, in a diffusion process, the expectations are zero for the higher than second-order terms.

In the multiallele, one-locus case, the change of variables $\tilde{p}_i = \sqrt{p_i}$ transforming the symplex Σ into a part of the hypersphere is shown (Section 11.2) to a give a simple approximation of the genetic drift process in small intervals of time.

The analysis of the diffusion model can sometimes be simplified by means of a random change of time along the process trajectories. The change does not affect the form of trajectories but does retard or accelerate the motion along them. Let us fix a trajectory and make the change of time for it, $\tau = \tau(\omega, t)$, according to the equation

$$\mathrm{d}\tau(\omega, t)/\mathrm{d}t = 1/g[\mathbf{x}_t(\omega)]\,, \tag{7.5}$$

where $g(\mathbf{x})$ is a positive function. Being defined so, this change will be random since there will be generally different values of $\mathbf{x}_t(\omega)$ in different trajectories at the same moment of time. As a result, we will have the diffusion process again, whose coefficients are related with the original ones by the following formulae:

$$\tilde{M}(\mathbf{p}) = M_i(\mathbf{p})/g(\mathbf{p}), \quad \tilde{V}_{ij}(\mathbf{p}) = V_{ij}(\mathbf{p})/g(\mathbf{p}) . \tag{7.6}$$

Let us consider the process of change in the frequency, p, of an allele invoked only by sampling fluctuations at the change of generation. The generating operator for this model will be represented by

$$\mathcal{A} = \frac{1}{2}\frac{p(1-p)}{2N}\frac{\partial^2}{\partial p^2} .$$

If $g(p)$ is taken equal to $p(1-p)/(2N)$, the random change of time will apparently transform the process into a Wiener one, the search for some of its characteristics being facilitated. Note that a random change of time can facilitate also the analysis of multidimensional sample fluctuations in a subdivided population (see the end of Section 13.8).

In a number of cases, the most interesting are the conditional characteristics of the process under the condition that a certain event takes place. When analyzing, for instance, the rate of gene substitution in the evolution process, it is important to know the mean fixation time under the condition that fixation takes place, rather than the mean absorption time (consisting of the fixation time and the mutant loss time). This can be reasoned, by the fact that, when comparing the protein amino-acid sequences for the organisms at different levels of organization, one can observe just the outcomes of fixation of the mutations occurred. A lost mutant leaves no trace in the amino-acid sequence, so that the data represent the conditional characteristics of the gene substitution process.

The first attempts to study conditional characteristics were referred to finding the conditional time for a neutral mutant fixation by means of the integral

$$\int_0^\infty t f(p, 1, t)\, dt = T(p)U_1(p) ,$$

where $T(p)$ is a mean fixation time under the fixation condition and $U_1(p)$ is a probability of fixation.

A general approach to this kind of problems is based on the concept of the conditional diffusion process under a corresponding condition (for instance, under the trajectory reaching a certain point in the boundary, and so on). If $f(p, x, t)$ designates the transition probability density for an unconditional process and $U(p)$ stands for the probability of the condition under which the process is considered, then the conditional density is equal to:

$$f^*(p, x, t) = f(p, x, t)U(x)/U(p) . \tag{7.7}$$

Let a one-dimensional process be considered. Recall that the drift coefficient corresponds to the mean increment, the diffusion coefficient to the mean square, while the means of higher powers of the increment during a time interval, t, can be neglected as $t \to 0$. Making use of this, let $U(x)$ be expanded into powers of the increment x-p so that the drift coefficient of the conditional process can be found as

$$M^*(p) = \lim_{t \to 0} \frac{1}{t} \int_0^1 f^*(p, x, t)(x - p)\, dx =$$

$$= \lim_{t \to 0} \frac{1}{t} \int_0^1 f(p, x, t) \frac{U(p) + U'(p)(x-p) + o(x-p)}{U(p)} (x - p)\, dx =$$

$$= M(p) + V(p) \frac{U'(p)}{U(p)} . \qquad (7.8)$$

Similarly, we have $V^*(x) = V(x)$.

In the case of a multidimensional conditional process, the same reason lead us to the conclusion that the diffusion matrix coincides with that of the unconditional process, while the drift coefficients have the following form:

$$M_i^*(\mathbf{p}) = M_i(\mathbf{p}) + \sum_j V_{ij}(\mathbf{p}) \frac{\partial U(\mathbf{p})/\partial p_j}{U(\mathbf{p})} . \qquad (7.9)$$

Having the diffusion process with coefficients (7.9), one can find various conditional characteristics of interest by the same standard methods as those applicable to an unconditional process. The conditional characteristics of the time to attain homozygosity as a result of sample fluctuations in gene frequencies are proved fairly useful in assessing the allele fixation time in the case of a two-allele locus and the times of consecutive allele losses in the multiallele case (see Section 11.4 and 11.5).

It is not always possible, especially in the multidimensional case, to solve the Kolmogorov equations by the separation-of-variables method considered in the beginning of this section. If, however, there exist a steady-state distribution, some other method can be used to find it. Normally, the habitat conditions of a natural population vary slowly enough to assume the population to be in a kind of equilibrium with its environment. The probability character of this equilibrium is expressed in a steady-state probability density function $f(\mathbf{x})$, whose finding is a simpler task than finding the fundamental solution. Since the derivative with respect to time equals zero in a steady state, we have the equation $\mathfrak{A}^* f = 0$ instead of (3.15). In the one-dimensional case this means that the steady-state flow of probability (3.16) is equal to zero, i.e. $f(x)$ satisfies the equation

$$M(x)f(x) - \frac{1}{2} \frac{d}{dx} [V(xf(x)] = 0 . \qquad (7.10)$$

A solution to (7.10) is given by

$$f(x) = \frac{C}{V(x)} \exp\left\{ \int^x \frac{2M(y)}{V(y)}\, dy \right\} , \qquad (7.11)$$

where constant C is to be determined from the normalizing condition: the integral of $f(x)$ over the space must be equal to unity.

It should be noted that the formal expression (7.11) does not always identify a steady-state distribution and to use (7.11) effectively some preliminary considerations of the process nature are needed.

In a multidimensional case, the existence of a steady-state distribution does not imply necessarily that the flow vector equals zero in any point of the space as a decrease in the density due to the flow in one direction can be well compensated by the flow in another coordinate.

Let a steady-state density be called a *potential density* if its flow vector is identically zero. Then $f(\mathbf{x})$ satisfies the following system of equations:

$$M_i(\mathbf{x})f(\mathbf{x}) - \frac{1}{2}\sum_j \frac{\partial}{\partial x_j}[V_{ij}(\mathbf{x})f(\mathbf{x})] = 0\,,\quad i = 1, 2,... \tag{7.12}$$

After dividing (7.12) by $f(\mathbf{x})$ and passing to the vector notation, we have

$$\text{grad } \ln f(\mathbf{x}) = \| V_{ij}(\mathbf{x}) \|^{-1}[2\mathbf{M}(\mathbf{x}) - \| \frac{\partial}{\partial x_j} V_{ij}(\mathbf{x}) \| \mathbf{e}]\,, \tag{7.13}$$

where $\mathbf{e}$ is the vector of the proper dimensionality whose each coordinate equals unity. The diffusion matrix is supposed to be non-singular. It follows that an explicit form of the steady-state density can be inferred from (7.13) if the coordinates of the gradient (7.13) comply with the condition that the mixed derivatives turn out equal when the order of differentiating $\ln f(\mathbf{x})$ is changed.

It is interesting to note that in a standard one-locus genetic model possessing a steady-state distribution there is a relation between the form of the steady-state density and the pattern of *dynamic* (freely speaking, *adaptive*) *landscape*, G, - i.e. the peaks and valleys G in the multidimensional space corresponding respectively to stable and unstable equilibrium states. The steady-state density concentrates mainly in the stable equilibrium points of the deterministic model (see Sections 12.6, 12.11).

This fact is the most evident in the case where the diffusion matrix is the identity one and the drift vector represents the gradient of some function $G(\mathbf{x})$. As follows from (7.13), the gradient of $\ln f(\mathbf{x})$ is equal to that of $G(\mathbf{x})$, i.e. $f(\mathbf{x}) = C \exp\{G(\mathbf{x})\}$. When the diffusion matrix $\| V_{ij}(\mathbf{x}) \|$ differs from the identity one, the drift is to be the gradient of $G(\mathbf{x})$ in the metrics defined by that matrix, i.e. the representation $\mathbf{M}(\mathbf{x}) = \|V_{ij}(\mathbf{x})\| \cdot \text{grad} G(\mathbf{x})$ must be true. Then it follows from (7.13) that $f(\mathbf{x}) = C \exp\{G(\mathbf{x})\}V(\mathbf{x})$, where the function $V(\mathbf{x})$ is to be specified by the terms containing the derivatives of $V_{ij}(\mathbf{x})$ in (7.13).

Thus, a complete correspondence between the steady-state density peaks and the stable equilibrium points takes place generally for the deterministic system modified by accounting for $V(\mathbf{x})$ (see (12.11.7)). Under a diffusion of small intensity, however, this modification is insignificant, while the contribution of $V(\mathbf{x})$ into the expression for a steady-state density can also be negligible (see Section 12.11).

10.8. Search for Moments of Some Functionals on Diffusion Processes

If we know the fundamental solution, $f(\mathbf{p}, \mathbf{x}, t)$, to the equations (6.5), then any characteristics of the process under concern can be found. But we can often dispense with more simple means. In the case of an absorption process, for example, where trajectories get eventually, with the unit probability, into the boundary $B(\Sigma)$, a class of problems arises, related with finding the expected value of an integral over trajectories. These include finding the probability of absorption in a particular region of the boundary, the mean absorption time, the expected value of a function on process states during the time until absorption, and so on.

Let $\tau(\omega)$ be a moment the trajectory hits the boundary $B(\Sigma)$ and let

$$U(\mathbf{p}) = E\left\{ \int_0^{\tau(\omega)} u[\mathbf{x}_t(\omega)]\, dt + h[\mathbf{x}_\tau(\omega)] | \mathbf{x}_0 = \mathbf{p} \right\} \tag{8.1}$$

be the expectation of a functional on the trajectories originating from $\mathbf{p}$. Then $U(\mathbf{p})$ can be rewritten in the form

$$U(\mathbf{p}) = \int_\Sigma u(\mathbf{x}) \int_0^\infty f(\mathbf{p}, \mathbf{x}, t)\, dt\, d\mathbf{x} + \int_{B(\Sigma)} h(\mathbf{x})) \int_0^\infty f(\mathbf{p}, \mathbf{x}, t)\, dt\, d\mathbf{x}\,. \tag{8.2}$$

The second term presents a surface integral of the first kind along the boundary $B(\Sigma)$.

Let operator $\mathfrak{A}$ be applied to both sides of (8.2), the permutability between $\mathfrak{A}$ and the integration being supposed. Recall that $\mathfrak{A}f = \partial f/\partial t$ by (6.5), so that

$$\mathfrak{A}U = \int_\Sigma u(\mathbf{x}) \int_0^\infty \frac{\partial f}{\partial t}\, dt\, d\mathbf{x} + \int_{B(\Sigma)} h(\mathbf{x}) \int_0^\infty \frac{\partial f}{\partial t}\, dt\, d\mathbf{x}\,.$$

As $\int_0^\infty \partial f/\partial t\, dt = f(\mathbf{p}, \mathbf{x}, \infty) - f(\mathbf{p}, \mathbf{x}, 0)$ and $f(\mathbf{p}, \mathbf{x}, t)$ is everywhere zero at the moment $t{=}\infty$, the first summand has this difference equal to $-f(\mathbf{p}, \mathbf{x}, t) = -\delta(\mathbf{x} - \mathbf{p})$, while in the second one it becomes zero since we have $\delta(\mathbf{x} - \mathbf{p})|_B = 0$ if $\mathbf{p} \notin B(\Sigma)$, and $\partial f/\partial t \equiv 0$ if $\mathbf{p} \in B(\Sigma)$. Thus,

$$(\mathfrak{A}U)(\mathbf{p}) = -u(\mathbf{p})\,,$$
$$U(\mathbf{p})|_{B(\Sigma)} = h(\mathbf{p})\,. \tag{8.3}$$

If a certain region of the boundary is inaccessible there is no need to specify the boundary condition for it.

If we set $u(\mathbf{p}) \equiv 0$ in (8.3) and consider $h(\mathbf{p})$ be equal to 1 when $\mathbf{p} \in B_1$(B_1 being the boundary region of interest) and $h(\mathbf{p}) = 0$ when $\mathbf{p} \in B(\Sigma) \backslash B_1$, then the expected value of the functional (8.1) will be equal to the probability that a trajectory hits B_1 before it reaches any other point of the boundary. In the case of a one-dimensional process (describing, for instance, the behavior of an allele concentration in [0, 1]), Equation (8.3) determines the allele fixation probability when $h(0) = 0$ and $h(1) = 1$, and the probability of the allele being lost when $h(0) = 1$ and $h(1) = 0$ (see Sections 11.4, 12.2).

By solving (8.3) in an arbitrary interval $(p_1, p_2) \subseteq (0, 1)$ with $h(p_1) = 0$ and $h(p_2) = 1$, we obtain the probability that a trajectory reaches p_2 before it reaches p_1.

To find the expected time of being within (0,1) one should set $u(p) \equiv 1$ and $h(p) \equiv 0$ (see Section 11.5). If $u(p) = 2p(1-p)$ and $h(p) = 0$, the solution to (8.3) represents the mean number of heterozygotes in the whole course of the population existence till the moment of absorption.

If we now consider a multidimensional process with absorption (that describes, for instance, the one-locus case with n alleles $\{A_i\}$), then a trajectory, having reached a point within B_1, the boundary region corresponding to loss of allele A_1, does not remain in this point but continues its moving along the region B_1. If we set $u(\mathbf{p}) \equiv 0$ in (8.3), $h(\mathbf{p})=1$ for any $\mathbf{p} \in B_1$ and $h(\mathbf{p})=0$ for any $\mathbf{p} \in B(\Sigma) \backslash B_1$, the solution of (8.3) will determine the probability that allele A_1 be lost first. By setting $h(\mathbf{p})$, for any $\mathbf{p} \in B(\Sigma)$, equal to the probability that another allele, say A_2, be fixed in a trajectory originating from a state of n -1 alleles, one can find the fixation probability for allele A_2 in a trajectory originating from a state where all n alleles are present. A proper form of the function $h(\mathbf{p})$ being chosen, the probabilities can be found that an allele of interest will be lost second, third, etc. (see Section 11.4). Similarly, one can pose the problems of searching for the expected times to lose one, two, or more alleles, and to reach homozygosity, finally.

In terms of a penalty function, we can also determine the further moments of the path integral of a function $g(\mathbf{x})$. Let, for example,

$$u(\mathbf{x}) = ng(\mathbf{x})E\left\{\left[\int_0^{\tau} g(\mathbf{x}_t)\,dt\right]^{n-1} \Big| \mathbf{x}_{t=0}=\mathbf{x}\right\} .$$

This function makes the following probability sense to the solution of (8.3):

$$U(\mathbf{p}) = E\left\{\int_0^{\tau} ng(\mathbf{x}_t)E\left\{\left[\int_0^{\tau} g(\mathbf{x}_{t'})\,dt'\right]^{n-1} \Big| \mathbf{x}_{t'=0}=\mathbf{x}_t\right\} dt \Big| \mathbf{x}_{t=0}=\mathbf{p}\right\} . \tag{8.4}$$

Note that the conditional expectation in (8.4) (conditioned with $\mathbf{x}_t$) can be treated as the mean value over all 'tails' of the trajectory passing through point $\mathbf{x}_t$ at moment t. Thus, from the Markov property of the diffusion process, it follows that

$$U(\mathbf{p}) = E\left\{\int_0^{\tau(\omega)} ng[\mathbf{x}_t(\omega)]\left[\int_0^{\tau(\omega)} g[\mathbf{x}_{t''}(\omega)]\,dt'\right]^{n-1} dt \Big| \mathbf{x}_{t=0} = \mathbf{p}\right\} .$$

Since, in a continuous trajectory ω, we have

$$ng(\mathbf{x}_t)\left[\int_{\tau}^{\tau(\omega)} g[\mathbf{x}_t(\omega)]\,dt\right]^{n-1} = -\frac{d}{dt}\left[\int_{\tau}^{\tau(\omega)} g[\mathbf{x}_{t'}(\omega)]\,dt'\right]^{n} ,$$

the expression (8.4) takes eventually the form

$$U(\mathbf{p}) = E\left\{\int_0^{\tau(\omega)} -\frac{d}{dt}\left[\int_t^{\tau(\omega)} g[\mathbf{x}_{t'}(\omega)]\,dt'\right]^{n} dt \Big| \mathbf{x}_{t=0} = \mathbf{p}\right\} = \tag{8.5}$$

$$= E\left\{\left[\int_0^{\tau(\omega)} [g[\mathbf{x}_t(\omega))]\, dt\right]^n \Big| \mathbf{x}_{t=0} = \mathbf{p}\right\}.$$

Hence, the n-order moment, M_n, of the path integral of a function $g(\mathbf{x})$ can be successively found from the following differential equations:

$$(\mathfrak{A} M_n)(\mathbf{p}) = -\, ng(\mathbf{p})\, M_{n-1}(\mathbf{p})\,.$$
$$M_n(\mathbf{p})|_{B(\Sigma)} = 0\,. \tag{8.6}$$

Calculating the expected value of path integral can be done by means of the Green function interpretable in probability terms as the density function for the time the process sojourns in points within Σ until the moment it reaches an absorbing boundary. For a point $\mathbf{y}$ in Σ, this sojourn time density, $\Phi(\mathbf{p}, \mathbf{y})$, under condition that a trajectory comes out of the point $\mathbf{p}$, is defined by

$$\Phi(\mathbf{p}, \mathbf{y}) = \int_0^{\infty} f(\mathbf{p}, \mathbf{y}, t)\, dt\,. \tag{8.7}$$

On the other hand, $\Phi(\mathbf{p}, \mathbf{y})$ is equal to the expected value of the following path integral:

$$\int_0^{\tau(\omega)} \delta[\mathbf{x}_t(\omega) - \mathbf{y}\,]\, dt\,,$$

where $\tau(\omega)$ designates a random moment of reaching the boundary. According to (8.3), $\Phi(\mathbf{p}, \mathbf{y})$ is to comply with the equation

$$\mathfrak{A}\Phi = -\,\delta(\mathbf{p} - \mathbf{y})\,,$$
$$\Phi|_{B(\Sigma)} = 0\,; \tag{8.8}$$

and is called the *Green function* for Equation (8.8).

Let us define operator G on a function $u(\mathbf{p})$ to be

$$(Gu)(\mathbf{p}) = -\int_{\Sigma} \Phi(\mathbf{p}, \mathbf{y}) u(\mathbf{y})\, d\mathbf{y}\,. \tag{8.9}$$

By (8.7) this expression can be rewritten as

$$(Gu)(\mathbf{p}) = -\int_{\Sigma} u(\mathbf{y}) \int_0^{\infty} f(\mathbf{p}, \mathbf{y}, t)\, dt\, d\mathbf{y} = -\,U(\mathbf{p})\,, \tag{8.10}$$

where

$$U(\mathbf{p}) = E\left\{\int_0^{\tau(\omega)} u[\mathbf{x}_t(\omega)]\, dt\, |\mathbf{x}_{t=0} = \mathbf{p}\right\}.$$

According to (8.3) the function U must comply with the equation $\mathfrak{A} U = -\, u$ and $U(\mathbf{y}) = 0$ if $\mathbf{y} \in B(\Sigma)$. On the other hand, $Gu = -U$ as follows from (8.10). Hence,

$$\mathfrak{A}Gu = -\mathfrak{A}U = u\,. \tag{8.11}$$

So operator G is the inverse to $\mathfrak{A}$ and, from the Green function, we can easily obtain expectations of integrals along trajectories.

10.9. An Approach to Searching for the Mean of a Function Defined on States of a Process

Recall that, according to (3.10), we have

$$\lim_{\tau \to 0} \frac{1}{\tau}[T_{t+\tau} - T_t] = \begin{cases} \mathfrak{A}T_t, \\ T_t\mathfrak{A}. \end{cases}$$

Then, for a function $u(\mathbf{x})$ it follows that

$$\frac{\mathrm{d}}{\mathrm{d}t} E_t\{u(\mathbf{x})\} = T_t\mathfrak{A}u = E_t\{(\mathfrak{A}u)(\mathbf{x})\}\,,$$

$$E_0\{u(\mathbf{x})\} = u(\mathbf{p})\,, \tag{9.1}$$

where

$$E_t\{u(\mathbf{x})\} = E\{u(\mathbf{x}_t) | \mathbf{x}_0 = \mathbf{p}\} = (T_t\mathbf{u})(\mathbf{p})\,.$$

In general, the Equation (9.1) gives almost nothing to searching for the expectation of $u(\mathbf{x})$ since there is the unknown expectation of $\mathfrak{A}u$ in its right-hand side. In a number of genetic models, however, the equation can be useful. The matter is that in some conditions operator $\mathfrak{A}$ maps a polynomial into a polynomial of the same power. This enables one to search for a solution to certain ordinary differential equations, or systems of the equations (under corresponding functions $u(\mathbf{x})$) instead of solving the partial differential equation (3.11) for T_tu.

It should be noted, however, that formal inferring from (9.1) may lead us to incorrect results. Let, for example, a process with absorption be under study and the function u be the mean absorption time. As shown in Section 10.8, $\mathfrak{A}u=-1$, hence $T_t\mathfrak{A}u\equiv-1$, i.e. the right-hand side of (9.1) is identically equal to -1. It follows that the value of $E_t\{u(\mathbf{x})\}$ inferred from (9.1) tends to $-\infty$ as $t\to\infty$. But since, with unit probability, the process comes to the boundary where $u=0$, the expectation $E_t\{u(\mathbf{x})\}$ tends to zero as $t\to\infty$, so that the solution of (9.1) makes no sense.

Let us investigate the conditions in which the Equation (9.1) is applicable. Let $g(\mathbf{x})$ be a sufficiently smooth function of states of the process. We consider first a one-dimensional case, where the diffusion takes place on the interval [0, 1], the process being specified by its infinitesimal variance, $V(x)$, and drift, $M(x)$. Also, we assume the possibility of absorption in the interval bounds. It is clear that

$$E_t\{g(x)\} = \int_0^1 g(x)f(p, x, t)\,\mathrm{d}x + g(0)U_0(p, t) + g(1)U_1(p, t)\,,$$

where U_0 and U_1 represent the probabilities of absorption up to moment t respectively in the left and the right bounds of the interval [0, 1]. By differentiating both sides of this equality with respect to t, we have

$$\frac{d}{dt}E_t\{g(x)\} = \int_0^1 g(x)\frac{\partial}{\partial t}f(p, x, t) + $$

$$+ g(0)\frac{\partial}{\partial t}U_0(p, t) + g(1)\frac{\partial}{\partial t}U_1(p, t)\,. \tag{9.2}$$

Recall that by (3.17) $\frac{\partial}{\partial t}f(p, x, t) = -\frac{\partial}{\partial x}P(p, x, t)$, where

$$P(p, x, t) = f(p, x, t)M(x) - \frac{1}{2}\frac{\partial}{\partial x}[f(p, x, t)V(x)]$$

represents the probability flow in a point x. By means of the flow, the right-hand side of equality (9.2) can be continued in the following way:

$$= -\int_0^1 g(x)\frac{\partial}{\partial x}P(p, x, t)\,dx - g\,(0)P(p, 0, t) + g(1)P(p, 1, t)\,.$$

Integrating further by parts, we have

$$= -g(x)P(p, x, t)\Big|_{x=0}^{1} + \int_0^1 \Big\{f(p, x, t)M(x) -$$

$$-\frac{\partial}{\partial x}\Big[f(p, x, t)\frac{1}{2}V(x)\Big]\Big\}\frac{dg(x)}{dx}dx - g(0)P(p, 0, t) + g\,(1)P(p, 1, t)\,.$$

After cancelling the terms with flows in the boundary points and integrating by parts the term $\frac{\partial}{\partial x}[f(p, x, t)1/2V(x)]$, we arrive at

$$= \int_0^1 \Big[\frac{1}{2}V(x)\frac{d^2g(x)}{dx^2} + M(x)\frac{dg(x)}{dx}\Big]f(p, x, t)\,dx -$$

$$-\frac{1}{2}V(x)\frac{dg(x)}{dx}f(p, x, t)\Big|_{x=0}^{1} =$$

$$= \int_0^1 (\mathfrak{A}g)(x)f(p, x, t)\,dx - \frac{1}{2}V(x)f(p, x, t)\frac{dg(x)}{dx}\Big|_{x=0}^{1} =$$

$$= E_t\{(\mathfrak{A}g)(x)\}\,,$$

provided that $V(x)\,dg(x)/dx$ and $(\mathfrak{A}g)(x)$ both are zero in the limit as x tends to zero or to one, the boundary values $f(p, x, t)\Big|_{x=0}^{1}$ being supposed finite. Otherwise, the limit of

$V(x)f(p, x, t)\, dg(x)/dx$ should be considered. Note that the limit of $V(x)f(p, x, t)$ must equal zero since $f(p, x, t)$ would otherwise be non-integrable near the boundaries.

To make a passage to an arbitrary dimension, K, we apply the mathematical induction. Let (9.1) be known to be true for $K=m$. Then let us prove that, in genetic models with a diffusion matrix of the form (6.2), the Equation (9.1) is true for $K=m+1$ too, and derive the corresponding constraints on the function $g(\mathbf{x})$.

The expectation $E_t\{g(\mathbf{x})\}$ can be written in the form

$$E_t\{g(\mathbf{x})\} = \int_{\Sigma} g(\mathbf{x}) f(\mathbf{p}, \mathbf{x}, t)\, d\mathbf{x} + \\ + \int_0^t \int_{B(\Sigma)} (\mathbf{P}(\mathbf{p}, \mathbf{x}_\tau, \tau), \mathbf{n}(\mathbf{x}_\tau)) E_{t-\tau}\{g(\mathbf{x}_{t-\tau}) | \mathbf{x}_\tau\}\, dS\, d\tau . \tag{9.3}$$

Here τ is the moment a trajectory comes to a point $\mathbf{x}_\tau$ of the boundary $B(\Sigma)$; $\mathbf{P}(\mathbf{p}, \mathbf{x}_\tau, \tau)$ is the flow vector in the point $\mathbf{x}_\tau$ at the moment τ; $\mathbf{n}(\mathbf{x}_\tau)$ is the vector of the outward normal to the boundary at this point, $E_{t-\tau}\{g(\mathbf{x}_{t-\tau})|\mathbf{x}_\tau\}$ is the conditional expectation of $g(\mathbf{x}_t)$ under the condition that $\mathbf{x}_t = \mathbf{x}_\tau \in B(\Sigma)$ at the moment $t = \tau$.

Since the process in the boundary has the lesser dimensionality, the induction premise leads us to the following relation:

$$\frac{d}{dt} E_{t-\tau}\{g(\mathbf{x}_{t-\tau})|\mathbf{x}_\tau\} = E_{t-\tau}\{(\mathcal{Q} g)(\mathbf{x}_{t-\tau})|\mathbf{x}_\tau\} .$$

When $t = \tau$, the right-hand side is equal to $g(\mathbf{x}_\tau)$. Differentiating both parts of equality (9.3), we have

$$\frac{d}{dt} E_t\{g(\mathbf{x})\} = \frac{\partial}{\partial t} \int_{\Sigma} g(\mathbf{x}) f(\mathbf{p}, \mathbf{x}, t)\, d\mathbf{x} + \\ + \frac{\partial}{\partial t} \int_0^t \int_{B(\Sigma)} (\mathbf{P}(\mathbf{p}, \mathbf{x}_\tau, \tau), \mathbf{n}(\mathbf{x}_\tau)) E_{t-\tau}\{g(\mathbf{x}_{t-\tau})|\mathbf{x}_\tau\}\, dS\, d\tau . \tag{9.4}$$

The first summand is equal to

$$\frac{\partial}{\partial t} \int_{\Sigma} g(\mathbf{x}) f(\mathbf{p}, \mathbf{x}, t)\, d\mathbf{x} = - \int_{\Sigma} g(\mathbf{x}) \left[\sum_i \frac{\partial}{\partial x_i} P_i(\mathbf{p}, \mathbf{x}, t) \right] d\mathbf{x}.$$

By the reasons which are similar to those in the proof of the Gauss-Ostrogradskii theorem, we have

$$= - \int_{B(\Sigma)} (\mathbf{P}(\mathbf{p}, \mathbf{x}, t), \mathbf{n}(\mathbf{x})) g(\mathbf{x})\, dS + \int_{\Sigma} (\mathbf{P}(\mathbf{p}, \mathbf{x}, t), \nabla g(\mathbf{x}))\, d\mathbf{x},$$

where the gradient of $g(\mathbf{x})$ is denoted by $\nabla g(\mathbf{x})$. Taking into consideration that the ith coordinate of the drift equals

$$P_i(\mathbf{p}, \mathbf{x}, t) = f(\mathbf{p}, \mathbf{x}, t)M_i(\mathbf{x}) - \frac{1}{2}\sum_j \frac{\partial}{\partial x_j}[f(\mathbf{p}, \mathbf{x}, t)V_{ij}(\mathbf{x})] ,$$

we transform, as before, the integral

$$\int_\Sigma (\mathbf{P}(\mathbf{p}, \mathbf{x}, t), \nabla g(\mathbf{x}))d\mathbf{x}$$

and continue the equality:

$$= - \int_{B(\Sigma)} (\mathbf{P}(\mathbf{p}, \mathbf{x}, t), \mathbf{n}(\mathbf{x}))g(\mathbf{x})\, dS -$$
$$- \int_{B(\Sigma)} \frac{1}{2}(\| V_{ij}(\mathbf{x}) \|\mathbf{n}(\mathbf{x}), \nabla g(\mathbf{x}))f(\mathbf{p}, \mathbf{x}, t)\, dS +$$
$$+ \int_\Sigma (\mathcal{Q} g)(\mathbf{x})f(\mathbf{p}, \mathbf{x}, t)\, d\mathbf{x} .$$

It is easy to see that, for a matrix with the entries $V_{ij}(\mathbf{x}) = x_i(\delta_{ij} - x_j)$, which appears in genetic models, the equality $\| V_{ij}(\mathbf{x}) \|\mathbf{n}(\mathbf{x}) = 0$ holds everywhere in $B(\Sigma)$ because, in each hyperplane $x_i = 0$, any coordinate of the normal vector equals zero excluded the ith one, while the ith column of the diffusion matrix turns into zero, too. In the hyperplane $\Sigma x_i = 1$, the coordinates of the normal vector are all identical, whereas the sum of entries along any row of the diffusion matrix is equal to zero.
Now let us consider the second summand in (9.4). It can be represented as

$$\int_{B(\Sigma)} (\mathbf{P}(\mathbf{p}, \mathbf{x}, t), \mathbf{n}(\mathbf{x}))g(\mathbf{x})\, dS + \int_0^t \int_{B(\Sigma)} (\mathbf{P}(\mathbf{p}, \mathbf{x}_\tau, \tau), \mathbf{n}(\mathbf{x}_\tau))\frac{d}{dt}E_{t-\tau}\{g(\mathbf{x}_{t-\tau})|\mathbf{x}_\tau\}\, dS\, d\tau .$$

The conditional expectation under the integral sign in the second term meets the induction premise. Also, the terms containing the flows to the boundary at the moment t must be canceled. After all the above expressions being substituted into (9.4), we arrive at

$$\frac{d}{dt}E_t\{g(\mathbf{x})\} =$$
$$\int_\Sigma (\mathcal{Q} g)(\mathbf{x})f(\mathbf{p}, \mathbf{x}, t)\, d\mathbf{x} +$$
$$+\int_0^t \int_{B(\Sigma)} (\mathbf{P}(\mathbf{p}, \mathbf{x}_\tau, \tau), \mathbf{n}(\mathbf{x}_\tau))E_{t-\tau}\{(\mathcal{Q} g)(\mathbf{x}_{t-\tau})|\mathbf{x}_\tau \}\, dS\, d\tau -$$
$$- \int_{B(\Sigma)} \frac{1}{2}(\| V_{ij}(\mathbf{x}) \|\mathbf{n}(x), \nabla g(\mathbf{x}))f(\mathbf{p}, \mathbf{x}, t)\, dS = E_t\{(\mathcal{Q} g)(\mathbf{x})\} ,$$

provided that

$$\lim_{\mathbf{x}\to\mathbf{x}_0\in B(\Sigma)} (\| V_{ij}(\mathbf{x}) \| \mathbf{n}(\mathbf{x}), \nabla g(\mathbf{x})) = 0 \,,$$

$$\lim_{\mathbf{x}\to\mathbf{x}_0\in B(\Sigma)} (\mathfrak{A} g)(\mathbf{x}) = 0 \,, \tag{9.5}$$

the function $f(\mathbf{p}, \mathbf{x}, t)$ being supposed finite on $B(\Sigma)$. But if $f(\mathbf{p}, \mathbf{x}, t)$ is unbounded near $B(\Sigma)$, the limits (9.5) should be considered together with $f(\mathbf{p}, \mathbf{x}, t)$ as a co-factor.

In the case of the narrow-sense random genetic drift process considered in the next chapter, the moments of the process are the most easy obtained from Equation (9.1) since the drift equals zero in this model, while the operator $\mathfrak{A}$ does not raise the order of a polynomial under concern. The situation is similar if we consider a model with a linear drift caused, for instance, by mutation or migrations in a subdivided population (see Chapter 13), the ordinary differential equations being similarly applicable to analysis of the moments dynamics.

As regards the incorrect application of Equation (9.1) exemplified in the beginning of the Section, the reason is that the conditions (9.5) are broken in that example, namely,

$$\lim_{\mathbf{x}\to\mathbf{x}_0\in B(\Sigma)} (\mathfrak{A} g)(\mathbf{x}) = -1 \neq 0 \,.$$

Sometimes, to solve Equation (9.1) and verify its correctness by substitution into (3.11) may be easier than to examine the conditions (9.5) and to analyze the behavior of $f(\mathbf{p}, \mathbf{x}, t)$ near boundaries.

10.10. Notes and Bibliography

Section 10.1.

Probabilistic approaches to study of genetic problems are presented in the book:

Moran, P.A.P.: 1962, *The Statistical Processes of Evolutionary Theory*, Clarendon Press, Oxford; London, Oxford Univ. Press, VII + 200 pp.

A short elementary introduction is given by:

Li, C.C.: 1976, *First Course in Population Genetics*, Boxwood Press, Pacific Grove, California.

The ideas of S. Wright, who is one of the founders of mathematical genetics, are presented in four volumes of his monograph:

Wright, S.: 1968, *Evolution and the Genetics of Populations.*

Vol. I. Genetic and Biometric Foundations. – Chicago: Univ. of Chicago Press, 1968, 469 pp.

Vol. II. The Theory Gene Frequencies. – Chicago: Univ. of Chicago Press, 1969, 511 pp.

Vol. III. Experimental Results and Evolutionary Deduction. – Chicago: Univ. of Chicago Press, 1977, 614 pp.

Vol. IV. Variability Within and Among Natural Populations. Univ. of Chicago Press, Chicago, London, 1978, 580 pp.

Significant contribution into study of stochastic genetic models was made by the authors of the book:

Crow, J.F. and Kimura, M.: 1970, *An Introduction to Population Genetics Theory*, New York: Harper and Row.

Devoted entirely to stochastic models is the monograph by:

Maruyama, T.: 1977, *Stochastic Problems in Population Genetics*. Lecture Notes in Biomathematics, 17 -Berlin: Springer-Verlag.

Section 10.3

Rigorous presentation of foundations to the diffusion process theory can be found in the two successive books:

Gikhman, I.I. and Skorohod, A.V.: 1969, *Introduction to the Theory of Random Processes*, W.B. Saunders Co., Philadelphia, XIII + 516 pp.;

Gikhman, I.I. and Skorohod, A.V.: 1972, *Stochastic Differential Equations*, Springer-Verlag, Berlin, New York, VIII + 354 pp.

See also:

Gardiner, C.W.: 1983, 1985, *Handbook of Stochastic Methods for Physics, Chemistry and the Natural Sciences*, Springer-verlag (Springer Series in Synergetics, Vol. 13), Berlin e.a., 444 pp.

The model of discrete diffusion was considered in the book by:

Nevelson, M.B. and Hasminskii, R.Z.: 1972, *Stochastic Approximation and Recurrent Estimation*, Nauka, Moscow, 304 pp. (in Russian).

Section 10.4.

A number of papers was devoted to the proof of convergence to a diffusion process, for example:

Guess, H.A.: 1973, On the weak convergence of Wright - Fisher models, *Stochastic Processes and Their Applications*, **1**, No. 3, pp. 287–306;

Ethier, S.N.: 1979, Limit theorems for absorption times of genetic models, *Ann. Probab.* **7**, No. 4, pp. 622–638;

Norman, M.F.: 1975, Diffusion approximation of non-Markovian processes, *Ann. Probab.* **3**, No. 2, pp. 358–364,

the last one featuring a consideration of a diffusion approximation for the model of a single-locus, bisexual population.

The presentation follows the scheme of the work:

Passekov, V.P.: 1981, Effects of genetic drift on dynamics of the genotype and phenotype variability in subdivided populations. In: Svirezhev, Y.M. and V.P. Passekov (eds.,), *Mathematical Models in Ecology and Genetics*. Nauka, Moscow, pp. 148–173 (in Russian).

The notion of effective size was analyzed by M. Kimura and J.F. Crow in their works:

Kimura, M. and Crow, J.F.: 1963, The measurement of effective population number, *Evolution* **17**, No. 3, pp. 279–288;

Crow, J.F. and Kimura, M.: 1972, The effective number of population with overlapping generations: a correction and further discussion, *Amer. J. Hum. Genet.* **24**, No. 1, pp. 1–10.

Calculation of the drift and diffusion coefficients in case where the intensity of selection varies randomly (with regard to autocorrelation) or seasonally and where the population size is variable too, is presented in the paper:

Karlin, S. and Levikson, B.: 1974, Temporal fluctuations in selection intensities: case of small population size, *Theor. Pop. Biol.* **6**, No. 3, pp. 383–412.

Section 10.5.

Investigation of boundaries for one-dimensional diffusion processes was first carried on by W. Feller:

Feller, W.: 1954, Diffusion processes in one dimension, *Trans. Amer. Math. Soc.* **77**, 1-31.

The classification cited in the Section is taken from:

Gikhman, I.I. and Skorohod, A.V.: 1972, *Stochastic Differential Equation*, Springer-Verlag, Berlin, New-York, VIII + 354 pp.

The modification for boundary examination in case of genetic diffusion processes was proposed in the paper:

Voronka, R. and Keller, J.B.: 1975, Asymptotic analysis of stochastic models in population genetics, *Math. Biosci.* **25**, No. 3,4, p. 331–362.

Section 10.7.

Transformations of random processes are described in the monograph:

Dynkin, E.B.: 1965, *Markov Processes*. Academic Press, New York, Vols. 1–2 (365 pp.; 274 pp.), and the handbook:

Prokhorov, Y.V. and Rozanov, Y.A.: 1973, *Theory of Probabilities* (2nd ed.), Nauka, Moscow, 494 pp. (in Russian).

Conditional diffusion processes were introduced into genetic models by:

Ewens, W.: 1973, Conditional diffusion processes in population genetics, *Theor. Pop. Biol.* **4**, No. 1, pp. 21–30;

Narain, P.: 1974, The conditional diffusion equation and its use in population genetics, *J. Roy. Statist. Soc.* **B36**, No. 2, pp. 258–266.

Diffusion in the Riemannian space was studied by A.N. Kolmogorov:

Kolmogoroff, A.: 1937, Zum Umkehrbarkeit der statistischen Naturgesetze, *Math. Ann.* **115**, No. 5, pp. 766–772,

where steadiness conditions were also considered.

Section 10.8.

A rigorous derivation of equations to determine characteristics of distribution of a functional on a process with absorption can be found in the above-mentioned book:

Gikhman, I.I. and Skorohod, A.V.: 1969, *Introduction to the Theory of Random Processes*, W.B. Saunders Co., Philadelphia, XIII + 516 pp.

Application of the Green function and its calculation under various patterns of boundaries in genetic models are in the monograph by:

Maruyama, T.: 1977, *Stochastic Problems in Population Genetics*. Lecture Notes in Biomathematics, 17. – Berlin: Springer–Verlag, 245 pp.

Section 10.9.

The approach applied here is valid under the conditions whose derivation follows the note:

Passekov, V.P.: 1975, An approach to study diffusion processes in genetics. In: *Application of statistical methods in problems of population genetics*, issue 49. Interdept. Laboratory of Statistical Methods, Moscow State University Press, Moscow, pp. 63-68 (in Russian),

which presents the findings of the work:

Passekov, V.P.: 1971, *Genetic Drift and Some Microtaxonomic Problems in Anthropology*. Synopsis of the thesis for Candidate of Science Degree in Biology. Moscow State University, Moscow, 24 pp.

Chapter 11

Random Genetic Drift in the Narrow Sense

11.1. The Kolmogorov Equations for a Single-Locus Model of Random Genetic Drift

By the genetic drift, or more strictly, by the *random genetic drift in the narrow sense* one usually means a random process of variation in gamete concentrations due to the effects of sampling alone at the change of the generations. Initially, the biologist who had paid attention to this phenomenon stressed the important role the drift played in reaching the genetic homogeneity under considerable variations in the population size (causing cancellation of some genetic variants when the size decreases), or under the presence of rare genes (which may happen to be absent in the next generation by pure chance). The situation is however the same when the population size is constant and the gene concentrations are arbitrary in the population.

Let us first consider the case of a single autosomal locus having n alleles $\{A_i\}$ in a diploid population of constant size N.

The sampling fluctuations of gamete frequencies (i.e. of allele frequencies in the single-locus case) have no preference in their directions, so that the regular shifts from the initial values of frequencies $\{p_i\}$ are equal to zero, but the variance of the frequency of an allele, say A_i, is proportional to $p_i(1-p_i)$. This is based on the fact that sampling the gametes randomly results in a polynomial distribution (with the covariance matrix of the form (10.6.2)). Under the proper choice of the time unit (that is one generation in the Fisher-Wright model and N birth-death events in the Moran model), the generating operator $\mathfrak{a}$ for the genetic drift diffusion process takes on the form

$$\mathfrak{a} = \frac{1}{2} \sum_{i,j=1}^{n-1} \frac{p_i(\delta_{ij} - p_j)}{2N} \frac{\partial^2}{\partial p_i \partial p_j} \tag{1.1}$$

in a multiallele case. The summation in (1.1) is taken from 1 to $n-1$, not to n, since there is no need to consider the variation in the nth allele concentration. The matter is that the sum of all frequencies amounts to 1 and the concentrations of any $(n-1)$ alleles completely determine the rest one (for instance, p_n). In the diallele case, expression (1.1) turns into

$$\mathfrak{A} = \frac{1}{2}\frac{p(1-p)}{2N}\frac{\partial^2}{\partial p^2}. \tag{1.1a}$$

Note that, due to the sampling nature of the genetic drift process, its regularities do not change when a certain allele is considered to have no distinction from some other ones (which is equivalent to considering a single artificial, 'combined' allele whose concentration equals the sum of those of the non-distinct alleles composing it). This signifies that the results inferred from a one-dimensional, two-dimensional, etc., model (for instance, the probabilities of allele loss or fixation) still remain valid for models of higher dimensionalities too, under the proper interpretation of the allele frequencies.

The genetic drift process proceeds in the following way. Random walking of gene frequencies takes place inside Σ until the trajectory reaches a boundary (corresponding to the loss of an allele). Thus, either the absorption occurs in the corresponding homozygote state (if there were two alleles only) or the diffusion proceeds on the corresponding hyperplane, governed by the operator (1.1) with the state coordinates referred to the rest of the alleles. The loss of one more allele occurs further, and so on up to the moment of absorption in one of the verteces of simplex Σ.

In a multidimensional case, operator $\mathfrak{A}^*$, the one of the forward equation, has the following form:

$$\mathfrak{A}^* = \frac{1}{2}\sum_{i,j=1}^{n-1}\frac{\partial^2}{\partial x_i\,\partial x_j}\left[\frac{x_i(\delta_{ij}-x_j)}{2N}\cdots\right], \tag{1.2}$$

and in the one-dimensional case:

$$\mathfrak{A}^* = \frac{1}{2}\frac{\partial^2}{\partial x^2}\left[\frac{x(1-x)}{2N}\cdots\right]. \tag{1.2a}$$

11.2. Approximating the Random Genetic Drift Process within Small Intervals of Time

In many studies there often arise a need to analyze the asymptotic properties of the genetic drift process when the time intervals (measured in generations) are relatively small. The need is dictated by the stress the modern theory of evolution makes on micro-evolutionary processes as well as by the fact that a genetic drift process, in its pure form, can not proceed too long due to the pressures inherent in a natural population such as that of selection, mutation, or migration from adjacent populations. In typical cases, the effects of selection (in its weak form) and mutation pressures can be neglected in a small time interval, and fairly regular is that the case where the migration effects are negligibly small, too, in that period of time. Also, the exact solutions which are known for the probability density as a function of the initial point and the time moment, have the form (like the most of solutions to partial differential equations) of an eigenfunction series (of a special kind, in addition) and look fairly complicated. This makes them difficult to deal with.

It is desirable, therefore, to find a convenient approximation to the genetic drift process in a small interval of time, that could essentially simplify an analysis of real data. As early as 1922, R. Fisher proposed a transformation possessing the desired properties in the case of a single two-allele locus. It was the first work where an equation of the diffusion type had been introduced into mathematical genetics. This had been done even before the corresponding branch of probability theory was built up and foundations of the diffusion process theory were developed.

In the contemporary terms, that transformation has the following sense. A change of variables is to be found such that, in the process of genetic drift in the concentration of an allele, whose probability density obeys (when the time unit equals one generation) the differential equation:

$$\frac{\partial}{\partial t} f(p, x, t) = \frac{1}{2} \frac{p(1-p)}{2N} \frac{\partial^2}{\partial p^2} f(p, x, t) . \tag{2.1}$$

the diffusion coefficient be constant in time and independent of the space coordinate.

If $g(p)$ is a twice continuously differentiable function, then the random process $g[x(t)]$ will be of the diffusion type and its coefficients can be found from (10.7.3). Thus, the diffusion coefficient equals $\frac{p(1-p)}{2N}\left[\frac{dg(p)}{dp}\right]^2$, while the drift one equals $\frac{1}{2}\frac{p(1-p)}{2N}\frac{d^2g(p)}{dp^2}$. If we want the diffusion coefficient to be constant, the desired transformation can be found from the following equation:

$$dg(p)/dp = [p(1-p)]^{-1/2}. \tag{2.2}$$

The equation can be satisfied with the function $\arccos(1-2p)$, the R. Fisher's transformation that was found by him from another considerations, or with $\arcsin\sqrt{p}$ (to within multiplication by a constant factor).

By setting $\theta = \arccos(1-2p)$ we can conclude that the probability density function for θ obeys the differential equation

$$\frac{\partial}{\partial t} f(\theta_0, \theta, t) = \frac{1}{4N} \frac{\partial^2}{\partial \theta^2} f(\theta_0, \theta, t) + \frac{1}{4N} \frac{\partial}{\partial \theta}[\cot \theta f(\theta_0, \theta, t)] , \tag{2.3}$$

i.e., although the diffusion coefficient is constant for the process $\theta(t)$, the drift appears which depends on the space coordinate θ.

Note that, for an interval of time t (measured in generations) which is small relative to the population size N, neglecting the drift will not result in any substantial distortion since variation in θ is to be determined mainly by the diffusion. The sum of deviations in θ which occur at the change of generations and have almost the same distributions, will have approximately normal distribution with the variance proportional to t. Although the transformation $\theta = \arccos(1-2p)$ does not reduce the random genetic drift to a Wiener process, it does simplify considerably the analysis of gene frequencies behavior in small intervals of time.

R. Fisher proposed the following generalization of the above formula. Let $(p_1,..., p_n)$ be the initial concentrations for a genetic process with n alleles, $A_1,..., A_n$. Then at a time moment t the state of the population relative to the initial point in the n-dimensional space whose ith axis represents the square root of the allele A_i concentration, can be described by the unit length vector, $(\sqrt{x_1(t)},\ldots,\sqrt{x_n(t)})$, of the transformed allele concentrations. The end point of this vector lies on the surface of the unit-radius hypersphere in the orthant of positive semi-axes of the n-dimensional space. A deviation of the concentrations from their initial values will be indicated by the angle, θ, between the vectors $(\sqrt{x_1(t)},\ldots,\sqrt{x_n(t)})$, and $(\sqrt{p_1},\ldots,\sqrt{p_n})$:

$$\theta(t) = \arccos\left(\sum_{i=1}^{n}\sqrt{x_i(t)}\sqrt{p_i}\right). \tag{2.4}$$

By the change-of-variables formulae (10.7.4) for the case of transformation $\tilde{p}_i=\sqrt{p_i}$, $i=1,\ldots, n$ the coefficients of the generating operator will be equal to:

$$M_i(\tilde{\mathbf{p}}) = -\frac{1}{16N}\frac{1-\tilde{p}_i^2}{\tilde{p}_i},\; V_{ij}(\tilde{\mathbf{p}}) = \frac{(\delta_{ij}-\tilde{p}_i\tilde{p}_j)}{8N}. \tag{2.5}$$

As well as in the one-dimensional case, the drift can be neglected in a small period of time. Roughly speaking, the diffusion deviations are proportional to $\sqrt{t}$, while the shift invoked by drift is proportional to t and can be neglected for small time intervals.

The diffusion matrix (without the co-factor $1/8N$) can be written in the form $\mathbf{I}-\tilde{\mathbf{p}}\tilde{\mathbf{p}}^T$, where $\mathbf{I}$ is the identity matrix of the $n\times n$ dimension. Since $\sum_{i=1}^{n}\tilde{p}_i^2=1$, vector $\tilde{\mathbf{p}}$, the normal vector to the hypersphere surface, is the eigenvector of the diffusion matrix associated with the zero eigenvalue. This confirms the fact the diffusion takes place on the sphere. The rest eigenvalues are equal to one, the eigenvectors, $\tilde{\mathbf{x}}$, being represented by any vector lying in the plane tangent to the hypersphere at the point $\tilde{\mathbf{p}}$ (since $(\mathbf{I}-\tilde{\mathbf{p}}\tilde{\mathbf{p}}^T)\tilde{\mathbf{x}}=\mathbf{I}\tilde{\mathbf{x}}=\tilde{\mathbf{x}}$). This means that the diffusion is isotropic in the hypersphere. Within a small period of time t the diffusion matrix is practically constant and equal to its value at the initial time moment. If, therefore, we introduce in the tangent plane the orthonormal system of coordinates consisting of the $(n-1)$ eigenvectors, then the diffusion matrix will be close to the identity one, the distribution of the transformed gene frequencies be approximated by the normal one, and the squared distance from the initial point be distributed in accordance with $(t/(8N))\chi^2_{n-1}$ where χ^2_{n-1} designates the chi-squared distribution with $n-1$ degrees of freedom. For a small t (and a consequently small deviation from the initial point) the tangent plane distance is equivalent to the angle (2.4). Hence, asymptotically as $t\to 0$, we have

$$(8N/t)\theta^2(t)\sim\chi^2_{n-1} \tag{2.6}$$

regardless of the initial, point.

Though formula (2.6) is valid for any internal initial point, the period of time where the approximation of the θ^2 distribution is effective, depends on the drift value that has been neglected in the derivation of (2.6). As can be seen from (2.5), the drift depends upon the state point and if one of the initial state coordinates tends to zero, the same drift coordinate increases infinitely. Thus, the approximation (2.6) should better be used only when gene frequencies are not too small. But if the number of alleles is great, all the frequencies are clearly unable to be much above zero. In such a case, several small frequencies can be united into one (the genetic drift regularities being not changed by indistinctness among certain alleles).

Due to the approximation of θ's distribution being so simple, one can easily write out a distribution of the 'angle distances' of the (2.4) type between isolated populations of the same origin as well as develop a statistical technique to treat the problem, typical, for instance, in ethnic studies, of reconstructing the genealogical tree for the origin of congeneric populations.

It is interesting to see whether the theoretical findings on divergence of gene frequencies from the initial point are in agreement with real data on human populations when the situation is somehow close to the above-described model of genetic drift in the narrow sense. In the case of a human population the model premises have apparently never been absolutely true, for neither time intervals, but under small deviations the essential features of the process must be quite ameanable to the theoretical analysis. Thus, one may hope for certain stability in predicted behavior of a population under small perturbations of the model premises. This permits studying real situations on the grounds considered above.

It may be appropriate here to cite the analogy with technical branches of science, where in use are such idealized notions as those of the incompressible fluid, of a body with point-concentrated mass, etc., and material entities are commonly likened to fairly approximate schemes. These approximate methods, nevertheless, give a potential to solve practical problems, thus enduring verification in practice. In biological cases, however, the practical verification of theoretical models faces more difficulties since we cannot always ascertain for sure that the major assumptions of the model are correct in the case under concern. Thus, the following example, concerning the isolation by religious causes of the Dunker sect in U.S.A., is given mostly to illustrate an approach to analyzing the effects of the population size being limited. These effects require the actual population size to be corrected by the variance effective one (see Section 10.4), the temporal variations in the population size to be taken into account, the data on several loci to be combined, and so on.

The information given below is taken from the classical work of B. Glass *et al.* (1952) on studying genetic drift. The religious isolate of Dunkers (a sect of German Baptist located) was in Pennsylvania, U.S.A. At the time of census it numbered 298 persons (adults and the children aged 3 to 21) who met all of the isolate-belonging conditions.

The sect was established in 1708 in Germany, from which 28 persons emigrated to Pennsylvania in 1719. Later on one more group joined them, whose number is not exactly known but should probably be about few hundred. Most of the new-comers were natives of the same region in Germany. In 1881 the sect disintegrated into three groups, and one of them gave rise to the present isolate.

So, during more than two centuries the sect members were forming a religious isolate and 70 years before the time of examination there was a sharp split that resulted in the part of the population which has generated the group under study. A careful investigation has revealed that approximately one fifth of the population leaved the isolate during the life-span of three generation, while the total size remained stable. This size was generally constant since 1881.

Direct observations showed that parents the individuals aged 1 to 28 had 90 presents belonging to isolate. This figure was proposed by the authors to be an estimate of the effective population size. The life-span of a generation was defined to be 28 years (26 years for women, and 30 for men). Immigration was also noted (a gene flow of 10% or more per generation). This violates the assumptions of the narrow-sense genetic drift model, but we may believe the shift to be insignificant at the early stage. Surveyed were 77.5% of the persons who met the isolate-membership requirements (the entire sample consisted of 265 individuals, of which 231 fell under the definition of isolate membership).

Serologic examinations of the ABO, MN, and Rh systems gave the results cited below (shown in the table are estimates of gene concentrations).

ABO system

Alleles \ Populations	Germany (1939)	Dunkers	U.S.A (1939)
I^A	0.2862	0.3778	0.2583
I^B	0.0743	0.0253	0.0409
I^O	0.6395	0.5969	0.7008

MN system

Alleles \ Populations	Germany (1939)	Dunkers	U.S.A (1939)
M	0.548	0.655	0.540
N	0.452	0.345	0.460

Rh system

Alleles \ Populations	England	Dunkers	U.S.A
rh	0.1510	0.1113	0.1448
rh'	0.0077	0	0.0107
rh''	0.0094	0	0.0056
rh'''	0.0002	0	0.0001
Rh_0	0.0206	0.0097	0.0225
Rh_1	0.5340	0.5790	0.5358
Rh_2	0.1408	0.1550	0.1473
Rh_{12}	0.1363	0.1450	0.1332

The corresponding data on Germany and U.S.A. are shown for comparison. For lack of data on the Rh system in Germany, cited are those on England.

In the systems examined, significant differences are noticeable between the population of Dunkers and those of U.S.A. or Germany. The authors explained these differences by the effects of random genetic drift. Assuming this explanation to be adequate, let us try to estimate the divergence time that were sufficient to cause so certain differences between gene concentrations of the isolated group (of Dunkers) and their initial values (which, in the first approximation, may be considered equal to the estimates of the gene frequencies in the population of Germany (of England in the case of Rh system), the frequencies being supposed stable during the whole period of Dunker's isolation.

In the Dunker population three alleles of the Rh system have zero concentrations. Hence, the question arises about the pattern of the θ distribution in this case. To avoid this difficulty we use the possibility to combine formally the alleles rh', rh'', rh''', and Rh_0, treating them as some new allele whose frequency equals the sum of the respective concentrations.

Also, we should know the effective size (see Section 10.4) of the isolate population during the divergence time. For our purposes (to estimate the period of isolation) it will be sufficient to find the harmonic mean of the effective size during this period, that should stand for the size N in (2.6) when the size is variable in time. B. Glass et al. proposed to take 90 people as an estimate of the isolate effective size during the 70 years preceding the time of examination. Before this period the effective size was at least three or four times more. Thus, the effective size was equal to 90 within about 1/3 of the isolation period and roughly to 300 within 2/3 of the period. Hence, the harmonic mean is equal to $(\frac{1}{3}\cdot\frac{1}{90}+\frac{2}{3}\cdot\frac{1}{300})^{-1}\approx 170$.

Finally, since the genetic systems under concern are not linked, it follows from the linkage equilibrium assumption that the sum

$$\frac{8N}{t}\sum_i \theta_i^2,$$

where θ_i designate the angle deviation in the i-th system, has the chi-square distribution whose number of degrees of freedom equals to the total number of the alleles under study minus the number of the systems. This holds due to the fact that the sum of independent random variables having chi-square distributions has also the chi-square distribution whose number of degrees of freedom equals to the sum of those for the summands.

The calculations result in the following. In the ABO system (with two independent alleles) the squared distance θ_1^2 equals 0.0204, and in the MN system (one independent allele) θ_2^2=0.0121. In the Rh system (four independent alleles, the rh', rh'', rh''' and Rh_0 being formally treated as one allele) we have the squared distance θ_3^2 equal to 0.0136.

The Rh system features a too small value of the distance per allele. As can be shown by finding the confidence intervals, however, such difference between the distances may be well observed in the genetic drift model under the given number of alleles.

So,

$$\sum_{i=1}^{3}\theta_i^2 = 0.046 .$$

The number, m, of all the independent alleles is equal to seven (the total number of alleles minus the number of systems). Hence,

$$\frac{8N}{t}\sum_{i=1}^{3}\theta_i^2 = \frac{1360}{t}0.046 \sim \chi_7^2 .$$

Omitting the time-independent terms, we have the logarithmic likelihood function equal to

$$-\frac{m}{2}\ln t - \frac{8N}{2t}\sum_i \theta_i^2,$$

whereby the maximum likelihood estimate for the time of divergence of the isolate genetic composition from its initial state will be

$$\hat{t} = \frac{8N\sum_{i=1}^{3}\theta_i^2}{m} = \frac{1360 \times 0.046}{7} \approx 8.9 \text{ generations}$$

If the time is measured in years, then

$$\hat{t} \approx 249 \text{ years} .$$

So, the point estimate of the divergence time appears to be in good agreement with the historical evidence. Calculation of the confidence intervals, however, shows this agreement to be rather a 'good luck'. To estimate the divergence time more definitely we need a greater number of independent alleles.

Generalization of the problem to estimate the time of divergence of the population genetic composition from its initial state leads us to the problem of the origin of several populations. In this problem individuals of the present-day groups are supposed to be descendants of a common ancestor population. The course of the descent from the ancestor in common is described by an unknown dichotomous tree of consecutive divisions (and isolations) of the descendant populations. By using an approximation of the distance between contemporary populations, one can evaluate the divergence time for each branching in the tree as well as the pattern of branching, but these applied topics go beyond the scope of the present book.

11.3. Asymptotics of the Fundamental Solution for the Random Genetic Drift Process When $t \to \infty$

Investigation of boundary points in the one-dimensional genetic drift process (see Section 10.5) has shown the boundaries to be absorbing. The solution to the forward Kolmogorov equation by the Fourier method can be represented by the series in characteristic functions with the coefficients decreasing exponentially in time. When $t \to \infty$ the probability density function is asymptotically determined by the principal term in the expansion, that decreases at rate λ_{max}, the smallest one in absolute values:

$$f(p, x, t) \sim f_a(p, x) \exp\{\lambda_{max} t\} . \tag{3.1}$$

Here $f_a(p, x)$ stands for the characteristic function corresponding to λ_{max} and specifying the asymptotically invariable form of the density function. From (10.3.15) and (3.1) it follows that

$$\frac{\partial}{\partial t} f(p, x, t) \begin{cases} = (\mathfrak{A}^* f)(p, x, t), \\ \underset{\text{asymp.}}{\sim} \lambda_{max} f(p, x, t), \end{cases} \tag{3.2}$$

whereby we have (by omitting the exponential):

$$(\mathfrak{A}^* f_a)(p, x) - \lambda_{max} f_a(p, x) = 0 . \tag{3.3}$$

Note that λ_{max} can be easily found by the method presented in Section 10.9. According to this method the expectation of a 'good enough' function $g(x)$ (i.e. one satisfying (10.9.5)) obeys the equation

$$\frac{d}{dt} E_t\{g(x)\} = E_t\{(\mathfrak{A}\, g)(x)\} . \tag{3.4}$$

As the asymptotic density decreases at the rate λ_{max}, while being invariable in its form, the same is the rate of decrease, for instance, in the expectation of the relative number, $2x(1-x)$, of heterozygotes in the population. The function $2x(1-x)$vanishes at the boundary points, so that the variation in the expected number of heterozygotes is determined only by the dynamics of density $f(p, x, t)$ in (0, 1). By the Equation (3.4), we have

$$\frac{d}{dt} E_t\{2x(1-x)\} = E_t\left\{\frac{x(1-x)}{4N} \frac{d^2}{dx^2} 2x(1-x)\right\} = -\frac{1}{2N} E_t\{2x(1-x)\} ,$$

$$E_0\{2x(1-x)\} = 2p(1-p) , \tag{3.5}$$

hence it follows that $\lambda_{max} = -1/(2N)$. Substitution of $\lambda_{max} = -1/(2N)$ into (3.3) results in the following equation for $f_a(p, x)$:

$$\frac{1}{2} \frac{x(1-x)}{2N} \frac{d^2}{dx^2} f_a(p, x) + \frac{1-2x}{4N} \frac{d}{dx} f_a(p, x) = 0 . \tag{3.6}$$

From integrating the Equation (3.6) we infer that only the constant $f_a(p)$ can be a unique solution having no negative values. Since in asymptotics we have

$$E_t\{2x(1-x)\} \sim \int_0^1 2x(1-x) f_a(p)\, e^{-t/(2N)}\, dx = 2 f_a(p) \frac{1}{6} e^{-t/(2N)}, \tag{3.7}$$

it follows from solving (3.5) that $f_a(p) = 6p(1-p)$. Therefore, when $t \to \infty$, we have

$$f(p, x, t) \sim 6p(1-p)\, e^{-t/(2N)} . \tag{3.8}$$

In the case of $n>2$ alleles we can find in a similar way the asymptotic rate of decrease in the probability that n alleles are present in the population. To do this we may consider the behavior of the expected product of allele frequencies $x_1, x_2,..., x_n$. The product itself vanishes at boundaries of symplex Σ, i.e. the expected product varies at the rate λ_{max}. On the other hand, by Equation (10.9.1) we have

$$\frac{d}{dt}E_t\left\{\prod_{i=1}^{n} x_i\right\} = E_t\left\{\frac{1}{2}\sum\sum_{i\neq j} -\frac{x_i x_j}{2N}\frac{\partial^2}{\partial x_i\,\partial x_j}\prod_{m=1}^{n} x_m\right\} =$$

$$= -\frac{n(n-1)}{4N}E_t\left\{\prod_{m=1}^{n} x_m\right\} . \tag{3.9}$$

Consequently $\lambda_{max}=-n(n-1)/(4N)$ and the asymptotic probability that all n alleles coexist in the population decreases very rapidly, being roughly proportional to the squared number of alleles for a large n.

As regards the asymptotic form of the probability density function, it does not depend, as well as in the one-dimensional case, upon the current values of alleles frequencies. According to Kimura's findings the asymptotic density in the simplex face that corresponds to the presence of k alleles with current coordinates x_i (where $\sum_{i=1}^{k} x_i=1$), is equal to

$$f(p_1,..., p_{n-1}, x_1,..., x_k, t)\sim(2k-1)!\left(\prod_{i=1}^{k} p_i\right)\exp\left\{-\frac{k(k-1)}{4N}\right\} . \tag{3.10}$$

11.4. Boundary Attainment Probabilities

Recall that, by the results of Section 10.6, the expected 'penalty', $U(\mathbf{p})$, on a process trajectory (being equal to $u(\mathbf{x})$ in a current state $\mathbf{x}\in\Sigma$ and $h(\mathbf{x}_B)$ in a point $\mathbf{x}_B$ of the absorbing boundary) obeys the equation

$$(\mathfrak{A}\, U)(\mathbf{x}) = -\, u(\mathbf{p}),\quad U(\mathbf{p})|_{B(\Sigma)}=h(\mathbf{p}) .$$

If we are interested in the probability of absorption in a boundary point $\mathbf{x}_B$, then we obviously have $u(\mathbf{x}) \equiv 0$, $h(\mathbf{x}_B) = 1$, $h(\mathbf{x}) = 0$, $\mathbf{x} \in B(\Sigma)$, $\mathbf{x}\neq\mathbf{x}_B$. To find the mean time to attain a boundary we should set $u(\mathbf{x})\equiv 1$, $h(\mathbf{x})\equiv 0$. Since it is possible to analyze the behavior of an allele frequency in the genetic drift process separately from the rest of the alleles, one can find the fixation probability, $U_1(p)$, for an allele with an initial concentration p from the equation:

$$\frac{1}{2}\frac{p(1-p)}{2N}\frac{d^2}{dp^2}U_1(p) = 0,$$
$$u_1(0) = 0,\ U_1(1) = 1 . \tag{4.1}$$

Its solution is know to be

$$U_1(p) = p,\ U_0(p) = 1 - U_1(p) = 1 - p , \tag{4.2}$$

where U_0 designates the loss probability for the allele. Note that these probabilities coincide exactly with the absorption probabilities in the corresponding Markov chain model.

Since by (10.3.20) the time derivative of probability of fixation up to moment t is equal to the flow value at the point $x=1$, it follows from the asymptotic density form (3.8) that

$$\frac{\partial}{\partial t} U_1(p, t) \sim \frac{1}{2}\frac{\partial}{\partial x}\left[-6p(1-p)\exp\left\{-\frac{t}{2N}\right\}\frac{x(1-x)}{2N}\right]\Bigg|_{x=1} =$$

$$= -\,6p(1-p)\exp\{-t/(2N)\}(-1/(4N))$$

as $t \to \infty$. Hence, taking (4.2) into account, we arrive to the well-known asymptotic expression for the allele fixation probability:

$$U_1(p, t) \sim p - 3p(1-p)\exp\{-t/(2N)\}\,. \tag{4.3}$$

Similarly,

$$U_0(p, t) \sim 1 - p - 3p(1-p)\exp\{-t/(2N)\}\,. \tag{4.4}$$

In the case of multiple alleles it is interesting to find not only the fixation or loss probabilities of an allele but also the probabilities that the allele is the first, the second, etc., lost, and, finally, that the alleles are lost in a certain order. Referring to the interpretation of these probabilities as the expected 'penalties' at the moment of getting to the boundary (see Section 10.8), we conclude that they must satisfy the equation

$$(\mathcal{Q} U)(\mathbf{p}) = 0\,.$$

If we consider the probability that an allele, say A_1 is the first lost, then the boundary conditions will be everywhere zero except the hyperplane $p_1 = 0$, where the probability be equal to one. In general, the probability, $U_{j(i)}(\mathbf{p})$, that an allele A_j is the ith lost ($i>1$) obeys the equation

$$(\mathcal{Q} U_{j(i)})(\mathbf{p}) = 0\,,$$
$$U_{j(i)}(\mathbf{p})\big|_{B(\Sigma)} = U_{j(i-1)}(\mathbf{p})\,, \tag{4.5}$$

i.e. the boundary attainment 'penalty' equals the probability that the allele is the (i-1)th lost (since one allele has been already lost).

Similar are the boundary conditions to determine the probability that several alleles are lost in a given sequence, the boundary 'penalty' being equal to the loss probability for a corresponding residue of the sequence.

One may solve the equation (4.5) starting with (4.1) and increasing successively the number of alleles. The values of U that have been derived in the n-allele case, give the boundary conditions for the case of (n+1) alleles.

For the genetic drift process, however, the procedure can be considerably simplified due to the symmetric pattern in which the operator $\mathcal{Q}$ coefficients depend on p_i variables. Thus, by making use of the formulae for the union-of-events probabilities, we can obtain results for a multiallele case, following the arguments of R.A. Littler and originating essentially from the results of the one-dimensional model (with two alleles).

For example, the probability of the allele A_j being the first lost can be represented in the following form:

$$U_{j(1)} = 1 - P\{\bigcup_{i \neq j} \{A_i \text{ is lost before } A_j\}\} =$$

$$= 1 - (\sum_{i \neq j} P\{A_i \text{ is lost before } A_j\} -$$

$$- \sum_{i_1 < i_2 \neq j} P\{A_{i_1}, A_{i_2} \text{ are lost before } A_j\} + \ldots$$

$$\ldots + (-1)^{n-1} P\{\text{all of the allele except } A_j \text{ are lost}\}). \tag{4.6}$$

From the results of the two-allele case it is easy to find the probability that allele A_i will be lost before A_j (this can be obviously done by monitoring the process of variations in frequencies of the allele A_i and A_j with no attention to the rest ones). Let us make the transformation

$$q_i = \frac{p_i}{p_i + p_j}, \quad q_j = \frac{p_j}{p_i + p_j}, \quad q_k = p_k, \quad k \neq i, j \,. \tag{4.7}$$

By the change-of-variables formulae (10.7.4) we can find the infinitesimal characteristics for coordinates q_i and q_j:

$$V_{ii} = \frac{q_i(1-q_i)}{2N(p_i+p_j)}, \quad V_{ij} = -\frac{q_i q_j}{2N(p_i+p_j)},$$

$$V_{jj} = \frac{q_j(1-q_j)}{2N(p_i+p_j)}, \quad V_{ik} = V_{jk} = 0, \quad k \neq i, j, \tag{4.8}$$

$$M_i = M_j = 0 \,.$$

From (4.8) it follows that, in the block matrix of diffusion coefficients, the coordinates $\{q_i, q_j\}$ cover the submatrix of the (10.6.2) form, i.e. that of the same kind as in case of the genetic drift at a locus of two alleles with concentrations q_i and q_j, excepting the co-factor $1/(p_i + p_j)$ in the diffusion coefficients. Since the co-factor does not change any trajectory of these coordinates while modifying only the speed of movement, the probability of allele A_i being lost before A_j (i.e. of reaching the boundary $q_j = 1$) is, by (4.2), equal to q_j, i.e.

$$P\{A_i \text{ is lost before } A_j\} = p_j/(p_i + p_j) \,. \tag{4.9}$$

The probability (4.9) can be verified to obey the equation $\mathfrak{L}P=0$, and, on the boundary, turn into the proper probability of allele A_i being lost before A_j.

Note that the probability that a group of alleles, $A_{i_1}, A_{i_2}, \ldots, A_{i_k}$, is lost before allele A_j, can be also found (by using the possibility of making 'no distinction' between some alleles, see Section 11.1) as the probability that the artificially 'combined' allele of the concentration $p_{i_1}+p_{i_2}+\ldots+p_{i_k}$ will be lost before A_j:

$$P\{A_{i_1}, A_{i_2}, \ldots, A_{i_k} \text{ will be lost before } A_j\} = p_j/(p_{i_1}+p_{i_2}+\ldots+p_{i_k}+p_j) \,. \tag{4.10}$$

These probabilities satisfy the equation $\mathfrak{A} P=0$ and the corresponding boundary conditions.

After substituting the probability values (4.10) for the probabilities in (4.6), we have

$$U_{j(1)} = 1 - \sum_{\substack{i=1 \\ i\neq j}}^{n} \frac{p_i}{p_i+p_j} + \sum_{\substack{i_1, i_2 \\ i_1<i_2}} \frac{p_j}{p_{i_1}+p_{i_2}+p_j} - \dots -(-1)^{n-1} p_j . \tag{4.11}$$

It can be verified that $\mathfrak{A} U_{j(1)}=0$ and the zero boundary conditions hold everywhere except the hyperplane $p_j = 0$, where $U_{j(1)}=1$.

In the case of three alleles we have $p_1=1-p_2-p_3, p_1+p_2=1-p_3$, and $p_1+p_3=1-p_2$, so that

$$U_{1(1)} = 1 - \frac{p_1}{p_1+p_2} + \frac{p_1}{p_1+p_3} + p_1 = p_2 p_3 \left(\frac{1}{1-p_2} + \frac{1}{1-p_3} \right) ,$$

$$U_{2(1)} = p_1 p_3 \left(\frac{1}{1-p_1} + \frac{1}{1-p_3} \right) , \tag{4.12}$$

$$U_{3(1)} = p_1 p_2 \left(\frac{1}{1-p_1} + \frac{1}{1-p_2} \right) .$$

The probability of allele A_j being the kth lost cane be found in a similar way:

$U_{j(k)} = 1 - P\{\text{there are } k \text{ alleles } A_{i_1},\dots, A_{i_k} \text{ lost before } A_j\}$.

The probability that the allele $A_n, A_{n-1},\dots, A_2$ will be lost exactly in this order equals

$$\prod_{i=1}^{n} \left(\frac{p_i}{\sum_{k=i}^{n} p_k} \right) = \prod_{i=1}^{n} \left(\frac{p_i}{\sum_{k=1}^{i-1} p_k} \right) .$$

11.5. Characteristics of the Boundary Attainment Time

By using the possibility to analyze the genetic drift behavior of any allele at a multiallelic locus separately from the rest ones, we have the following equation for $T(p)$, the mean time till the moment of absorption (i.e. that of either fixation or loss) of an allele with initial concentration p:

$$\frac{1}{2} \frac{p(1-p)}{2N} \frac{d^2 T(p)}{dp^2} = -1 , \tag{5.1}$$

$$T(0) = T(1) = 0 .$$

The proper solution will be

$$T(p) = -4N[p \ln p + (1-p) \ln (1-p)] . \tag{5.2}$$

The mean absorption time increases linearly with the population size N and varies as a function of the initial concentration p. It reaches its maximum value of 2.76 N

generations at $p = 0.5$ and decreases symmetrically with any deviation from this initial concentration.

In the case of two allele, losing one of them means attaining the homozygosity. One should clearly expect an increase in the attainment time when the number of alleles increases, since losing one of them in this case does not yet result in genetic homozygosity of the population. In the case of n alleles the mean homozygosity attainment time (i.e. the time to lose $(n-1)$ alleles) turns out equal to

$$T(\mathbf{p}) = -4N \sum_{i=1}^{n} (1-p_i) \ln (1-p_i) . \tag{5.3}$$

For the notation uniformity and convenience, the independent variable p_n also participates in this formula. The mean time has its maximum equal to

$$-4Nn(1-1/n) \ln (1-1/n)$$

when all of the n initial concentrations are the same, the maximum tending to $4N$ as $n \to \infty$.

The easiest way to derive (5.3) goes through using the concept of the conditional diffusion process introduced in Section 10.7. Let us consider the conditional average fixation time for an allele with initial concentration p under the condition of fixing that very allele (the probability, $U_1(p)$, of this event being equal to p). As follows from Section 10.7, the conditional process differs from the unconditional one by the additional drift equal to

$$V(p)U_1'(p)/U_1(p) .$$

The conditional time $T_1(p)$ thus satisfies the equation

$$\frac{1}{2}\frac{p(1-p)}{2N}\frac{d^2T_1(p)}{dp^2} + \frac{1-p}{2N}\frac{dT_1(p)}{dp} = -1 , \tag{5.4}$$

$$T_1(1) = 0 .$$

The solution within the set of bounded functions is given by

$$T_1(p) = -4N\frac{1-p}{p} \ln (1-p) . \tag{5.5}$$

Similarly, the mean loss time for an allele, $T_0(p)$, can be found under the condition that it is lost:

$$\frac{1}{2}\frac{p(1-p)}{2N}\frac{d^2T_0(p)}{dp^2} - \frac{p}{2N}\frac{dT_0(p)}{dp} = -1 , \tag{5.6}$$

$$T_0(0) = 0 .$$

Within the set of bounded functions, Equation (5.6) is satisfied with

$$T_0(p) = -4N\frac{p}{1-p}\ln p\,. \tag{5.7}$$

In a multiallele case one of the mutually exclusive events takes place inevitably, with the unit probability: a homozygoes state with one of the alleles (the fixed one) is attained. Since, on the average, it takes $T_1(p_i)$ generations to fix an allele A_i of the initial concentration p_i, the event occurring with probability p_i, the mean time to reach homozygosity (to lose all but one alleles) equals the sum of products $p_iT_1(p_i)$, i.e. the expression (5.3).

It is known that, in the conditional process under the condition for an allele being fixed, the mean squared fixation time for the allele can be obtained from equation (10.8.6), i.e. from the equation

$$\frac{1}{2}\frac{p(1-p)}{2N}\frac{d^2T_{1,2}(p)}{dp^2} + \frac{1-p}{2N}\frac{dT_{1,2}(p)}{dp} = -2T_1(p)\,, \tag{5.8}$$

which is complied with the solution given by

$$T_{1,2}(p) = 32N^2\left[\frac{\pi^2}{6} + \frac{1-p}{p}\ln(1-p) - \sum_{j=1}^{\infty}\frac{p^j}{j^2}\right]. \tag{5.9}$$

Hence, the mean squared time for the population to come into a homozygous state, being equal to the sum of products $p_iT_{1,2}(p_i)$, equals

$$32N^2\left[\frac{\pi^2}{6} + \sum_{i=1}^{n}(1-p_i)\ln(1-p_i) - \sum_{i=1}^{n}\sum_{j=1}^{\infty}\frac{p_i^{j+1}}{j^2}\right].$$

The further moments of the homozygosity attainment time can be found in a similar way, by means of the conditional diffusion process characteristics, the analytical expressions being fairly tedious. Examples of the mean and variance as well as those of the skewness and excess are given in Figures 34 and 35 and in the table below.

Figure 34 shows the following characteristics of the time to attain homozygosity: (*1*)

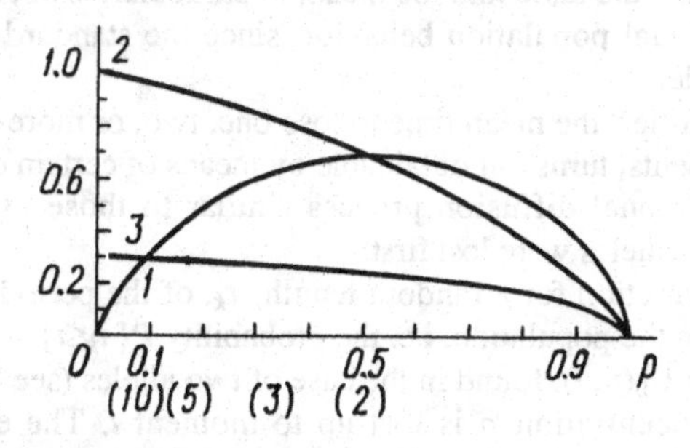

Fig. 34. Characteristics of the homozygosity attainment time.

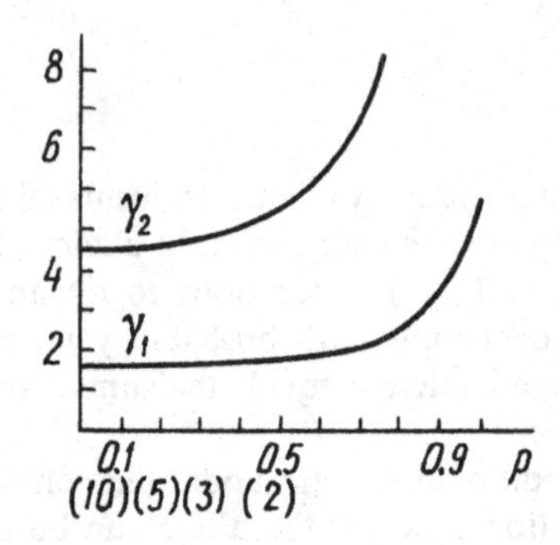

Fig. 35. The skewness (μ_1) and exess (μ_2) coefficients for the distribution of the allele fixation time conditioned by no allele loss.

the mean homozygosity attainment time in the case of two alleles, the mean (*2*) and variance (*3*) of an allele fixation time under the condition that the allele is not lost. The time is counted along the ordinate axis, the scale unit being equal to $4N$ generations (N stands for the size of a diploid population), the initial concentration, p, of the allele under concern in counted along the abscissa axis. When p varies from 0 to 0.5, the curves *2* and *3* represent the mean homozygosity attainment time also for the case of n (indicated by the digits in parentheses along the abscissa) mutliple alleles of equal initial concentrations.

Shown in Figure 35 are plots of the skewness (γ_1) and excess (γ_2) coefficients for the distribution of the allele fixation time conditioned on its fixation as functions of the allele concentration p (measured along the abscissa). When p varies from 0 to 0.5, the curves represent the characteristics of the homozygosity attainment time also for the case of n (the numbers in parentheses) multiple alleles of equal initial concentrations.

Given in the table are the first moments (M_i), the skewness and the excess coefficients (γ_1 and γ_2) for the conditional time till fixation of a neutral mutant (i.e.until homozygosity is reached in a population with equal initial allele frequencies) as functions of its initial frequency p (or of the total number, n, of the alleles with frequencies $1/n$). The upper line of the heading shows the n values, the lower line the p values. It can be seen from the Figures and the table that the mean, in particular, is not an enough reliable characteristic of individual population behavior, since the standard deviation has the same order of magnitude.

As shown by R.A. Littler, the mean time to lose one, two, or more of the n alleles, as well as the higher moments, turns out obtainable by means of certain characteristics of a one-dimensional conditional diffusion process similar to those used in finding the probabilities that certain alleles were lost first.

The probability distribution for a random length, τ_k, of the period after which there are k alleles remained in the population, i.e. the probability $P\{\tau_k \le t\}$, can be expressed in terms of the probability $U_0(p, t)$, found in the case of two alleles (see Section 11.8), that an allele of initial concentration p is lost up to moment t. The event $\tau_k \le t$ means occurrence of at least $n-k$ such events as loss of one of the n alleles up to moment t. The occurrence probability of at least $(n-k)$ events of the n ones is known to be

	lim ... $n\to\infty$ $p\to 0$	50 0.02	25 0.04	10 0.10	5 0.20	3 0.33	2 0.50	– 0.60	– 0.70	– 0.80	– 0.90
M_1	1.000	0.990	0.980	0.948	0.893	0.811	0.693	0.611	0.516	0.402	0.256
M_2	1.29	1.270	1.250	1.188	1.083	0.936	0.739	0.613	0.479	0.336	0.178
M_3	2.13	2.092	2.053	1.935	1.737	1.468	1.122	0.909	0.691	0.467	0.238
M_4	4.41	4.330	4.245	3.988	3.558	2.980	2.250	1.808	1.362	0.912	0.459
γ_1	1.67	1.670	1.671	1.678	1.701	1.763	1.909	2.055	2.278	2.660	3.508
γ_2	4.51	4.537	4.540	4.564	4.658	4.923	5.627	6.418	7.785	10.512	18.280

$$S_{n-k} - \binom{n-k}{1} S_{n-k+1} + \binom{n-k+1}{2} S_{n-k+2} - \ldots + (-1)^{n-(n-k)} \binom{n-1}{k} S_n ,$$

where S_i designates the sum of probabilities of all possible intersections of i events from the n ones.

The simultaneous occurrence of i events, each being a loss of one allele, is equivalent to loss of the 'artificial' allele whose initial concentration equals the sum of initial frequencies, $\{p_{i_m}\}$, of the lost alleles. The probability of this intersection is equal to $U_0(\Sigma_{m=1}^{i} p_{i_m}, t)$, so that

$$P\{\tau_k \leq t\} = \sum_{i=1}^{k} (-1)^i \binom{n-k-1+i}{i} \sum_{\{i_m\}} U_0 (\sum_{m=1}^{i} p_{i_m}, t) =$$

$$= \sum_{l=1}^{k} (-1)^{k-l} \binom{n-l-1}{k-l} \sum_{\{i_m\}} U_1 (\sum_{m=1}^{l} p_{i_m}, t) \tag{5.10}$$

The latter form of expression in (5.10) is obtained as a result of substituting l for $(k-i)$ and taking into account that the loss of $n-k+i$ alleles is equivalent to reaching the unitary value by the total concentration of the rest $(k-i)$ alleles, i.e. fixation of the additional 'artificial' allele. The probability of fixation up to moment t of the 'artificial' allele composed by l alleles with initial concentrations p_{i_m}, is denoted by $U_1(\Sigma_{m=1}^{l} p_{i_m}, t)$. Summation of the U_0 and U_1 terms takes place over all possible choices of $n-k+i$ (or l) alleles out of the n ones.

When the distribution function is known, one can find moments of any order for the time until the population has k alleles rested. The moments are readily expressed in terms of those for the one-dimensional process. Actually, by differentiating both sides of (5.10) with respect to t, multiplying them by t^m, and integrating over t from 0 to ∞ we will have the moment of mth order in the left-hand side, while in the right-hand side, instead of U there will be products of the loss (or fixation) probabilities of 'artificial' alleles (with corresponding initial concentrations) by the conditional m-order moments of the loss (or fixation) time for those alleles. Consequently, the moments of the allele loss (fixation) time, which in general require partial differential equations to be solved, in the genetic drift case can be found from the ordinary differential equations for conditional characteristics of the two-allele process.

By means of (5.6) we have the following expression for the mean time to lose $n-k$ alleles (i.e. until the population will have k alleles rested):

$$E\{\tau_{k,n}\} = -4N \sum_{i=1}^{k} (-1)^{k+i} \binom{n-1-i}{k-i} \sum_{\{j_m\}} (1-p_{j_1}-\ldots-p_{j_i}) \ln (1-p_{j_1}-\ldots-p_{j_i}) . \tag{5.11}$$

It can be shown that

$$\mathcal{Q} E\{\tau_{k,n}\} = -1, \quad E\{\tau_{K,n}\}|_{B(\Sigma)} = E\{\tau_{k-1,n-1}\} . \tag{5.12}$$

These conditions can be verified immediately, by taking into account that

$$\mathcal{Q}\{4N\sum_{\{j_m\}}(1-p_{j_1}-\ldots-p_{j_i})\ln(1-p_{j_1}-\ldots-p_{j_i})\}=\binom{n-1}{i-1}$$

and that the equality

$$(-1)^{k-1}\sum_{i=0}^{k-1}(-1)^i\binom{n-2-i}{k-1-i}\binom{n-1}{i}=1$$

is true, ensuring from comparison of the coefficients at t^k in the identity $(1+t)^{n-1}/(1+t)^{n-k} = (1+t)^{k-1}$. At the boundary of Σ (where concentration of one of the alleles becomes zero) the quantity

$$\Sigma(1-p_{j_1}-\ldots-p_{j_i})\ln(1-p_{j_1}-\ldots-p_{j_i})$$

referred to as $\Sigma(i, n)$ below, turns into

$$\Sigma(i, n-1)+\Sigma(i-1, n-1)$$

from which the boundary conditions (5.12) readily follow.

The pattern of successive loss of alleles for large n and equal initial concentrations is such that there are k alleles ($k<<n$) rested in the population in $4N/k$ generations on the average. When the initial concentration of any allele equals $1/n$, all the terms in $\Sigma(i, n)$, corresponding to sets of i alleles chosen from the n ones, turn into $(1-i/n)\ln(1-i/n)$. The total number of these sets is equal to the number of ways to choose i of the n alleles, i.e. $\binom{n}{i}$. Therefore,

$$E\{\tau_{k,n}\}=-4N\sum_{i=1}^{k}(-1)^{k+i}\binom{n-1-i}{k-i}\binom{n}{i}(1-\frac{i}{n})\ln(1-\frac{i}{n})=$$

$$=-(-1)^k 4N\binom{n-1}{k}\sum_{i=1}^{k}(-1)^i\binom{k}{i}\ln(1-\frac{i}{n})=$$

$$=(-1)^k 4N\binom{n-1}{k}\sum_{i=1}^{k}(-1)^i\binom{k}{i}\left(\frac{i}{n}+\frac{i^2}{2n^2}+\ldots+\frac{i^k}{kn^k}+\ldots\right). \tag{5.13}$$

If we differentiate both sides of the identity

$$(1-t)^k=\sum_{i=0}^{k}(-t)^i\binom{k}{i}$$

j times with respect to t and set $t = 1$, then we have

$$\frac{d^j}{dt^j}(1-t)^k=\sum_{i=0}^{k}(-1)^i\binom{k}{i}i(i-1)\ldots(i-k+1)=\begin{cases}0, & j\neq k,\\ (-1)^k k!, & j=k.\end{cases}$$

By letting j be sequentially equal to 1, 2,..., we obtain the zero sum of terms with i^m ($m< k$) in (5.13) and the value $(-1)^k 4N(-1)^k\binom{n-1}{k}k!/(kn^k)$ of those with i^k, whereby

$$E\{\tau_{k,n}\} \underset{n\to\infty}{\rightarrow} 4N/k\,. \tag{5.14}$$

Behavior of the higher moments can be studied similarly.

11.6 Probability Density Function for the Sojourn Time and the Age of an Allele

In Section 10.8 the probability density function for the time the process sojourns in points of Σ is shown to be an important characteristic of the process, which permits easy determination of expected path integrals of a given function on process states. The density value, $\Phi(p, y)$, at point y (if the initial state was p) can be treated as the expected 'penalty' over trajectories for the 'penalty' function $\delta(x\text{-}y)$. In the two-allele case, therefore, $\Phi(p, y)$ for the genetic drift process can be found from (10.8.8) as the solution to the equation

$$\frac{1}{2}\frac{p(1-p)}{2N}\frac{d^2}{dp^2}\Phi(p, y) = -\,\delta(p-y)\,, \tag{6.1}$$

satisfying the boundary conditions

$$\Phi(0, y) = \Phi(1, y) = 0\,.$$

Hence,

$$\frac{d}{dp}\Phi(p, y) = -\int^{p} \frac{4N\delta(x-y)}{x(1-x)}\,dx = \begin{cases} c, & p<y; \\ -\dfrac{4N}{y(1\text{-}y)} + c, & p\geq y. \end{cases}$$

Recall that a definite integral of the product of a continuous function $g(x)$ by $\delta(x-y)$ equals zero if the upper limit of integration is less than y, and equals $g(y)$ if the limit exceeds y. Therefore, the anti-derivative of $4N\delta(x-y)/[x(1-x)]$ is a step-function with a break at point x=y, the height of the step being equal to $4N/[y(1-y)]$.
After integrating once more, we have

$$\Phi(p, y) = \begin{cases} cp + a; & p<y; \\ -\dfrac{4N}{y(1-y)}p + cp + b, & p\geq y. \end{cases}$$

From the boundary condition $\Phi(0, y)$=0 it follows that a=0. Since the sojourn time density $\Phi(p, y)$ must be continuous at point y, we have the equality

$$cy = -\frac{4N}{y(1-y)}y + cy + b,$$

which yields b=$4N/(1-y)$. The value of c is then found from the second boundary condition

$$-\frac{4N}{y(1-y)}+c+\frac{4N}{1-y}=0$$

to be $c=4N/y$. Finally, the solution to (6.1) can be written in the following form:

$$\Phi(p,y)=\begin{cases}4Np/y, & p<y;\\ 4N(1-p)/(1-y), & p\geq y;\end{cases} \tag{6.2}$$

Integrating $\Phi(p, y)$ from $y=p$ to 1, we have the expected time the trajectory spends in the region where the concentration of an allele under concern exceeds its initial value, being equal to $(-4Np \ln p)$. Similarly, we have the mean time spent in $(0, p)$ equal to $-4N(1-p) \ln (1-p)$, so that, consisting of these two summands, the mean time to reach homozygosity is

$$T(p)=\int_0^1 \Phi(p,y)\,dy=-4N(1-p)\ln(1-p)-4Np\ln p$$

in complete accordance with (5.2).

Related with the time the process stays in Σ is the problem of finding the expected age, $A(p, x)$, of an allele with an initial concentration p and a current one x. Let $B(p, x)$ be the product of the mean age of an allele with the frequency x by the density function of the sojourn time at state x. Then

$$B(p,x)=\int_0^\infty tf(p,x,t)\,dt. \tag{6.3}$$

and

$$A(p,x)=B(p,x)/\int_0^\infty f(p,x,t)\,dt=B(p,x)/\Phi(p,x),$$

i.e. $A(p, x)$ represents the mean time of passage (but not of the first passage) through x if the initial state was p. Let us apply operator $\mathfrak{A}$ to both sides of (6.3); we then obtain that

$$\mathfrak{A}B(p,x)=\int_0^\infty t\mathfrak{A}f(p,x,t)\,dt=\int_0^\infty t\frac{\partial}{\partial t}f(p,x,t)\,dt=$$

$$tf(p,x,t)\Big|_0^\infty-\int_0^\infty f(p,x,t)\,dt=\Phi(p,x)$$

since $tf(p,x,t)\Big|_0^\infty=0$. For the random genetic drift process in the single two-allele locus case, the operator $\mathfrak{A}$ is defined by formula (1.1a), so that $B(p, x)$ satisfies the equation

$$\frac{1}{2}\frac{p(1-p)}{2N}\frac{d^2}{dp^2}B(p, x) = -\,\Phi(p, x)\ ,$$

$$B(0, x) = B(1, x) = 0\ . \qquad (6.4)$$

The boundary conditions are defined by those for the sojourn time (6.1), since $B(p, x)$ is the product of the (finite-valued) mean age by the sojourn time density function.

After substituting the (6.2) value of $\Phi(p, x)$ into Equation (6.4), we obtain the unique solution satisfying the continuity (and the continuity-of-derivative) restriction at point y and the zero boundary conditions:

$$B(p, x) = \begin{cases} -(4N)^2\left[\dfrac{(1-p)\ln(1-p)}{x} + \dfrac{p}{x} + \dfrac{p\ln x}{1-x}\right], & p<x; \\ -(4N)^2\left[\dfrac{p\ln p}{1-x} + \dfrac{1-p}{1-x} + \dfrac{(1-p)\ln(1-x)}{x}\right], & p\geq x. \end{cases} \qquad (6.5)$$

Following T. Maruyama's approach, we find then the mean age of an allele with an initial concentration p and a current one x, equal to

$$A(p, x) = \begin{cases} -4N\left[\dfrac{(1-p)\ln(1-p)}{p} + \dfrac{x\ln x}{1-x} + 1\right], & p<x; \\ -4N\left[\dfrac{p\ln p}{1-p} + \dfrac{(1-x)\ln(1-x)}{x} + 1\right], & p\geq x. \end{cases} \qquad (6.6)$$

In the biological literature, a low concentration of one of the allele under concern is sometimes considered to be an argument in favour of its recent origin from a single mutation. Calculations shows, however, that the notion of 'recent', when applied to the mean age of a low-concentration allele, is poorly correlated with smallness of time in a common sense. For example, the mean age of an allele with concentration 0.1 is roughly equal to $4N$ generations. The life-time of a human generation is usually not less than 25 years. If the (effective) population size is 100, then the mean age of a neutral mutant with concentration 0.1 has a value about 10000 years.

To determine the mean age for a small x, one may use the well-known approximation of (6.6) when $p<x$:

$$A(p, x) \sim -\,4Nx\ln x/(1-x)\ . \qquad (6.7)$$

The characteristics considered in this Section (viz. the sojourn time density function and the allele age) can be defined for a conditional process as well, under the condition of the allele loss or fixation. The generating operator for the process is then to be properly modified (see Section 10.7).

When mutation pressure is weak, the characteristics described can be treated as certain approximations for a more general situation, i.e. that with mutating alleles. The assumption should be made, however, that the mutation probability is negligibly small in the course of reaching 'absorption' states.

11.7 Moments of the Random Genetic Drift Process

From the results presented in Section 10.3 it follows that the mathematical expectation of a function on process states obeys the backward Kolmogorov equation (10.3.11). For a genetic drift process, however, a number of characteristics can be found much more easily, by the method described in Section 10.9. The problem is simplified due to the fact that operator $\mathcal{Q}$ of the form (1.1) maps a polynomial into that of the same power, so that we have to solve ordinary differential equations instead of those in partial derivatives. Further simplification arise from the possibility to combine artificially several allele frequencies into one, still preserving the correctness of the conclusion for the original model as well. This results in reducing dimensionality of the problem and we obtain known findings in dynamics of the moments for the genetic drift process in the most simple way.

Let us, for example, investigate the behavior of the expected concentration, $E_t\{x_i\}$, by application of (3.4) to the one-dimensional process (1.1a), with the allele A_i, to which the original process is reduced:

$$\frac{d}{dt}E_t\{x_i\} = E_t\left\{\frac{x_i(1-x_i)}{4N}\frac{d^2x_i}{dx_i^2}\right\} = 0\,,$$

$$E_0\{x_i\} = p_i\,. \tag{7.1}$$

This equation is satisfied with the function

$$E_t\{x_i\} \equiv p_i\,, \tag{7.2}$$

i.e. frequencies of the allele are invariable on the average.

Consider also some properties of the population genetic structure which are referred to its heterozygosity. Under condition that the allele frequencies were equal to $\{p_i\}$ in the parent population, the number of heterozygotes, $H_{ij}(\mathbf{p})$, with the ith and jth alleles in the offspring population, equals, on the average,

$$E\{H_{ij}\} = 2p_ip_j\,,\, i \neq j \tag{7.3}$$

by the Hardy-Weinberg law, due to the independence in parent gamete combinations. If, therefore, the value of p_i and p_j in the parent population are governed by some probability distribution function, the unconditional expectation of the number of the heterozygotes in the offspring population is to be $E\{2p_ip_j\}$ Since the time (in generations) and concentrations vary continuously in the diffusion model, we may consider the quantity $2p_ip_j$ to characterize the number of heterozygotes in the population with current concentrations p_i and p_j.

To find $E_t\{H_{ij}\}$ let us use the Equation (3.4):

$$\frac{d}{dt}E_t\{H_{ij}\} = E_t\{\mathcal{Q}\, H_{ij}\} = -\frac{1}{2N}E_t\{H_{ij}\}\,, \tag{7.4}$$

$$E_0\{H_{ij}\} = 2p_ip_j = H_{ij}^0\,.$$

The well-known result follows from here, depending neither on a number of other alleles nor upon their concentrations:

$$E_t\{H_{ij}\} = 2p_i p_j \exp\left\{-\frac{t}{2N}\right\} = H_{ij}^0 \exp\left\{-\frac{t}{2N}\right\}. \tag{7.5}$$

Let us agree that H_{ii}=$2p_i(1\text{-}p_i)$. Then $E_t\{H_{ii}\}$ complies with (7.5). If we define the total population heterozygosity as $H=\sum\sum_{i<j} H_{ij}$, then, by (7.5), we will have

$$E_t\{H\} = H^0 \exp\left\{-\frac{t}{2N}\right\}$$

independently of the number of alleles under concern.

Thus, $E_t\{H\}\to 0$ as $t\to\infty$. It is clear that the number of heterozygotes tends to zero on each particular trajectory too, with the probability 1 (since H does not take on any negative values). In a random-mating population this can be true only if the population becomes totally homozygous, so that, in the genetic drift process, fixation of one of the alleles and loss of the rest ones occur inevitably.

Recall that the expected concentration of each allele is constant for any t and equal to its initial value (7.2). Let U_i denote the fixation probability of the ith allele (its concentration being equal to 1 at fixation and to 0 at its loss). In the limit, the expected value of the concentration (which is always equal to p_i) must be determined as

$$p_i = U_i{\cdot}1 + (1 - U_i){\cdot}0 = U_i\ . \tag{7.6}$$

Thus, one more of the well-known results has been obtained: the fixation probability of an allele is equal to its initial concentration.

The number of heterozygotes characterizes the genetic variability in the population. This genetic variability diminishes in the genetic drift process at the average rate $1/(2N)$ of its current value per generation. Eventually, the variability vanishes once the population reaches a complete genetic homogeneity. It is interesting to find the integral average of the variability in the course of reaching homozygosity. To do this, we integrate both sides of the Equation (7.4) for $E_t\{H_{ij}\}$ along the t-axis from 0 to ∞:

$$\int_0^\infty \frac{\mathrm{d}}{\mathrm{d}t} E_t\{H_{ij}\}\,\mathrm{d}t = -\frac{1}{2N}\int_0^\infty E_t\{H_{ij}\}\,\mathrm{d}t.$$

Since the integral in the left side equals $E_\infty\{H_{ij}\}-H_{ij}^0$, the term $E_\infty\{H_{ij}\}$=0 being equal to zero by (7.5), we have the average heterozygosity in the whole course of the drift process to be equal to

$$\int_0^\infty E_t\{H_{ij}\}\,\mathrm{d}t = 2NH_{ij}^0 \tag{7.7}$$

and correspondent with the known results.

By (7.2) the expected values of the allele concentrations are constant in time. But there are random oscillations on trajectories near these values. For the variance of a concentration over process trajectories we have the following differential equation

$$\frac{\mathrm{d}}{\mathrm{d}t}E_t\{[x_i - E_t\{x_i\}]^2\} = E_t\{\mathfrak{A}[x_i - E_t\{x_i\}]^2\} = \tag{7.8}$$

$$= E_t\{\frac{1}{2N}x_i(1-x_i)\} = \frac{1}{2N}p_i(1-p_i)\exp\left\{-\frac{t}{2N}\right\},$$

$$E_0\{[x_i - E_0\{x_i\}]^2\} = 0\,.$$

We make use of the formula (7.5) for H_{ii} here. The known solution to (7.8) is

$$E_t\{[x_i - E_t\{x_i\}]^2\} = \left(1 - \exp\left\{-\frac{t}{2N}\right\}\right)p_i(1-p_i)\,. \tag{7.9}$$

The following is an evident remark concerning interpretation of the formula (7.5) that characterizes the expected heterozygosity in the population. The formula contains no current values of allele concentrations, but only their initial values, which are impossible to determine in a study of the population genetic structure at time moment t. Since the genetic structure formation is modelled by independent random sampling of gametes, the current average number of heterozygotes is only defined by the allele concentrations in the parent population, in accordance with the formula (7.3) for any time moment t. Therefore, it is impossible to infer any conclusion about duration of the genetic drift process (and the related value of the inbreeding rate) from a study of heterozygosity in a locus under concern at a particular time moment.

It is clear from (7.2) that $E\{\mathbf{x}(t+\tau)|\mathbf{x}(t)\}=\mathbf{x}(t), \tau \geq 0$. Making use of this fact, let us find the correlation function of the process. By using the complete probability formula and taking the constant $\mathbf{x}(t)$ out of the conditional expectation sign, we have:

$$\{\mathbf{x}(t)\mathbf{x}^T(t+\tau)\} = E\{\mathbf{x}(t)E\{\mathbf{x}^T(t+\tau)|\mathbf{x}(t)\}\} = E\{\mathbf{x}(t)\mathbf{x}^T(t)\}\,, \tag{7.10}$$

where $\mathbf{x}$ denotes a column vector and $\mathbf{x}^T$ a row vector. Hence, the correlation function of the process takes on the matrix form:

$$\mathbf{K}(t_1, t_2) = E\{\mathbf{x}(\min\{t_1, t_2\})\mathbf{x}^T(\min\{t_1, t_2\})\} - \mathbf{p}\mathbf{p}^T = \tag{7.11}$$

$$= \| k_{ij}(t_1, t_2) \|\,,$$

where

$$k_{ij}(t_1, t_2) = \left(1 - \exp\left\{\frac{-\min\{t_1, t_2\}}{2N}\right\}\right)(\delta_{ij}p_i - p_j)\,.$$

It follows from (7.2) that expected increments during any intervals of time are zero, so that the covariance of the increments on disjoint time intervals (t_1, t_2) and (t_3, t_4) is equal to

$$\mathrm{cov}\{x_i(t_2) - x_i(t_1)\,, x_j(t_4) - x_j(t_3)\} =$$

$$= E\{x_i(t_2)x_j(t_4) - x_i(t_2)x_j(t_3) - x_i(t_1)x_j(t_4) + x_i(t_1)x_j(t_3)\}\,.$$

To be definite, we put $t_1<t_2<t_3<t_4$. By (7.10)

$$E\{x_i(t)x_j(t')\} = E\{x_i(\min\{t, t'\}x_j(\min(t, t'\})\} .$$

Therefore, the expectations of the terms like $x_i(t')x_j(t'')$ are mutually cancelled and the covariance equals zero. So, the genetic drift process is a process with uncorrelated increments.

By using (7.9) and (7.11) we find the normalized correlation function, $\|\rho_{ij}(t_1, t_2)\|$, to be

$$\rho_{ij}(t_1, t_2) = \begin{cases} \left[\dfrac{1-\exp\{-\min\{t_1, t_2\}/(2N)\}}{1-\exp\{-\max\{t_1, t_2\}/(2N)\}}\right]^{1/2}, & i=j; \\ \left[\dfrac{1-\exp\{-\min\{t_1, t_2\}/(2N)\}p_ip_j}{1-\exp\{-\max\{t_1, t_2\}/(2N)\}(1-p_i)(1-p_j)}\right]^{1/2}, & i\neq j. \end{cases}$$

11.8. Fundamental Solution to the Kolmogorov Equations

Following M. Kimura, we consider the two-allele case. In accordance with (1.2a), the forward equation has the form

$$\frac{\partial}{\partial t}f(p, x, t) = \frac{1}{2}\frac{\partial^2}{\partial x^2}\left[\frac{x(1-x)}{2N}f(p, x, t)\right],$$

$$f(p, x, 0) = \delta(x-p) . \tag{8.1}$$

Application of the Fourier method results in a solution of the form

$$f(p, x, t) = \sum_{n=1}^{\infty} C_nX_n(x)\, e^{-\lambda_n t},$$

where C_n are constants, λ_n are eigenvalues, and each function $X_n(x)$ satisfies the ordinary differential equation

$$x(1-x)\frac{d^2X_n}{dx^2} + 2(1-2x)\frac{dX_n}{dx} - (2-4N\lambda_n)X_n = 0 . \tag{8.2}$$

This equation is a particular case of the hypergeometric equation

$$x(1-x)\frac{d^2X}{dx^2} + [\gamma-(\alpha+\beta+1)x]\frac{dX}{dx} - \alpha\beta X = 0 \tag{8.3}$$

with $\gamma=2$, $\alpha+\beta=3$, $\alpha\beta=2-4N\lambda$, i.e.

$$\alpha = \left(3+\sqrt{1+16N\lambda}\right)/2,\quad \beta = \left(3-\sqrt{1+16N\lambda}\right)/2 .$$

Note that the flow values at the bounds x=0 and x=1 must be finite. By (10.3.16) and (8.1) these values are equal to $-f(p, 0,t)$ and $f(p, 1,t)$ respectively. The solution of (8.2) should, therefore, be also finite in those points. Of two independent solutions to the Equation (8.3), only one given by the hypergeometric function $F(\alpha, \beta, 2, x)$ is finite at x=0. We apply the formula relating a value of F near the singular point x=0 to that near the singular point x=1:

$$F(\alpha, \beta, 2, x) = \frac{\Gamma(2)\Gamma(2-\alpha-\beta)}{\Gamma(2-\alpha)\Gamma(2-\beta)} F(\alpha, \beta, -1+\alpha+\beta, 1-x) + $$
$$+ \frac{\Gamma(2)\Gamma(\alpha+\beta-2)}{\Gamma(\alpha)\Gamma(\beta)} (1-x)^{2-\alpha-\beta} F(2-\alpha, 2-\beta, 3-\alpha-\beta, 1-x) .$$

Since

$$F(\alpha, \beta, \gamma, x) = 1 + \frac{\alpha\beta}{\gamma} x + \frac{\alpha(\alpha+1)\beta(\beta+1)}{2!\, \gamma(\gamma+1)} x^2 + \ldots,$$

$F(\alpha, \beta, 2, x)$ remains finite as $x \to 1$ only when β equals zero or a negative integer and (as $\alpha+\beta=3$) $2-\alpha$ is negative integer, too. Then λ can clearly take on the following values only:

$$\lambda_n = n(n+1)/(4N), \quad n = 1, 2, \ldots . \tag{8.4}$$

The corresponding eigenfunctions are:

$$X_n = F(2+n, 1-n, 2, x), \quad n = 1, 2, \ldots . \tag{8.5}$$

It is now convenient to pass from the hypergeometric function to the Gegenbauer ones, T^1_{n-1}:

$$T^1_{n-1}(y) = \frac{n(n+1)}{2} F\left(n+2, 1-n, 2, \frac{1-y}{2}\right),$$

where y=1-2x. Thus,

$$X_n(x) = T^1_{n-1}(y)$$

and the solution to (8.1) can be rewritten as

$$f(p, x, t) = \sum_{n=1}^{\infty} C_n T^1_{n-1}(y) \exp\left\{\frac{-n(n+1)t}{4N}\right\}. \tag{8.6}$$

The constants C_n can be found from the initial condition

$$f(p, x, 0) = \sum_{n=1}^{\infty} C_n T^1_{n-1}(y) = \delta(x-p) . \tag{8.6a}$$

Since the Gegenbauer functions, weighted by $(1-y^2)$, are orthogonal in the interval $(-1, 1)$, i.e.

$$\int_{-1}^{1} (1-y^2)T^1_m(y)T^1_{n-1}(y)\,dy = \frac{2n(n+1)}{2n+1}\delta_{m,n-1},$$

multiplication of both sides of (8.6a) by $(1-y^2)T^1_{n-1}(y)$ and integration over the interval (-1, 1) result in

$$2[1-(1-2p)^2]T^1_{n-1}(1-2p) = C_n\frac{2n(n+1)}{2n+1}.$$

Hence,

$$C_n = 4p(1-p)\frac{2n+1}{n(n+1)}T^1_{n-1}(1-2p).$$

Finally, the solution to (8.1) can be written in the form

$$f(p,x,t) = \frac{(2n+1)[1-(1-2p)^2]}{n(n+1)}T^1_{n-1}(1-2p)\times$$
$$\times T^1_{n-1}(1-2x)\exp\left\{\frac{-n(n+1)t}{4N}\right\} \tag{8.7}$$

or, by means of the hypergeometric functions,

$$f(p,x,t) = p(1-p)\sum_{n=1}^{\infty} n(n+1)(2n+1)F(1-n,n+2,2,p)\times$$
$$\times F(1-n,n+2,2,x)\exp\{-n(n+1)t/(4N)\} =$$
$$= 6p(1-p)\exp\left\{-\frac{t}{2N}\right\} + 30p(1-p)(1-2p)(1-2x)\exp\left\{-\frac{3t}{2N}\right\} + \ldots \tag{8.8}$$

It is clear that, as $t\to\infty$,

$$f(p,x,t) \sim 6p(1-p)\exp\{-t/(2N)\},$$

which is in accord with the result (3.8) obtained before. The calculations show that this asymptotic approximation is correct for $t \geq 2N$ when $p=0.5$ (and about one half of all trajectories reach the boundaries). But if $p=0.1$, then the time must be more than $4N$–$5N$ generations, when 90% of trajectories is now terminated with absorption.

By integrating the flows in accordance with (10.3.19) and (10.3.20) or by solving the backward Kolmogorov equation, one can find the fixation (U_1) or loss (U_0) probabilities till a moment t for the allele under concern:

$$U_1(p,t) = p + \sum_{n=1}^{\infty}(2n+1)p(1-p)(-1)^n\times$$
$$\times F(1-n,n+2,2,p)\exp\{-n(n+1)t/(4N)\}, \tag{8.9}$$

$$U_0(p,t) = 1-p+\sum_{n=1}^{\infty}(2n+1)p(1-p)(-1)^n\times$$

$$\times F(1 - n, n+2, 2, 1 - p) \exp\{-n(n + 1)t/(4N)\} . \tag{8.10}$$

By means of a biorthogonal polynomial system on Σ one may succeed in finding the fundamental solution even for an arbitrary number of alleles, the solution having a highly tedious form though. Therefore, to solve the problems considered above, it is reasonable to use the techniques capable of yielding the results in the most simple way.

11.9 A Random Genetic Drift Model with Two Loci

Now we pass to analyzing the genetic drift behavior of frequencies of the gametes classified with respect to two autosomal loci. While the random variation in gamete frequencies at the change of generation occurs, as before, due to the sampling nature of the offsrpring population formation (i.e. due to an undirected process), the drift coefficients will no longer be zero in the diffusion model. Gametes of one type can spring up from those of other types as a result of combining alleles from different gametes of the diploid parent into a gamete of the offspring. This phenomenon occurs due to recombination process when both loci are in one linkage group or due to independent segregation chromosomes, otherwise. Mathematically, the both cases can be described in the same way, by means of parameter r, the occurrence probability of a recombinant gamete.

Let there be n_1 alleles at the first locus and n_2 alleles at the second one. By $\Gamma_{i_1k_2}$ we designate a gamete carrying the i_1th allele at the first locus and the k_2th allele at the second one, and by $p_{i_1k_2}(x_{i_1k_2})$ the initial (current) frequency of this gamete in the population. The gamete $\Gamma_{i_1j_2}$ can be produced by recombination $\Gamma_{i_1k_2}$ and $\Gamma_{l_1j_2}$ having arbitrary k_2 and l_1. Under the Hardy-Weinberg principle the probability of the genotype $\Gamma_{i_1k_2}\Gamma_{l_1j_2}$ occurrence in the population is $p^2_{i_1k_2}$ when $i_1=l_1$ and $k_2=j_2$, and $2p_{i_1k_2}p_{l_1j_2}$ otherwise (with $p_{i_1k_2}$ denoting a concentration of gamete $\Gamma_{i_1k_2}$ in the population). In the case of recombination the genotype under concern yields the gamete $\Gamma_{i_1k_2}$ with the unit probability when $i_1=l_1$ and $k_2=j_2$, and with the probability 1/2 otherwise. Thus, the probability of $\Gamma_{i_1j_2}$ occurrence is equal (by the arbitrariness of k_2 and l_1) to

$$\sum_{k_2=1}^{n_2}\sum_{l_1=1}^{n_1} rp_{i_1k_2}p_{l_1j_2} = rp_{i_1}p_{j_2},$$

where

$$p_{i_1} = \sum_{k_2=1}^{n_2} p_{i_1k_2}, \quad p_{j_2} = \sum_{l_1=1}^{n_1} p_{l_1j_2}.$$

Here p_{i_1} and p_{j_2} denote the frequencies of the i_1th and j_2th alleles at the first and second loci respectively. In the absence of recombination (the probability of this event being equal to $1-r$), the concentration of any gamete remains clearly unchanged. Treated deterministically, the probabilities of genotypes and gametes should coincide with their frequencies. Therefore, the concentration of gamete $\Gamma_{i_1j_2}$ after recombination will equal

$$\tilde{p}_{i_1j_2} = (1-r)p_{i_1j_2} + rp_{i_1}p_{j_2}\,.$$

The correspondent component of the drift vector in the diffusion model will consequently be

$$M_{i_1j_2} = -r(p_{i_1j_2} - p_{i_1}p_{j_2}) = -\,rD_{i_1j_2} \tag{9.1}$$

The generating operator for the two-locus genetic drift process has the form

$$\mathfrak{A} = \frac{1}{2}\sum_{i_1k_2}\sum_{l_1j_2} \frac{p_{i_1k_2}(\delta_{i_1l_1}\delta_{k_2j_2} - p_{l_1j_2})}{2N} \frac{\partial^2}{\partial p_{i_1k_2}\,\partial p_{l_1j_2}} - r\sum_{i_1j_2} D_{i_1j_2}\frac{\partial}{\partial p_{i_1j_2}}, \tag{9.2}$$

where $D_{i_1j_2}$ is found from (9.1) to be

$$D_{i_1j_2} = p_{i_1j_2} - p_{i_1}p_{j_2} \tag{9.3}$$

and is called *a coefficient of linkage disequilibrium.* If we represent each gamete as a random integer-valued vector whose coordinates, ξ_{1i} and ξ_{2j}, take on values 1 or 0 in the presence or absence of the correspondent alleles at the first and second loci, then $D_{i_1j_2}$ will represent the covariance of ξ_{1i} and ξ_{2j}. The value of $D_{i_1j_2}$ shows a deviation from independence in combinations of alleles at different loci in the gamete.

The two-locus model of genetic drift still preserves the useful property to be invariant under non-distinction of several gamete types. One may sum, for example, frequencies of the gametes containing a number of non-distinct alleles at one of the loci and consider them to be a new, 'artificial' allele. The dynamic behavior in such a 'combined' model is determined by a generating operator of the (9.2) type. When all the alleles at one of the loci are considered non-distinct, the model reduces to the single-locus one with a generating operator of the (1.1) type.

Making use of this property of the genetic drift process, we may simplify the study of coefficients $D_{i_1j_2}$'s behavior. To do so, it is sufficient to consider only the following four gamete types: $\Gamma_{i_1j_2}$, $\Gamma_{i_1\bar{j}_2}$, $\Gamma_{\bar{i}_1j_2}$, $\Gamma_{\bar{i}_1\bar{j}_2}$, where a bar above an allele number indicates that the allele is absent in the gamete. We denote the frequencies of these gametes respectively by p_1, p_2, p_3, and p_4. Then the more usual expressions spring up for $\{D_{i_1j_2}\}$:

$$D_{i_1j_2} = p_1p_4 - p_2p_3 = D,$$

$$D_{\bar{i}_1j_2} = D_{i_1\bar{j}_2} = -\,D,\;\; D_{\bar{i}_1\bar{j}_2} = D\,,$$

and the operator (9.2) takes on the form:

$$\mathfrak{A} = \frac{1}{4N}\sum_{i,\,j=1}^{3} p_i(\delta_{ij} - p_j) - rD\left(\frac{\partial}{\partial p_1} - \frac{\partial}{\partial p_2} - \frac{\partial}{\partial p_3}\right). \tag{9.4}$$

The expectation $E_t\{D_{i_1j_2}\}$ can be found from Equation (3.4) as

$$\frac{d}{dt}E_t\{D_{i_1j_2}\} = E_t\{\mathcal{Q}D_{i_1j_2}\} = -\left(\frac{1}{2N}+r\right)E_t\{D_{i_1j_2}\}\ ,$$

$$E_0\{D_{i_1j_2}\} = D^0_{i_1j_2}\ . \tag{9.5}$$

The known solution to this equation is given by

$$E_t\{D_{i_1j_2}\} = D^0_{i_1j_2}\exp\left\{-\left(\frac{1}{2N}+r\right)t\right\}\ . \tag{9.6}$$

It differs from the solution (9.1.14) to the deterministic model by the term $1/(2N)$ in the exponential, which is fairly insignificant. In the limit as $t\to\infty$, the expectation of $D_{i_1j_2}$ equals zero.

As shown in Section 11.4, the homozygosity will be reached with the unit probability at each locus, so that, in the two-locus model, the process comes inevitably to fixation of one of the gametes. The fixation probability for $\Gamma_{i_1j_2}$ is clearly equal to $E_\infty\{x_{i_1j_2}\}$. From Equation (3.4) and expression (9.6) it follows that

$$\frac{d}{dt}E_t\{x_{i_1j_2}\} = E_t\{\mathcal{Q}x_{i_1j_2}\} = E_t\{-rD_{i_1j_2}\} =$$

$$= -rD^0_{i_1j_2}\exp\left\{-\left(\frac{1}{2N}+r\right)t\right\}\ ,$$

$$E_0\{x_{i_1j_2}\} = p_{i_1j_2}\ . \tag{9.7}$$

The solution to (9.7) is given by

$$E_t\{x_{i_1j_2}\} = p_{i_1j_2} - \left(1-\exp\left\{-\left(\frac{1}{2N}+r\right)t\right\}\right)\frac{2Nr}{1+2Nr}D^0_{i_1j_2}\ . \tag{9.8}$$

In the limit as $t\to\infty$, we obtain the known expression for the probability, $U_{i_1j_2}$, of the gamete $\Gamma_{i_1j_2}$ fixation:

$$U_{i_1j_2} = p_{i_1j_2} - \frac{2Nr}{1+2Nr}D^0_{i_1j_2}\ . \tag{9.9}$$

Since the limiting genetic state of the population will be completely homogeneous, the coefficient $D_{i_1j_2}$ vanishes eventually along any trajectory of the process. It is interesting to find the total of the expected values of this coefficient in the course of reaching the genetic homogeneity. Integration of both sides of equation (9.5) along the t-axis from 0 to ∞ yields

$$\int_0^\infty \frac{d}{dt}E_t\{D_{i_1j_2}\}\,dt = -\left(\frac{1}{2N}+r\right)\int_0^\infty E_t\{D_{i_1j_2}\}\,dt.$$

Since the integral in the left side equals $E_\infty\{D_{i_1j_2}\}-D^0_{i_1j_2}$, while the value of $E_\infty\{D_{i_1j_2}\}$ being zero by (9.6), we have the expected covariance of the allele in the whole course of genetic drift process equal to

$$\int_0^\infty E_t\{D_{i_1j_2}\}\,dt = \frac{2N}{1+2Nr} D^0_{i_1j_2} \,. \tag{9.10}$$

We emphasize that the formula (9.6) showing the expected covariance of the allele at different loci involves no current concentrations of the alleles or gametes but their (non-observable in an examination) initial values. It is thus impossible to make a conclusion about the duration of the genetic drift process from a study of interlocus disbalance in a single population.

11.10 Notes and Bibliography

Section 11.1.
A diffusion equation was first applied to a study of the genetic drift process by R. Fisher in his paper:
Fisher R.A.: 1922, On the dominance ratio, *Proc. Roy. Soc. Edinb.* **42**,.321–341,
where the independent variable was represented by the function, arccos (1-2p), of the gene frequency p.
The drift coefficient was written down with an error that was corrected in the further monograph:
Fisher R.A.: 1930, *The Genetical Theory of Natural Selection*. Oxford: Clarendon Press.

Section 11.2.
The proof presented for the approximation of the angle distance θ follows the paper::
Malyutov, M.B. and Passekov, V.P.: 1971, *On the Reconstruction of the Genealogical Tree of Isolated Populations*. Interdept. Laboratory of Statistical Methods, Moscow State University, preprint No. 19, 52 pp. (in Russian, with English summary),
where the drift in the Dunkers isolate was studied; see also:
Malyutov, M., Passekov, V., and Rychkov, Yu.: 1972, On the reconstruction of evolutionary trees of human populations resulting from random genetic drift. In: Weiner, J.S., and J. Huizinga (eds.), *The Assesment of Population Affinities in Man*. Clarendon Press, Oxford, pp. 48–71.
The data on blood groups in the isolate of Dunkers were obtained in:
Glass B., Sacks M., Jahn E., and Hess C.: 1952, Genetic drift in a religious isolate: an analysis of the causes of variation in blood group and other gene frequencies in small populations, *Amer. Natur.* **86**, No. 828, pp. 145–159.
Based on that approximation, there are several methods to analyze the origin of related populations, which are surveyed in:
Passekov, V.P.: 1978, *Rodstvo i geneticheskaya blizost populyatsij (Kinship and genetical similarity of populations)*. Itogi Nauki i Techniki, VINITI, USSR Acad. Sci., Moscow, 'Mathematical Biology and Medicine' Series, Vol. 1, pp. 166–209 (in Russian).

Section 11.3.
The asymptotics of the fundamental solution as $t\to\infty$ in the multidimensional case were studied by M. Kimura:
Kimura M.: 1955, Random genetic drift in multi-allelic locus, *Evolution* **9**, No. 4, 419–435.

Section 11.4.
The fixation and loss probabilities for alleles at a multi-allele locus were considered by Littler and Good in a model of neutral mutations:
Littler, R.A. and Good, A.J.: 1978, Ages, extinction times and first passage probabilities for a multi-allele diffusion model with irreversible mutation, *Theor. Pop. Biol.* **13**, No. 2, 214–225,
from which the results cited in the Section follow.

Section 11.5.
The mean absorption time for a diallelic locus was obtained by A.N. Kolmogorov; the result, however was not published but was cited in a footnote at the paper by A.A. Malinovsky:

Malinovsky, A.A.: 1947, *Biologicheskie i sotsialnye faktory v proiskhozhdenii rasovykh razlichiy u cheloveka.* (*Biological and social factors of racial differentiation in man*). Priroda, No. 7, pp. 40–48 (in Russian).

The homozygosity attainment time in the multi-allele case (its first four moments) was studied in:

Passekov, V.P.: 1974, Zamechaine otnositelno opredeleniya pervykh momentov vremeni dostizhenii nejtralnogo lokusa (A note on derivation of first moments for the homozygosity attainment time at a neutral locus of a finite population), – *Genetika*, **10**, No. 2, pp. 162–170 (in Russian).

The presentation of methods to determine the characteristics of the time to lose (to fix) a number of alleles follows the paper by R. Littler quoted above and the paper:

Littler, R.A.: 1975, Loss of variability at one locus in a finite population, – *Math. Biosci.* **25**, N. 1-2, pp. 151–163.

The mean time to lose a number of alleles was determined from equation (5.12) in the note:

Passekov V.P.: 1978, *Srednee vremya uteri allelej v resultate gennogo dreifa v konechnoj populatsii* (*The mean alleles loss time in the genetic drift process in a finite population*). In: Doklady MOIP. Obscaya biologiya, 1976. Sektsiya antropologii, biofiziki, vitaminologii, genetiki, gerontologii, gistologii i embriologii, istorii estestvoznaniya, Komissiya po primeneniyu matematiki v biologii Moskovskogo obsciestva isptatelei prirody (MOIP Reports. General Biology, 1976. Sections of Anthropology, Biophysics, Vitaminology, Genetics, Histology and Embryology, and Natural Sciences History, Commission on Application of Mathematics in Biology of the Moscow Society of Naturalists).Moscow State University, pp. 218–220 (in Russian)

Section 11.6.

The derivation of the sojourn time and allele age density functions follows the work:

Maruyama, T.: 1974, The age of an allele in a finite population, *Genetical Res.* **23**, No. 2, pp. 137–143.

Section 11.7.

The approach in use was substantiated in the note:

Passekov V.P.: 1975, *Odin podkhod k issledovaniju protsessov diffuzii v genetike* (*An approach to the investigation of diffusion processes in genetics*), Interdept. Laboratory of Statistical Methods, Moscow State University (Moscow, USSR), 49, pp. 63–68 (in Russian).

Section 11.8.

The fundamental solution in the two-allele case was obtained by M. Kimura in:

Kimura M.: 1955, Solution of a process of random genetic drift with a continuous model, *Proc. Nat. Acad. Sci. U.S.A*, **41**, No. 3, pp. 144–150.

In the multi-allele case, the solution was obtained by R. Littler and E. Fackerell in:

Littler R.A. and Fackerell E.D.: 1975, Transition densities for neutral multi-allele diffusion models.*Biometrics*, 31, No. 1, pp. 117–123.

In a different way, the problem was solved in the paper:

Griffiths R.C.: 1979, A transition density expansion for a multi-allele diffusion model, *Adv. Appl. Probab.* **11**, No. 2, pp. 310–325.

The approach to study the expectation of the linkage disequilibrium coefficient was presented in the paper:

Ohta T.: 1974, Linkage disequilibrium and associative overdominance due to random genetic drift, *Japanese J. Genetics*, **46**, No. 3, pp. 195–206.

Chapter 12

Properties of Single-Locus Models under Several Microevolutionary Pressures

12.1. Kolmogorov Equations in Case of Several Microevolutionary Conditions

The narrow-sense genetic drift model considered above is a kind of starting or reference point in a study of the effect a microevolutionary pressure has on the fate of a population. This role is similar to that of the random mating (panmixia) model among deterministic models of population genetics.

Effects of other microevolutionary factors, besides of random fluctuations in gamete frequencies at the change of generation, are included, as was shown in Section 10.4, into the drift coefficients of a diffusion model (provided the factors themselves have no stochastic features). The transfer to diffusion models means the transfer from a discrete time scale to a continuous one. Therefore, the influence of deterministic factors are described simpler than in discrete models, the order the factors act is irrelevant, the combined effect being reduced to mere summation of effects by individual factors (e.g. selection, mutations, migrations, recombinations, etc.) acting at a proper stage of the population life-span. If, for instance, the increment of concentration p at the ith stage is equal to $\varepsilon f_i(p)$ (where f_i is a sufficiently 'good' function, $\varepsilon \sim 1/N$ and N is a population size), then the total increment during the entire life-span can be written as

$$\Delta p = \varepsilon f_1(p) + \varepsilon f_2[p + \varepsilon f_1(p)] +$$
$$+ \varepsilon f_3\{[p + \varepsilon f_1(p) + \varepsilon f_2[p + \varepsilon f_1(p)]\} + \ldots = \varepsilon \sum_i f_i(p) + o(\varepsilon)$$

and, in the limit as $N \to \infty$, the terms corresponding to $o(\varepsilon)$ are negligible.

The components f_i are usually assumed the same as those in deterministic models considered in Part I.

If, for example, the fitness of the genotype composed by gametes Γ_i and Γ_j is equal to a constant w_{ij} showing the selection pressure, then the ith component of the drift coefficient (for the concentration p_i of the ith gamete) equals

$$M_i^{(1)}(\mathbf{p}) = p_i[w_i(\mathbf{p}) - w(\mathbf{p})] \tag{1.1}$$

where $w_i(\mathbf{p})=\Sigma_{j=1}^n w_{ij}p_j$ is interpreted as the fitness of the ith of n gametes and $w(\mathbf{p})=\Sigma_{i,j=1}^n w_{ij}p_ip_j$ as the average fitness of the population.

Sometimes, the effect of selection under these conditions is described by the drift components in the form:

$$M_i^{(1)}(\mathbf{p}) = p_i[w_i(\mathbf{p}) - w(\mathbf{p})]/w(\mathbf{p}) \tag{1.2}$$

indicating the origin of the diffusion model from the discrete process.

In general, however, fitness values w_{ij} are not constant but depend on time moment, genetical structure of the population, etc. (see Section 12.8).

Migration effects are usually described by the 'island' model of S. Wright. Assumed in the model, there is a flow of migrants of constant intensity m from a large external (mainland) population were all gamete frequencies q_i are constant. The (island) population under concern is assumed invariable in size, i.e. regulated by some, e.g. ecological, mechanism or by emigration flow of the proper intensity. As a result of the migrations, the concentration of the ith gamete becomes equal to $mq_i+(1-m)p_i$ and the corresponding component of the drift coefficient (the increment in the concentration) is

$$M_i^{(2)}(\mathbf{p}) = m(q_i - p_i)\,. \tag{1.3}$$

Transitions between alleles caused by mutations are described by a stochastic matrix $\|\mu_{ij}\|$ whose entries μ_{ij} are interpreted as probabilities that allele A_j mutates into A_i. The product $\mu_{ij}p_j$ then represents the contribution from mutation of the jth allele type into the i-th one. As a result of mutation the frequency of allele A_i will, therefore, equal $\Sigma_{j=1}^n \mu_{ij}p_j$ (note that the sum includes both the contribution by allele A_n, whose concentration is taken as a dependent variable, and that by the allele A_i itself; $\mu_{ii}=1-\Sigma_{i,\,j\neq i}\mu_{ij}$ is interpreted as a probability that allele A_i has no mutation). This results in variation in concentration of the allele A_i (or of the ith gamete type if gametes are classified by a single locus) and the corresponding component of the drift being both equal to

$$M_i^{(3)}(\mathbf{p}) = \sum_{j=1}^{n} \mu_{ij}p_j - p_i\,. \tag{1.4}$$

As was shown in Section 11.9, the drift coefficient for gamete concentrations (when gametes are classified with respect to two loci) takes on the form

$$M_{i_1j_2}^{(4)}(\mathbf{p}) = r(1|2)(p_{i_1j_2} - p_{i_1}p_{j_2}) \tag{1.5}$$

due to a recombination with probability $r(1|2)$. Here the double subscript i_1j_2 referes to a gamete having the i_1th allele at the first locus and the j_2th allele at the second one, $p_{i_1j_2}$ is a concentration of this gamete, and p_{i_1}, p_{j_2} are concentrations of the alleles i_1 and j_2 respectively.

Reasoning along similar lines, we can also find the drift coefficient arising from joint action of inbreeding and selection, from some forms of selection depending on the genetic structure of the population, and so on. These situations are considered below.

The generating operator of a diffusion process corresponding to a certain combination of microevolutionary factors, has the following form:

$$\mathcal{A} = \frac{1}{2}\sum_{i,j} \frac{p_i(\delta_{ij} - p_j)}{2N} \frac{\partial^2}{\partial p_i \partial p_j} + \sum_i M_i(\mathbf{p}) \frac{\partial}{\partial p_i} \tag{1.6}$$

where N stands, as before, for the size of a diploid population, $M_i(\mathbf{p})$ are drift coefficients representing the sums of expressions of the (1.1)–(1.5) forms, each summand corresponding to one of the microevolutionary factors from the combination under concern.

The operator (1.6) can be considered as an operator with a small parameter $\varepsilon=1/(2N)$ at the diffusion coefficients:

$$\mathcal{A} = \frac{1}{2}\varepsilon \sum_{i,j} V_{ij}(\mathbf{p}) \frac{\partial^2}{\partial p_i \partial p_j} + \sum_i M_i(\mathbf{p}) \frac{\partial}{\partial p_i} . \tag{1.7}$$

Then it represents a small random perturbation of the dynamical system

$$dp_i/dt = M_i(\mathbf{p}) , \quad i = 1, 2, \ldots . \tag{1.8}$$

The notation form (1.7), with a small parameter ε, is useful in comparing asymptotic (as $\varepsilon \to 0$) results of the diffusion model with findings for the unperturbed dynamical system (1.8) (see Section 12.5). However, the findings, which are formulated below in terms of the process coefficients V_{ij} and M_i, do not require the smallness of random perturbations and are valid for a diffusion process in general.

The correspondence between a dynamical system (1.8) and its small diffusion disturbance (1.7) should be regarded in the sense that, for any finite interval of time, the random process trajectory deviates arbitrarily little from the deterministic one, with a probability arbitrarily close to unit, provided that ε is chosen sufficiently close to zero.

12.2. Probabilities of Allele Fixation

Note first of all that in a finite population, any form of selection with constant fitness coefficients leads inevitably to the population homozygosity. Since the change in genetic structure of a population under selection can be caused by differential contribution of various genotypes to the next generation, the selection acts upon the structure only when the latter is polymorphic and there are options to select. Therefore, the coefficient of the drift by selection is zero in homogeneous, homozygous states. Under this condition, as shown in Section 10.5, the genetic homogeneity is to be reached in the population in the course of time due to loss or fixation of alleles (the boundaries are capturing ones).

Let us investigate the influence of selection on allele fixation and loss probabilities. In the two-allele case, the mean fitness of a population can be shown (from the unit sum of all allele frequencies) to have the form

$$w(p) = w_{11}p^2 + w_{12}2p(1-p) + w_{22}(1-p)^2 , \tag{2.1}$$

where p is a concentration of the given (first) allele. With $\partial/\partial p = -\partial/\partial(1-p)$ in mind, it can be readily verified that the drift coefficient (1.2) admits the notation in the form

$$M(p) = p[\,w_1(p) - w(p)] \,/\, w(p) = p\frac{1}{2w(p)}\left\{\frac{\partial w}{\partial p} - \left[p\frac{\partial w}{\partial p} + (1-p)\frac{\partial w}{\partial(1-p)}\right]\right\} \quad (2.2)$$
$$= \frac{1}{2}p(1-p)\frac{1}{w(p)}\frac{dw(p)}{dp}$$

proposed since by S. Wright. As w depends linearly on fitness values $\{w_{ij}\}$, the drift value will not change when all the fitnesses are multiplied or divided by the same positive constant. In particular, $\{w_{ij}\}$ can be interpreted as probabilities that individuals are alive till a reproductive age and production of progeny. This property of the drift coefficients shows that different levels of selection hardiness (indicated by a measure of deviation of $\{w_{ij}\}$ from zero) are associated with the same random process of variation in gene frequencies. Being evaluated from the dynamics of allele proportions, the efficiency of selection is not defined by total elimination of individuals but is defined rather by their differential survival, i.e. by relations between fitness values $\{w_{ij}\}$. Owing to this fact, one can achieve certain simplicity in analytical derivation, for instance, by setting one of the fitnesses equal to unit or by making some other pertinent normalization of fitness values.

The fixation probability, $U_1(p)$, of the allele with initial concentration p (in terms of penalty functions it can be interpreted as the mean payment for the trajectory, the penalty being equal to zero inside (0, 1) and to 1 upon getting in the point x=1) satisfies the backward Kolmogorov equation

$$(\mathfrak{A}U_1)(p) = \frac{1}{2}\frac{p(1-p)}{2N}\frac{d^2U_1(p)}{dp^2} + \frac{1}{2}p(1-p)\frac{d\ln w(p)}{dp}\frac{dU_1(p)}{dp} = 0\,, \quad (2.3)$$
$$U_1(0) = 0,\ U_1(1) = 1\,.$$

After dividing both sides of (2.3) by $p(1-p)[dU_1(p)/dp]\,/(4N)$, we obtain the equation for $d/dp\ \ln U_1(p)$, from which it follows that $d/dp\ U_1(p) = Cw(p)^{-2N}$. Taking the boundary conditions into account, we find the known expression for the fixation probability:

$$U_1(p) = \int_0^p w(x)^{-2N}\,dx \,/ \int_0^1 w(x)^{-2N}\,dx\,. \quad (2.4)$$

Considered below are several particular cases of the formula (2.4).

Let fitness to be additive, i.e. $w_{ij} = s_i + s_j$. If we group the terms of (2.1) containing s_1 and those containing s_2, then the mean fitness will have the following form:

$$w(p) = 2[s_1 p + s_2(1-p)] = 2s_2(1+sp) = 2w_h(p)\,,$$

where $w_h(p)$ denotes the mean fitness of a haploid population with the same frequencies of the alleles whose fitness are equal to s_1 and s_2; $s = (s_1 - s_2)/s_2$ is a selection coefficient. Substitution of $w(p)$ into (2.4) yields proper integrals which result in

$$U_1(p) = [1-(1+sp)^{-(2N-1)}]/[1-(1+s)^{-(2N-1)}]\,. \quad (2.5)$$

It can be easily seen that, if the selection coefficient s is positive (i.e. selection favors the allele under concern), then the allele fixation probability is greater than p, its fixation probability in the neutral (i.e. random genetic drift) case. For a small s, by expanding the numerator and denominator of (2.5) into the power series up to the second-order terms in s, we obtain the following approximate expression for the fixation probability:

$$U_1(p) \sim p\,\frac{1-2Nsp}{1-2Ns} \sim p + 2Nsp(1-p)\,,$$

the product Ns being supposed small too.

When the fitnesses are multiplicative, i.e. $w_{ij}=s_i s_j$, it can be easily verified that

$$w(p) = [s_1 p + s_2(1-p)]^2 = s_2^2(1+sp)^2 = [w_h(p)]^2,$$

where $w_h(p)$ stands for the mean fitness of the haploid population, $s=(s_1-s_2)/s_2$ is a selection coefficient. This case is clearly equivalent to the previous one with a doubled drift coefficient, corresponding to the double increase in the population size (this follows also from (2.4)).

The general case of selection, unfortunately, does not admit any simple expression for the allele fixation or loss probabilities. An analogy, however, can be seen here between properties of the deterministic model and the diffusion one: if, for any non-trivial initial state, fixation of the allele occurs in the deterministic case, then its fixation probability in the diffusion model will be greater than that under the allele neutrality. To demonstrate this, let us substitute $\tilde{U}_1(p)=p$ into operator $\mathfrak{A}$ as a test function. We have

$$\mathfrak{A}p = \frac{1}{2}p(1-p)\frac{d}{dp}\ln w(p)\,.$$

Hence, by results presented in Section 10.8, the function $\tilde{U}_1(p)=p$ can be interpreted as the expected penalty till the moment of absorption, which is equal to $-1/2x(1-x)\mathrm{d}\ln w(x)/\mathrm{d}x$ at a point x, plus the expected penalty upon reaching a boundary: the penalty equals unit when reached is the point $x=1$, and equals zero otherwise. The second summand is clearly equal to the allele fixation probability, $U_1(p)$. Note further that the quantity $1/2x(1-x)\,\mathrm{d}/\mathrm{d}x \ln w(x)$ is a rate of allele frequency change under selection pressure in the corresponding deterministic model. The mean value of this rate, let it be denoted by E_1, is therefore considered as the mean value of selection pressure. The corresponding summand of the penalty function then equals $-E_1$, so that

$$p = U_1(p) - E_1\,. \tag{2.6}$$

It follows that the expected selection pressure till absorption is equal to the increment of the allele fixation probability as compared with the neutrality case. If $E_1$is positive, then $U_1(p)>p$.

Let the fitness coefficients comply with the condition that

$$w_{11} \geq w_{12} \geq w_{22}\,. \tag{2.7}$$

where at least one of the inequalities is strict. Note that the dominant and recessive types of allele interaction turn out to be particular cases of this scheme. If a concentration of the first allele equals p, then that of the second equals $1-p$, so that, when $p \neq 0,1$, we have:

$$dw(p)/dp = 2p(w_{11} - 2w_{12} + w_{22}) + 2(w_{12} - w_{22}) \geq$$
$$\geq 2p(-w_{12} + w_{22}) + 2(w_{12} - w_{22}) = 2(w_{12} - w_{22})(1-p) \geq 0, \quad (2.8)$$

where at least one of these inequalities must be strict since $p<1$ and the condition (2.7) holds. By the fundamental theorem of natural selection the mean fitness increases with time and, by (2.8), the same must be true for the concentration p (because of $dw/dt=(dw/dp)(dp/dt)$). Thus, for the deterministic model, we have obtained the known result: condition (2.7) guarantees fixation of the allele. At the same time, the condition (2.8) provides that the drift coefficient

$$M(p) = \frac{1}{2}p(1-p)\frac{d}{dp}\ln w(p)$$

is positive in (0, 1). Since E_1 represents the expected value of the function $M(p)$, it must be positive too and the inequality $U_1(p)>p$ actually follows from (2.6).

If we change the inequalities (2.7) into the contrary ones (which would correspond to loss of the allele in the deterministic model), the fixation probability will be apparently less than that in the neutral case.

In the deterministic model, of the most interest is a situation where the fitness of heterozygotes is superior than that of homozygotes (*overdominance*), guaranteeing a stable polymorphism in the population. In this case the drift is directed to the polymorphic equilibrium state p^*, i.e. it changes its sign in (0, 1). From (2.4) it can be easily seen that $U_1(p)$ increases monotically with p since the sign of its derivative coincides with that of $w(p)^{-2N}$, while the mean fitness $w(p)$ is positive. At the same time, the sign of the second derivative is opposite to that of $dw(p)/dp$ or, by (2.2), to the sign of $M(p)$. Therefore, the second derivative of $U_1(p)$ is negative at the left of the deterministic polymorphic equilibrium point p^* and positive at the right of p^*, the p^* itself being a point of inflection. The plot of $U_1(p)$ resembles an inverted S-shaped curve.

Shown in Figure 36 are the allele fixation probabilities (along the ordinate axis) for a finite-sized population as functions of the initial concentration p (along the abscissa axis): (*1*) the fixation probability in the absence of selection, and (2) the fixation probability under overdominance selection pressure. The population size is $N=15$, the fitness of each homozygote equals 1, that of the heterozygote equals 1.1.

If the curve intersects the bisectrix of the first quadrant (which represents the plot of the neutral allele fixation probability), then the p-coordinate of the intersection point divides the interval (0, 1) into two parts. When the initial concentration p lies in the left part, the allele fixation probability is greater than in the neutral case; but if p belongs to the right part, the fixation is more probable in the absence of selection.

This pattern is in agreement with the intuitive idea that in the left the drift 'helps' the allele frequency to increase (and to be fixed eventually) but 'hampers' it in the right. The situation takes place when the homozygote fitnesses are equal (or in general close

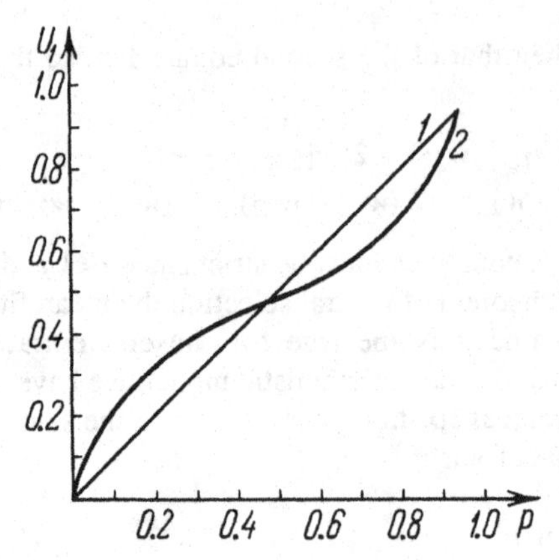

Fig. 36. Allele fixation probabilities in the absence of selection (*1*) and under overdominance conditions (2).

enough) to each other. Under overdominance, in fact, the mean fitness attains its maximum inside (0, 1) and its minima at the boundaries (the minimum is assumed to be $w(0)=w(1)$). By the mean-value theorem the denominator of the expression (2.4) for $U_1(p)$ can be written in the form $w(\tilde{p})^{-2N}$ where $\tilde{p}\in(0,1)$. Hence, $w(\tilde{p})>\{w(0),w(1)\}$. When written down by the Taylor formula for p close enough to zero, the numerator of (2.4) yields

$$U_1(p) = \int_0^p w(x)^{-2N}\,dx \Big/ \int_0^1 w(x)^{-2N}\,dx \sim \left[\frac{w(0)}{w(\tilde{p})}\right]^{-2N} p\,.$$

In case p is close to unit, we have

$$U_1(p) \sim \frac{w(\tilde{p})^{-2N} + w(1)^{-2N}(p-1)}{w(\tilde{p})^{-2N}}\,.$$

In both cases the coefficient at p is equal to $[w(x_B)/w(\tilde{p})]^{-2N}$, i.e. greater than unit as $w(p)$ reaches its minimum at the bounds of (0, 1). Since $U_1(p)$ is convex upwards at the left bound and downwards at the right one, the plot of $U_1(p)$ lies above the bisectrix in the left (enters the point (0, 0) with a tangent coefficient more than unit) and below the bisectrix in the right, the point of their inersection must therefore exists.

If we consider the case of lowered heterozygote fitness, with the mean fitness maximum attained at the boundary, then $U_1(p)$ will be convex downwards in the left and upwards in the right. When fitnesses of the homozygotes are close to each other, the interval (0, 1) can be divided into two parts of which the left one features the allele fixation probability less than in the neutral case (since the drift 'hampers' increase in concentration) and the right part features the probability that is greater.

When the drift in a diffusion model has the form (1. 1) without the normalizing denominator $w(p)$, it can be rewritten as

$$M(p) = \frac{1}{2}p(1-p)\frac{d}{dp}\, w(p) \,. \tag{2.9}$$

Note that the drift coefficient (2.9) will not change if all fitnesses are increased (or decreased) by a constant. Then the mean fitness will increase (or decrease) by the same constant, which will then vanish after differentiation. Therefore, the same random process of variation in gene frequencies appears to be associated with selection processes of different levels of hardiness, the efficiency of selection being determined by differences in the fitness of genotypes.

By solving the backward Kolmogorov equation (2.3) with the drift coefficient (2.9) we obtain the known expression for the allele fixation probability:

$$U_1(p) = \int_0^p e^{-2Nw(x)}\, dx \Big/ \int_0^1 e^{-2Nw(x)}\, dx. \tag{2.10}$$

In a particular case the fitnesses can be additive, i.e. $w_{ij}=s_i+s_j$. Due to the possibility to measure the fitness up to an additive constant, we may set $s_2=0$ (then the new value of s_1 will be equal to $s=s_1+s_2$). The mean fitness of the population will then have especially simple form

$$w(p) = 2sp = 2w_h(p) \,,$$

where $w_h(p)$ is the mean fitness of the corresponding haploid population. After inserting this expression of $w(p)$ into (2.10) we have

$$U_1(p) = (1 - e^{-4Nsp})/(1 - e^{-4Ns}) \,. \tag{2.11}$$

For small values of Ns the fixation probability can be approximated, as usual, by

$$U_1(p) \sim p + 2Nsp(1-p) \,.$$

As previously, there is no simple expression for the fixation probability in the general case of selection. Its increment, however, as compared with the neutrality case, still equals the expected value of selection pressure till the absorption moment. Thus, by reasoning along similar lines, the qualitative pattern of behavior in fixation probabilities can be shown to be the same as in situation considered above.

Generally, if the drift is written in the form

$$M(p) = \frac{1}{2}p(1-p)\frac{d}{dp}G(p) \,,$$

where $G(p)$ is not necessarily the mean fitness (the representation is always possible in the one-dimensional case, the function G being definable by formula (2.14)), then $G(p)$ sets up a qualitative pattern of behavior in the corresponding deterministic model, while defining the 'adaptive' surface (see Section 12.6) whose points of maximum concur with stable equilibrium states. The fixation probability in the diffusion model is still defined by the formula (2.10) where the function $w(p)$ is replaced by $G(p)$. The relation is also retained between the pattern of the 'adaptive' surface (the curve in the two-allele case) and the allele fixation probability.

As an example of this situation we may consider the case of selection in an inbred population. Recall that the heterozygote frequency then equals $2p(1-p)(1-F)$, while the frequency of each homozygous class is higher than that under panmixia by the quantity $Fp(1-p)$ where F denotes the coefficient of inbreeding. The population thus can be imagined as consisting of two parts. The first part (whose contribution into the total population equals $1-F$) is a common, random-mating, diploid population, where genotype frequencies are governed by the Hardy-Weinberg law. The second part (whose contribution equals F) consists exclusively of homozygous individuals whose concentrations are equal to frequencies of the correspondent alleles. It can be treated as a 'haploid' population with the allele fitnesses that are equal to those of the correspondent homozygotes. The drift coefficient will be equal to the weighted average of the drift from the diploid and haploid components:

$$M(p) = p\left[w_1^F(p) - w^F(p) \right] =$$

$$= p(1-p)\left[\frac{1}{2}\frac{\mathrm{d}}{\mathrm{d}p}(1-F)w(p) + \frac{\mathrm{d}}{\mathrm{d}p}Fw_h(p) \right] =$$

$$= \frac{1}{2}p(1-p)\frac{\mathrm{d}}{\mathrm{d}p}G(p)\,.$$

In this notation, $w_1^F(p)=(1-F)w_1(p)+Fw_{1h}(p)$ is a fitness of the given (first) allele consisting of its fitness in the diploid, $w_1(p)=w_{11}p+w_{12}(1-p)$, and the haploid, $w_{1h}(p)\equiv w_{11}$, parts of the population. Similarly, the mean fitness

$$w^F(p) = (1-F)w(p) + Fw_h(p)$$

consists of the value in the diploid ($w(p)$ is to be found by (2.1)) and the haploid, $w_h(p)=w_{11}p+w_{22}(1-p)$, components. The coefficient at $(1-F)$ will therefore be the common drift (2.2) from the diploid model with random mating, while that at F can be easily shown to be $\mathrm{d}w_h(p)/\mathrm{d}p$. As the final result, we have

$$G(p) = (1-F)w(p) + 2Fw_h(p)\,. \tag{2.12}$$

Note that $G(p)$ differs from the mean fitness by the multiplier 2 at $w_h(p)$. If fitnesses are additive, then $w=2w_h$ and $G=2w_h=w$, i.e. under the additivity condition the inbreeding does not have any effect on model coefficients. For a general form of selection, one should substitute $G(p)$ for $w(p)$ in (2.10) to determine the allele fixation probability $U_1(p)$; if G generates a stable polymorphic equilibrium p^* in the deterministic model, the plot of $U_1(p)$ then has inflection at this point and so on.

Along similar lines, we may find the function G associated with certain types of the frequency-dependent selection, which are considered below.

In terms of the drift and diffusion coefficients the allele fixation probability can be generally written in the following form:

$$U_1(p) = \int_0^p \exp\left\{-\frac{1}{\varepsilon}G(x)\right\} \mathrm{d}x \Big/ \int_0^1 \exp\left\{-\frac{1}{\varepsilon}G(x)\right\} \mathrm{d}x, \tag{2.13}$$

where

$$G(x) = \int^{x} \frac{2M(y)}{V(y)} dy = \int^{x} \frac{2M(y)}{y(1-y)} dy, \quad \varepsilon = \frac{1}{2N} . \tag{2.14}$$

Unfortunately, there are practically no findings on absorption probabilities for multidimensional processes (multiallelic or multilocus diffusion models).

12.3. Characteristics of the Homozygosity Attainment Time

When analyzing the mean homozygosity attainment time, we fail to derive a simple expressions even for the cases of additive or multiplicative fitnesses. In case of overdominance, the intuition prompts us to believe that the mean boundary attainment time should be greater than in the neutrality case since the drift is directed to an inner point, the deterministic polymorphic equilibrium state, and prevents the process from reaching a boundary. This is actually true under equal (sufficiently close to each other in general) fitnesses of homozygotes. To prove, let us consider the equation that governs the mean homozygosity attainment time, $T(p)$, i.e. the expectation of the penalty function (the right side of the equation $(\mathfrak{A}T)(p)=-h(p)$ taken with the opposite sing) being equal to unit inside (0, 1) and to zero at the boundary:

$$(\mathfrak{A}T)(p) = \frac{1}{2}\frac{p(1-p)}{2N}\frac{d^2T(p)}{dp^2} + \frac{1}{2}p(1-p)\frac{dw(p)}{dp}\frac{dT(p)}{dp} = -1 ,$$

$$T(0) = T(1) = 0 . \tag{3.1}$$

Insert the function

$$\tilde{T}(p) = -4N[p \ln p + (1-p) \ln (1-p)] ,$$

the mean homozygosity attainment time under the neutrality condition, into operator $\mathfrak{A}$ as a test function. Then the term with the second derivative turns into -1, since it corresponds to the neutrality operator, while

$$d\tilde{T}/dp = 4N \ln[(1-p)/p] .$$

Function $\tilde{T}(p)$ is consequently equal to the expected time the process stays in (0, 1), $T(p)$,plus the expected (till the absorption) values of the penalty, that, at a point x, equals $-1/2x(1-x)dw(x)/dx4N \ln[(1-x)/x]$. Let the second expectation be denoted by E; then

$$\tilde{T}(p) = T(p) + E .$$

Since $\ln [(1-x)/x]$ is positive when $x<1/2$, and negative when $x>1/2$ (i.e. its sign concurs with that of the drift, $1/2x(1-x)\, dw(x)/dx$, in the overdominance case under concern), it follows that E is negative as an expectation of the negative (excepting the point $x=1/2$) penalty function.

Therefore, $T(p)$, the mean heterozygosity attainment time, is greater than that in the neutrality case, $\tilde{T}((p)$.

If the fitness of homozygotes is lower than those of homozygotes (which are assumed equal), the drift and ln $[(1-x)/x]$ are opposite in sign. The value of E is therefore positive and, on the average, it takes less time to reach homozygosity than under the neutrality conditions, the conclusion being foreseeable since the drift is directed to the nearest boundary. It is paradoxically that, even under overdominance conditions, the mean homozygosity attainment time can be shown to be less than in the neutrality case if the homozygote fitnesses are distinct so as the deterministic equilibrium point lies outside the interval (0.2, 0.8). This indicates inadequacy of straightforward, heuristic conclusions originating from deterministic analogies.

In terms of the drift and diffusion coefficients, the mean absorption time is generally represented in the following way:

$$T(p) = \frac{1}{\varepsilon}\left[-\int_0^p Q(x)\int_0^x \frac{2\mathrm{d}y}{V(y)Q(y)}\,\mathrm{d}x + \frac{\int_0^1 Q(x)\int_0^x \frac{2\mathrm{d}y}{V(y)Q(y)}\,\mathrm{d}x}{\int_0^1 Q(x)\,\mathrm{d}x}\int_0^p Q(x)\,\mathrm{d}x \right], \tag{3.2}$$

where $Q(x)$ is defined by $Q(x) = \exp\{-G(x)/\varepsilon\}$.

The density function, $\Phi(p, x)$ of the time the process sojourns in point $x \in (0, 1)$ if starting from p, does not admit any simple expression in genetic models lacking the assumption of allele neutrality. The function is to be found from the equation

$$\frac{1}{2}\frac{p(1-p)}{2N}\frac{\mathrm{d}^2}{\mathrm{d}p^2}\Phi(p, x) + M(p)\frac{\mathrm{d}}{\mathrm{d}p}\Phi(p, x) = -\,\delta(p - x), \tag{3.3}$$

$$\Phi(0, x) = \Phi(0, 1) = 0\,.$$

Both bounds of the interval (0, 1) are supposed to be absorbing boundaries.

In terms of the process coefficients, the solution to (3.3) can be written in the following form (integration constants being determined from the boundary conditions with regard for continuity of $\Phi(p, x)$):

$$\Phi(p, x) = \begin{cases} \dfrac{4Ne^{G(x)/(2N)}}{x(1-x)}\,\dfrac{I(1) - I(x)}{I(1)}\,I(p), & p<x, \\[2ex] \dfrac{4Ne^{G(x)/(2N)}}{x(1-x)}\left[\dfrac{I(1) - I(x)}{I(1)}\,I(p) - I(p) + I(x)\right], & p\geq x, \end{cases}$$

where

$$I(y) = \int_0^y \exp\{-G(z)/(2N)\,\mathrm{d}z,\quad G(x) = \int_0^x \frac{2M(y)}{y(1-y)}\,\mathrm{d}y.$$

Note that $\exp\{-G(x)/(2N)\}/I(1)=dU_1(x)/dx$, where the fixation probability $U_1(x)$ is defined by formula (2.13), and $I(y)/I(1)=U_1(y)$. By using the relation $U_0(y)=1-U_1(y)$ for the loss probability of the allele, we rewrite the formula for the sojourn time density function in terms of the loss and fixation probabilities:

$$\Phi(p, x) = \begin{cases} 4N \dfrac{U_0(x)U_1(p)}{x(1-x)U_1'(x)}, & p<x, \\ 4N \dfrac{U_1(x)U_0(p)}{x(1-x)U_1'(x)}, & p\geq x. \end{cases} \tag{3.4}$$

Recall that, according to statement (10.7.7), the sojourn time density $\Phi^*(p, x)$ conditioned, for instance, on fixation of the allele, differs from the unconditional density by the multiplier $U_1(x)/U_1(p)$ (the multiplier will be equal to $U_0(x)/U_0(p)$ under condition of allele loss). As was remarked by T. Maruyama and M. Kimura, the density function of the time the process sojourn in states greater than an initial one, conditioned on allele fixation, turns out equal to that in the states lesser than initial, conditioned on allele loss. In fact, when inferring the density conditioned on fixation from the upper expression for $\Phi(p, x)$ in (3.4) and the density conditioned on loss from the lower one, we multiply the former by $U_1(x)/U_1(p)$ and the latter by $U_0(x)/U_0(p)$ and see the results being equal to the same function $4NU_0(x)U_1(x)/[x(1-x)\, U'_1(x)]$. This is true under any form of selection or other microevolutionary pressures resulting jointly in non-zero values of allele fixation or loss probabilities. It is interesting to note that the conditional density function of sojourn time does not depend on the initial state.

By means of $\Phi(p, x)$, the mean absorption time can be represented as a sum of the mean time the trajectory spends in the region where the allele concentration is less than initial, and the mean time spent in the complement to the region:

$$T(p) = 4NU_0(p) \int_0^p \frac{U_1(x)}{x(1-x)U_1'(x)}\, dx + 4NU_1(p) \int_p^1 \frac{U_0(x)}{x(1-x)U_1'(x)}\, dx\,. \tag{3.5}$$

12.4. Steady-State Probability Density Function for the Case of a Single Diallelic Locus

As was noted above, any microevolutionary conditions which define the drift being equal to zero at the boundaries, are incapable of sustaining the polymorphism endlessly in a finite-sized population. But if the drift at the boundaries is directed inside the interval (0, 1), then there exists (see Section 10.5) a probability distribution of population states, invariable in time (steady-state) and persisting infinitely long. Such a pattern of the drift can be caused, for instance, by effects of migrations from a polymorphic source or mutability of alleles. The state probability density function, $f(x)$, evolves usually to the steady-state one from any initial distribution. The steady-state distribution may be regarded as a probabilistic analogue to the equilibrium in the deterministic case.

Having the zero derivative with respect to time, the steady-state density function must satisfy the equation

$$(\mathfrak{A}^*f)(x) = \frac{1}{2}\frac{d^2}{dx^2}\left\{ \frac{x(1-x)}{2N} f(x)\right\} - \frac{d}{dx}[M(x)f(x)] = 0\,. \tag{4.1}$$

Since the flow of probability is absent in the steady state, the steady-state density can be found by setting the flow expression (10.3.16) equal to zero:

$$\frac{1}{2}\frac{d}{dx}\left[\frac{x(1-x)}{2N} f(x)\right] - M(x)f(x) = 0\,. \tag{4.2}$$

From this equation it follows that

$$f(x) = \frac{C}{x(1-x)} \exp\left\{2N \int^{x} \frac{2M(y)}{y(1-y)}\, dy\right\}, \tag{4.3}$$

where the constant C is determined by the condition that the integral of density over the interval (0, 1) equals unit. The multiplier $2N$ in the exponential function is the inverse to the coefficient $\varepsilon=1/(2N)$ indicating the intensity of random perturbations. The small parameter ε is separated from the diffusion coefficient to make the asymptotic study of the steady-state density function more convenient when the intensity of random perturbations tends to zero.

Recall that in genetic models the drift coefficient $M(y)$ is usually represented by the sum of contributions, $M^{(i)}(y)$, indicating effects of various microevolutionary factors. Since an integral of a sum equals the sum of the integrals, the contribution of the ith factor into the steady-state density is associated with the co-factor

$$\exp\left\{ 2N \int^{x} \frac{2M^{(i)}(y)}{y(1-y)}\, dy\right\} = \exp\,\{2NG_i(x)\}, \tag{4.4}$$

where

$$G_i(x) = \int^{x} \frac{2M^{(i)}(y)}{y(1-y)}\, dy\,. \tag{4.5}$$

The co-factor

$$\exp\{\,-\ln x\, - \ln\,(1-x)\} = 1/[x(1-x)]$$

is then related to the influence of genetic drift in the narrow sense when it is treated separately. This co-factor can be found by solving formally the Equation (4.2) with $M(y)\equiv 0$. Although the result makes no sense of the steady-state density (giving an additional warning against formal interpretation of a solution to Equation (4.2) as a steady-state distribution in case of arbitrary coefficients of the diffusion process), it indicates, nevertheless, the effect of the drift when other factors are also taken into account to provide the existence of a steady-state solution.

In general, if a steady-state density function is found for a combination of microevolutionary factors, then any additional factor results in a new multiplier of the form (4.4), i.e. there is no need to search for the entire steady-state density anew, but just determine the corresponding co-factor. If we succeed in determining, by merely formal reasons, the co-factors of the (4.4) type for a number of conceivable effects, then the steady-state density for an arbitrary combination of effects turn out mere multiplication of the co-factors corresponding to these effects (the existence problem, of course, must be solved independently).

Let us find, for example, co-factors which are associated with selection, mutation, and migrations' effects (the genetic drift effect, as remarked above, brings about the term $1/[x(1-x)]$). In Section 12.2 the drift coefficient due to selection was written down via $w(y)$, the mean fitness of the population, in the form

$$M^{(1)}(y) = \frac{1}{2} y\,(1-y)\,\frac{\mathrm{d}}{\mathrm{d}y}\,\ln w(y)\,,$$

which is appropriate for further considerations. Substitution of $M^{(1)}(y)$ into (4.4) results in the following expression:

$$\exp\{2NG_1(x)\} = \exp\{4N\frac{1}{2}\ln w(x)\} = w^{2N}(x)\,. \tag{4.6}$$

If the drift due to selection is written in the form

$$M^{1a}(y) = \frac{1}{2} y(1-y)\frac{\mathrm{d}}{\mathrm{d}y} w(y)\,,$$

then

$$\exp\{2NG_{1a}(x)\} = \exp\{2Nw(x)\}\,. \tag{4.7}$$

The joint action of random genetic drift and selection eventually leads the population to homozygosity. Migrations, bringing various types of alleles, are the factor that permits the population to sustain its polymorphism and provides the existence of a steady-state probability distribution. In the island model, the intensity of the interchange flow of migrants between the population ('island') and the outer source (with constant allele frequencies q and $1-q$) is assumed equal to a constant m. For the diallelic case the drift coefficient due to migrations (1.3) can be conveniently rewritten in the following form:

$$M^2(y) = m(q-y) = \frac{1}{2} y(1-y)\frac{\mathrm{d}}{\mathrm{d}y} 2m[q\ln y + (1-q)\ln(1-y)]\,.$$

Inserting this expression into (4.4), we find readily the corresponding co-factor for the steady-state probability density function:

$$\exp\{2NG_2(x)\} = x^{4Nmq}(1-x)^{4Nm(1-q)}\,. \tag{4.8}$$

Mutation is another factor providing the existence of a steady-state distribution. Let μ_{21} designates the probability that the allele in question undergoes mutation into the complement one and μ_{12} the probability of mutation in the inverse way. The drift coefficient (1.4) then takes on the form

$$M^{(3)}(y) = (1 - \mu_{21})y + \mu_{12}(1 - y) =$$
$$= \frac{1}{2}y(1 - y)\frac{d}{dy} 2[\mu_{21} \ln (1 - y) + \mu_{12} \ln y] .$$

Obtained from (4.4) and (4.5), the co-factor in the steady-state density function will be clearly equal to

$$\exp\{2NG_3(x)\} = x^{4N\mu_{12}}(1-x)x^{4N\mu_{21}} . \quad (4.9)$$

From these examples it can be seen that the drift coefficient due to the influence of the ith factor, $M^{(i)}(y)$, is to be written in the form

$$M^{(i)}(y) = y(1 - y)\frac{M^{(i)}(y)}{y(1-y)} = \frac{1}{2}y(1 - y)\frac{d}{dy} G_i(y) , \quad (4.10)$$

where, as before,

$$G_i(x) = \int^x \frac{2M^{(i)}(y)}{y(1-y)} dy.$$

Finally, the steady-state density function caused by several microevolutionary factors takes on the following form

$$f(x) = \frac{C}{x(1-x)} \prod_i \exp\{2NG_i(x)\} = \frac{C}{x(1-x)} \exp\{2NG(x)\} , \quad (4.11)$$

where $G(x)=\Sigma_i G_i(x)$. For example, when those factors are genetic drift in the narrow sense, selection, mutation, and migrations, considered along the above schemes, the steady-state density function will equal, as is known,

$$f(x) = Cw^{2N}(x)x^{4N(mq+\mu_{12})-1}(1 - x)^{4N[m(1-q)+\mu_{21}]-1} . \quad (4.12)$$

If the effects of mutation, or migrations, or even selection are neglected, the respective co-factors ought to be omitted in the expression of the steady-state density function.

12.5. Investigation of the Steady-State Probability Density Function for a Single Diallelic Locus

In the absence of selection the steady-state density function

$$f(x) = Cx^{4N(mq+\mu_{12})-1}(1 - x)^{4N[m(1-q)+\mu_{21}]-1} \quad (5.1)$$

is that of the beta-distribution with parameters a=$4N(mq+\mu_{12})$ and b=$4N[m(1-q)+\mu_{21}]$. The constant C is known to be determined from the equality

$$C^{-1}=\int_0^1 x^{a-1}(1-x)^{b-1}\,dx=B(a,b)\,, \tag{5.2}$$

where $B(a, b)$ can be expressed via the gamma-function as

$$B(a,b)=\Gamma(a)\Gamma(b)/\Gamma(a+b)\,. \tag{5.3}$$

Thus,

$$f(x)=\frac{\Gamma[4N(m+\mu_{12}+\mu_{21})]}{\Gamma[4N(mq+\mu_{12})]\Gamma[4N(m(1-q)+\mu_{21})]}\times$$

$$\times\, x^{4N(mq+\mu_{12})-1}(1-x)^{4N[m(1-q)+\mu_{21}]-1}\,. \tag{5.4}$$

The form of distribution $f(x)$ can be studied without the constant C, i.e. by analyzing the function $x^{a-1}(1-x)^{b-1}$. If $a<1$ (or $b<1$), then $f(x)$ infinitely increases near the left (or the right) boundary. When both a and b exceed unit, the density curve is one-vertex, having the maximum at the point

$$x_{\max}=\frac{a-1}{a+b-2}=\frac{4N(mq+\mu_{12})-1}{4N(m+\mu_{12}+\mu_{21})-2}\,.$$

If we consider the corresponding deterministic model without any perturbations by random effects,

$$dx/dt=m(q-x)+\mu_{12}-(\mu_{21}+\mu_{12})x, \tag{5.5}$$

then its stable equilibrium state appears to be

$$x^*=(mq+\mu_{12})/(m+\mu_{12}+\mu_{21}). \tag{5.6}$$

It can be easily seen that for a large population size N the maximum of the steady-state density function turns out practically at the point of stable deterministic equilibrium x^*. From (5.3) it follows that $\int_0^1 xf(x)\,dx$, the expectation for the beta-distribution, is equal to $B(a+1,b)/B(a,b)=a/(a+b)$ and coincides with the stable deterministic equilibrium point for any N. Similarly, the variance of the beta-distribution can also be expressed in terms of its parameters by the formula:

$$\sigma^2=ab/[(a+b)^2(a+b+1)]\,. \tag{5.7}$$

Since both a and b have the order of magnitude of $O(N)$, we have $\sigma^2=O(1/N)$. Thus, the variance in possible concentrations tends to zero when the population size increases, i.e. the density function shrinks to the deterministic equilibrium state.

Higher moments of beta-distribution can be found by the formula

$$E\{x^n\}=B(a+n,b)/B(a,b)\,,$$

where $B(a, b)$ can be expressed in terms of the gamma-function by formula (5.3).

Under selection pressure the steady-state probability distribution has a more complicated form and is no longer a beta-distribution. The normalizing constant C, highly tedious in its form, can be calculated from the condition that the integral of the density function over (0, 1) equals unit, i.e.

$$C^{-1} = \int_0^1 w(x)^{2N} x^{4N(mq+\mu_{12})-1} (1-x)^{4N[m(1-q)+\mu_{21}]-1} dx.$$

To calculate the integral at the right, recall that by (2.1) $w(x)$ is a polynomial in x and $(1-x)$. Raised to the power $2N$, it yields a sum of the terms like

$$\frac{(2N)!}{n_1!\, n_2!\, n_3!} w_{11}^{n_1} (2w_{12})^{n_2} w_{22}^{n_3} x^{2n_1+n_2} (1-x)^{n_2+2n_3}. \tag{5.8}$$

A contribution of any such term into the integral can be readily determined by formula (5.3) as it corresponds (without constants) to $\int_0^1 x^{k_1-1} (1\text{-}x)^{k_2-1} dx = B(k_1, k_2)$ for some k_1 and k_2. Thus,

$$C^{-1} = \sum \frac{(2N)!}{n_1!\, n_2!\, n_3!} w_{11}^{n_1} (2w_{12})^{n_2} w_{22}^{n_3} \frac{B(a+2n_1+n_2,\, b+n_2+2n_3)}{B(a,\, b)}, \tag{5.9}$$

where summation is performed over all triples of non-negative integers n_1, n_2, n_3 such that $n_1+n_2+n_3=2N$; a and b are equal, as before, to $4N(mq+\mu_{12})$ and $4N[m(1-q)+\mu_{21}]$, respectively.

Remark that the steady-state density function does not depend on hardiness of selection (if the hardiness is judged by deviation from zero in fitness coefficients w_{ij}). Indeed, multiplication of all the coefficients w_{ij} by a positive constant d will result in the co-factor $w^{2N}(x)$ increased d^{2N} times. Simultaneously, the normalizing constant C will decrease d^{2N} times (since the sum of exponents in the product (5.8) of fitness coefficients w_{ij} equals $2N$). Hence, by cancelling d^{2N}, we have the steady-state density unchanged.

According to (2.1) the mean fitness function $w(x)$ represents a quadratic trinomial. Its plot on [0, 1], being therefore a part of a parabola, is concave when the coefficient at x^2 is negative (this means that the heterozygote fitness is greater than the average of homozygote fitnesses). This case the curve $w(x)$ has only one vertex (the vertex being located strictly inside the interval (0, 1) under the overdominance condition). Double differentiation then shows that the plot of $2N \ln w(x)$ is also concave. If a and b exceed unit, then $\ln[x^{a-1}(1-x)^{b-1}]$ is a concave function too. Consequently, the logarithm of the steady-state density function (4.12) is concave and the steady-state distribution has a one-vertex density function.

Recall that in a general case the steady-state probability density function (4.11) has the form

$$f(x) = \frac{C}{x(1-x)} [\exp\{G(x)\}]^{2N},$$

where $G(x)$ corresponds to the joint action of microevolutionary factors considered. Since the co-factor $1/[x(1-x)]$ tends to infinity at boundaries and is not integrable on (0, 1), the function $\exp\{G(x)\}$ must converge to zero as x approaches a boundary to provide the integrability of $f(x)$. The rate at which $[\exp\{G(x)\}]^{2N}$ converges to zero obviously increases when the population size N does, and the contribution of the co-factor $1/[x(1-x)]$ into the steady-state density becomes vanishing at the boundaries as compared with that of $\exp\{2NG(x)\}$. This contribution is even less significant at a distance from the boundaries, where the function $1/[x(1-x)]$ is finite. Therefore, asymptotically for large values of N, the form of the steady-state density function is given by $\exp\{2NG(x)\}$. Moreover, if the function $G(x)$ has its own maximum at point x^*, then the asymptotic ratio of the steady-state density at x^* to its value at any other point x, $[\exp\{G(x^*)\}/\exp\{G(x)\}]^{2N}$, increases ad infinitum as $N\to\infty$. Thus, the steady-state density concentrates further at point x^* and it can be strictly shown to represent the delta-function $\delta(x-x^*)$ in the limit.

12.6. Steady-State Density Function and the Adaptive Landscape in the Two-Allele Case

According to the results presented above, the functions $G_i(x)$ and $G(x)=\Sigma_i G_i(x)$ determine to a considerable degree the form of the steady-state density function, which coincides with that of the function $C \exp\{2NG(x)\}$ asymptotically as $N\to\infty$. These functions are also important in calculating the allele fixation probabilities and the mean homozygosity attainment time. It would be convenient if the same functions could characterize, to some extent, also the deterministic models of population genetics. Fortunately, it turns out to be just the case, the relation between the stochastic model and the deterministic one being intuitively expected and quite visible in this situation.

Recall that a function $M^{(i)}(x)$ participating in the formula (4.5) for $G_i(x)$ represents the right-hand side of the Equation (1.8) defining an unperturbed dynamical system. A diffusion model springs up as a result of small random perturbations introduced into a deterministic scheme. According to the notation (2.2) for coefficient $M^{(i)}(x)$, a deterministic model to describe the influence of the ith microevolutionary factor takes on the form

$$\frac{dx}{dt} = M^{(i)}(x) = x(1-x)\frac{d}{dx}\frac{1}{2}G_i(x) \,. \tag{6.1}$$

Note that the function $G_i(x)$ is monotone non-decreasing along trajectories of (6.1):

$$\frac{d}{dt}G_i[x(t)] = \frac{1}{2}x(1-x)\left[\frac{d}{dx}G_i(x)\right]^2 \geq 0 \,, \tag{6.2}$$

since $x(1-x)>0$ in (0, 1). From (6.2) it can be shown that functions $G_i(x)$ define an 'adaptive landscape' for variations in gene frequencies in the corresponding dynamic model.

The term 'adaptive landscape' should not be treated in a mere biological sense, as a topography of the fitness, but in a wider sense, as a landscape where trajectories of the dynamical system, speaking teleologically, tend to occupy the peak, the highest point, that corresponds to a (local, may be) maximum of the function $G_i(x)$. Thus, the entire adaptive landscape characterizes globally the dynamics of the population genetic structure under the corresponding pressure. On the landscape, an inner point of equilibrium for Equation (6.1) coincides with a critical point of the function $G_i(x)$, the maximum being associated with a stable equilibrium and minimum with an unstable one, so that the pattern of $G_i(x)$ gives a qualitative insight into the behavior of solutions to (6.1). By means of functions $G_i(x)$ one can study, for example, the Lyapunov stability of equilibrium points x^* for the Equation (6.1), using $G_i(x^*)-G_i(x)$ as a Lyapunov function. The landscape in the two-allele case is merely a curve, namely, the plot of function $G_i(x)$.

In continuous-time genetic models, the right-hand side of a differential equation for a model with a joint action of several microevolutionary factors is represented by the sum where each term corresponds to the respective factor. Therefore,

$$\frac{dx}{dt} = \frac{1}{2}x(1-x)\frac{d}{dx}\sum_i G_i(x) = \frac{1}{2}x(1-x)\frac{d}{dx}G(x), \tag{6.3}$$

where $G(x)=\Sigma_i G_i(x)$. Obviously, $G(x)$ is monotone non-decreasing on trajectories of equation (6.3) and

$$\frac{d}{dt}G[x(t)] = \frac{1}{2}x(1-x)\left[\frac{d}{dx}G(x)\right]^2 \geq 0. \tag{6.4}$$

Thus, the function $G(x)$ defines the adaptive landscape for the case of joint action of several microevolutionary factors. Given the functions of the adaptive landscape, in other words, the objective functions $G_i(x)$ for each separate factor, the total objective function for any combination of them can be determined by mere summation of the adaptive landscape functions for all the factors entering the combination chosen. This greatly simplifies the analysis of joint influence exerted by several causes of change in the population genetic structure.

The notion of objective function introduced above may be regarded as a generalization of the Wright's adaptive topography principle and Fisher's fundamental theorem of natural selection. These author's findings were mostly concerned with the behavior of the population fitness, which, unlike the objective function, is readily interpretive in biological terms. This advantage, however, caused by the interpretation of the mean population fitness $w(x)$ as a per capita rate of population increase, is seeming to a certain extent. If, in fact, the fitness equals the logarithmic rate of population increase, it results in the exponential change (increasing infinitely or decreasing to zero) in the population size, which has little in common with biological reality. It is also known that inclusion of several microevolutionary causes besides selection results normally in breaking the monotone pattern of the mean fitness behavior. Free of this shortcoming, the objective functions preserve nevertheless an important (in the case of selection) property of giving insight into the pattern of possible changes in the population genetic structure.

The relation of objective functions with the form of the steady-state density function for population states is another important property of those functions. Roughly speaking, the population state looks so as if it were 'smeared' around the objective functions' peaks. If an objective function is chosen to be an argument of a monotone increasing function, the latter can itself be treated as an adaptive landscape function. Therefore, $\exp\{G(x)\}$ or $\exp\{2NG(x)\}$ could be taken instead of $G(x)$. According to (4.11) the steady-state density function differs from the objective function $\exp\{2NG(x)\}$ by the co-factor $1/[x(1-x)]$, i.e. is mostly determined by the function $G(x)$.

As was shown at the end of the previous section, the relative contribution of the co-factor $1/[x(1-x)]$ becomes vanishing for large N, the steady-state density function is asymptotically proportional to the objective function and concentrated about its peaks, which concur with maxima of $G(x)$. These maxima are attained at points corresponding to stable equilibrium states in the unperturbed dynamical system. Thus, small random perturbations of the dynamical system bring about the result anticipated by intuition: 'smearing' the population state about stable equilibrium points. Finally, in the limit as $N \to \infty$, the steady-state density concentrates entirely in the stable deterministic equilibrium state (if the state is unique) and equilibrium findings in the diffusion model coincide with those in the deterministic one.

12.7. Derivation of a Steady-State Density Function in the Case of Multiple Alleles

If there may be n alleles at a single autosomal locus, the equation for a steady-state probability density function for genetic states of a population takes on the following form:

$$\mathfrak{a}^* f = \frac{1}{2} \sum_{i,j=1}^{n-1} \frac{\partial^2}{\partial x_i \, \partial x_j} \left[\frac{x_i(\delta_{ij} - x_j)}{2N} f \right] - \sum_{i=1}^{n-1} \frac{\partial}{\partial x_i} [M_i(\mathbf{x}) f] = 0 . \tag{7.1}$$

In contrast to the diallelic case, we can no longer assert the steady-state flow vector of probability to be zero for any drift coefficients. Quite possible is a situation where the circulation takes place but the density still remains invariable in each point, as flows in different coordinate axes' directions compensate for each other (for instance, under mutations of the type $A_i \to A_{i+1} \to \ldots$ closed into a cycle). In this case we have to solve the Equation (7.1), for instance, by separation of variables.

In the important particular case where the flow equals zero, the problem is much simpler, however. By equating the flow coordinates with zero we have the following system of equations (see Section 10.7).

$$M_i(\mathbf{x}) f(\mathbf{x}) - \frac{1}{2} \sum_{j=1}^{n-1} \frac{\partial}{\partial x_j} \left[\frac{x_i(\delta_{ij} - x_j)}{2N} f(\mathbf{x}) \right] = 0 , \quad i = \overline{1, n-1} . \tag{7.2}$$

After dividing both sides of each equation by $f(\mathbf{x})$ and differentiating the terms under the summation sign, we come to the system of inhomogeneous linear algebraic equations for the gradient of the logarithmic steady-state density function:

$$\sum_{j=1}^{n-1} \frac{x_i(\delta_{ij}-x_j)}{2N} \frac{\partial}{\partial x_j} \ln f(\mathbf{x}) = 2\, M_i(\mathbf{x}) - \frac{1-nx_i}{2N},\quad i = \overline{1, n-1}\ . \tag{7.3}$$

The matrix of this linear system is represented by that of diffusion coefficients, whose reciprocal matrix is known to have the form

$$\left[\frac{1}{2N}\left\| x_i(\delta_{ij}-x_j)\right\|\right]^{-1} = 2N\left\|\frac{\delta_{ij}}{x_i}+\frac{1}{x_n}\right\|, \tag{7.4}$$

where $x_n = 1 - \Sigma_{i=1}^{n-1} x_i$.

The formal solution to the system (7.3) looks as

$$\text{grad} \ln f(\mathbf{x}) = 2\,N\left\|\frac{\delta_{ij}}{x_i}+\frac{1}{x_n}\right\|\left[2M(\mathbf{x}) - \frac{\mathbf{e}-n\mathbf{x}}{2N}\right], \tag{7.5}$$

where $M(\mathbf{x})$ stands for the drift vector and $\mathbf{e}$ for the $(n-1)$-dimensional vector of unit coordinates. When the solution (7.5) meets the condition of mixed derivative invariance, it is a gradient indeed.

Laying out becomes simple if we note that for any vector $\mathbf{z}$ of $(n-1)$ dimensions

$$(\|\delta_{ij}/x_i + 1/x_n\|\mathbf{z})_i = z_i/x_i - z_n/x_n\ ,$$

where z_n denotes the value of $-\Sigma_{i=1}^{n-1} z_i$. Remark that this notation has a fairly transparent sense. If the $(n-1)$-dimensional vector $\mathbf{z}$ represents the right-hand side of differential equations for the dynamical system of gamete frequencies' changes, then it can be complimented with the coordinate z_n corresponding to the dependent concentration. As the sum of all frequencies is identically equal to unit, the sum of coordinate derivatives in the 'complemented' dynamical system is identically zero, i.e. $z_n = -\Sigma_{i=1}^{n-1} z_i$. Since the choice of a independent variable is conventional, z_n is determined by the same regularities (of selection, mutation, migrations, etc.) as the rest of the coordinates and can be written down immediately, with no use summing the rest coordinates.

Thus, the solution (7.5) can be rewritten in the coordinate-wise form:

$$(\text{grad} \ln f(\mathbf{x}))_i = 4N\left[\frac{M_i(\mathbf{x})}{x_i} - \frac{M_n(\mathbf{x})}{x_n}\right] - \left(\frac{1}{x_i} - \frac{1}{x_n}\right). \tag{7.6}$$

The term $1/x_i - 1/x_n$ clearly meets the mixed derivatives invariance condition. The term is caused by the effect of genetic drift in the narrow sense considered separately and can be obtained formally, by solving equation (7.3) with $M(\mathbf{x}) \equiv 0$. Under this condition, the expression for $\ln f(\mathbf{x})$ will be

$$-\sum_{i=1}^{n} \ln x_i = -\ln\left(\prod_{i=1}^{n} x_i\right) = -\ln V(\mathbf{x})$$

where $V(\mathbf{x})$ designate the determinant of the diffusion matrix (without the multiplier $1/(2N)$).

This result, as in the two-allele case, makes no sense of the logarithmic steady-state density function since it leads the function to the non-integrability over the state space Σ. If, however, $M(\mathbf{x})\not\equiv 0$, so that the steady-state density does exist, then it has the co-factor appearing due to the 'random genetic drift' cause:

$$\exp\{-\ln V(\mathbf{x})\} = x_1^{-1}x_2^{-1}\dots x_n^{-1}\,. \tag{7.7}$$

In general, when the right-hand side of (7.6) is representable in the form of a sum of gradients of some functions, the steady-state density will equal the product of exponentials of functions times a normalizing constant.

In genetic models the drift vector $\mathbf{M}(\mathbf{x})$ is usually equal to a sum of vectors $\mathbf{M}^{(i)}(\mathbf{x})$ caused by different factors of microevolution. If for any of them the gradient of some function $G_i(\mathbf{x})$ can be found from equations

$$\frac{\partial}{\partial x_j}G_i(\mathbf{x}) = 2\left[\frac{M_j^{(i)}(\mathbf{x})}{x_j} - \frac{M_n^{(i)}(\mathbf{x})}{x_n}\right],\ j=\overline{1,n-1}\,. \tag{7.8}$$

then the steady-state density function can be written as the normalized product of all $\exp\{2NG_i(\mathbf{x})\}$times $\Pi_{i=1}^n x_i^{-1}$. In a complete analogy with the two-allele case, the steady-state density for any combination of microevolutionary factors (admitting the existence of a steady-state distribution) is determined merely by multiplying out all the co-factors $\exp\{2NG_i\}$ involved in the combination under concern.

12.8. Contribution to the Steady-State Density Caused by Selection

We consider a contribution to the steady-state probability density function caused by different forms of selection. By (1.2) the vector of a drift coefficients due to individuals elimination under constant genotypes fitness coefficients has coordinates

$$M_i(\mathbf{x}) = x_i(w_i(\mathbf{x}) - w(\mathbf{x}))/w(\mathbf{x})\,.$$

This expression can be easily shown be true also when genotype fitness coefficients, w_{ij}, depend upon the vector of gamete frequencies, $\mathbf{x}$. As before, we have

$$w_i(\mathbf{x}) = \sum_{j=1}^n w_{ij}(\mathbf{x})x_j,\quad w(\mathbf{x}) = \sum_{i,j=1}^n w_{ij}(\mathbf{x})x_ix_j\,.$$

Let the contribution to the steady-state density function that is caused by the selection factor be denoted by $G_1(\mathbf{x})$. Then the ith component of the function $G_1(\mathbf{x})$ gradient is equal by (7.8) to

$$\frac{\partial}{\partial x_i}G_1(\mathbf{x}) = 2\,\frac{w_i(\mathbf{x})-w_n(\mathbf{x})}{w(\mathbf{x})} = \frac{\partial}{\partial x_i}\ln w(\mathbf{x})\,, \tag{8.1}$$

where fitnesses w_{ij} are assumed constant. Evidently,

$$G_1(\mathbf{x}) = \ln w(\mathbf{x})\,. \tag{8.2}$$

If the drift due to selection is written without the normalizing multiplier $1/w(\mathbf{x})$, then

$$G_{1a}(\mathbf{x}) = w(\mathbf{x}) , \tag{8.3}$$

i.e. in a multi-allele case function $G_1(\mathbf{x})$ have the same form as in the diallelic one. In the (8.3) case, however, the fitness is measured rather differently than in (8.2). Note that under weak election pressure (when $w_{ij}=1+m_{ij}, m_{ij}=O(1/N)$) we have $w^{2N}(\mathbf{x})\sim[1+m(x)]^{2N}\sim\exp\{2N\, m(\mathbf{x})\}$, where $m(\mathbf{x})=\Sigma_{i,j}m_{ij}x_ix_j$ is the mean fitness of the population measured by Malthusian parameters m_{ij}. Since $\ln[1+m(\mathbf{x})]\sim m(\mathbf{x})$, the function $G_1(\mathbf{x})\sim G_{1a}(\mathbf{x})$ but the mean fitness, although denoted by $w(\mathbf{x})$ in (8.3), is now measured by means of Malthusian parameters corresponding to the deterministic population dynamics in the continuous time.

Following S. Wright, we assume the dependence of the fitness upon the population genetic structure to have the form

$$w_{ij}= w_{ij}(\mathbf{x}) = \Phi(\mathbf{x})\upsilon_{ij} .$$

Then, after writing the drift coefficient down with the normalizing multiplier $1/w(\mathbf{x})$, we obtain

$$G_{1b}(\mathbf{x}) = \ln \upsilon (\mathbf{x}), \quad \upsilon (\mathbf{x}) = \sum_{i,j=1}^{n} \upsilon_{ij}x_ix_j , \tag{8.4}$$

as the function $\Phi(\mathbf{x})$ cancels out of the drift expression (1.2).

In case the dependence of fitness upon the genetic structure is of the type

$$w_{ij}(\mathbf{x}) = \upsilon_{ij}- \Phi(\mathbf{x})$$

and the drift (1.1) lacks normalization, the function $\Phi(\mathbf{x})$ also cancels out and

$$G_{1c}(\mathbf{x}) = \upsilon (\mathbf{x}) , \tag{8.5}$$

where $\upsilon(\mathbf{x})$ is defined in (8.4).

The way the fitness is known from experiments to depend on genetic composition of the population can be specified also in the following approach. Let us assume that pair-wise, triple-wise, etc. interactions of individuals have an effect on the fitness of genotypes involved in the interaction. The probability that a number of genotypes interact with each other can be assumed equal to the product of their frequencies. Then the fitness coefficients are representable in the following form

$$w_{ij}(\mathbf{x}) = w_{ij} + \varepsilon_2 w_{ij}^{(2)}(\mathbf{x}) + \varepsilon_3 w_{ij}^{(3)}(\mathbf{x}) +\ldots+\varepsilon_m w_{ij}^{(m)}(\mathbf{x}) + \Phi (\mathbf{x}) , \tag{8.6}$$

where taken into account are interactions up to the mth order; w_{ij} is a constant indicating the genotype A_iA_j fitness in the absence of influence from other individuals; a coefficient $w_{ij}^{(k)}(\mathbf{x})$ indicates the A_iA_j fitness at the interaction of k individuals:

$$w_{ij}^{(k)}(\mathbf{x}) = \sum_{1\le i_1, j_1;\ldots; i_{k-1}, j_{k-1}\le n} w_{ij,\, i_1j_1,\ldots,\, i_{k-1}j_{k-1}} \times x_{i_1}x_{j_1}\ldots x_{i_{k-1}}x_{j_{k-1}} \tag{8.7}$$

A constant $w_{ij,\, i_1j_1,\ldots,\, i_{k-1}j_{k-1}}$ can be interpreted as the fitness of the genotype A_iA_j among genotypes $\{A_{i_1}A_{j_1},\ldots,A_{i_{k-1}}A_{j_{k-1}}\}$, a coefficient ε_k indicates the intensity of k-

order interactions, $\Phi(\mathbf{x})$ is a function of gamete frequencies. All the interactions are further assumed symmetric, i.e. the constants $w_{ij,\, i_1j_1,\ldots,\, i_{k-1}j_{k-1}}$ be invariant under any permutation of genotype subscripts and gamete subscripts within a genotype. Moreover, any differences among these constants are assumed small, the assumption making valid the hypothesis of independent random combination of gametes in the genotype.

By using the representation (8.6) of $w_{ij}(\mathbf{x})$ in $w_i(\mathbf{x})$ and by (7.8) the function $G_{1d}(\mathbf{x})$ can be shown to obey the equations

$$\partial G_{1d}(\mathbf{x})/\partial x_i = 2[w_i(\mathbf{x}) - w_n(\mathbf{x})]\ ,$$

where the corresponding expression for $G_{1d}(\mathbf{x})$ is given by

$$G_{1d}(\mathbf{x}) = w^{(1)}(\mathbf{x}) + \frac{1}{2}\varepsilon_2 w^{(2)}(\mathbf{x}) + \ldots + \frac{1}{m}\varepsilon_m w^{(m)}(\mathbf{x})\ , \tag{8.8}$$

the function

$$w^{(k)}(\mathbf{x}) = \sum_{i,j=1}^{n} w_{ij}^{(k)}(\mathbf{x}) x_i x_j$$

is interpreted as the mean fitness in k-order interactions of individuals, and $w^{(1)}(\mathbf{x})$ is a usual fitness defined by constants w_{ij}.

Suppose now that the random mating assumption is violated and consider the effect of selection under inbreeding with a coefficient F. The population can then be considered to consist of the following two parts. Within the first part individuals mate randomly, the contribution of this part to the total population being equal to $1-F$. The second part is totally inbred and composed exclusively by homozygotes. It can be conventionally thought of being a 'haploid' population with the fitness coefficients of the alleles equal to those of the corresponding homozygotes. The second part's contribution into the total population equals F. Now, in the complete analogy to the diallelic case, the drift represents a weighted average of the drifts for each of the two parts:

$$M_i(\mathbf{x}) = x_i\{(1-F)[w_i(\mathbf{x}) - w(\mathbf{x})] + F[w_{ii} - w_h(\mathbf{x})]\}\ ,$$

where $w_h(\mathbf{x})=\Sigma_{i=1}^{n} w_{ii} x_i$ stands for the mean fitness of the 'haploid' population. Function G for the first summand differs from the function (8.3) corresponding to selection under random mating by the multiplier $(1-F)$. The second summand yields the function that differs by the multiplier F from one corresponding to selection in a haploid population, i.e. from $2w_h(\mathbf{x})$ as can be easily seen. Finally, when selection and inbreeding are taken into account, we have

$$G_{1e}(\mathbf{x}) = (1-F)w(\mathbf{x}) + 2Fw_h(\mathbf{x}) \tag{8.9}$$

as in the two-allele case (2.12). For the zero coefficient of inbreeding the function (8.9) reduces to the panmixia case (8.3); for the complete inbreeding ($F=1$) we have $G_{1e}(\mathbf{x})=2w_h(\mathbf{x})$.

12.9. Contribution Caused by Migrations and Mutations. The General Form of a Steady-State Density Function

In a multi-allele case the random genetic drift and selection lead a finite population eventually to a homozygote state (it can be readily verified that formal solutions (7.5) are non-integrable over the state space Σ in this case). When migrations from a polymorphic source are taken into account, the convergence to a steady-state distribution takes place for any initial state of the population.

If the migration exchange with an external population, where allele frequencies q_i are constant, proceeds at a time-invariable rate m and migration does not depend on the genotype, then by (1.3) the drift vector equals $m(\mathbf{q}-\mathbf{x})$ and the function $G_2(\mathbf{x})$ that defines the contribution caused by migrations can be found from Equations (7.8) which reduce to

$$\partial G_2(\mathbf{x})/\partial x_i = 2m(q_i/x_i - q_n/x_n)\ . \tag{9.1}$$

The solution is given by

$$G_2(\mathbf{x}) = 2m \sum_{i=1}^{n} q_i \ln x_i\ . \tag{9.2}$$

From experimental data, however, migration probabilities are known to depend on the genotype of migrants. Let the 'island' population be regulated by emigration such that the population size remains constant under the immigration flow with intensity m and let the emigration potential of the genotype A_iA_j be denoted by P_{ij} (i.e.the frequency of the genotype among all emigrants is proportional to the product of P_{ij} times the concentration of A_iA_j in the whole population. The vector of drift coefficients caused by the immigration inflow with constant allele frequencies q_i has clearly the following coordinates:

$$M_i(\mathbf{x}) = m\left[q_i - x_i - x_i\left(\sum_{j=1}^{n} P_{ij}x_j - \sum_{i,j=1}^{n} P_{ij}x_ix_j\right)\right]. \tag{9.3}$$

According to (7.8) the corresponding function G_{2a} must obey the equations

$$\partial G_{2a}(\mathbf{x})/\partial x_i = 2m(q_i/x_i - q_n/x_n) - 2m[P_i(\mathbf{x}) - P_n(\mathbf{x})]\ , \tag{9.4}$$

where $P_i(\mathbf{x}) = \Sigma_{j=1}^{n} P_{ij}x_j$.

It can be seen from (9.4) that $G_{2a}(\mathbf{x})$ includes a summand $G_2(\mathbf{x})$ showing the immigration and a function of the same type as $G_{1a}(\mathbf{x})$ caused by selection effects. This could be certainly expected since in the model the emigration is equivalent to elimination of individuals. On the whole,

$$G_{2a}(\mathbf{x}) = 2m \sum_{i=1}^{n} q_i \ln x_i - mP(\mathbf{x})\ , \tag{9.5}$$

where

$$P(\mathbf{x}) = \sum_{i,j=1}^{n} P_{ij} x_i x_j \,. \tag{9.6}$$

By the similarity with the selection case, this result can be generalized to the situation where the emigration probability depends on the population genetic composition, for instance, in a mode like (8.7). The dependence of immigration probabilities upon genotypes can be also included.

Besides migrations, there is another factor that provides existence of a steady-state distribution, namely, the mutability of alleles. According to (1.4), the drift coefficient for the concentration of the ith allele due to mutations is equal to

$$M_i(\mathbf{x}) = \sum_{k=1}^{n} \mu_{ik} x_k - x_i \,, \tag{9.7}$$

where μ_{ij} is a probability that allele A_j mutates into A_i. The function $G_3(\mathbf{x})$ that corresponds to the mutation pressure must, therefore, obey the equations

$$\frac{\partial}{\partial x_i} G_3(\mathbf{x}) = 2\left(\sum_{k=1}^{n} \mu_{ik}\, x_k / x_i - \sum_{k=1}^{n} \mu_{nk} x_k / x_n \right). \tag{9.8}$$

Let us verify whether the mixed derivatives are equal:

$$\frac{\partial^2}{\partial x_i\, \partial x_j} G_3(\mathbf{x}) = 2\left(\frac{\mu_{ij} - \mu_{in}}{x_i} - \frac{\mu_{nj} - \mu_{nn}}{x_n} + \frac{\sum_{k=1}^{n} \mu_{nk} x_k}{x_n^2} \right).$$

$$\frac{\partial^2}{\partial x_j\, \partial x_i} G_3(\mathbf{x}) = 2\left(\frac{\mu_{ji} - \mu_{jn}}{x_j} - \frac{\mu_{ni} - \mu_{nn}}{x_n} + \frac{\sum_{k=1}^{n} \mu_{nk} x_k}{x_n^2} \right).$$

It is clear that, under an arbitrary pattern of mutations, there exists no function $G_3(\mathbf{x})$ satisfying the Equation (9.8), i.e. the probability flow will be non-zero for the steady-state density. For the mixed derivatives to be equal it is necessary and sufficient that $\mu_{ij} = \mu_{in}$ for any j and i $(i \neq j)$. This means that the probability of allele A_j mutation into A_i (the intensity of reverse mutations) is the same for all j. Let it be denoted by μ_i (note that in general the value of $\mu_i = \mu_{ij} (i \neq j)$ depends on subscript i). As matrix $\|\mu_{ij}\|$ is stochastic in columns, its diagonal entries can be expressed by

$$\mu_{ii} = 1 - \sum_{\substack{j=1 \\ j \neq i}}^{n} \mu_j \,.$$

In this scheme, independent mutability parameters are presented by intensities of reverse mutations μ_i. Let μ designate their total intensity:

$$\mu = \sum_{i=1}^{n} \mu_i \, .$$

Then from (9.7) we have the following expression for the drift coefficients due to mutations:

$$M_i(\mathbf{x}) = \mu_i (1 - x_i) = (1 - \sum_{\substack{j=1 \\ j \neq i}}^{n} \mu_j) x_i - x_i = \mu_i - \mu x_i \, . \tag{9.9}$$

Hence, the function $G_3(\mathbf{x})$ corresponding to the mutability effect is to be found, in accordance with (7.8), from the equations

$$\partial G_3(\mathbf{x})/\partial x_i = 2(\mu_i/x_i - \mu_n/x_n) \, . \tag{9.10}$$

The solution to (9.10) is obviously presented by

$$G_3(\mathbf{x}) = 2 \sum_{i=1}^{n} \mu_i \ln x_i \, . \tag{9.11}$$

Now, the functions $G_i(\mathbf{x})$ have been obtained from Equations (7.8) for each factor of microevolution. As a result of combined action of these factors, the steady-state density function takes on the form

$$f(\mathbf{x}) = C\left[\prod_{j=1}^{n} x_j^{-1}\right] \exp\left\{2N \sum_i G_i(\mathbf{x})\right\}.$$

If, for example, the population undergoes mutation, selection and migrations of one of the types considered, then

$$f(\mathbf{x}) = C \exp\{2N[(1 - F)w(\mathbf{x}) + 2Fw_h(\mathbf{x}) + mP_F(\mathbf{x})]\} \prod_{i=1}^{n} x_i^{4N(mq_i + \mu_i) - 1} \, . \tag{9.12}$$

Here F denotes the coefficient of inbreeding, $w(\mathbf{x})$ the mean fitness, $w_h(\mathbf{x})$ the mean fitness of the inbred part of the population, m the intensity of migrations, $P_F(\mathbf{x})$ the mean migration activity of the (9.6) type but with genotype concentrations defined with regard for F, $\{q_i\}$ the allele frequencies among immigrants, μ_i the probability of mutation from an arbitrary allele into allele A_i.

When the effect of some microevolutionary cause is not taken into account (or has another form of expression), then the respective co-factor is to be omitted in the steady-state density function (or modified by one of the formulae proposed). If $F=\mu_i=0$ migration activity is the same for different genotypes, and fitness coefficients w_{ij} are independent of the genetic structure, then we obtain the known formula of Wright:

$$f(\mathbf{x}) = Cw^{2N}(\mathbf{x}) \prod_{i=1}^{n} x_i^{4Nmq_i - 1} \tag{9.13}$$

where the drift vector due to selection is taken with regard to the normalizing factor and Equation (1.2).

12.10. Investigation of the Steady-State Probability Density Function for Concentrations of Multiple Alleles. A Multi-Locus Case

When the migration activity of individuals is independent of their genotypes and there is no selection, the steady-state density function has the following form:

$$f(\mathbf{x}) = C\prod_{i=1}^{n} x_i^{4N(mq_i+\mu_i)-1} = C\prod_{i=1}^{n} x_i^{a_i-1}. \tag{10.1}$$

It is the density function for the Dirichlet distribution with parameters $\{a_i\}$. The constant C is determined from the condition that the integral of the density function over Σ is equal to unit, and is known to admit an expression in terms of the gamma-function:

$$C^{-1} = \int_{\Sigma}\left[\prod_{i=1}^{n-1} x_i^{a_i-1}\right]\left(1-\sum_{i=1}^{n-1} x_i\right)^{a_n-1} dx = D(a_1,\ldots,a_n) = \prod_{i=1}^{n}\Gamma(a_i)/\Gamma\left(\sum_{i=1}^{n} a_i\right). \tag{10.2}$$

Hence,

$$f(\mathbf{x}) = \frac{\Gamma\left[4N\left(m+\sum_{i=1}^{n}\mu_i\right)\right]}{\prod_{i=1}^{n}\Gamma[4N(mq_i+\mu_i)]}\prod_{i=1}^{n} x_i^{4N(mq_i+\mu_i)-1}. \tag{10.3}$$

We use here the restriction $\Sigma_{i=1}^{n} q_i=1$ on the sum of allele frequencies (in the outer source of immigrants). If some of the parameters, say a_i, is less than one, then the density function tends to infinity near the boundary $x_i=0$; in case where all the parameters a_i are greater than one, the function turns into zero at boundaries. The distribution then has a uni-modal pattern due to the concavity of its density function (the matrix of second derivatives is negative definite on Σ).

Examining the concentration distribution of one of the alleles (for instance, A_i), we find it to be a beta-distribution, with the parameters $a=a_i$ and $b=\Sigma_{j=1}^{n} a_j-a_i$, i.e. we have a diallelic system with direct mutations of intensity $\mu-\mu_i$ and reverse ones with intensity μ_i. The migration proceeds from an external population which is diallelic too (the second allele corresponds to the union of all the alleles different from A_i). If we make no distinction among alleles within some arbitrary alleles groups (which is possible in some experimental techniques, for example, in the electrophoresis, where non-distinct are the alleles determining protein molecules of the same charge), then new, 'artificial' alleles (corresponding to groups of 'no distinction') will have the Dirichlet distribution again.

Let the ith group (i.e. the new allele A_i^*) be formed by uniting alleles $A_{i_1},\ldots,A_{i_k}$. The corresponding Dirichlet distribution will then have the parameter $a_i^*=\Sigma_{j=1}^{k} a_{i_j}$, which means grouping the same alleles in the outer source of migrants and summing the probabilities of mutation into the new allele. For example, the probability that some (may be, 'artificial') alleles mutates into allele $\overset{*}{A_i}$ will equal $\overset{*}{\mu_i}=\Sigma_{j=1}^{k}\mu_{i_j}$. When treated separately, the distribution for an 'artificial' (as well as an 'actual') allele is again a beta-distribution with corresponding parameters. These distributions were studied in the two allele case (see Section 12.5) and the conclusions that were made before (about the expectation, the variance, and the relation to the deterministic equilibrium state) are still valid in the case under concern.

In particular, the expected concentration of an allele is equal (with regard for (10.2)) to

$$E\{x_i\} = D(a_1 ,..., a_i + 1,..., a_n)/D(a_1,..., a_i ,..., a_n) =$$

$$= a_i / \sum_{i=1}^{n} a_i = (mq_i + \mu_i) / \left(m + \sum_{i=1}^{n} \mu_i \right) = \frac{mq_i+\mu_i}{m+\mu_i+v_i}. \tag{10.4}$$

We use here the property of the gamma-function to meet the condition $\Gamma(a+1)=a\Gamma(a)$ and we designate by v_i the value of $\Sigma_{j=1}^{n}\mu_j\text{-}\mu_i$ (corresponding to the total intensity of direct mutations into any other allele). In this notation, the result concurs completely with the expectation in the two-allele case where the intensity of direct mutations is equal to v_i and that of reverse mutations to μ_i. At the same time, the deterministic analogue of the diffusion model appears to be

$$\frac{dx_i}{dt} = m(q_i - x_i) + \mu_i \sum_{\substack{j=1 \\ j \neq i}}^{n} x_j - x_i \sum_{\substack{j=1 \\ j \neq i}}^{n} \mu_j = m(q_i - x_i) + \mu_i - (\mu_i + v_i)x_i \, . \tag{10.5}$$

The system of ordinary differential equations is clearly seen to split into individual equations, each corresponding entirely to the diallelic case. The stable equilibrium state of this system coincides with the expectation (10.4) of the steady-state density function.

Moments of the higher orders for the Dirichlet distribution can be found, as before, by means of (10.2):

$$E\left\{ x_1^{n_1} x_2^{n_2} \ldots x_n^{n_n} \right\} = D(a_1 + n_1,..., a_n + n_n)/D(a_1,..., a_n) \, . \tag{10.6}$$

For example, the variance of any concentration has an order of $O(1/N)$ and the distribution shrinks to the deterministic equilibrium point as N increases.

Under selection pressure with drift coefficients of the (1.2) form, there appears the co-factor $w^{2N}(\mathbf{x})$ in the steady-state density function, which no longer yields a Dirichlet distribution. The constant C can nevertheless be found in the same way as in the two-allele case: raised to the power, $w^{2N}(\mathbf{x})$ represents a sum of terms having the form of $\Pi_{i=1}^{n} x_i^{n_i}$ with coefficients depending on fitness values $\{w_{ij}\}$. How much the integral of such a term contributes into C^{-1} can be determined from (10.2) and the expression for C can thus be obtained.

If $w(\mathbf{x})$ is a concave function, then, as well as in the two-allele case, the steady-state distribution will have only one vertex when inequality a_i>1 holds for all i.

As well as in the case of two alleles, the steady-state density function does not depend on hardiness of selection. This should be understood in the sense that the density will not change if all fitness coefficients are multiplied by the same constant.

In a general case the steady-state distribution for a large population size N is determined mainly by the function $G(\mathbf{x})$ since the contribution by the co-factor $\Pi_{i=1}^{n} x_i^{-1}$ becomes negligibly small. The greater the population size, the stronger the density concentrates around its maximum points, the stable equilibrium states of the deterministic model. If $G(\mathbf{x})$ is a concave function, the steady-state density will be the delta-function $\delta(\mathbf{x}-\mathbf{x}^*)$ in the limit, the point $\mathbf{x}^*$ being the (unique) stable equilibrium state of the deterministic model.

The next step in the study of steady-state distribution is naturally a transition to the multi-locus case. In this case the mean fitness function $w(\mathbf{x})$ is defined by fitness coefficients depending on genotype throughout all the loci. The population state should be represented by a vector of concentrations of various gamete types (or of allele frequencies and linkage disequilibrium characteristics). The allele frequencies will generally not be sufficient to define the genotype concentrations. The diffusion matrix, as before, has the form (7.4) due to the polynomial pattern of gamete sampling in the random mating hypothesis. The drift caused by selection or migrations also coincide in its form with the proper expression in the single-locus, multi-allele case. The new point in the multi-locus case is the occurrence of recombinations.

In the simplest example of two diallelic loci there are gametes of the four possible types, whose concentrations can be denoted by x_1, x_2, x_3, and x_4 including a dependent variable. Here x_1 corresponds to the gamete A_1B_1, x_2 to A_1B_2, x_3 to A_2B_1, and x_4 to A_2B_2, the A_i representing an allele at the first locus, B_i at the second one (i=1,2). Let $D(\mathbf{x})$ designates the linkage disequilibrium coefficient for alleles A_1 and B_1:

$$D(\mathbf{x}) = x_1x_4 - x_2x_3 .$$

Then the drift vector components (1.5) can be written (see (11.9.4)) in the following form:

$$M_i(\mathbf{x}) = (-1)^{i+\delta_{i3}} rD(\mathbf{x}),\ i = 1, 2, 3,$$

where δ_{i3} is the Kronecker symbol, r is the interlocus recombination probability.

Equations (7.8) takes on the form

$$\partial G(\mathbf{x})/\partial x_i = 2rD(\mathbf{x})[(-1)^{i+\delta_{i3}}/x_i - 1/x_4],\quad i = 1, 2, 3, \tag{10.7}$$

and have no solution in this case since the mixed derivative invariance condition does not hold. Hence, the flows of steady-state probability density will be non-zero. No analytical expression is known for the steady-state distribution of gamete frequencies classified with respect to two or more loci.

12.11. Steady-State Density and Objective Functions in Case of Multiple Alleles

As well as in the diallelic case, the functions $G_i(\mathbf{x})$ and $G(\mathbf{x})=\Sigma_i G_i(\mathbf{x})$ define principally the form of the steady-state density function (almost completely when the population size N is large). At the same time, they play an important role in studying respective unperturbed deterministic models in case of two alleles. The relation noted above between deterministic and diffusion models turns out valid for multi-allele loci too.

In order to see the role of functions $G_i(\mathbf{x})$ in the deterministic case, let us consider unperturbed system of differential equations governing the dynamics of gene frequencies x_j under the action of the ith microevolutionary factor:

$$dx_j/dt = M_j^{(i)}(\mathbf{x}), \; j=\overline{1, n} \; . \tag{11.1}$$

As the sum of all allele concentrations is identically equal to one, the sum of all right-hand sides in (11.1) is identically zero and only n-1 first equations are enough to be considered: at any time moment we have $x_n(t)=1-\Sigma_{j=1}^{n-1}x_j(t)$.

We introduce a function $\tilde{G}(x_1, ..., x_{n-1}, x_n)$, assuming it to obey the equations

$$\partial\tilde{G}_i(\mathbf{x})/\partial x_j = 2M_j^{(i)}(\mathbf{x})/x_j, \; j=\overline{1, n} \; . \tag{11.2}$$

Then (11.1) can be written in the following way:

$$dx_j/dt = \frac{1}{2}x_j\partial\tilde{G}_i(\mathbf{x})/\partial x_j, \; j=\overline{1, n} \; . \tag{11.3}$$

It is immediately seen that critical points of the function $\tilde{G}_i(\mathbf{x})$ correspond to equilibrium states of system (11.1). Maxima of $\tilde{G}_i(\mathbf{x})$ are clearly associated with stable equilibrium states as x_j are positive (when an internal state is under concern) and the dynamics of deviations from the equilibrium state are determined by the matrix of second derivatives of $\tilde{G}_i(\mathbf{x})$ (for simplicity the matrix being supposed non-singular). When a maximum of $\tilde{G}_i(\mathbf{x})$ lies on the boundary of Σ, the corresponding stable equilibrium will be at the boundary too, the condition holding automatically that the deviations do not lead the system out of Σ.

Besides being useful in the local stability analysis, the function $\tilde{G}_i(\mathbf{x})$ characterizes also some global features in behavior of the system (11.1) trajectories: $\tilde{G}_i(\mathbf{x})$ is monotone non-decreasing along those trajectories. To prove, let us differentiate $\tilde{G}_i[\mathbf{x}(t)]$ with respect to t and with regard to (11.2). We have

$$\frac{d}{dt}\tilde{G}_i[\mathbf{x}(t)] = 2\sum_{j=1}^{n}[M_j^{(i)}(\mathbf{x})]^2/x_j \geq 0 \; ,$$

since concentrations x_j are non-negative. The derivative becomes zero only when all $M_j^{(i)}(\mathbf{x})$ are equal to zero, i.e. in the state of equilibrium. The function $\tilde{G}_i(\mathbf{x})$ defines an adaptive landscape for dynamics in the population genetic composition. It was a curve in the two-allele case, and now it is a hypersurface, whose pattern permits judging on the behavior of system (11.1) trajectories: the movement proceeds in the direction to the, 'goal' i.e. the increase in $\tilde{G}_i(\mathbf{x})$, to one of the hypersurface peaks.

In these heuristic considerations the dependent variable x_n was used as equally well as the rest ones. In fact, we must analyze $\tilde{G}_i$ (x) on the symplex Σ, where

$$x_n = 1 - \sum_{j=1}^{n-1} x_j, \text{ i.e.}$$

$$\tilde{G}_i(x_1, ..., x_{n-1}, x_n) = G_i(x_1, ..., x_{n-1}).$$

The correspondence between the vectors $(x_1,..., x_{n-1}, x_n)$ and $(x_1,...,x_{n-1})$ is one-to-one in this case and they can be designated by the same letter **x**.

By (11.2) we have on Σ

$$\frac{\partial G_i(\mathbf{x})}{\partial x_j} = \frac{\partial \tilde{G}_i(\mathbf{x})}{\partial x_j} - \frac{\partial \tilde{G}_i(\mathbf{x})}{\partial x_n} = 2\left[\frac{M_j^{(i)}(\mathbf{x})}{x_j} - \frac{M_n^{(i)}(\mathbf{x})}{x_n}\right], \; j = \overline{1, n-1}. \tag{11.4}$$

Since $\Sigma_{j=1}^{n-1} M_j^{(i)}(\mathbf{x}) = -M_n^{(i)}(\mathbf{x})$ (as the sum of right-hand sides of system (11.1) must be zero), we obtain:

$$\frac{d}{dt} G_i[\mathbf{x}(t)] = 2\sum_{j=1}^{n-1} [M_j^{(i)}(\mathbf{x})/x_j - M_n^{(i)}(\mathbf{x})/x_n] M_j^{(i)}(\mathbf{x}) =$$

$$= 2\sum_{j=1}^{n-1} [M_j^{(i)}(\mathbf{x})]^2/x_j + 2[M_n^{(i)}(\mathbf{x})]^2/x_n \geq 0. \tag{11.5}$$

Thus, $G_i(\mathbf{x})$ is the object function for the system (11.1) reduced to n -1 equations.

Note that the function $\tilde{G}_i(\mathbf{x})$, though found by means of Equation (11.4), is not yet bound to obey the Equations (11.2). Its derivatives differ from $2M_j^{(i)}(\mathbf{x})/x_j$ by a function $\Phi(\mathbf{x})$ (the same for all j), which cancels out when substituted into (11.4). It can be further shown that

$$\Phi(\mathbf{x}) = -\sum_{j=1}^{n} x_j \frac{1}{2} \partial \tilde{G}_i(\mathbf{x})/\partial x_j,$$

where $\Phi(\mathbf{x})$ is the normalizing function that provides invariance of the state space Σ:

$$\frac{dx_j}{dt} = x_j\left[\frac{\partial}{\partial x_j}\frac{1}{2}\tilde{G}_i(\mathbf{x}) - \sum_{k=1}^{n} x_k \frac{\partial}{\partial x_k}\frac{1}{2}\tilde{G}_i(\mathbf{x})\right], j = \overline{1, n}$$

the change in $\tilde{G}_i$ (x) being monotone along any trajectory of the system.

So, if we find a function $G_i(\mathbf{x})$ satisfying the system (11.4) of partial derivatives equations, then it will define the adaptive landscape for the dynamics in the population genetic composition caused by the ith factor of microevolution in accordance with Equations (11.1). But the system (11.4) coincide with system (7.8), which determines a contribution into the steady-state density function caused by the same microevolutionary factor.

Thus, the object function of the deterministic model determines, as well as it does in case of two alleles, the form of the steady-state distribution in the diffusion model.

Although the equation to find the function $G_i(\mathbf{x})$ in the diallelic case (following form (4.5)),

$$dG_i(x)/dx = 2M^{(i)}(x)/[x(1-x)], \tag{11.6}$$

differs from (11.4) in its form, it can be written down in a similar way by means of trivial transformations. To do so, we recall that $x=x_1$, $M_1(x)-M_2(x)$ and $x_2=1-x_1=1-x$, so that the Equation (11.6) takes on the form

$$\frac{dG_i(x)}{dx} = 2\left[\frac{M_1^{(i)}(x)}{x} - \frac{-M_1^{(i)}(x)}{1-x}\right] = \frac{2M^{(i)}(x)}{x(1-x)},$$

which coincides with (11.4).

At the same time, the diallelic case is distinct principally from that of multiple alleles. Whatever may be the terms forming the decomposition of the drift coefficient into components caused by various microevolutionary factors in a model of two alleles, the objective function can be found from (11.6) for each term. Unfortunately, it is not the case for a multi-dimensional system, which appeared already in the examples with general pattern of mutations and with recombination between two linked loci. Within the diffusion model this distinction corresponds to the fact that the probability flow in the diallelic (i.e. one-dimensional) case is always zero at a steady state, while in the multi-dimensional case the steady-state circulation is quite possible.

Thus, as well as in the case of two alleles, a function $G_i(\mathbf{x})$ obeying (11.4) is the 'objective' function in the deterministic analysis of the effect caused by the ith factor of microevoultion: the evolution proceeds in such a way that, speaking teleologically, increases the current value of $G_i(\mathbf{x})$. The objective function in the case of an arbitrary combination of microevolutionary factors can be obtained by mere summation of adaptive landscape functions over all the factors of the combination under concern. Stable deterministic equilibrium states correspond to peaks of the adaptive landscape surface. Simultaneously, the same functions $G_i(\mathbf{x})$ define essentially the form of the steady-state probability density function in the respective diffusion model: population states are 'smeared' over stable equilibria of the deterministic model. When the population size increases, the steady-state density concentrates more and more about stable equilibria of the deterministic model. While these conclusions are valid in the two-allele case, roughly speaking, for any kind of influence on the population, they are no longer true in case of multiple alleles.

Note that, for moderate values of population size N, the deterministic model of the form

$$\frac{dx_j}{dt} = M_j^{(i)}(\mathbf{x}) - \frac{1-nx_j}{4N}, j = \overline{1, n-1}, \tag{11.7}$$

gives better correspondence with the diffusion one than the model (11.1). This correspondence should be understood in the sense that in a finite interval of time the stochastic trajectory comes out of a narrow tube surrounding the trajectory of (11.7) with less probability than of a tube surrounding the trajectory of (11.1). Also, the steady-state probability density function will be defined by a corresponding object function of the model (11.7) completely rather than just asymptotically. The additional component (with the coefficient $1/(4N)$) appears in the right-hand side of (11.7) due to the fact that the diffusion matrix of the stochastic model differs from the identity one. As a result, some additional 'forces' spring up in the deterministic model modification, which push the population towards boundaries of the state space Σ but vanish in the center of Σ. Due to singularity of the diffusion matrix on $B(\Sigma)$, the pressure caused by the additional component becomes infinite at boundaries, but its contribution is small in the rest of the state space because of the multplier $1/(4N)$.

12.12. Relation of Objective Functions to the Sphere Motion Potential. Mechanical Interpretation of Single-Locus Genetic Processes in Terms of Motion in a Force Field

The relation noted above between the form of steady-state density function and the behavior in the corresponding deterministic model is caused by the fact the drift vector represents the gradient of function $G/2$ in a metrics defined by the diffusion matrix. We may thus hope to obtain, by a change of variables, the most simple form of the deterministic model equations, where the right-hand side (according to the drift vector under the diffusion perturbation) represents the gradient of function $Q=cG$ (constant $c>0$) taken with the minus sign. The behavior of deterministic trajectories is geometrically obvious in this case, being defined by the surface of the potential function Q and resembling the motion of a small ball rolling on the surface: stable equilibrium states correspond to 'wells', while unstable ones to 'peaks'.

The potential gives a global picture of the deterministic model: all the state space is partitioned into domains of attraction to stable equilibrium points (when, for instance, the potential surface has a finite number of isolated critical points); the motion proceeds orthogonally to level surfaces of the potential function; the potential is monotone non-increasing and reaches its minimum at stable equilibrium points; while proceeding to a minimum, the movement follows to that one of possible directions which gives the maximal fall in the potential function.

The most simple change of variables resulting in a potential model is one given by $\tilde{x}_j=\tilde{x}_j(x_j)$, $j=\overline{1, n}$. Let the motion equations of a deterministic model for an n-allele locus take on the form (11.3), i.e. let there be a function $\tilde{G}(\mathbf{x})=\tilde{G}(x_1, ..., x_n)$ such that the equalities

$$\frac{dx_j}{dt} = x_j \frac{\partial}{\partial x_j} \frac{1}{2} \tilde{G}(\mathbf{x}), \; j = \overline{1, n}, \tag{12.1}$$

hold. We attempt to identify the pattern of the functional dependence $\tilde{x}_j(x_j)$ which results in the 'potential' form of Equations (12.1) in new variables. It is clear from (12.1) that

$$\frac{d\tilde{x}_j}{dt} = \frac{d\tilde{x}_j}{dx_j}\frac{dx_j}{dt} = \frac{1}{2}\frac{d\tilde{x}_j}{dx_j} x_j \frac{\partial \tilde{G}(\mathbf{x})}{\partial x_j}, \; j = \overline{1, n}. \tag{12.2}$$

The change $\tilde{x}_j(x_j)$ must be a one-to-one correspondence (for instance, $\tilde{x}_j$ may strictly increase with x_j). The 'potential' form requirement means that

$$\frac{d\tilde{x}_j}{dt} = -\frac{\partial Q}{\partial \tilde{x}_j} = c\frac{\partial \tilde{G}(\tilde{\mathbf{x}})}{\partial \tilde{x}_j} = c\frac{\partial \tilde{G}(\tilde{\mathbf{x}})}{\partial x_j}\frac{dx_j}{d\tilde{x}_j}, j = \overline{1, n}. \tag{12.3}$$

By virtue of the monotonicity in $\tilde{x}_j$ we have $dx_j/d\tilde{x}_j=[d\tilde{x}_j/dx_j]^{-1}$. Substituting this expression into Equations (12.2) reveals them to be coincident with (12.3) provided that coincident are the coefficients at $\partial\tilde{G}(\mathbf{x})/\partial x_j$, i.e. the equality (with $c = 1/8$)

$$(d\tilde{x}_j/dx_j)^2 = 1/(4x_j) \tag{12.4}$$

must hold. The solution to this equation is evidently

$$\tilde{x}_j = \sqrt{x_j}, \tag{12.5}$$

the change of all other variables being similar.

Thus, if we choose the function $Q=-G/8$ as a potential, then the dynamic equations are written down in new variables as the gradient descent equations:

$$d\tilde{x}_j/dt = -\partial Q(\tilde{\mathbf{x}})/\partial \tilde{x}_j, \ j=\overline{1, n}, \tag{12.6}$$

i.e. the change of variables (12.5) brings about equations of the potential motion.

However, as was noted above, in the remark followed formula (11.5), the equations of, for instance, single-locus models must be actually written not in the form (12.1) but rather in the modified one:

$$\frac{dx_j}{dt} = x_j\left[\frac{\partial}{\partial x_j}\frac{1}{2}\tilde{G}(\mathbf{x}) - \sum_{k=1}^{n} x_k\frac{\partial}{\partial x_k}\frac{1}{2}\tilde{G}(\mathbf{x})\right], j=\overline{1, n}, \tag{12.7}$$

with regard to the normalizing function preserving the state space invariance. Clearly, the change of variables (12.5) maps simplex Σ to a part of the n-dimensional hypersphere in the domain of positive semi-axes. The system of Equations (12.7) than takes on the following form:

$$\frac{d\tilde{x}_j}{dt} = -\left[\frac{\partial Q(\tilde{\mathbf{x}})}{\partial \tilde{x}_j} - \tilde{x}_j\sum_{k=1}^{n}\tilde{x}_k\frac{\partial Q(\tilde{\mathbf{x}})}{\partial \tilde{x}_k}\right], \ j = \overline{1, n}, \tag{12.8}$$

which is different from the potential motion equations (12.6). But (12.8) does define a potential motion, though on the hypersphere surface rather than the whole state space. The gradient is determined under condition that increments must not lead the system out of the hypersphere (i.e. differentials lie in the tangent plane). Geometrically, this means that the conditional gradient, $\mathbf{V}^c$, is a projection of the full space gradient, ∇Q onto the plane tangent to the hypersphere at the point under the concern. The conditional gradient lies evidently in the plane spanning the gradient $\nabla Q(\tilde{\mathbf{x}})$ and the vector normal to the tangent (i.e. the radius vector $\tilde{\mathbf{x}}=(\tilde{x}_1,\ldots,\tilde{x}_n)$). Therefore, it can be decomposed by these two vectors provided they are non-collinear at the point under concern (from geometrical reasons it is clear that points of collineation are stationary in the surface motion, i.e. the conditional gradient should be set zero at such points):

$$\mathbf{V}^c = \nabla Q(\tilde{\mathbf{x}}) + \alpha\tilde{\mathbf{x}} .$$

Lying in the tangent plane, the conditional gradient is orthogonal to the normal vector $\tilde{\mathbf{x}}$: $(\mathbf{V}^c(\tilde{\mathbf{x}}),\tilde{\mathbf{x}}) = 0$, so that $\alpha\ -(\nabla Q(\tilde{\mathbf{x}}),\tilde{\mathbf{x}})/(\tilde{\mathbf{x}},\tilde{\mathbf{x}})$. Since $(\tilde{\mathbf{x}},\tilde{\mathbf{x}})=1$, in the coordinate-wise notation we have

$$V_j^c(\tilde{\mathbf{x}}) = [\nabla Q(\tilde{\mathbf{x}})]_j - \left[\sum_{k=1}^{n} \tilde{x}_k \frac{\partial Q(\tilde{\mathbf{x}})}{\partial \tilde{x}_k}\right]\tilde{x}_j, \tag{12.9}$$

i.e. there is the coordinate of the conditional gradient of potential $Q(\tilde{\mathbf{x}})$ in the right-hand side of dynamic Equations (12.8).

The potential hypersurface defining the trajectory behavior should be respectively treated over the phase space that is represented by the part of the hypersphere.

If the dynamic equations are written down as the gradient descent Equations (12.6), then the motion trajectory coincides with that of a unit-mass point moving in a force field. To prove, let us differentiate both sides of (12.6) with respect to t:

$$\frac{d^2\tilde{x}_j}{dt^2} = \sum_k \frac{\partial^2}{\partial\tilde{x}_j\,\partial\tilde{x}_k} Q \frac{d\tilde{x}_k}{dt} = \sum_k \frac{\partial^2 Q}{\partial\tilde{x}_k\,\partial\tilde{x}_j}\frac{\partial Q}{\partial\tilde{x}_k} =$$

$$= \frac{1}{2}\frac{\partial}{\partial\tilde{x}_j}\sum_k\left(\frac{\partial Q}{\partial\tilde{x}_k}\right)^2 = \frac{1}{2}\frac{\partial}{\partial\tilde{x}_j}\sum_k\left(\frac{d\tilde{x}_k}{dt}\right)^2, \; j = \overline{1,n} . \tag{12.10}$$

Thus, if T designates the kinetic energy,

$$T = \frac{1}{2}\sum_k\left(\frac{d\tilde{x}_k}{dt}\right)^2 = \frac{1}{2}\sum_k\left(\frac{\partial Q}{\partial\tilde{x}_k}\right)^2,$$

and the force function is taken to be $U = -T$, where T is a function on the phase space defined by (12.6), then Equations (12.10) are written down as classical mechanics equations for the motion in a potential force field:

$$d^2\tilde{x}_j/dt^2 = -\,\partial U/\partial\tilde{x}_j, \; j = \overline{1,n} . \tag{12.11}$$

But in the study of gene frequencies' dynamics the motion equations differ from (12.6) since trajectories must pertain to the surface of the unit radius hypersphere. Hence, there must be a reaction force in the dynamic equations besides the active ones, which can be decomposed into the tangent and normal (to the sphere) components. In order that the mass point could not leave the surface, the reaction force must neutralize the normal component of active forces. Also, reaction forces prevent the point from being 'teared' off the surface by centrifugal forces. This component of reaction forces coincides with the centripetal force, which is known to equal $-V^2\tilde{\mathbf{x}}$ at the point $\tilde{\mathbf{x}}$ of the unit radius sphere, the squared velocity V^2 being defined as $(\mathbf{V}^c,\mathbf{V}^c)$ where $\mathbf{V}^c$ being given by formula (12.9). Pertaining to the sphere, any turn in the trajectory is defined by the projection of active forces on the plane tangent to the sphere. We may say, therefore, that, given a force field and the condition of mass point moving on the hypersphere, only the tangent component of active forces and the centripetal component of constraint forces must enter the motion equation in place of full active forces (defined by the field). In contrast to equations of mechanics, the centripetal component of the constraint force is now easily determined from (12.8).

Let us consider what the mechanical analogue to the force field motion looks like for the system (12.8). Relying on (12.11), we may expect the force function for the hypersphere motion to be definable by the kinetic energy T_c corresponding to the velocity (12.9) in the plane tangent to the hypersphere:

$$T_c = \frac{1}{2}\sum_k\left(\frac{d\tilde{x}_k}{dt}\right)^2 = \frac{1}{2}\sum_k (V_k^c)^2. \tag{12.12}$$

To prove this, let us differentiate both sides of (12.8) with respect to t as it was done in studying system (12.6):

$$\frac{d^2\tilde{x}_j}{dt^2} = \sum_k \left(\frac{\partial V_j^c}{\partial \tilde{x}_k}\right)V_k^c = \left(\mathbf{V}^c, \nabla V_j^c - \frac{\partial \mathbf{V}^c}{\partial \tilde{x}_j} + \frac{\partial \mathbf{V}^c}{\partial \tilde{x}_j}\right) =$$

$$= \left(\mathbf{V}^c, \nabla V_j^c - \frac{\partial \mathbf{V}^c}{\partial \tilde{x}_j}\right) + \frac{\partial T_c}{\partial \tilde{x}_j}, \quad j = \overline{1, n}.$$

Note that, if the difference $\nabla V_j^c - \partial\mathbf{V}^c/\partial\tilde{x}_j$ is written out by formula (12.9), the terms with coordinates $\partial^2 Q/(\partial\tilde{x}_k\partial\tilde{x}_j), k=\overline{1, n}$ H, cancel out and the difference $(\tilde{\mathbf{x}},\nabla Q)\nabla\tilde{x}_j$-$(\tilde{\mathbf{x}},\nabla Q)\partial\tilde{\mathbf{x}}/\partial\tilde{x}_j$ vanishes, while the term $-\tilde{\mathbf{x}}\partial(\tilde{\mathbf{x}},\nabla Q)/\partial x_j$ can be omitted as vector $\tilde{\mathbf{x}}$ is orthogonal to $\mathbf{V}^c$. Hence,

$$\frac{d^2\tilde{x}_j}{dt^2} = \frac{\partial T_c}{\partial \tilde{x}_j} - \tilde{x}_j(\mathbf{V}^c, \nabla(\tilde{\mathbf{x}}, \nabla Q)) = \frac{\partial T_c}{\partial \tilde{x}_j} - \tilde{x}_j(\tilde{\mathbf{x}}, \nabla T_c) - \tilde{x}_j V^2, \tag{12.13}$$

where the relation

$$(\mathbf{V}^c, \nabla(\tilde{\mathbf{x}}, \nabla Q)) = \sum_k V_k^c \frac{\partial}{\partial \tilde{x}_k}\left(\sum_m \tilde{x}_m \frac{\partial Q}{\partial \tilde{x}_m}\right) = (\mathbf{V}^c, \nabla Q) + \sum_k V_k^c \sum_m \tilde{x}_m \frac{\partial^2 Q}{\partial \tilde{x}_m\, \partial \tilde{x}_k}$$

is taken into account, the first term being equal to V^2 as ∇Q differs from $\mathbf{V}^c$ with a summand orthogonal to $\mathbf{V}^c$. Furthermore,

$$\sum_k V_k^c \sum_m \tilde{x}_m \frac{\partial^2 Q}{\partial \tilde{x}_m\, \partial \tilde{x}_k} =$$

$$= \sum_m \tilde{x}_m \sum_k V_k^c \frac{\partial}{\partial \tilde{x}_m}\left[\frac{\partial Q}{\partial \tilde{x}_k} - \tilde{x}_k(\tilde{\mathbf{x}}, \nabla Q) + \tilde{x}_k(\tilde{\mathbf{x}}, \nabla Q)\right] =$$

$$= (\tilde{\mathbf{x}}, \nabla T_c) + \sum_m \tilde{x}_m \sum_k V_k^c \frac{\partial}{\partial \tilde{x}_m} [\tilde{x}_k(\tilde{\mathbf{x}}, \nabla Q)].$$

Note that the last term of this expression equals zero because summing up (over k) the terms with the factor $\partial(\tilde{\mathbf{x}},\nabla Q)/\partial\tilde{x}_m$ (that is taken out of the summation sign) yields the inner product $(\mathbf{V}^c, \tilde{\mathbf{x}})$ of orthogonal vectors. The same product arises as a result of summing up (over m) the terms with derivatives $\partial\tilde{x}_k/\partial\tilde{x}_m$.

Thus, the formula (12.13) is proved valid, which defines the motion on the surface of the unit radius hypersphere under the action of potential forces with the potential $U_c = -T_c$: the two first terms of (12.13) represent the projection of active forces on the plane tangent to the hypersphere, while the last term equals the centripetal component of bond reaction forces. We may use, therefore, the whole store of classical mechanics techniques to study systems (12.11) and (12.13).

In particular, genetic models under concern comply with variational principles of mechanics. For example, the integral, least-action principle of Hamilton is valid for the motion in a force field: the minimal value of the functional

$$\mathcal{J} = \int_{t_0}^{t_1} L(t)\,\mathrm{d}t$$

is reached on the true trajectory. Here the initial and the final points of trajectories under examination are fixed as well as (arbitrary) moments of time t_0 and t_1; L is the Lagrange function given by the difference between the kinetic, T_c, and the potential, U_c, energies.

In our case, under condition that the motion proceeds on a surface specified by the constraint equation $\phi(\tilde{\mathbf{x}})=0$, we have:

$$\tilde{L}(t) = T_c - U_c + \lambda(t)\phi\,,$$

$$T_c = \frac{1}{2}\sum_k \left(\frac{\mathrm{d}\tilde{x}_k}{\mathrm{d}t}\right)^2,$$

$$U_c = -\frac{1}{2}\sum_j \left[\frac{\partial Q}{\partial \tilde{x}_j} - \tilde{x}_j(\tilde{\mathbf{x}}, \nabla Q)\right]^2 = -\frac{1}{2}V^2[\tilde{\mathbf{x}}(t)]\,,$$

$$Q = -\frac{1}{8}G\,. \tag{12.14}$$

Here $\phi(\tilde{\mathbf{x}}) = \Sigma_j \tilde{x}_j^2 - 1$ as $\tilde{\mathbf{x}}$ lies on the hypersphere, λ is a Lagrange indefinite multiplier. Finally

$$\mathcal{J} = \int_{t_0}^{t_1} \left[\frac{1}{2}\sum_j \left(\frac{\mathrm{d}\tilde{x}_j}{\mathrm{d}t}\right)^2 + \frac{1}{2}V^2(\tilde{\mathbf{x}}) + \lambda(t)\left(\sum_j \tilde{x}_j^2 - 1\right)\right] \mathrm{d}t. \tag{12.15}$$

The Lagrange indefinite mutliplier must satisfy the condition

$$\lambda(t)\nabla\phi = -V^2\tilde{\mathbf{x}} - \left(\tilde{\mathbf{x}}, \nabla\frac{1}{2}V^2\right)\tilde{\mathbf{x}}|_t, \tag{12.16}$$

where the first term equals the centripetal component of bond reaction forces and the second one neutralizes the normal (to the surface) component for the force function U_c's gradient; its coordinates are determined by formula (12.9).

It can be directly verified that the necessary conditions of $\mathcal{J}$ having an extremum, namely, the Euler equations, hold in this case owing to the motion equations (12.13):

$$\frac{d}{dt}(\partial\tilde{L}/\partial\dot{\tilde{x}}_j) = \partial\tilde{L}/\partial\tilde{x}_j, \; j = 1,n. \tag{12.17}$$

Also, the Legendre strong condition holds: the matrix of second derivatives, $\|\partial^2\tilde{L}/(\partial\dot{\tilde{x}}_i\,\partial\dot{\tilde{x}}_j)\|$, is positive definite (it is readily seen to be the identity matrix). This is known to be sufficient for the true trajectory value of $\mathcal{J}$ being less than the value of $\mathcal{J}$ on any, arbitrary close (with its derivative) trajectory when t_1 is near enough to t_0.

The minimal value of $\mathcal{J}$ can be easily calculated. On a true trajectory the integrand of (12.15) turns into $V^2 = \Sigma_i \dot{\tilde{x}}_i^2$ (the coefficient at λ being equal to zero). Hence,

$$\mathcal{J} = \int_{t_0}^{t_1} \sum_j (\dot{\tilde{x}}_j)^2\, dt = \int_{t_0}^{t_1} \sum_j \left[\frac{\partial Q}{\partial\tilde{x}_j} - (\tilde{\mathbf{x}}, \nabla Q)\tilde{x}_j\right]\dot{\tilde{x}}_j\, dt =$$

$$= \int_{t_0}^{t_1} \sum_j \left(\frac{\partial Q}{\partial\tilde{x}_j}\right)\dot{\tilde{x}}_j\, dt - \int_{t_0}^{t_1} (\tilde{\mathbf{x}}, \nabla Q)\frac{1}{2}\sum_j \frac{d\tilde{x}_j^2}{dt}\, dt = Q(\tilde{\mathbf{x}}_1) - Q(\tilde{\mathbf{x}}_0), \tag{12.18}$$

since $\Sigma_j(\partial Q/\partial\tilde{x}_j)\dot{\tilde{x}}_j = dQ/dt$ and also $d(\Sigma_j\tilde{x}_j^2)/dt = d(\Sigma_j x_j)/dt \equiv 0$ as the sum of allele frequencies. $x_j = \tilde{x}_j^2$ is identically equal to unit.

As well as any mechanical motion that complies with a variational principle, the results of this section can be reformulated in terms of the motion along the shortest path in a Riemannian space, which is the analogue to the straight line in a common Euclidean space. An example of such a space was presented in Section 4.11, where considered was a particular case of function G corresponding to the simplest form of selection with constant coefficients of genotype fitness.

The property of a path to be an extremal does not depend on the coordinate system chosen. The Euler equations may thus be readily rewritten in common coordinates, i.e. allele concentrations, by means of the Lagrange function in those coordinates.

Recall that the function G (and consequently Q) can be defined both individually for any factor of microevolution (various forms of selection coupled, may be, with inbreeding, several types of migrations, and mutation pressure) and for a joint action of any combination of these factors. Attractive feature of the latter case is the simplicity in finding the potential function that describes globally the model dynamics: the function is equal merely to the sum of potentials for all factors of a combination under concern. Respectively, the force function and the Lagrangian can be easily written down for the mechanical analogue of the genetic process.

12.13. Notes and Bibliography

Section 12.2.

Allele fixation probabilities were studied by M. Kimura for a single-locus models, the results being presented, for instance, in his survey:

Kimura, M.: 1970, Stochastic processes in population genetics, with special reference in distribution of gene frequencies and probability of gene fixation. In: Kojima Ken-ichi (ed.). *Mathematical Topics in Population Genetics*, Berlin: Springer-Verlag, pp. 178–209.

Section 12.3.

The posibility that the mean absorption time may decrease under the overdominance condition was revealed by:

Ewens, W.J. and Thomson, G.: 1970, Heterozygote selective advantage. *Ann. Hum. Genet.* 33, No. 4, pp. 365–376.

Various results concerning the sojourn time density function are summarized in the book:

Maruyama, T.: 1977, *Stochastic Problems in Population Genetics*, Berlin: Springer-Verlag, 254 pp.

Coincidence between the sojourn time density function conditioned on allele loss and that conditioned on allele fixation was shown in the paper:

Maruyama, T. and Kimura, M.: 1974, A note on the speed of gene frequency changes in reverse directions in a finite population, *Evolution*, 28, No. 1, pp. 161–163.

Section 12.4 to 11.

One of the pioneers of studying steady-state distributions in genetics was S. Wright, whose results are summarized in his monograph:

Wright, S.: 1969, *Evolution and Genetics of Populations. Vol. 2. The Theory of Gene Frequencies*, Chicago: Univ. of Chicago Press, 511 pp.

By means of the forward Kolmogorov equation, steady-state distributions were first studied in the paper:

Kolmogorov, A.N.: 1935, Deviation from the Hardy formula under partial isolation. *Doklady AN SSSR*. 3, No. 3, pp. 129–132 (in Russian).

The derivation of the steady-state density function in case of multiple alleles follows the papers:

Passekov, V.P.: 1977, *On finding the steady-state distribution of gene frequencies in Wright's island model*. Doklady MOIP, Obščaya biologiya (Reports of Moscow Soc. of Naturalists, General Biology), 1974, Nauka, Moscow, pp. 165–168 (in Russian).

Passekov, V.P.: 1975, Some steady-state distributions in genetics. In: *Applications of statistical methods in problems of population genetics*, issue 49. Interdept. Lab. of Statistical Methods, Moscow State University, pp. 13–18 (in Russian).

The relation between steady-state density functions and adaptive landscape functions was considered in the note:

Passekov, V.P.: 1978, On the relation between steady-state patterns of the gene frequencies' distribution and extensions of the Fisher fundamental theorem for a single multi-allele locus. Doklady MOIP, Obscaya biologiya (Reports of Moscow Soc. of Naturalists, General Biology), 1975. Moscow State Univ. Press, pp. 135–138 (in Russian).

Section 12.12.

For the particular form of the function G corresponding to selection which constant fitness coefficients Yu. M. Svirezhev has shown that population trajectories represent the steepest ascent pathes in a Riemannian space (see also Section 4.11):

Svirezhev, Yu.M.: 1972, Optimality principles in population genetics. In: *Studies in Theoretical Genetics*, Institute of Cytology and Genetics, Novosibirsk, pp. 86–102 (in Russian).

It is shown ibidem that the Euler equation for the Lagrange function

$$\sum_i \left[\frac{1}{2x_i} \left(\frac{dx_i}{dt} \right)^2 + \frac{1}{8} x_i (w_i - w)^2 \right]$$

holds on the true trajectory and that, under selection of the above-mentioned form, the trajectories on the unit radius hypersphere in the Euclidean space are those of the steepest ascent, too; see also:

Timofeeff-Ressovsky, N.V. and Svirezehev, Y.M.: 1970, Population genetics and optimal processes. *Genetika*, **6**, No. 1, pp. 155–166 (in Russian).

The gradient pattern of genetic process of variations in allele frequencies under selection pressure as a motion in a Riemannian space, as well as properties of this motion, in case of several loci (located in a single chromosome lacking multiple crossing-overs) were considered in the paper:

Shahshahani, S.: 1979, A new mathematical framework for the study of linkage and selection, *Memoirs of the American Methamatical Society*, **17**, No. 211, pp. 1–34,

see also:

Akin, E.: 1979, *The geometry of population genetics.* Lecture Notes in Biomathematics, 31, Springer, Berlin e.a., 205 pp.

Well-known is the fact the mean fitness increases under deterministic selection pressure, which is the Fisher fundamental theorem. The monotone behavior of the function G under the joint action of selection, mutation, migrations, etc., represents, in a certain sense, a generalization of this theorem. In the particular case of pair-wise interaction between selection and one of the other factors of microevolution, similar functions of a monotone pattern on process trajectories were found by Yu. M. Svirezhev for one diallelic locus:

Svirezhev, Yu. M.: 1974, Possible ways to generalize the Fisher fundamental theorem of natural selection. *Zurnal obščei bilogii* (*Journal of General Biology*), **35**, No. 4, pp. 590–599 (in Russian).

A general case of the joint action of selection, mutations, migrations, and inbreeding (as well as an arbitrary combination of some of these factors) on the dynamics of a multiple allele locus is considered in the note:

Passekov, V.P.: 1978, On the relation between steady-state patterns of the gene frequencies' distribution and extensions of the Fisher fundamental theorem for a single multi-allele locus. Doklady MIOP, Obsczya biologiya (Reports of Moscow Soc. of Naturalists, General Biology), 1975. Moscow State University Press, pp. 135–138 (in Russian).

where presented are expressions for the functions G_i and G in models of the dynamics in the non-transformed space Σ of allele frequencies.

The transformation of the space (resulting in gradient type equations) to analyze ecological competitive communities by using a complete analogy with genetic processes is proposed in the note:

Passekov, V.P.: 1981, Some variational principle in ecology and genetics. Doklady MOIP, Obščaya biologia (Reports of Moscow Soc. of Naturalists, General Biology), 1979. Nauka, Moscow, pp. 184–188 (in Russian),

where the mechanistic interpretation is given too. Proposed ibidem is an adaptive landscape function for a single-locus genetic models. Noted is the fact that mechanical analogues undergo modification due to the sum of allele frequencies being unit.

Chapter 13

Random Genetic Drift in Subdivided Populations

13.1. Generating Operator for the Random Genetic Drift Process in a Subdivided Finite-Sized Population with Migrations of the 'Island' Type

Natural populations are scarcely represented by a panmictic entity but rather by a collection of groups of individuals (subpopulations) which are linked one to another by migrations. Mating occurs mainly within a subpopulation, which is partly isolated from other groups. Isolation barriers of this kind arise in spreading of population over space (due to mere geographic barriers or isolation by distance).

For simplicity let us consider a system of M subpopulations, each having a size N invariable in time. The genetic structure of the system (under the assumption of random mating within subpopulations) can be characterized in the most complete way by frequencies of various gamete types within each of M groups. Integrated indices of genetic structure are given then by average (over subpopulations) gamete concentrations, i.e. their frequencies in the total population, by the portion of heterozygotes in the population, by average values of linkage disequilibrium coefficients, by indices of genetic variability among subpopulations, etc.

By means of such integrated characteristics we obtain an aggregated description for the genetic structure of the whole system, capable of determining the phenotypic variability,the heritability of quantitative characters, the response to selection pressure, and other properties of the system, which are important both in evolutionary and practical aspects.

In the case of one diallelic locus, such an integrated characteristic as the fraction of heterozygotes in a system of M equal-sized subpopulations, will be equal to

$$H = \frac{1}{M}\sum_{k=1}^{M} 2p^k(1-p^k) = 2\bar{p}(1-\bar{p}) - 2D(\mathbf{p}), \tag{1.1}$$

where p^k is the frequency of the allele under concern in the kth subpopulation, $\bar{p}=\Sigma_{k=1}^{M}p^k/M$ is its (average) concentration in the system, and $D(\mathbf{p})$ is the variance of frequencies p^k among subpopulations:

$$D(\mathbf{p}) = \frac{1}{M}\sum_{k=1}^{M}(p^k - \overline{p})^2 = \frac{1}{M}\sum_{k=1}^{M}(p^k)^2 - \overline{p}^2 . \qquad (1.2)$$

The formula (1.1), that relates the fraction, H, of heterozygotes in the system and the panmictic (under the random-mating assumption) heterozygosity $\overline{H}=2\overline{p}(1-\overline{p})$, is called the Wahlund formula.

By means of panmictic heterozygosity $\overline{H}$ formula (1.1) can be extended for the case of multiple alleles in the following way:

$$H_{ij} = \overline{H}_{ij} + 2\,\mathrm{cov}_{ij} . \qquad (1.3)$$

Here H_{ij} is the fraction of heterozygotes having alleles A_i and A_j relative to the system, $\overline{H}_{ij}$ is the heterozygosity under the random-mating assumption (i.e. in the absence of subdivision):

$$H_{ij} = \frac{1}{M}\sum_{k=1}^{M} 2p_i^k p_j^k , \quad \overline{H}_{ij} = 2\overline{p}_i\overline{p}_j , \quad i \neq j . \qquad (1.4)$$

The value of H_{ij} is determined by means of allele concentrations p_i^k in subpopulations, the superscript referring to the subpopulation number, while the subscript to the number of an allele. The value of $\overline{H}_{ij}$ is expressed in terms of the (average) allele concentrations in the system, $\overline{p}_i$,

$$\overline{p}_i = \frac{1}{M}\sum_{k=1}^{M} p_i^k . \qquad (1.5)$$

Finally, the covariance between the frequencies of alleles A_i and A_j is defined as

$$\mathrm{cov}_{ij} = \frac{1}{M}\sum_{k=1}^{M}(p_i^k - \overline{p}_i)(p_j^k - p_j) = \frac{1}{M}\sum_{k=1}^{M} p_i^k p_j^k - \overline{p}_i\overline{p}_j . \qquad (1.6)$$

The panmictic characteristic of the system heterozygosity, $\overline{H}$, and the actual one, H, are obtained by summing $\overline{H}_{ij}$, or H_{ij}, over all possible heterozygote types A_iA_j, being thus related by the equality

$$H = \overline{H} + 2\mathrm{cov}(\mathbf{p}) . \qquad (1.7)$$

Here cov(**p**) is the total covariance among all kinds of pairs of (different) alleles. In case of two alleles (the situation can be always considered diallelic formally, by defining the combined allele which is complementary to the given one) the formula (1.7) reduces back to (1.1):

$$H = \overline{H} - 2D(\mathbf{p}) . \qquad (1.8)$$

The panmictic ('speculative') heterozygosity $\overline{H}_{ij}$ together with the true heterozygosity H_{ij} characterize the genetic structure of the system. If, for example, H_{ij} becomes zero while $\overline{H}_{ij}$ being positive, then allele A_i is lost in certain part of subpopulations, while A_j is lost in the rest part of them. The same situation in H and $\overline{H}$ means fixation of different alleles in subpopulations. Generally, if H_{ij} and $\overline{H}_{ij}$ are known, we can find from (1.3) and (1.8) the variance and covariances of alleles among subpopulations and thus get a general view of the system heterogeneity.

A complete genetic characteristic of the system is given by the vector of frequencies of various gamete types in subpopulations. Variations in these frequencies occur as a result of the random genetic drift process described earlier, as well as mutation process, and migrations, both outside and inside ones (among subpopulations). In accordance with the general scheme of deviations from panmixia considered in Part I, the effect of subdivision can be described by a stochastic matrix whose entries represent probabilities that mating results in a union of gametes from different subpopulations. These probabilities can be determined from the pattern of migrations and we make the following assumptions concerning this pattern.

The intensity of migration exchange between an arbitrary pair of subpopulations is supposed independent of the pair and equal to m_1. We are interested in the case of weak migratory flows, since an intensive exchange of migrants brings the system nearer to the panmictic entity studied earlier. After migrations take place, the random mating occurs within each subpopulation (independently of others).

This scheme fits formally into the island migration model, which admits the following interpretation, for instance. Suppose that there is a system with an infinite number of subpopulations of the same size and the subpopulations make up a single pool of migrants before mating. Gene frequencies are constant in this pool unless the system as a whole undergoes a permanent influence (for example, if a steady-state probability distribution is reached among states of subpopulations). It is this pool (the 'mainland') from which the 'reverse' migration proceeds into the 'islands'.

An essential difference between this island model and the scheme under concern springs up from the assumption that the number, M, of subpopulations is finite. As a result, the average system characteristics 'drift' in some way and the genetic homogeneity of the whole system is eventually reached. If, however, some genes are brought to the system of M subpopulations by migrations from an outer polymorphic source, then the system average characteristics and gamete frequencies in subpopulations undergo random fluctuations as before, but eventually reached is now a non-trivial steady-state distribution and the limiting genetic structure will be polymorphic.

We consider at first the behavior of the system genetic structure with respect to a single autosomal locus with n alleles. Since mating processes within subpopulations are independent, the diffusion matrix for this model takes on a block diagonal form, each block corresponding to a generating operator of the (11.1.1) form for the narrow-sense genetic drift process within a respective subpopulation.

Let the intensity of migration exchange between subpopulations be denoted by m_1. The contribution of migrants to a concentration p_i^k is clearly equal to

$$m_1 \sum_{l \neq k} p_i^l = m_1 M \overline{p}_i - m_1 p_i^k \ .$$

Hence, the average increment in the coordinate p_i^k as a result of migrations inside the system is given by

$$M_{ik}^{(1)}(\mathbf{p}) = [1 - m_1(M-1)]p_i^k + m_1M\overline{p}_i - m_1p_i^k - p_i^k =$$
$$= (m_1M\,\overline{p}_i - m_1p_i^k) - m_1(M-1)p_i^k = m_1M(\overline{p}_i - p_i^k)\,, \qquad (1.9)$$

i.e. the drift coefficient is equal to the difference between the contributions by immigrants (the term $m_1M\overline{p}_i$ -$m_1p_i^k$)) and the diminution caused by emigrations to other M-1 subpopulations. Along with migrations among subpopulations, we consider also the migration exchange with the outer source, where the frequencies of alleles are constant. Let the intensity of migrations of this kind (being supposed equal for all of the subpopulations) be denoted by m and the allele frequencies in the outer source by q_i, $i=\overline{1, n}$. Then the drift coefficients due to this factor will equal

$$M_{ik}^{(2)}(\mathbf{p}) = m(q_i - p_i^k)\,. \qquad (1.10)$$

for the i-th allele's frequency in the k-th subpopulation.

Finally, we introduce mutation transitions among alleles by the scheme presented in Section 12.9. Let μ_i denote, as before, the intensity of mutations into allele A_i (μ_i being supposed independent of the type of an allele mutating into A_i) and let μ denote the total intensity of mutations:

$$\mu = \sum_{i=1}^{n} \mu_i\,.$$

Then, by (12.9.9), the drift component due to irreversible mutations is to be

$$M_{ik}^{(3)}(\mathbf{p}) = \mu_i - \mu p_i^k \qquad (1.11)$$

for the coordinate p_i^k .

If μ_i are put zero, then formula (1.11) determines irreversible mutations, the value of μ being positive and interpretable now as a total intensity of mutations into new, unique alleles. The scheme of irreversible mutations is based on modern knowledge of structure of the gene that represents a very long (up to several hundred) sequence of nucleotide pairs. A mutation change in any pair is able to modify the product encoded by the gene, so that the potential number of various alleles (i.e. different sequences) is highly great, practically infinite. It is reasonable, therefore, to assume that any new mutation yields a new unique allele which has not yet been present in the population.

With regard for all microevolutionary factors considered, the generating operator for a diffusion process of variations in frequencies of alleles at one locus in a system of subpopulations can be written down in the following form:

$$\mathfrak{a} = \sum_{k=1}^{M}\left[\frac{1}{2}\sum_{i,j=1}^{n-1}\frac{p_i^k(\delta_{ij}-p_j^k)}{2N}\frac{\partial^2}{\partial p_i^k\,\partial p_j^k} + \sum_{i=1}^{n-1} M_{ik}(\mathbf{p})\frac{\partial}{\partial p_i^k}\right] = \sum_{k=1}^{M}\mathfrak{a}_k\,, \qquad (1.12)$$

where

$$M_{ik}(\mathbf{p}) = m_1M(\overline{p}_i - p_i^k) + m(q_i - p_i^k) + \mu_i - \mu p_i^k\,. \qquad (1.13)$$

In the two-allele case the generating operator appears somewhat simpler:

$$\mathfrak{A} = \sum_{k=1}^{M} \left\{ \frac{1}{2} \frac{p^k(1-p^k)}{2N} \frac{\partial^2}{\partial (p^k)^2} + [m_1 M(\bar{p} - p^k) + m(q - p^k) + \mu_{12} - \mu p^k] \frac{\partial}{\partial p^k} \right\}. \quad (1.14)$$

Here μ_{12} represents the intensity of (reverse) mutations into a given allele from the complementary one.

It is clear how the operator $\mathfrak{A}^*$ looks in the situations under concern, and the probability density function, f, for subpopulation states in the system obeys both the forward and backward Kolmogorov equations

$$\partial f/\partial t = \mathfrak{A}^* f, \quad \partial f/\partial t = \mathfrak{A} f.$$

13.2. Dynamics of Expected Allele Frequencies in a Subdivided Population

We investigate the behavior of the first moments of allele concentrations in the whole system and in each individual subpopulation by using the approach presented in Section 10.9. Assuming conditions (10.9.5) to hold, we will search for expectations of some functions $g(\mathbf{x})$ on process states by using equations of the following form:

$$\frac{d}{dt} E_t\{g(\mathbf{x})\} = E_t\{(\mathfrak{A} g)(\mathbf{x})\}. \quad (2.1)$$

If, for example, $g(\mathbf{x}) = \bar{x}_i$, we have

$$\frac{d}{dt} E_t\{\bar{x}_i\} = E_t\left\{ \sum_{k=1}^{M} \mathfrak{A}_k \bar{x}_i \right\} =$$

$$= E_t\left\{ m_1 M \sum_{k=1}^{M} (\bar{x}_i - x_i^k) \frac{1}{M} + m \sum_{k=1}^{M} (q_i - x_i^k) \frac{1}{M} + \mu_i - \right.$$

$$\left. - \mu \sum_{k=1}^{M} x_i^k \frac{1}{M} \right\} = m q_i + \mu_i - (m + \mu) E_t\{\bar{x}_i\}, \quad (2.2)$$

as $\Sigma_{k=1}^{M} (\bar{x}_i - x_i^k) = 0$. The solution to this equation with the initial condition $E_0\{\bar{x}_i\} = \bar{p}_i$ is evidently given by

$$E_t\{\bar{x}_i\} = \frac{m q_i + \mu_i}{m + \mu} + \left(\bar{p}_i - \frac{m q_i + \mu_i}{m + \mu} \right) e^{-(m+\mu)t}. \quad (2.3)$$

If the intensities of mutation and external migrations are set zero in the solution (2.3), i.e. the genetic drift in a subdivided population is considered in the narrow sense, then $E_t\{\bar{x}_i\} \equiv \bar{p}_i$ as in the case of random mating (cf. (11.7.2)).

When there are no migrations but mutations have the irreversible nature, we obtain

$$E_t\{\bar{x}_i\} = p_i e^{-\mu t}, \quad (2.4)$$

i.e. the mean frequency of the ith allele converges exponentially to zero at the rate of irreversible mutations μ. The result is also true for an undivided population with random mating.

If there exist mutation transitions among alleles given by pattern (1.11) but external migrations are absent, then, in the limit as $t \to \infty$, the expected frequency of the ith allele will be equal to μ_i/μ. For an arbitrary time moment we have

$$E_t\{\overline{x_i}\} = \frac{\mu_i}{\mu} + \left(\overline{p_i} - \frac{\mu_i}{\mu}\right)e^{-\mu t}. \tag{2.5}$$

In formulae (2.3) to (2.5), there is no coefficient characterizing the intensity of migrations among subpopulation within the system. Therefore, the results concerning expected concentrations remain valid when the system either falls into totally disconnected isolates or lacks any subdivision at all, being overall panmictic.

We analyze next the dynamics of expected allele frequencies in individual subpopulations. From (2.1) it follows that

$$\frac{d}{dt}E_t\{x_i^k\} = E_t\{m_1 M(\overline{x_i} - x_i^k) + \mu_i - \mu x_i^k + m\,(q_i - x_i^k)\}\,.$$

By substituting for $E_t\{\overline{x_i}\}$ its corresponding value from (2.3), we obtain the following linear inhomogeneous equation:

$$\frac{d}{dt}E_t\{x_i^k\} = (mq_i + \mu_i)\left(1 + \frac{m_1 M}{m+M}\right) + m_1 M\left(\overline{p_i} - \frac{mq_i+\mu_i}{m+\mu}\right)e^{-(m+\mu)t} - (m_1 M + m + \mu)E_t\{x_i^k\}\,, \tag{2.6}$$

$$E_0(x_i^k\} = p_i^k\,.$$

The solution to this equation is given by

$$E_t\{x_i^k\} = \frac{mq_i+\mu_i}{m+\mu} + \left(\overline{p_i} - \frac{mq_i+\mu_i}{m+\mu}\right)e^{-(m+\mu)t} + (p_i^k - \overline{p_i})e^{-(m_1 M+m+\mu)t}\,. \tag{2.7}$$

If mutation and external migrations are 'switched off' then solution (2.7) takes on the form of

$$E_t\{x_i^k\} = \overline{p_i} + (p_i^k - \overline{p_i})e^{-m_1 M t}\,, \tag{2.8}$$

i.e. the allele frequencies in subpopulations converge, due to intermixing, to the initial average concentrations in the system. If we take irreversible mutations into account, the expression (2.8) must be multiplied by $e^{-\mu t}$. The time period for the expected concentrations to become almost equal in subpopulations has by (2.4) an order of $1/(m_1 M)$, while the time for allele disappearance has by (2.4) an order of $1/\mu$. If μ is considerably less than $m_1 M$, the homogeneity of the expected concentrations will be reached in the system before any alleles be lost.

In the absence of external migrations the irreversible mutation pressure leads all (initially present) alleles to disappearance from each subpopulation. Migrations from an outer polymorphic source brings about the same limiting expectations of allele frequencies in any subpopulation, $(mq_i+\mu_i)/(m+\mu)$, which are fairly close to the allele frequencies, q_i, in the outer source when $m>>\mu$ (the intensity of mutations has an order of magnitude 10^{-5}- 10^{-7}).

Note also that the behavior of mathematical expectations of the average (over all the subpopulations) allele frequencies (2.3) and concentrations within each subpopulation (2.7) coincides with temporal dynamics of proper solutions in the deterministic model defined by ordinary differential equations. Some dispersion, however, exists there about the deterministic paths due to random deviations from expected characteristics in the population genetic composition. By this reason, for example, the expectation of a genetic structure index which depends on the second and higher-order moments of concentrations, is distinct from the corresponding expression in the deterministic model.

13.3. Behavior of Expected Heterozygosity Indices

The level of heterozygosity is an important index of the population genetic structure, defined in terms of the second moments of gene concentrations. Under the assumption of random mating within subpopulations, the fraction of heterozygotes with alleles A_i and A_j in the system is determined by formula (1.4):

$$H_{ij} = \frac{1}{M}\sum_{k=1}^{M} 2p_i^k\, p_j^k .$$

The behavior of heterozygosity in case of panmixia was studied in Section 11.7. Let $\overline{p_i}$ and $\overline{p_j}$ denote concentrations of alleles A_i and A_j respectively at the initial time moment. If there are neither external migrations nor mutation in the system, then it follows from (11.7.5) that

$$E_t\{H_{ij}\} = E_t\{2\overline{x_i}\,\overline{x_j}\} = 2\overline{p_i}\,\overline{p_j}\ \exp\{-t/(2MN)\}, \tag{3.1}$$

where MN represents the total population size.

To study the influence that the subdivision of the population exerts upon the course of random genetic drift process (without mutation and external migrations) and behavior of the expected heterozygosity, we note first that

$$\mathfrak{A}_k H_{ij} = -\frac{1}{4N}\,\frac{4p_i^k p_j^k}{M} + m_1 M\left(\overline{p}_i\frac{2p_j^k}{M} + \overline{p}_j\frac{2p_i^k}{M}\right) - 2m_1 M\frac{2p_i^k p_j^k}{M}.$$

Similarly,

$$\mathfrak{A}_k\overline{H}_{ij} = \mathfrak{A}_k 2\overline{p}_i\,\overline{p}_j = -\frac{1}{4N}\,\frac{4p_i^k p_j^k}{M^2} + m_1 M\left[(\overline{p}_i - p_i^k)\frac{2\overline{p}_j}{M} + (\overline{p}_j - p_j^k)\frac{2\overline{p}_i}{M}\right].$$

Remark that the expression in square brackets vanishes when summed over k. Applying now equation (2.1) to the functions H_{ij} and $\overline{H}_{ij}$ and utilizing the equality $\mathfrak{a}=\Sigma_{k=1}^{M}\mathfrak{a}_k$, we obtain readily a homogeneous system of linear differential equations to find the expectations $E_t\{H_{ij}\}$ and $E_t\{\overline{H}_{ij}\}$. Summing up the equations for various combinations of (different) subscripts i and j shows that the equations for the expected total heterozygosities, H and $\overline{H}$, have the same form as those for heterozygotes of the A_iA_j type:

$$\frac{d}{dt}E_t\{H\} = -\left(\frac{1}{2N} + 2m_1M\right)E_t\{H\} + 2m_1ME_t\{\overline{H}\},$$
$$\frac{d}{dt}E_t\{\overline{H}\} = -\frac{1}{2MN}E_t\{H\};$$
$$E_0\{H\} = H^0,\ E_0\{\overline{H}\} = \overline{H}^0. \tag{3.2}$$

The characteristic equation for system (3.2) is clearly

$$\lambda^2+\left(\frac{1}{2N} + 2m_1M\right)\lambda+\frac{m_1}{N} = 0. \tag{3.3}$$

If there were no subdivision, then by (3.1) the rate of decrease in heterozygosity would be equal to $1/(2MN)$. In the case under concern this rate (being equal to the maximum non-zero eigenvalue of operator (1.12)) equals asymptotically the greatest root of Equation (3.3). Let this root be represented in the form of $\lambda_{max}=-\nu/(2MN)$. Then the influence of subdivision can be measured by how far the value of ν deviates from unit. This value obeys evidently the equation

$$\nu^2 - M(2KM+1)\nu + 2KM^2 = 0, \tag{3.4}$$

where K designates the number of alleles brought in by internal migrations from one subpopulation into another: $K=2m_1N$. P. Moran used Equation (3.4) as an approximating one for the subdivision scheme with small values of m_1 in case of discrete time. But we have derived the equation as an exact one and this approach enables us to study both the asymptotic rate, λ_{max}, of decreases in genetic variability and the behavior of the expected heterozygosity on any interval of time.

Calculating the roots of Equation (3.4) we find the minimum value of ν (corresponding to the maximum of λ) to be close to 1 (regardless of M) when $K\geq 1$, and the second value of ν to be substantially more. Therefore, the expected heterozygosity behavior fairly soon becomes definable by the total size, MN, of subpopulations as if there were no subdivision. Thus, an exchange of one migrant per generation between any pair of subpopulations is sufficient to provide that the asymptotic decrease in heterozygosity be practically independent of the population subdivision.

The solution to (3.2) has the following form:

$$E_t\{H\} = \frac{\lambda_1H^0+2m_1M\overline{H}^0}{\lambda_1-\lambda_2}e^{\lambda_1 t} - \frac{\lambda_2H^0+2m_1M\overline{H}^0}{\lambda_1-\lambda_2}e^{\lambda_2 t},$$

$$E_t\{\overline{H}\} = -\frac{\lambda_2\overline{H}^0+H^0/(2MN)}{\lambda_1-\lambda_2}\, e^{\lambda_1 t} + \frac{\lambda_1\overline{H}^0+H^0/(2MN)}{\lambda_1-\lambda_2}\, e^{\lambda_2 t}. \tag{3.5}$$

Comparing the values of $E_t\{H\}$ (obtained from (3.5)) for the subdivided population with those obtained by (3.1) for the panmictic case, when both taken with the same initial conditions, reveals a great deal of similarity between them, not only asymptotically but also for any time moment, provided the number of migrants per generation between any pair of subpopulations has an order of unit or more. Shown in Figure 37 are the dynamics of the expected numbers of heterozygotes in the undivided (H_Π) and the subdivided populations of the same total size and the same initial values of gene frequencies. Time is measured along the abscissa axis, the unit corresponding to $4N$ generations (where N is the total size of the diploid population). The values of H_Π, H, and $\overline{H}$ are normalized by means of division by the constant, the number of heterozygotes corresponding to the initial allele concentrations in the panmictic case. The number of subpopulations equals 5, the mean number of migrants per generation equals 0.1: (a) there was no distinction in gene frequencies between any subpopulations at the initial time moment; (b) the initial number of heterozygotes is zero in the population because of fixing different alleles in subpopulations.

With migrations of this intensity, the influence of subdivision upon the the dynamics of the heterozygote numbers can be neglected, the conclusion being fairly unexpected since intuition, relied upon common sense, supposes the intermixing to be more intensive.

Under the same initial conditions, the expected number of heterozygotes in the subdivided population is somewhat less than in the panmictic one during a fairly long period of time (about $1.5N$ generations in magnitude). The situation then changes and the expected number of heterozygotes becomes less in the absence of subdivision. In the limit as $t \to \infty$, the number of heterozygotes will be zero on each trajectory with the unit probability. Therefore, the homozygosity with one of possible alleles will be enevitably attained.

Despite the difference between the curves of expected heterozygosities in the panmictic and the subdivided populations, their integral values in the course of reaching the genetic homogeneity will be the same in the absence of initial genetic differences. The simplest way to find this integral value is to integrate both sides of the second of Equations (3.2) over t from zero to infinity. After doing this, we have

$$\int_0^\infty E_t\{H\}\,dt = 2MN\overline{H}^0, \tag{3.6}$$

as $E_\infty\{\overline{H}\}=0$. If $\overline{H}^0 = H^0$ at the initial time moment, then subdivision has no effect on the total expected number of heterozygotes in the entire course of reaching homozygosity (cf. with (11.7.7)).

But the mean time to reach homozygosity, $T(\mathbf{p})$, will be greater in the subdivided population than that in the panmictic one. To demonstrate this, consider the equation for $T(\mathbf{p})$ in case of a diallelic locus:

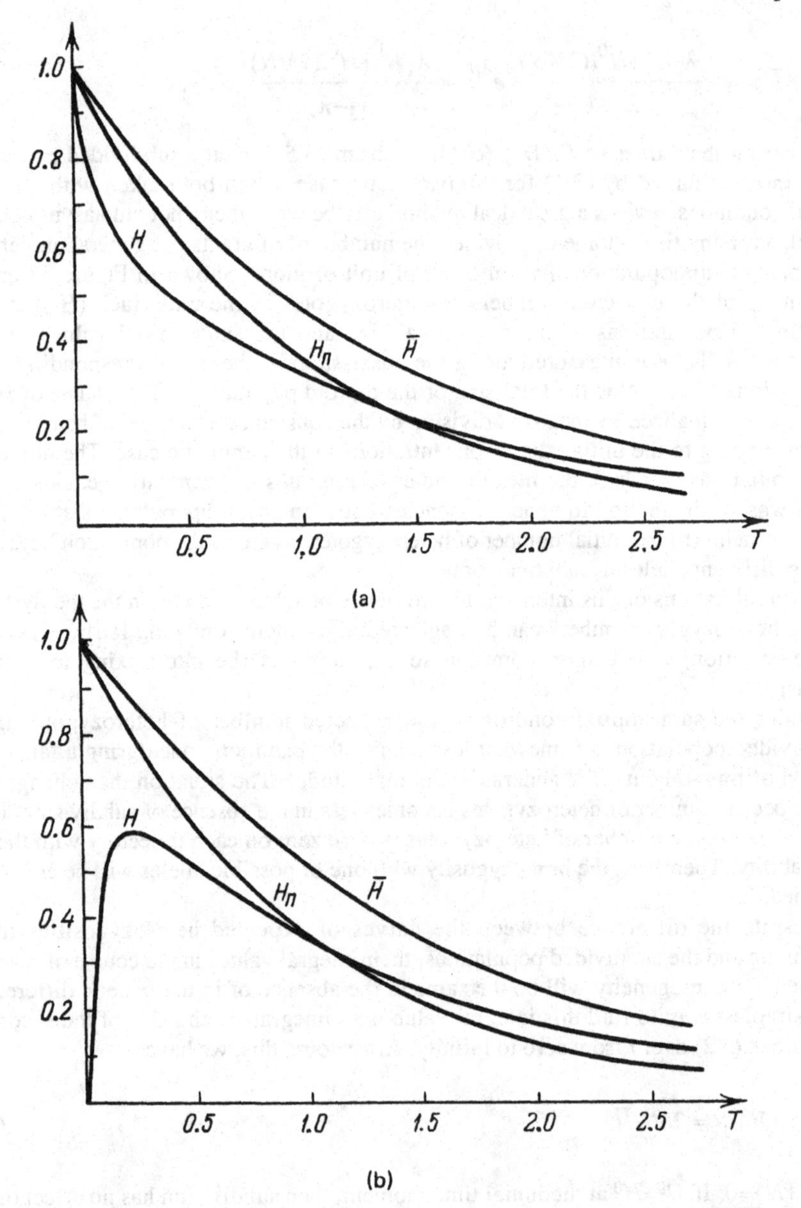

Fig. 37. The curves of dynamics of the expected heterozygote numbers in an undivided (H_{Π}) and a subdivided populations.

$$(\mathfrak{Q}T)(\mathbf{p}) = \sum_{k=1}^{M}\left[\frac{1}{2}\frac{p^k(1-p^k)}{2N}\frac{\partial^2 T(\mathbf{p})}{\partial(p^k)^2} + m_1 M(\bar{p} - p^k)\frac{\partial T(\mathbf{p})}{\partial p^k}\right] = -1\,,$$

$$T(\mathbf{p}) = 0, \text{ if } \bar{p} = 0 \text{ or } \bar{p} = 1\,. \tag{3.7}$$

If there were no subdivision in the system, then by (11.5.2) the mean time as a function of initial allele frequencies would equal $-4MN[\bar{p}\ \ln \bar{p} + (1-\bar{p})\ln(1-\bar{p})]$, since the initial concentration of the allele in the system would be $\bar{p}$. Let this function, $\tilde{T}$, be substituted in Equation (3.7) as a trial function:

$$(\mathfrak{Q}\tilde{T})(\mathbf{p}) = -4MN\sum_{k=1}^{M}\left\{\frac{1}{2}\frac{p^k(1-p^k)}{2N}\frac{1}{M^2\bar{p}(1-\bar{p})} + m_1 M(\bar{p} - p^k)\left[\frac{\ln\bar{p} - \ln(1-\bar{p})}{M}\right]\right\} = -1 + \frac{D(\mathbf{p})}{\bar{p}(1-\bar{p})}\,. \tag{3.8}$$

We have used here the fact the terms with m_1M vanish when summed over k, while $\Sigma_k p^k(1-p^k)$ is expressed by the Wahlund formula (1.1). By (10.8.3) the function $\tilde{T}(\mathbf{p})$ can be represented in terms of the penalty on trajectories as the expectation of a penalty function that equals unit in any point of the state space (i.e. as the mean homozygosity attainment time $T(\mathbf{p})$) plus the expectation, which we denote by $-E_F$, of the penalty that equals $-D(\mathbf{p})/[\bar{p}(1-\bar{p})]$. Obviously, $-E_F<0$ as the expectation of a function that is almost everywhere negative. Thus,

$$T(\mathbf{p}) = \tilde{T}(\mathbf{p}) + E_F > \tilde{T}(\mathbf{p})\,.$$

The term E_F can be interpreted as the expected (over trajectories) value of the empirical coefficient of inbreeding that is defined by the Wahlund formula (1.1):

$$H = \frac{1}{M}\sum_{k=1}^{M} 2x^k(1-x^k) = 2\,\bar{x}\,(1-\bar{x}^{\,k}) - 2D(\mathbf{x}) = 2\bar{x}\,(1-\bar{x})\,(1-F)\,.$$

Formulae (3.5) remain valid if $\overline{H}_{ij}$ and H_{ij} are considered instead of $\overline{H}$ and H (under corresponding initial conditions). Therefore, the expected value of covariance (1.6) between alleles A_i and A_j at time t can be determined by means of formulae (1.3) and (1.8):

$$E_t\{\mathrm{cov}_{ij}\} = \frac{1}{2}[E_t\{H_{ij}\} - E_t\{\overline{H}_{ij}\}]\,.$$

The proper expressions appear especially simple if there is no genetic difference among subpopulations at the initial moment: i.e. $H_{ij}^0 = \overline{H}_{ij}^0$. Then, by taking into account that $\lambda_1+\lambda_2 = -1/(2N) - 2m_1M$ in accordance with (3.3), we have the following expression for the expected variance of the ith allele:

$$E_t\{D_i\} = \frac{1}{4N}\left(1 - \frac{1}{M}\right)H_{ii}^0\,\frac{\exp\{\lambda_1 t\} - \exp\{\lambda_2 t\}}{\lambda_1 - \lambda_2}\,. \tag{3.9}$$

Here the value $H_{ii}^0 = \overline{H}_{ii}^0$ is defined to be $2\overline{p}_i\,(1-\overline{p}_i)$, which corresponds to the share of all possible heterozygote types having allele A_i (or to the formal treatment of the system as a diallelic one). From (3.9) it is clear that the intergroup variance deviates in the course of time from its zero initial value but then approaches asymptotically to zero again (because of the whole system's tendency to genetic homogeneity).

Similar is the behavior of expected covariance between alleles, $E_t\{\mathrm{cov}_{ij}\}$, whose values can be expressed by the formula (3.9) if we substitute H_{ij}^0 for H_{ii}^0 and change the sign of the right side into the opposite one.

Note that the present formulae for the behavior of the expectations of heterozygosity values, variances, and covariances among alleles can be easily modified for the case of irreversible mutations with an intensity μ. In this case the system of equations can be obtained by application of (2.1) to the functions H_{ij} and $\overline{H}_{ij}$ (or H and $\overline{H}$) with m and μ_i being set zero in operator $\mathfrak{a}$ (1.12)–(1.13). Then the system of differential equations with constant coefficients to determine, for instance, $E_t\{H\}$ and $E_t\{\overline{H}\}$ will have the following form:

$$\frac{d}{dt}E_t\{H\} = -\left(\frac{1}{2N} + 2m_1M + 2\mu\right)E_t\{H\} + 2m_1ME_t\{\overline{H}\}\,,$$

$$\frac{d}{dt}E_t\{\overline{H}\} = -\frac{1}{2MN}E_t\{H\} - 2\mu E_t\{\overline{H}\}\,. \tag{3.10}$$

The coefficient matrix of this system differs from that of system (3.2) by the quantity 2μ subtracted from its each diagonal entry. Hence it follows immediately that the characteristic roots $\tilde{\lambda}_i$ for Equations (3.10) differ from the respective roots λ_i for system (3.2) by the quantity 2μ::$\tilde{\lambda}_i = \lambda_i - 2\mu$, $i=1, 2$. The solution to (3.10) for the expectation of H, for example, takes on the form

$$E_t\{H\} = C_1e^{\tilde{\lambda}_1 t} + C_2e^{\tilde{\lambda}_2 t}\,.$$

With regard for the initial conditions, the constants C_1 and C_2 must obey the system of linear algebraic equations

$$\begin{bmatrix} H^0 \\ (H_\mu^0)' \end{bmatrix} = \begin{Vmatrix} 1 & 1 \\ \tilde{\lambda}_1 & \tilde{\lambda}_2 \end{Vmatrix} \begin{bmatrix} C_1 \\ C_2 \end{bmatrix}\,.$$

Note that, by (3.10), in case of irreversible mutations, the derivative of the mean heterozygosity with respect to t at t=0, $(H_\mu^0)'$, is less than the derivative $(H^0)'$ in the case of no mutations (3.2) by the quantity $2\mu H^0$. At the same time, by expressing $\tilde{\lambda}_i$ in terms of λ_i we obtain

$$(H_u^0)' = \tilde{\lambda}_1 C_1 + \tilde{\lambda}_2 C_2 = \lambda_1 C_1 + \lambda_2 C_2 - 2\mu H^0\,,$$

since $C_1+C_2=H^0$. Thus, if irreversible mutations are 'switched on' at the same level of initial heterozygosity H^0, then the coefficients C_i at $\exp\{\lambda_i t\}$ and $\exp\{\tilde{\lambda}_i t\}$ in the solutions to (3.2) and (3.10) obey the same equations. Hence, the expressions for $E_t\{H\}$ and $E_t\{\overline{H}\}$ in case of irreversible mutations coincide with the formulae (3.5) if the latters are multiplied by the function $\exp\{-2\mu t\}$. The expressions for expected variances and covariances of allele frequencies in the system are to be modified similarly.

But if we consider the case of reversible mutations and/or external migrations, then the approach used above to find mathematical expectations of the heterozygosity values H and $\overline{H}$ leads now to an inhomogeneous system of linear differential equations with constant coefficients. The characteristic values of this system, $\tilde{\lambda}_i$, are expressed in terms of those of system (3.2), λ_i, by the formula $\tilde{\lambda}_i=\lambda_i-2(m+\mu)$. The explicit solutions to the equations look too tedious to be cited here.

In the limit as time tends to infinity, the expectations of heterozygosity characteristics converge to some non-zero value (in contrast to the case of random genetic drift with migrations among subpopulations and a possibility of irreversible mutations). For example, the limiting expected fraction of heterozygotes will be equal to

$$\frac{2N(m^2H_q+2H_{q\mu}+H_\mu)}{(m+\mu)\left[m+\mu+4(m+\mu)^2N+m_1(1+4(m+\mu)MN)\right]},$$

where $H_q=\sum\sum_{i\neq j}q_iq_j$ is the fraction of heterozygotes in the outer source, $H_{q\mu}=\sum\sum_{i\neq j}q_i\mu_j$ and $H_\mu=\sum\sum_{i\neq j}\mu_i\mu_j$.

13.4. Dynamics of Expected Indices of Linkage Disequilibrium in Case of Two Loci

When studying the behavior of gamete frequencies in a system of subpopulations with gametes classified with respect to two autosomal loci, we should take into account, as well as in the single-locus case, the influence of diffusion (sampling effects at the change of generation), migrations, and an additional effect of recombinations. The later causes a shift in the coordinate $p^k_{i_1j_2}$ (the frequency within the kth subpopulation of the gamete having allele A_{i_1} at the first locus and B_{j_2} at the second) of the form (see Section 11.9):

$$M^{(4)}_{i_1j_2,k}=-rD^k_{i_1j_2}\,,\quad D^k_{i_1j_2}=p^k_{i_1j_2}-p^k_{i_1}\,p^k_{j_2} \tag{4.1}$$

Here $D^k_{i_1j_2}$ denotes the coefficient of linkage disequilibrium (11.9.3) between the alleles A_{i_1} and B_{j_2} in the kth subpopulation, $p^k_{i_1}$ and $p^k_{j_2}$ are the frequencies of these alleles in the subpopulation.

Let $\overline{p}_{i_1j_2}$ denote the concentration of the gamete $\Gamma_{i_1j_2}$ (carrying alleles A_{i_1} and B_{j_2}) in the system of M subpopulations:

$$\overline{p}_{i_1j_2}=\frac{1}{M}\sum_{k=1}^{M}p^k_{i_1j_2}\,. \tag{4.2}$$

Then the generating operator for the random drift at two loci in the system of subpopulations with regards for migrations and recombinations can be written in the following way:

$$\mathfrak{a} = \sum_{k=1}^{M} \left\{ \frac{1}{2} \sum_{i_1 j_2} \sum_{l_1, m_2} \frac{p_{i_1 j_2}^k (\delta_{i_1 l_1} \delta_{j_2 m_2} - p_{l_1 m_2}^k)}{2N} \frac{\partial^2}{\partial p_{i_1 j_2}^k \partial p_{l_1 m_2}^k} + \right.$$

$$\left. + \sum_{i_1 j_2} M_{i_1 j_2, k}(\mathbf{p}) \frac{\partial}{\partial p_{i_1 j_2}^k} \right\} = \sum_{k=1}^{M} \mathfrak{a}_k , \tag{4.3}$$

where

$$M_{i_1 j_2, k}(\mathbf{p}) = m_1 M (\bar{p}_{i_1 j_2} - p_{i_1 j_2}^k) + m(q_{i_1 j_2}^k - p_{i_1 j_2}) - r D_{i_1 j_2}^k . \tag{4.4}$$

In analogy with single-locus indices of heterozygosity, we introduce the average disequilibrium among subpopulations with respect to alleles A_{i_1} and B_{j_2} :

$$D_{i_1 j_2} = \frac{1}{M} \sum_{k=1}^{M} (p_{i_1 j_2}^k - p_{i_1}^k \, p_{j_2}^k) = \frac{1}{M} \sum_{k=1}^{M} D_{i_1 j_2}^k . \tag{4.5}$$

This expression can be written down differently, by means of the gamete and allele frequencies in the whole system:

$$D_{i_1 j_2} = \bar{p}_{i_1 j_2} - \bar{p}_{i_1} \bar{p}_{j_2} - \mathrm{cov}_{i_1 j_2} , \tag{4.6}$$

where $\bar{p}_{i_1}$ and $\bar{p}_{j_2}$ denotes the (average) concentrations of alleles A_{i_1} and B_{j_2} respectively at the first and second loci in the system of subpopulations:

$$\bar{p}_{i_1} = \frac{1}{M} \sum_{k=1}^{M} p_{i_1}^k , \; \bar{p}_{j_2} = \frac{1}{M} \sum_{k=1}^{M} p_{j_2}^k . \tag{4.7}$$

The covariance in frequencies of these alleles at different loci is defined as

$$\mathrm{cov}_{i_1 j_2} = \frac{1}{M} \sum_{k=1}^{M} (p_{i_1}^k - \bar{p}_{i_1})(p_{j_2}^k - \bar{p}_{j_2}) = \frac{1}{M} \sum_{k=1}^{M} p_{i_1}^k p_{j_2}^k - \bar{p}_{i_1} \bar{p}_{j_2} . \tag{4.8}$$

Let us introduce another index of disequilibrium in combinations of alleles in gametes, $\bar{D}_{i_1 j_2}$, coinciding with panmictic disequilibrium defined in (11.9.3) if we 'forget' the subdivision of the total population and use the allele and gamete concentrations throughout it:

$$\bar{D}_{i_1 j_2} = \bar{p}_{i_1 j_2} - \bar{p}_{i_1} \bar{p}_{j_2} = D_{i_1 j_2} + \mathrm{cov}_{i_1 j_2} . \tag{4.9}$$

Note that the generating operator (1.12) – (1.13) possesses the property to be invariant under non-distinction of some gamete types (for instance, of the gametes that carry certain subset of alleles at one of the loci). Utilizing this property, we may treat both loci formally as if they were diallelic ones. The part $\mathfrak{a}_k$ of the generating operator (corresponding to the k-th subpopulation) will then be written down in the form (11.9.4) with the superscript k appearing in variables. Also, (11.9.4) is to be modified by the drift coefficients caused by effects of migrations.

Let the behavior of the expected indices of disequilibrium, $D_{i_1j_2}$ and $\overline{D}_{i_1j_2}$, be considered in case of no external migrations. To do this, we use the possibility to treat both loci as diallelic ones with the alleles A_{i_1} and non-A_{i_1} at the first locus and B_{j_2} and non-B_{j_2} at the second one. Applying Equation (2.1) to the functions $D_{i_1j_2}$ and $\overline{D}_{i_1j_2}$, we obtain a system of linear homogeneous differential equations to determine the expectations. To simplify laying out, we note that

$$\mathfrak{A}_k D_{i_1j_2} = \mathfrak{A}_k D^k_{i_1j_2}/M = [-(1/(2N)+r)\, D^k_{i_1j_2} + m_1 M\,(\cdots)]/M,$$

where the first summand appears by (11.9.5) as a result of operation by the part $\mathfrak{A}_k$ coinciding with (11.9.4), while the second shows the influence of migrations among subpopulations. Eventually, the system takes on the following form:

$$\begin{aligned}
&\frac{d}{dt} E_t\{D_{i_1j_2}\} = -\left(\frac{1}{2N} + r + 2m_1 M\right) E_t\{D_{i_1j_2}\} + 2m_1 M E_t\{\overline{D}_{i_1j_2}\},\\
&\frac{d}{dt} E_t\{\overline{D}_{i_1j_2}\} = -\left(\frac{1}{2MN} + r\right) E_t\{D_{i_1j_2}\},\\
&E_0\{D_{i_1j_2}\} = D^0_{i_1j_2},\ E_0\{\overline{D}_{i_1j_2}\} = \overline{D}^0_{i_1j_2}.
\end{aligned} \tag{4.10}$$

Remark on the following analogy with the single-locus case. If we denote by Λ_N the greatest eigenvalue of the generating operator for the random genetic drift process in a panmictic diploid population of size N (it will be $-1/(2N)$ in case of one locus and $\Lambda_N = -1/(2N)-r$ in case of two loci), then the coefficient matrices of systems (3.2) and (4.10) will have the same form in terms of Λ. The coefficients of the first equation take on the form $\Lambda_N - 2m_1M$ and $2m_1M$, while that of the second equals Λ_{MN}, the greatest eigenvalue of the random genetic drift generating operator under the assumption of panmixia in the system whose total size equals MN.

Therefore, the solutions to systems (3.2) and (4.10) take on the same form as functions of Λ_N, Λ_{MN}, initial conditions, time, and the roots of the characteristic equations which can be rewritten in the form

$$\lambda^2 - (\Lambda_N - 2m_1M)\lambda - 2m_1 M \Lambda_{MN} = 0.$$

For example, the expected indices of disequilibrium appear to be

$$\begin{aligned}
&E_t\{D_{i_1j_2}\} = \frac{\lambda_1 D^0_{i_1j_2} + 2m_1 M \overline{D}^0_{i_1j_2}}{\lambda_1 - \lambda_2} e^{\lambda_1 t} - \frac{\lambda_2 D^0_{i_1j_2} + 2m_1 M \overline{D}^0_{i_1j_2}}{\lambda_1 - \lambda_2} e^{\lambda_2 t},\\
&E_t\{\overline{D}_{i_1j_2}\} = -\frac{\lambda_2 \overline{D}^0_{i_1j_2} - \Lambda_{MN} D^0_{i_1j_2}}{\lambda_1 - \lambda_2} e^{\lambda_1 t} + \frac{\lambda_1 \overline{D}^0_{i_1j_2} - \Lambda_{MN} D^0_{i_1j_2}}{\lambda_1 - \lambda_2} e^{\lambda_2 t},
\end{aligned} \tag{4.11}$$

where $\Lambda_{MN} = -(1/(2MN)+r)$ and λ_1, λ_2 are the roots of the characteristic equation

$$\lambda^2 + (1/(2N) + r + 2m_1M)\lambda + 2m_1M(1/(2MN) + r) = 0\,. \quad (4.12)$$

The solutions for $E_t\{H_{ij}\}$ and $E_t\{D_{i_1j_2}\}$ have the same form but the characteristic roots appearing in the notation must be found from different equations.

Calculation of the roots to Equation (4.12) and explicit solutions (4.11) shows that, when the linkage is tight (the parameter Nr is small) and migrations are not too weak, the curves of the expected indices of disequilibrium in case where the population is subdivided are fairly close to those in the panmictic case. But the increase in parameter Nr and/or the decrease in the mean number of migrants per generation result already in considerable difference between the pattern of dynamics in the subdivided population and that in the panmictic one. The general picture is such that quantities $D_{i_1j_2}$ of the subdivided population first are less in the mean than those of the panmictic population, but afterwards the situation changes to the opposite (yet the indices $\overline{D}_{i_1j_2}$ and $\overline{H}_{ij}$ always exceeding in the mean the respective values in case of panmixia).

Shown in Figure 38 are the dynamics of the expected disequilibrium with respect to two loci in an undivided D_{Π} and a subdivided populations of the same size and the same initial gamete frequencies. Time is measured along the abscissa axis, one unit corresponding to $4N$ generations (where N is a size of the diploid population). The values of D_{Π}, D, and $\overline{D}$ are normalized by means of division by a constant (the initial value of the disequilibrium corresponding to the undivided, panmictic population). The number of subpopulations equals 5, the mean number of migrants per generation equals 0.1, the product of the recombination coefficient time the double size of the population equals 0.03:

(a) there were no differences among subpopulations in their gamete frequencies at the initial moment of time;

(b) there was zero disequilibrium D in the population at the initial moment as a result of, for instance, fixation of different gametes in subpopulations.

Despite the difference in the pattern of dynamics of the genetic composition in the subdivided and the panmictic populations, the integral value of the expected indices of disequilibrium $D_{i_1j_2}$ (i.e. covariances of alleles at different loci among subpopulations), accumulated in the course of reaching homozygosity, will be the same provided there are no differences among subpopulations at the initial moment. This can be easily shown by integrating the second of the equations in system (4.10) over t from zero to infinity (with regard for the equality $E_\infty\{\overline{D}_{i_1j_2}\}=0$). If follows that

$$\int_0^\infty E_t\{D_{i_1j_2}\}\,dt = \frac{2MN}{1+2MNr}\,\overline{D}^0_{i_1j_2}\,, \quad (4.13)$$

which coincides with the formula (11.9.10) for the panmictic case provided $D^0_{i_1j_2} = \overline{D}^0_{i_1j_2}$. The latter condition holds, for instance, in the absence of any initial genetic differences among subpopulations of the system. Thus, the mean integral disequilibrium index in the course of random drift, (4.13), and the heterozygosity index (3.6) in the absence of initial differentiation in the system are determined by the same formulae as in case of panmixia. While, however, the heterozygosity index H shows an actual fraction

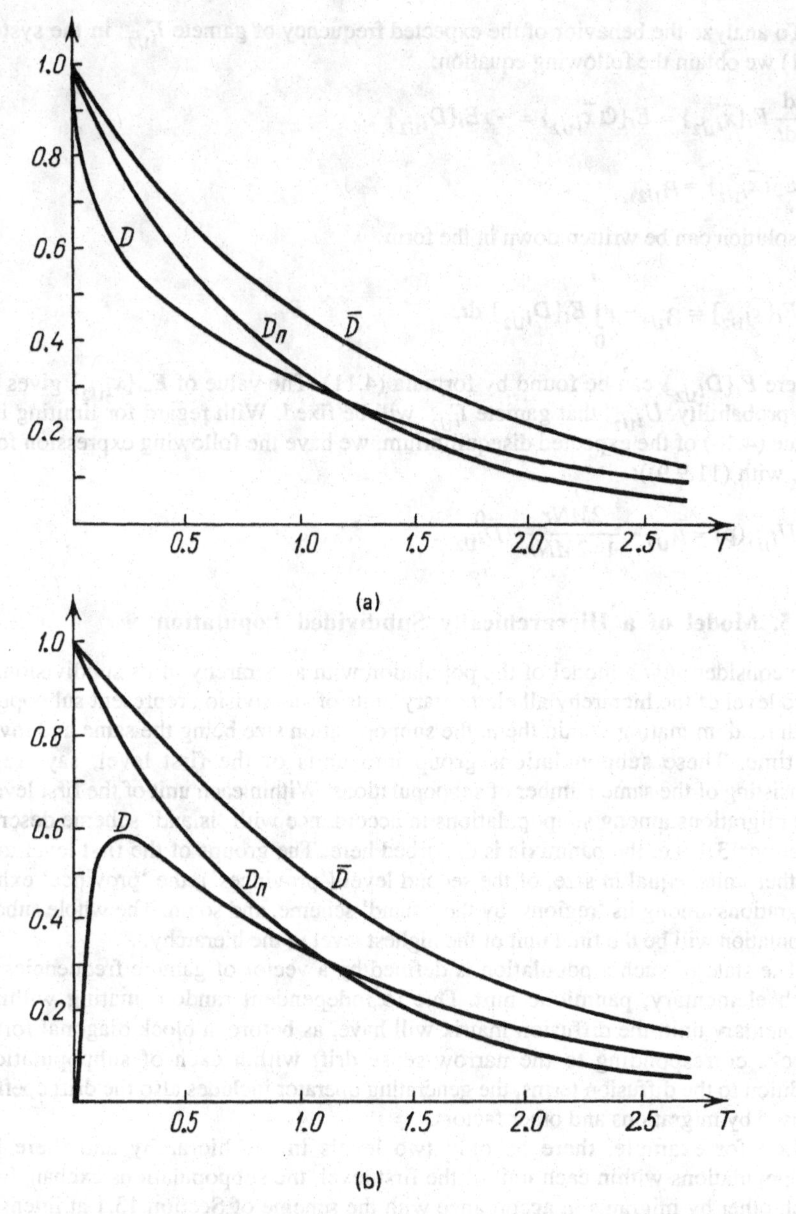

Fig. 38. The curves of dynamics of the expected disequilibrium with respect to two loci in an undivided (D_Π) and a subdivided populations.

of heterozygotes in the total population, the index D is an average covariance among alleles per subpopulation rather than the covariance of alleles in gametes of the system.

To analyze the behavior of the expected frequency of gamete $\Gamma_{i_1j_2}$ in the system, by (2.1) we obtain the following equation:

$$\frac{\mathrm{d}}{\mathrm{d}t}E_t\{\bar{x}_{i_1j_2}\} = E_t\{\mathfrak{a}\bar{x}_{i_1j_2}\} = -rE_t\{D_{i_1j_2}\},$$

$$E_0\{\bar{x}_{i_1j_2}\} = \bar{p}_{i_1j_2}. \tag{4.14}$$

Its solution can be written down in the form

$$E_t\{\bar{x}_{i_1j_2}\} = \bar{p}_{i_1j_2} - r\int_0^t E_t\{D_{i_1j_2}\}\,\mathrm{d}t, \tag{4.15}$$

where $E_t\{D_{i_1j_2}\}$ can be found by formula (4.11). The value of $E_\infty\{\bar{x}_{i_1j_2}\}$ gives clearly the probability, $U_{i_1j_2}$, that gamete $\Gamma_{i_1j_2}$ will be fixed. With regard for limiting integral value (4.13) of the expected disequilibrium, we have the following expression for $U_{i_1j_2}$ (cf. with (11.9.9)):

$$U_{i_1j_2}(\mathbf{p}) = \bar{p}_{i_1j_2} - \frac{2MNr}{1+2MNr}\,\bar{D}^0_{i_1j_2}\ . \tag{4.16}$$

13.5. Model of a Hierarchically Subdivided Population

We consider now a model of the population with a hierarchy in its subdivision. In the zero level of the hierarchy all elementary units of subdivision represent subpopulations with random mating within them, the subpopulation size being the same and invariable in time. These subpopulations group into units of the first level, say 'regions', consisting of the same number of subpopulations. Within each unit of the first level there are migrations among subpopulations in accordance with 'island' scheme described in Section 13.1, i.e. the panmixia is disturbed here. The groups of the first level make up further units, equal in size, of the second level ('provinces'), the 'province' exhibiting migrations among its 'regions' by the 'island' scheme, and so on. The whole subdivided population will be the final unit of the highest level in the hierarchy.

The state of such a population is defined by a vector of gamete frequencies within each elementary, panmictic unit. Due to independent random mating within each elementary unit, the diffusion matrix will have, as before, a block diagonal form with blocks corresponding to the narrow-sense drift within each of subpopulations. In addition to the diffusion terms, the generating operator includes also the drift coefficients caused by migrations and other factors.

Let, for example, there be only two levels in the hierarchy and there be M_1 subpopulations within each unit of the first level, the subpopulations exchanging with each other by migrants in accordance with the scheme of Section 13.1 at intensity m_1. The contributions of migrants into the drift coefficient for p_i^k, the concentration of the ith allele in the kth subpopulation, will be equal as above to

$$m_1(M_1\bar{p}_i^1(k) - p_i^k),$$

where $\bar{p}_i^1(k)$ designates the concentration of the ith allele in that unit of the first hierarchical level (denote it by k_1) which includes the kth subpopulation. Simultaneously, the emigrants to (M_1-1) subpopulations cause a decrease by $m_1(M_1-1)p_i^k$ in the drift component for the kth subpopulation.

Let the whole population consist of M_2 units of the first level. The exchange of migrants proceeds at intensity m_2 among subpopulations of various units of that level. These migrants contribute

$$m_2 \sum_{j, j \notin k_1} p_i^j = m_2 M_1 M_2 \bar{p}_i - m_2 M_1 \bar{p}_i^1(k)$$

into the drift component, where $\bar{p}_i$ is a concentration of the ith allele in the total population. Also, the emigration to (M_2-1) units of the first level (each consisting of M_1 subpopulations) decreases the drift component for the k-th subpopulation by $m_2 M_1(M_2-1)p_i^k$. As the final result, the drift coefficient will be equal, as well as in formula (1.9), to the difference between the contribution by immigrants and the diminution caused by emigration:

$$\begin{aligned} M_{ik}(\mathbf{p}) &= m_1[M_1 \bar{p}_i^1(k) - p_i^k] - m_1(M_1-1)\, p_i^k + \\ &+ m_2 M_1 [M_2 \bar{p}_i - \bar{p}_i^1(k)] - m_2 M_1 (M_2-1) p_i^k = \\ &= M_1(m_1 - m_2)[\bar{p}_i^1(k) - p_i^k] + M_1 M_2 m_2 (\bar{p}_i - p_i^k)\,. \end{aligned} \tag{5.1}$$

Consider now the general case with L levels in the hierarchy. Let M_l be the number of units of the $(l-1)$th level included in each unit of the lth level (the quantity $M(l) = \Pi_{j=1}^{l} M_j$ showing the total number of elementary subpopulations in this unit). Denote by m_l the intensity of migration exchange among subpopulations from various units of the $(l-1)$th hierarchical level, by $\bar{p}_i^l(k)$ the (average) concentration of the ith allele in the unit of the lth level that contains the kth subpopulation:

$$\bar{p}_i^l(k) = \frac{1}{M(l)} \sum_{j \in k_l} p_i^j\,, \tag{5.2}$$

by k_l the unit itself. Then the contribution by the immigrants into the concentration of allele A_i in the subpopulation k (of the zero level) due to the 'gene flow' of intensity m_l from the subpopulations not entering into the group k_{l-1} will be equal to

$$m_l M(l) \bar{p}_i^l(k) - m_l M(l-1)\, \bar{p}_i^{l-1}(k)\,. \tag{5.3}$$

At the same time, the emigration from subpopulation k proceed into other (not containing it) (M_l-1) units of the $(l-1)$th level. The proportion of emigrants is equal to

$$m_l M(l-1)\,(M_l-1) = m_l[M(l) - M_k(l-1)]\,. \tag{5.4}$$

The mean increment in coordinate p_i^k is determined, as well as in (1.9), in the form of the difference between the contribution by immigrants (5.3) and the diminution by emigrants (5.4), multiplied by p_i^k. Summing over all of L levels of the hierarchy, we obtain the following expression for the drift coefficient:

$$M_{ik}(\mathbf{p}) = \sum_{l=1}^{L} m_l\{M(l)[\bar{p}_i^l(k) - p_i^k] - M(l-1)[\bar{p}_i^{l-1}(k) - p_i^k]\} = \tag{5.5}$$

$$= \sum_{l=1}^{L} M(l)(m_l - m_{l+1})[\bar{p}_i^l(k) - p_i^k],$$

where $m_{L+1}=0$. When $L=1$, formula (5.5) reduces to (1.9) as $\bar{p}_i^0(k)=p_i^k$ and second term in braces vanishes; when $L=2$ (5.5) coincides with (5.1).

So, in the absence of mutations and external migrations, the generating operator of the genetic drift process at a single autosomal locus with n alleles for the hierarchically subdivided population can be written down in the following way:

$$\mathfrak{A} = \sum_{k=1}^{M(L)} \left[\frac{1}{2} \sum_{i=1}^{n-1} \sum_{j=1}^{n-1} \frac{p_i^k(\delta_{ij} - p_j^k)}{2N} \frac{\partial^2}{\partial p_i^k \partial p_j^k} + \sum_{i=1}^{n-1} M_{ik}(\mathbf{p}) \frac{\partial}{\partial p_i^k} \right],$$

where $M_{ik}(\mathbf{p})$ is given by formula (5.5) and N represents the size of each elementary, panmictic subpopulation (of the zero level).

In order to investigate the effect of the hierarchy in subdivision on the behavior of the expectations of relative numbers of heterozygotes with alleles A_i and A_j,

$$H_{ij} = \frac{1}{M(L)} \sum_{k=1}^{M(L)} 2p_i^k p_j^k,$$

we introduce the following set of functions $\overline{H}_{ij}^l$, $l=\overline{1,L}$, $i \neq j$:

$$\overline{H}_{ij}^1 = \frac{M_1}{M(L)} \sum_{\dots} 2\bar{p}_i^1(\cdots)\bar{p}_j^1(\cdots),$$

$$\overline{H}_{ij}^l = \frac{M(l)}{M(L)} \sum_{\dots} 2\bar{p}_i^l(\cdots)\bar{p}_j^l(\cdots), \quad \overline{H}_{ij}^L = 2\bar{p}_i^L \bar{p}_j^L. \tag{5.6}$$

Summation in (5.6) for H_{ij}^l proceeds over all $M(L)/M(l)$ units of the lth level.

To find the mathematical expectations of the above functions, we apply the Equation (2.1) and obtain a system of linear differential equations with constant coefficients. In search of the expression for $\mathfrak{A}\overline{H}_{ij}^m$ appearing in (2.1), we consider first the value of operator $\mathfrak{A}$ on one of the summands entering the function $\overline{H}_{ij}^m$. Let us fix, for example, the group m_1, a unit of the mth level containing the first subpopulation, and consider the summand $2\bar{p}_i^m(1)\bar{p}_j^m(1)$. Then

$$\mathfrak{A}2\bar{p}_i^m(1)\bar{p}_j^m(1) = \frac{1}{M^2(m)} \sum_{k\in m_1} \left(-\frac{p_i^k p_j^k}{2N} \right) +$$

$$+ 2\sum_{l=1}^{L} M(l)(m_l - m_{l+1}) \sum_{k\in m_1} [\bar{p}_i^l(k) - p_i^k] \frac{2\bar{p}_j^m(1)}{M(m)}. \tag{5.7}$$

Here the first term appears due to the diffusion part of operator $\mathfrak{A}$, while the second due to the drift. It has multiplier 2 since differentiating $\overline{p}_i^m(1)\overline{p}_j^m(1)$ with respect to both first and second co-factors yields eventually the same contribution into (5.7).

Note that, when $m \geq l$, the sum over k in the second term of (5.7) equals zero, representing the sum of deviations in $\{p_i^k\}$ from their average value $\overline{p}_i^l(k)$. When $m<l$, this sum is equal to

$$2\overline{p}_i^l(1)\overline{p}_j^m(1) - 2\overline{p}_i^m(1)\overline{p}_j^m(1)\,. \tag{5.8}$$

Besides group m_1, other units of the mth level contribute also to $\overline{H}_{ij}^m$. To account for these contributions we have to sum up expressions (5.8) over all $M(L)/M(m)$ units on the mth level, which results in $(\overline{H}_{ij}-\overline{H}_{ij}^m)M(L)/M(m)$. Consequently,

$$\mathfrak{A}\overline{H}_{ij}^m = -\frac{1}{2M(m)N}H_{ij} - \left[\sum_{l=m+1}^{L} 2M(l)(m_l - m_{l+1})\right]\overline{H}_{ij}^m + \sum_{l=m+1}^{L} 2M(l)(m_l - m_{l+1})\overline{H}_{ij}^l\,. \tag{5.9}$$

Instead of $\overline{H}_{ij}^l$ we may consider the functions $\overline{H}^l$ resulting from summation of $\overline{H}_{ij}^l$ over all possible types of 'heterozygotes' (over superscripts i,j, $i\neq j$). As operator $\mathfrak{A}$ is linear, the value of $\mathfrak{A}\overline{H}^m$ equals the linear combination of functions $\overline{H}^l$ with coefficients appearing in (5.9). Denote the value $2M(l)(m_l - m_{l+1})$ by $m(l)$. Then the system of differential equations to find the mathematical expectations of functions H and $\{\overline{H}^l\}$ can be written down in the following form:

$$\frac{d}{dt}E_t\{H\} = -\left[\frac{1}{2N} + \sum_{l=1}^{L} m(l)\right]E_t\{H\} = \sum_{l=1}^{L} m(l)E_t\{\overline{H}^l\}\,,$$

$$\frac{d}{dt}E_t\{\overline{H}^m\} = -\frac{1}{2M(m)N}E_t\{H\} - \left[\sum_{l=m+1}^{L} m(l)\right]E_t\{\overline{H}^m\} + \sum_{l=m+1}^{L} m(l)E_t\{\overline{H}^l\}\,,$$

$$m = \overline{1, L-1},$$

$$\frac{d}{dt}E_t\{\overline{H}^L\} = -\frac{1}{2M(L)N}E_t\{H\}\,. \tag{5.10}$$

13.6. Investigation of the Asymptotic Rate of Decrease in Heterozygosity in the Hierarchical Model

The exact analytical solution to system (5.10) is not known and we have to use numerical methods for the investigation. Another approach supposes an approximation of solutions under the assumption that the size N of individual subpopulations is great enough. This approach permits a fairly easy determination of the asymptotic pattern in behavior of the heterozygosity in a subdivided population.

Let the coefficient matrix of system (5.10) be rewritten in the form $\mathbf{A}+\varepsilon\mathbf{B}$ where $\varepsilon = -1/(2N)$ and for $i,j=\overline{0, L}$

$$\mathbf{A}=\|a_{ij}\|,\quad a_{ij}=\begin{cases}0, & i<j;\\ -\sum_{l=i+1}^{L} m(l), & i=j;\\ m(j), & i>j;\end{cases} \tag{6.1}$$

$$\mathbf{B}=\|b_{ij}\|,\quad b_{ij}=\begin{cases}0, & j>1;\\ 1/M(i), & i=\overline{0,L},\ j=1,\ M(0)=1.\end{cases}$$

From this notation it is clear that the coefficient matrix can be treated as a perturbation of matrix **A** by addition of $\varepsilon\mathbf{B}$ and its eigenvalues are known from the perturbation theory to be representable in the form of power series in ε. Assuming the subpopulation size sufficiently great, we may confine these expansions to their first terms.

To find these terms, we note that matrix **A** is triangular. Hence, its eigenvalues coincide with its diagonal entries and, together with their left ($\mathbf{l}_i$) and right ($\mathbf{r}_i$) eigenvectors, are given by the formulae

$$\lambda_0=0,\ \mathbf{l}_0=\underbrace{(0,\ldots,\ 0,\ 1)}_{L+1},\ \mathbf{r}_0=(1,\ldots,1)^T;$$

$$\lambda_i=-\sum_{j=0}^{i-1} m(L-j),\ \mathbf{l}_i=(0,\ldots,1,\ -1,\underbrace{0,\ldots,\ 0}_{i}),$$

$$\mathbf{r}_i=(1,\ldots,1,\ \underbrace{0,\ldots,\ 0}_{i})^T,\ i=\overline{1,L-1};$$

$$\lambda_L=-\sum_{j=1}^{L} m(j)=-\sum_{j=0}^{L-1} m\,(L-j)\,,\ \mathbf{l}_L=(1,\ -1,\ 0,\ldots,0),\ \mathbf{r}_L=(1,\ 0,\ldots,0)^T. \tag{6.2}$$

We will look for the eigenvalues of the perturbed matrix in the form

$$\tilde{\lambda}_i=\lambda_i+\varepsilon\lambda_i^{(1)}+\varepsilon^2\lambda_i^{(2)}+\ldots$$

and the eigenvectors in the form

$$\tilde{\mathbf{l}}_i=\mathbf{l}_i+\varepsilon\mathbf{l}_i^{(1)}+\ldots\ \text{and}\ \tilde{\mathbf{r}}_i=\mathbf{r}_i+\varepsilon\mathbf{r}_i^{(1)}+\ldots.$$

By equating the coefficients at ε in the equality $(\mathbf{A}+\varepsilon\mathbf{B})\tilde{\mathbf{r}}_i=\tilde{\lambda}\,\tilde{\mathbf{r}}_i$, we have

$$\mathbf{B}\mathbf{r}_i+\mathbf{A}\mathbf{r}_i^{(1)}=\lambda_i^{(1)}\mathbf{r}_i+\lambda_i\mathbf{r}_i^{(1)}. \tag{6.3}$$

Multiplying both sides of (6.3) by $\mathbf{l}_i$ from the left and taking the equalities $\mathbf{l}_i\mathbf{A}=\lambda_i\mathbf{l}_i$ and $(\mathbf{l}_i,\mathbf{r}_i)=1$ into account, we find

$$\lambda_i^{(1)} = (\mathbf{l}_i,\mathbf{B}\mathbf{r}_i)/(\mathbf{l}_i,\mathbf{r}_i) = (\mathbf{l}_i,\mathbf{B}\mathbf{r}_i)\ . \tag{6.4}$$

If we multiply both sides of (6.3) by $\mathbf{l}_j, j \neq i$, from the left, then, taking the equality $(\mathbf{l}_j,\mathbf{r}_i)=0$ into account, we obtain

$$(\mathbf{l}_j,\mathbf{B}\mathbf{r}_i) = (\lambda_i - \lambda_j)(\mathbf{l}_j, \mathbf{r}_i^{(1)})\ . \tag{6.5}$$

To find the components $\mathbf{r}_j^{(1)}$ of the right eigenvectors $\mathbf{r}_j$, we represent them in the basis of vectors $\mathbf{r}_j$:

$$\mathbf{r}_i^{(1)} = \sum_{j=0}^{L} c_{ij}\mathbf{r}_j\ ,\ \ i=\overline{0, L}. \tag{6.6}$$

Multiplying (6.6) by $\mathbf{l}_j$ from the left, we find

$$(\mathbf{l}_j, \mathbf{r}_i^{(1)}) = c_{ij}(\mathbf{l}_j, \mathbf{r}_j) = c_{ij}\ .$$

Inserting here the value of $(\mathbf{l}_j,\mathbf{r}_i^{(1)})$ from (6.5), we can write down the following expression for c_{ij}:

$$c_{ij} = (\mathbf{l}_j, \mathbf{B}\mathbf{r}_i)/[(\lambda_i - \lambda_j)(\mathbf{l}_j, \mathbf{r}_j)] = (\mathbf{l}_j, \mathbf{B}\mathbf{r}_i)/(\lambda_i - \lambda_j),\ i \neq j \tag{6.7}$$

the coefficients c_{ii} still remaining undefined. To find them, suppose the vectors $\tilde{\mathbf{r}}_i$ be normalized such that $(\mathbf{l}_i,\tilde{\mathbf{r}}_i)=(\mathbf{l}_i,\mathbf{r}_i)=1$. Then

$$(\mathbf{l}_i\ , \tilde{\mathbf{r}}_i\ ) = (\mathbf{l}_i, \mathbf{r}_i + \varepsilon\mathbf{r}_i^{(1)} + \varepsilon^2\mathbf{r}_i^{(2)}+...) = (\mathbf{l}_i, \mathbf{r}_i) + \varepsilon(\mathbf{l}_i, \mathbf{r}_i^{(1)}) + \varepsilon^2...\ ,$$

from which it follows that $(\mathbf{l}_i, \mathbf{r}_i^{(1)})=0$. Since this inner product equals c_{ii} by virtue of decomposition (6.6), we have

$$c_{ii} = 0,\ \ i=\overline{0, L}. \tag{6.8}$$

By means of these results we may find the values of $\tilde{\lambda}_i$, $\tilde{\mathbf{r}}_i$, and $\tilde{\mathbf{l}}_i$ with an accuracy up to $o(\varepsilon^2)$ and so on. In particular, the value of $\lambda_i^{(2)}$ can be find from the equality $(\mathbf{l}_i,(\mathbf{A}+\varepsilon\mathbf{B})\tilde{\mathbf{r}}_i\ )=\tilde{\lambda}_i(\mathbf{l}_i,\tilde{\mathbf{r}}_i\ )$, so that the eigenvalues of the perturbed matrix are representable in the following way:

$$\tilde{\lambda}_i \sim \lambda_i + \varepsilon(\mathbf{l}_i, \mathbf{B}\mathbf{r}_i) + \varepsilon^2 \sum_{j \neq i} \frac{(\mathbf{l}_j,\mathbf{B}\mathbf{r}_i)(\mathbf{l}_i,\mathbf{B}\mathbf{r}_j)}{\lambda_i - \lambda_j}\ . \tag{6.9}$$

Coming back to analysis of the model for a hierachically subdivided population, suppose all the coefficients $m(l\,)$ be positive (corresponding to a reasonable assumption that the intensity of migrations decreases as the level number increases). Then $\lambda_0=0$ will be the greatest eigenvalue of matrix $\mathbf{A}$. By (6.1), (6.2), and (6.4) the perturbed eigenvalue will be equal to

$$\tilde{\lambda}_{\max} \sim -1/(2M(L)N) \tag{6.10}$$

up to $o(\varepsilon)$.

Note that $M(L)N$ is the total size of the subdivided population, i.e. in this approximation the asymptotic rate of reaching homozygosity, defined as $\tilde{\lambda}_{max}$, coincides with the rate in the panmictic population of the same size. We do not cite the approximate solution to system (5.10) as it is too cumbersome.

More accurate value of $\tilde{\lambda}_{max}$ can be determined by means of formula (6.9):

$$\tilde{\lambda}_{max} \sim 0 + \frac{1}{2N}(\mathbf{l}_0,\mathbf{B}\mathbf{r}_0) + \frac{1}{(2N)^2}\sum_{j=1}^{L}\frac{(\mathbf{l}_j,\mathbf{B}\mathbf{r}_0)(\mathbf{l}_0,\mathbf{B}\mathbf{r}_j)}{-\lambda_j} =$$

$$= -\frac{1}{2M(L)N} + \frac{1}{(2N)^2}\sum_{j=1}^{L}\frac{1/M(L-j)-1/M(L-j+1)}{M(L)\sum_{l=0}^{j-1}m(L-l)} \quad . \tag{6.11}$$

It can be seen from (6.11) that the asymptotic rate of reaching homozygosity in the subdivided population will be less than that in the panmictic one. Thus, 'subdividedness' is asymptotically equivalent to an increase in the total population size, though the change having the second order of magnitude in $1/N$. The most simple is the expression for the second approximation in case where all intensities, m_l, of migrations at different levels are equal to the same value m^*. In this case $m(l)=2M(l)(m_l-m_{l+1})=0$ for $l \le L-1$ and there is only one term rested in the sum over l in (6.11) (remind that $m_{L+1}=0$). Hence,

$$\tilde{\lambda}_{max} \sim -\frac{1}{2M(L)N} + \frac{1}{[2M(L)N]^2}\,\frac{M(L)-1}{2M(L)m^*} \ .$$

13.7. Model of Isolation by Distance

The model of migrations presented in the previous Section described some kind of uniform intermixing of all subpopulations, which were in the same conditions of migration exchange with respect to each other. This situation may take place actually for a small number of low-sized, for instance, island populations or, on the contrary, for several superpopulations (spread for, may be, the whole continents) like major human races. But if we consider a typical case where a significant number of subpopulations are scattered over a homogeneous space, it is natural to suppose the level of migration exchange to decrease as the distance of migration increases. The simplest mathematical scheme for this phenomenon of isolation by distance is a model where migration flows exist between neighboring populations only, with an intensity invariable in time and space.

Within the limits of this assumption, we consider a model of M subpopulations having the same, time-invariable size N and located along a one-dimensional 'area' (for example, a number of settlements along a river or a sea coasts). Let the subpopulations be numbered in the order they follow each other along the area and suppose each of the bound subpopulations to exchange migrants only with its (single) neighbor while the 'inner' ones with their neighbors from the left and the right, the intensity of exchange, m_1, being constant. Random mating occurs in each subpopulation (independently of others). In the diffusion model for this kind of subdivision, the state of the whole population is commonly represented by a vector, **p**, of gamete frequencies in elementary panmictic units. Its changes are described by a stochastic process whose generating operator is given by a block diagonal matrix of diffusion coefficients and by the drift coefficients associated with the effects of migrations and other factors. As before, the drift coefficient for the concentration of the *i*th gamete in the *k*th subpopulation caused by internal migrations is equal to the difference between the contribution by immigrants and diminution by emigrants:

$$M_{ik}(\mathbf{p}) = \begin{cases} m_1(p_i^2 - p_i^1), & k=1, \\ m_1(p_i^{k+1} + p_i^{k-1}) - 2m_1 p_i^k, & k=\overline{2,M-1}, \\ m_1(p_i^{M-1} - p_i^M), & k=M. \end{cases} \tag{7.1}$$

According to (7.1) the vector of drift due to migrations for the frequencies of *i*th gamete, $\mathbf{p}_i$ in subpopulations, can be written down in the form:

$$\mathbf{M}_i(\mathbf{p}) = m_1 \left\| \begin{matrix} -1 & 1 & & & & \\ 1 & -2 & 1 & & \mathbf{0} & \\ & \ddots & \ddots & \ddots & & \\ & & & & & \\ \mathbf{0} & & & 1 & -2 & 1 \\ & & & & 1 & -1 \end{matrix} \right\| \begin{bmatrix} p_i^1 \\ p_i^2 \\ \vdots \\ p_i^{M-1} \\ p_i^M \end{bmatrix} = \| m_{ij} \| \, \mathbf{p}_i \, . \tag{7.2}$$

In the study of the population genetic structure with respect to a single autosomal locus with *n* alleles, the generating operator for the genetic drift process in the absence of external migrations and mutations takes on the form (1.12) with drift coefficients (7.1) and (7.2) for $i=\overline{1,n-1}$.

Let us consider the behavior of the relative number of heterozygotes with alleles A_i and A_j in the *k*th subpopulation, that is equal to $2x_i^k(t)x_j^k(t)$, where $x_i^k(t)$ is the current (at moment *t*) value of allele concentration. To determine expectation of this number, we use Equation (2.1) but apply it directly to the functions $2x_i^k x_j^l$, that, making though less transparent sense, reduce to the heterozygosity when $k=l$. This results in the equation

$$\frac{\mathrm{d}}{\mathrm{d}t} E_t\{2x_i^k x_j^l\} = -\frac{\delta_{kl}}{2N} E_t\{2x_i^k x_j^k\} - m_1 E_t\{f_{kl}(\mathbf{x})\} , \tag{7.3}$$

where

$$f_{kl} = 2\,(x_i^{k+1} + x_i^{k-1} - 2x_i^k)x_j^l + 2\,(x_j^{l+1} + x_j^{l-1} - 2x_j^l)x_i^k ,$$
$$k, l = \overline{1, M}.$$

The expressions for f_{kl} are obviously modified in cases where one of the subscripts equals 1 or M. It becomes clear that if we have to analyze the behavior of the expected number of heterozygotes in a particular subpopulation k by means of Equation (2.1), then the functions of the form $x_i^k x_j^l$, $k,l=\overline{1,M}$ should be also included into analysis to get a closed system of differential equations.

Each of these functions can be treated as the (kl)th component of the vector $2\mathbf{x}_i \otimes \mathbf{x}_j$. Recall that the Kronecker product of vectors $\mathbf{x}_i$ and $\mathbf{x}_j$ (of matrices **A** and **B** in general) is defined as

$$\mathbf{x}_i \otimes \mathbf{x}_j = \begin{bmatrix} x_i^1 x_j^1 \\ \vdots \\ x_i^1 x_j^M \\ \vdots \\ x_i^M x_j^1 \\ \vdots \\ x_i^M x_j^M \end{bmatrix}, \quad \mathbf{A} \otimes \mathbf{B} = \left\| \begin{matrix} a_{11}\mathbf{B} & a_{12}\mathbf{B} & \cdots \\ a_{21}\mathbf{B} & a_{22}\mathbf{B} & \cdots \\ a_{31}\mathbf{B} & a_{32}\mathbf{B} & \cdots \\ \vdots & \vdots & \ddots \end{matrix} \right\|. \tag{7.4}$$

In what follows it will be convenient to index coordinates of the vector $\mathbf{x}_i \otimes \mathbf{x}_j$ by two, rather than one, numbers to make immediately clear what the coordinate means. If we rewrite Equations (7.3) for various values of k and l in the vector-matrix form with the left side being equal to $dE_t\{2\mathbf{x}_i \otimes \mathbf{x}_j\}/dt$, then the matrix of coefficients will have, a three-diagonal form with two more diagonals being shifted from the principle one by M entries in both directions. This suggests an idea that the matrix has a special structure and the direct examination proves it indeed that system (7.3) has the coefficient matrix of the form

$$\mathbf{A} - \frac{1}{2N}\mathbf{B}, \text{ where } \mathbf{A} = \| m_{ij} \| \otimes \mathbf{I} + \mathbf{I} \otimes \| m_{ij} \|, \tag{7.5}$$

matrix $\|m_{ij}\|$ is defined in (7.2), **I** is the identity matrix of dimension $M \times M$ and **B** is a diagonal matrix of dimension $M^2 \times M^2$ with units and zeros in its principal diagonal. If this diagonal is represented as the Kronecker product of two M-dimensional vectors whose elements are numbered by two superscripts (showing the correspondent numbers of coordinates from the first and second vectors of the product), then the units will correspond to superscripts of the form (i,i), $i=\overline{1,M}$.

Notation (7.5) shows the coefficient matrix of system (7.3) to represent the perturbation of matrix **A** by addition of $-\mathbf{B}/(2N)$, so that the perturbation effect can be considered for a great enough N by means of the first terms in the proper expansions of characteristic values and vectors. To find these terms, we have to know the eigenvalues of matrix **A** and their respective eigenvectors, which turn out easily expressible in terms of those of the migrational matrix $\|m_{ij}\|$ from (7.2). Recall that if $\{\lambda_i, \mathbf{y}_i\}$ and $\{\mu_j, \mathbf{z}_j\}$ are characteristic values and vectors of two respective matrices, then $\lambda_i\mu_j$ is known to represent an eigenvalue of the Kronecker product of these matrices with the eigenvector being represented by the Kronecker product $y_i \otimes z_j$. Since for the identity matrix any vector is a characteristic one corresponding to the unit characteristic value, the eigenvalues λ_{ij} of matrix **A** and its respective eigenvectors $\mathbf{e}_{ij}$ can be proved to be equal to

$$\lambda_{ij} = \lambda_i + \lambda_j \,,\ \mathbf{e}_{ij} = \mathbf{e}_i \otimes \mathbf{e}_j,\ i,j = \overline{1, M}\,. \tag{7.6}$$

where $\{\lambda_i, \mathbf{e}_i\}$ are eigenvalues and eigenvectors of matrix $\|m_{ij}\|$, namely,

$$\lambda_{i+1} = 2m_1\left(\cos\frac{\pi i}{M} - 1\right),$$

$$\mathbf{e}_{i+1}^T = \left(\cos\frac{\pi i}{2M},\ \cos\frac{3\pi i}{2M},\ldots,\ \cos\frac{(2M-1)\pi i}{2M}\right),$$

$$i = \overline{0, M-1}. \tag{7.7}$$

It follows that the greatest eigenvalue, λ_{00}, of matrix **A** will be zero (and for small enough perturbations it will bring about the greatest eigenvalue of matrix $\mathbf{A}-\mathbf{B}/(2N)$). The respective right (and left) eigenvector will be

$$\mathbf{e}_{00} = \mathbf{e}_1 \otimes \mathbf{e}_1 = (1,\ldots,1)^T \otimes (1,\ldots,1)^T.$$

Hence, according to (6.4) the first approximation for the (asymptotic) rate of reaching homozygosity will be equal to

$$\lambda_{\max} \sim -\frac{1}{2N}\,\frac{(\mathbf{e}_{00}, \mathbf{B}\mathbf{e}_{00})}{|\mathbf{e}_{00}|^2} = -\frac{1}{2N}\,\frac{M}{M^2} = -\frac{1}{2MN}\,. \tag{7.8}$$

Here the vector norm $|\ldots|$ is defined as the square root of its inner square and appears in formula (7.8) as the normalization of inner products among left and right eigenvectors is now absent in contrast to the assumptions made in (6.4). Thus, the fact the population is subdivided does not modify, in the first approximation, the rate of reaching homozygosity as compared with the case of panmixia in the population of the same size MN.

Due to the symmetry of matrix **A** its left and right eigenvectors are the same, so that the greatest eigenvalue of matrix $\mathbf{A}-\mathbf{B}/(2N)$, defined in the second approximation by formula (6.9), will be equal (with regard for normalization) to

$$\tilde{\lambda}_{\max} \sim -\frac{1}{2MN} + \left(\frac{1}{2N}\right)^2 \sum_{\substack{i,j=0 \\ (i,j)\neq(0,0)}}^{M-1} \frac{(\mathbf{e}_{00}, \mathbf{B}\mathbf{e}_{ij})^2}{|\mathbf{e}_{00}|^2\, |\mathbf{e}_{ij}|^2 (\lambda_{00} - \lambda_{ij})}\,. \tag{7.9}$$

Recall that $\mathbf{e}_{00}$ represents the M^2-dimensional vector of units, whereby

$$|\,\mathbf{e}_{00}\,|^2 = M^2\,.$$

Also, as $\mathbf{e}_{ij} = \mathbf{e}_i \otimes \mathbf{e}_j$, its norm is representable in the form

$$|\,\mathbf{e}_{ij}\,|^2 = (\mathbf{e}_i \otimes \mathbf{e}_j)^T (\mathbf{e}_i \otimes \mathbf{e}_j)\,.$$

Then, by the general property of the Kronecker product that $(\mathbf{A}\otimes\mathbf{B})(\mathbf{C}\otimes\mathbf{D})=\mathbf{AC}\otimes\mathbf{BD}$ provided the products **AC** and **BD** exist, we have

$$|\,\mathbf{e}_{ij}\,|^2 = (\mathbf{e}_i, \mathbf{e}_i)(\mathbf{e}_j, \mathbf{e}_j)\ .$$

Finally, when a vector is multiplied by a matrix **B** from the left, its coordinates that correspond to the diagonal entries with superscripts $(k,k), k=\overline{1, M}$, remain unchanged, while the rest ones vanish. Hence, multiplying this product by the vector of units, $\mathbf{e}_{00}^T$, from the left is equivalent to summing up the product coordinates thus obtained. Therefore, we have (with $e_i(k)$ denoting the k-th coordinate of vector $\mathbf{e}_i$)

$$(\mathbf{e}_{00}, \mathbf{B}\mathbf{e}_{ij}) = \sum_{k=1}^{M} e_i(k)e_j(k) = \delta_{ij}|\,\mathbf{e}_i\,|^2$$

by virtue of orthogonality between vectors $\mathbf{e}_i$ and $\mathbf{e}_j$ in (7.7). Having made all necessary simplifications in (7.9), we come to

$$\tilde{\lambda}_{\max} \sim -\frac{1}{2MN} + \frac{1}{16M^2N^2}\sum_{i=1}^{M-1}\frac{1}{m_1\left(1-\cos\dfrac{\pi i}{M}\right)}\ , \tag{7.10}$$

so that the rate of reaching homozygosity under isolation by distance is however less than that in the panmictic population of the same size.

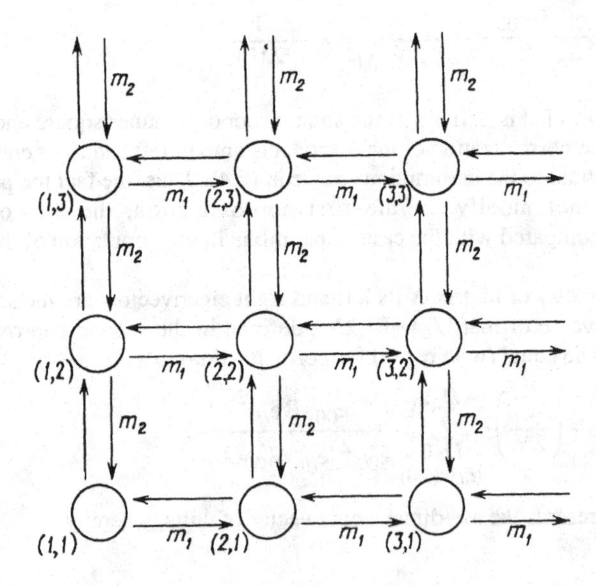

Fig. 39. The scheme of two-dimensional migrations in the model of isolation by distance.

In case where the subpopulations are distributed two-dimensionally on the plane (schematically, on a two-dimensional lattice of size $M_1 \times M_2$), we suppose that the pattern of migration exchange in the ith coordinate direction is in accordance with the model described above for one-dimensional migrations among M_i subpopulations with intensity m_i, $i=1,2$. Subpopulations will be numbered by the two superscripts indicating a position the subpopulation has in the projection to each of the axes (Figure 39). Let p_i^{kl} be the concentration of the ith allele in subpopulation kl ($k=\overline{1,M_1}$; $l=\overline{1,M_2}$). Then the drift coefficient in the coordinate p_i^{kl} of the diffusion model will equal the sum of the drifts along each axis of the form (7.1). It can be readily verified that the drift vector, caused by internal migrations, takes on the following form for the ith gamete frequency:

$$M_i(\mathbf{p}) = (\mathbf{I}_2 \otimes \| m_{ij}^1 \| + \| m_{ij}^2 \| \otimes \mathbf{I}_1)\mathbf{p}_i = \| m_{ij} \| \, \mathbf{p}_i, \tag{7.11}$$

where $\mathbf{I}_i$ is the identity matrix of dimension $M_i \times M_i$, $\|m_{ij}^k\|$ is the migration $M_k \times M_k$-matrix of the form (7.2) with the intensity of migrations denoted by m_k, and $\mathbf{p}_i$ is the vector of gamete frequencies in subpopulations. If $M_1=2$ and $M_2=3$, the migration matrix in (7.11) has the following form:

$$\begin{array}{c} \\ (11) \\ (21) \\ (12) \\ (22) \\ (13) \\ (23) \end{array}
\begin{array}{c} \begin{array}{cc:cc:cc} (11) & (21) & (12) & (22) & (13) & (23) \end{array} \\
\left\| \begin{array}{cc:cc:cc} \tilde{m} & m_1 & m_2 & 0 & & \\ m_1 & \tilde{m} & 0 & m_2 & & \mathbf{0} \\ \hdashline m_2 & 0 & \tilde{m} & m_1 & m_2 & 0 \\ 0 & m_2 & m_1 & \tilde{m} & 0 & m_2 \\ \hdashline & \mathbf{0} & m_2 & 0 & \tilde{m} & m_1 \\ & & 0 & m_2 & m_1 & \tilde{m} \end{array} \right\| \end{array},$$

where $\tilde{m} = -m_1 - m_2$.

The diffusion matrix for random genetic drift process in the two-dimensional model of migrations has a block diagonal pattern as before, with diagonal blocks corresponding to the sampling drift in individual subpopulations. In studies of the random genetic drift at a single autosomal locus with n alleles, the generating operator is determined by this block diagonal matrix of diffusion coefficients and by the drift coefficients of type (7.11).

If we study the behavior of heterozygosity in the two-dimensional model by means of equation (2.1), then, in order to obtain a closed system of differential equations, we have to consider functions of the form $2x_i^{kl} x_j^{mr}$ (in case where $k=m$ and $l=r$ they define the fraction of heterozygotes with alleles A_i and A_j in subpopulation (k, l) with current allele concentrations x_i^{kl} and x_j^{mr} respectively). The matrix of the linear system of differential equations then has the form (7.5) with $\|m_{ij}\|$ defined in (7.11). The system will not change if we consider all possible types of heterozygotes instead of a particular one with alleles A_i and A_j; thus the further conclusions are valid for the total population heterozygosity too. Eigenvalues of matrix $\|m_{ij}\|$ and their respective (7.6), (7.7) for matrices $\|m_{ij}^1\|$ and $\|m_{ij}^2\|$ of the form (7.2). Therefore, the non-zero eigenvalues of migration matrix in (7.11) will equal to

$$\lambda_{ij} = -2m_1\left(1-\cos\frac{\pi(i-1)}{M_1}\right) - 2m_2\left(1-\cos\frac{\pi(j-1)}{M_2}\right),$$

$$i=\overline{1,M_1};\, j=\overline{1,M_2};\, (i,j)\neq(1,1)\,. \tag{7.12}$$

The arguments, similar to those presented above for the one-dimensional case (which are actually true for the general case of symmetric migrations considered below), show that the second approximation to the rate of reaching homozygosity can be calculated by the formula

$$\lambda_{max} \sim -\frac{1}{2M_1M_2N} + \frac{1}{4M_1^2M_2^2N^2}\sum_{\substack{i=1\\(i,j)\neq(1,1)}}^{M_1}\sum_{j=1}^{M_2}\frac{1}{-2\lambda_{ij}}, \tag{7.13}$$

where λ_{ij} are determined in (7.12).

In case the distribution of subpopulations has an arbitrary dimensionality l in the model of isolation by distance, we have

$$\lambda_{max} \sim -\frac{1}{2N_T} + \frac{1}{4N_T^2}\sum_{\substack{i_1=1\\(i_1,\dots,i_l)\neq(1,\dots,1)}}^{M_1}\cdots\sum_{i_l=1}^{M_l}\left[\sum_{j=1}^{l}4m_{i_j}\left(1-\cos\frac{\pi(i_j-1)}{M_j}\right)\right]^{-1}, \tag{7.14}$$

where $N_T = N\prod_{i=1}^{l} M_i$ is the total size of a subdivided population.

13.8. Properties of the Random Genetic Drift Process in a Subdivided Population with Migrations of the General Type

Now we consider a system of M elementary subpopulations whose total size N_T is constant in time as well as their individual sizes (which may differ from each other). The diffusion process describing the changes in gamete frequencies within subpopulations has a block diagonal matrix of the diffusion coefficients and the drift vector defined by a migration matrix $\|m_{ij}\|$. Its entries are interpreted as relative intensities of migration flows from the ith subpopulations into the jth ones (in the discrete version the element m_{ij}, $i\neq j$, indicates a portion of migrants from subpopulation i among individuals of subpopulation j). The drift coefficient for coordinate p_i^k, the frequency of the ith gamete in the kth subpopulation, as defined is the increment in p_i^k caused by internal migrations:

$$M_{ik}(\mathbf{p}) = \sum_{\substack{j=1\\j\neq i}}^{M} m_{jk}p_i^j + \left(1-\sum_{\substack{j=1\\j\neq i}}^{M} m_{jk}\right)p_i^k - p_i^k = (\|m_{ij}\|^T\mathbf{p}_i)_k\,, \tag{8.1}$$

where $\mathbf{p}_i$ is the vector of the ith gamete frequencies in subpopulations, $\|m_{ij}\|$ is the migration matrix whose diagonal entries are set equal to

$$m_{jj} = -\sum_{i,\, i\neq j} m_{ij},\quad j=\overline{1,M}, \tag{8.2}$$

so that the sum of entries equals zero in each column of $||m_{ij}||$. (Matrix $||m_{ij}||$ is the continuous analogue to the so-called backward matrix of migrations, which corresponds to the dynamics of subpopulation sizes when the time direction is reversed in the discrete model).

The present model can be studied in two versions. The first one features constant sizes of subpopulations due to attainment of a migratory equilibrium. The vector of these sizes $\{N_i\}$ is then a (right) characteristic one for matrix $||m_{ij}||$, corresponding to λ=0. In the second version the sizes are constant owing to rapid regulation by some other (e.g. ecological) mechanisms rather than to migrations.

Suppose that we study the population genetic structure with respect to a single autosomal locus with n alleles. In this case the drift is completely defined by formula (8.1). We consider first the case where all subpopulations have the same size N. To analyze the behavior of heterozygosity, we introduce a set of functions $\{2x_i^k x_j^l\}$ in which the superscript at the allele concentration x_i^k refers to the number of a subpopulation while the subscript to the number of an allele, the functions determining the fraction of heterozygotes with alleles A_i and A_j in subpopulation k when $k=l$ and current allele concentrations are x_i^k and x_j^k. In the vector form this set can be written down as $2\mathbf{x}_i \otimes \mathbf{x}_j$ In order to see the behavior of the expected vector $2\mathbf{x}_i \otimes \mathbf{x}_j$, we use Equation (2.1). Note that

$$\mathfrak{a} x_i^k x_j^l = -\frac{\delta_{kl}}{2N} x_i^k x_j^l + x_i^k \ (|| m_{ij} ||^T \mathbf{x}_j)_l + x_j^l \ (|| m_{ij} ||^T \mathbf{x}_i)_k \tag{8.3}$$

as $\mathfrak{a} x_j^l = M_{jl}(\mathbf{x})$. It can be verified directly that the following vector-matrix notation form arises from (2.1) and (8.3) for the system of differential equations for $E_t\{2\mathbf{x}_i \otimes \mathbf{x}_j\}$:

$$\frac{\mathrm{d}}{\mathrm{d}t} E_t\{2\mathbf{x}_i \otimes \mathbf{x}_j\} = \left(\mathbf{A} - \frac{1}{2N}\mathbf{B} \right) E_t\{2\mathbf{x}_i \otimes \mathbf{x}_j\}, \tag{8.4}$$

where

$$\mathbf{A} = || m_{ij} ||^T \otimes \mathbf{I} + \mathbf{I} \otimes || m_{ij} ||^T$$

and $\mathbf{B}$ represents, as before, the diagonal matrix of dimension $M^2 \times M^2$ with units and zeros in its principal diagonal, the units corresponding to coordinates of the type $x_i^k x_j^k$, $k=\overline{1, M}$, when the matrix is multiplied by $\mathbf{x}_i \otimes \mathbf{x}_j$. Equation (8.4) is a linear homogeneous one with the coefficient matrix $\mathbf{A}$ perturbed by addition of $-\mathbf{B}/(2N)$. For N being large enough, the perturbation effect can be accounted for by the first terms of the proper expansions in powers of $1/(2N)$.

Recall that by (8.2) matrix $||m_{ij}||$ has zero sum of its (non-negative for $i \neq j$) entries in each of the columns. Hence, the vector $\mathbf{l}_0 = \mathbf{e}^T = (1,1,...,1)$ will be its left eigenvector corresponding to λ=0. By the Gershgorin theorem the eigenvalues λ of matrix $||m_{ij}||$ satisfy inequalities

$$| m_{ii} - \lambda | \leq \sum_{\substack{j=1 \\ j \neq i}}^{M} | m_{ji} |, \quad i = \overline{1, M}.$$

According to non-negativity of entries m_{ji} for $i{\neq}j$ and to the equality

$$-m_{ii} = \sum_{\substack{j=1 \\ j\neq i}}^{M} m_{ji} = a_i > 0 ,$$

we can rewrite the Gershgorin inequalities in the form

$$| a_i + \lambda | \leq a_i, \quad i = \overline{1, M}.$$

It is clear now that the real parts of all eigenvalues are non-positive. For the model robustness reason (i.e. the requirement for the change in its properties being small under small variations in parameters), we assume the eigenvalue λ=0 be unique. Let the right eigenvector corresponding to zero eigenvalue be denoted by $\mathbf{r}_0$. If we add $||m_{ij}||$ with matrix $a\mathbf{I}$ where $a{\geq}a_i$, $i=\overline{1, M}$, the sum will be a non-negative matrix whose eigenvectors will coincide with those of $||m_{ij}||$. By the Perron-Frobenius theorem, vector $\mathbf{r}_0$ can be chosen in a way such that all its coordinates be non-negative. The greatest eigenvalue λ_{00} of matrix $\mathbf{A}$ in (8.4) will be zero, the corresponding left and right vectors being equal to $\mathbf{L}_0=\mathbf{r}_0^T \otimes \mathbf{r}_0^T$ and $\mathbf{R}_0=\mathbf{l}_0^T \otimes \mathbf{l}_0^T$. For N being large enough, the perturbed value of λ_{00} will be still the greatest eigenvalue of $\mathbf{A}-\mathbf{B}/(2N)$ and equal, in the first approximation, to

$$\tilde{\lambda}_{\max} \sim -\frac{1}{2N} \frac{(\mathbf{B}\mathbf{R}_0, \mathbf{L}_0)}{(\mathbf{R}_0, \mathbf{L}_0)} = -\frac{1}{2N} \sum_{i=1}^{M} \left(\frac{r_0(i)}{\sum_{i=1}^{M} r_0(i)} \right)^2 . \tag{8.5}$$

We have taken here into account that if coordinates of vector $\mathbf{L}_0=\mathbf{r}_0^T \otimes \mathbf{r}_0^T$ are indexed by two numbers, then, owing to the fact the vector $\mathbf{R}_0$ consists of unit coordinates only, the following relations are true:

$$(\mathbf{B}\mathbf{R}_0, \mathbf{L}_0) = \sum_{i=1}^{M} L_0(i, i) = \sum_{i=1}^{M} r_0^2(i) ,$$

$$(\mathbf{R}_0, \mathbf{L}_0) = \sum_{i,j=1}^{M} L_0(i, j) = \sum_{i,j=1}^{M} r_0(i) r_0(j) = \left[\sum_{i=1}^{M} r_0(i) \right]^2 .$$

Due to the special choice of vector $\mathbf{r}_0$ all $r_0(i)$ ar non-negative (as well as the quantities $c_i=r_0(i)/\Sigma_{i=1}^M r_0(i)$). Obviously, $\Sigma_{i=1}^M c_i=1$. Under these constraints, it can be easily shown that the quantity $\Sigma_{i=1}^M c_i^2$ appearing in (8.5) takes on its maximum value when all c_i are equal to $1/M$. It is fulfilled automatically for a symmetric matrix of migrations $||m_{ij}||$, where $\mathbf{r}_0=\mathbf{l}_0^T$ (=$\mathbf{e}$). Thus, the first approximation for the rate of reaching homozygosity, $\tilde{\lambda}_{\max}$, under symmetric migrations will be equal to $-1/(2MN)$, i.e. to the value of this rate in the undivided, panmictic population of the same size. When there is no symmetry in migrations, the homozygosity is reached generally at a slower asymptotic rate than in case of symmetry.

In order to find the second approximation for the greatest eigenvalue of matrix $\mathbf{A}-\mathbf{B}/(2N)$ in (8.4), we have to know the spectral decomposition of $\|m_{ij}\|$. The corresponding formula looks to be the most simple in case of symmetric migrations. The right eigenvectors then coincide with the left ones $\{\mathbf{e}_i\}$, the vectors being orthogonal when corresponding to different eigenvalues. When the multiplicity of an eigenvalue is greater than unit, the corresponding eigenvectors can also be chosen orthogonal. In this case the second approximation looks especially simple. Denoting vector $\mathbf{e}_i \otimes \mathbf{e}_j$ by $\mathbf{E}_{ij}$ (but $\mathbf{E}_{00}=\mathbf{e}_1 \otimes \mathbf{e}_1$) and taking the normalization into account, we will have by (6.9)

$$\tilde{\lambda}_{\max} \sim -\frac{1}{2MN} + \frac{1}{(2N)^2} \sum_{\substack{i,j=1 \\ (i,j)\neq(1,1)}}^{M} \frac{(\mathbf{BE}_{ij},\mathbf{E}_{00})(\mathbf{BE}_{00},\mathbf{E}_{ij})}{(\mathbf{E}_{00},\mathbf{E}_{00})(\mathbf{E}_{ij},\mathbf{E}_{ij})(\lambda_{00}-\lambda_{ij})}. \tag{8.6}$$

Since, for any matrix $\|m_{ij}\|$, $\lambda_{00}=0$; $\mathbf{E}_{00}$ is the M^2-dimensional vector of units; $\lambda_{ij}=\lambda_i+\lambda_j$, and the eigenvectors of $\|m_{ij}\|$ are taken orthogonal, it follows that $(\mathbf{BE}_{ij}, \mathbf{E}_{00})=\delta_{ij}(\mathbf{e}_i,\mathbf{e}_i)$ and, after transforming (8.6) in analogy with the analysis of (7.9), we will have

$$\tilde{\lambda}_{\max} \sim \lambda_{00} + \frac{1}{2N}\lambda^{(1)} + \left(\frac{1}{2N}\right)^2 \lambda^{(2)} = -\frac{1}{2MN} - \frac{1}{(2MN)^2} \sum_{i=2}^{M} \frac{1}{2\lambda_i}. \tag{8.7}$$

The values of some λ_i may be equal. Since the greatest eigenvalue of $\|m_{ij}\|$ is zero, the values of λ_i $(i=\overline{2,M})$ in (8.7) are negative. It thus follows that the asymptotic rate of reaching homozygosity is lower in the subdivided population than in the panmictic one of the same size.

These results can be readily extended to the case where the subpopulations have different sizes N_i. The perturbation $(\tilde{\mathbf{B}})$ of matrix A then represents a diagonal matrix whose non-zero diagonal entries are equal to $-1/(2N_k)$ (in the place of the kth unit of matrix B). Hence, in case of symmetric migrations, where $\mathbf{l}_0=\mathbf{r}_0=\mathbf{e}=(1,\ldots 1)^T$, the first approximation yields

$$\tilde{\lambda}_{\max} \sim -\sum_{i=1}^{M} \frac{1}{M^2 2N_i} = -\frac{1}{2M\tilde{N}} \leq -\frac{1}{2M\overline{N}} = -\frac{1}{2N_T},$$

where $\tilde{N}=M/[\Sigma_{i=1}^{M} N_i^{-1}]$ is the harmonic mean of $\{N_i\}$, which is known to not exceed their arithmetic mean $\overline{N}$. The variability in subpopulation sizes under the constancy of their total size thus promotes the faster attainment of homozygosity. In calculating the second approximation, we have to substitute $\tilde{\mathbf{B}}$ into formula instead of $-\mathbf{B}/(2N)$.

Unequal sizes of subpopulations are possible for symmetric migrations if we adopt the hypothesis that size constancy is sustained by non-migratory mechanisms. In case of migration equilibrium the eigenvector $\mathbf{r}_0$ is proportioned to the vector of subpopulation sizes $\{N_i\}$. Thus, even for non-symmetric migrations there is no difference in the first approximation by (6.4) between the results for the subdivided and the panmictic populations $(L_{00}(i,j)=N_iN_j,\ R_{00}(i,j)=1)$:

$$\tilde{\lambda}_{\max} \sim \frac{-\sum_{i=1}^{M} R_{00}(i,i) L_{00}(i,i)/(2N_i)}{(\mathbf{L}_{00},\mathbf{R}_{00})} = -\sum_{i=1}^{M} \frac{N_i^2/(2N_i)}{N_T^2} = -\frac{1}{2N_T}.$$

As $\tilde{\lambda}_{\max}$ is negative for matrix $\mathbf{A}+\tilde{\mathbf{B}}$, it is clear that the number of heterozygotes in the system of subpopulations converges exponentially to zero. In spite of differences in the dynamics, the total expected number of heterozygotes in subpopulations accumulated in the course of reaching homozygosity turns out the same (when, for instance, there are no initial genetic differences among subpopulations) as that for the panmictic population. To prove this statement, we apply Equation (2.1) to the function $2\bar{x}_i\,\bar{x}_j$ where the bar above a symbol denotes averaging among subpopulations (their sizes being not supposed equal). For example,

$$\bar{x}_i = \sum_k x_i^k N_k / \sum_k N_k = \sum_k x_i^k N_k/N_T$$

represents the (average) concentration of the ith allele in the system of total size $N_T=\Sigma_k N_k$. Obviously,

$$\frac{d}{dt} E_t\{2\bar{x}_i\,\bar{x}_j\} = -\sum_k E_t\left\{\left(\frac{N_k}{N_T}\right)^2 \frac{2x_i^k x_j^k}{2N_k}\right\} +$$

$$+ E_t\left\{2\bar{x}_i \sum_k (\|m_{ij}\|^T \mathbf{x}_j)_k \frac{N_k}{N_T} + 2\bar{x}_j \sum_k (\|m_{ij}\|^T \mathbf{x}_i)_k \frac{N_k}{N_T}\right\} = -\frac{1}{2N_T} E_t\{H_{ij}\}, \quad (8.8)$$

where $H_{ij}=\Sigma_k 2x_i^k x_j^k N_k/N_T$ is a fraction of heterozygotes in the system. In writing down the drift terms, we have used formula (8.1); under the hypothesis of migration equilibrium in subpopulation sizes, all the coordinates of $\|m_{ij}\|\mathbf{N}$ are equal to zero as vector $\mathbf{N}=(N_1,..., N_M)^T$ is the characteristic one of $\|m_{ij}\|$ with $\lambda=0$. If we integrate both sides of (8.8) over t from zero to infinity and take into account that $E_\infty\{2\bar{x}_i\,\bar{x}_j\}=0$ due to the population being homozygous in the limit, then we have

$$\int_0^\infty E_t\{H_{ij}\}\,dt = 2N_T\bar{H}_{ij}^0, \quad (8.9)$$

where $\bar{H}_{ij}^0=2\bar{p}_i\,\bar{p}_j$, $\bar{p}_i$ representing the initial concentration of the ith allele in the system. If, for instance, there are no genetic differences among subpopulations at the initial moment, the following relation holds:

$$\bar{H}_{ij}^0 = H_{ij}^0 = \sum_{k=1}^{M} 2p_i^k p_j^k N_k/N_T$$

and the expression (8.9) coincides with (11.7.7), i.e. with that for the panmictic population.

However, the mean time to attain homozygosity in a subdivided population will exceed the time for the panmictic population of the same size by a quantity which is equal to the average value of the empirical coefficient of inbreeding along the whole trajectory. For the case of unequal subpopulation sizes it can be shown that the empirical coefficient, F_i, of inbreeding in the ith allele having concentration p_i^k in the kth subpopulation, can be determined from the Wahlund formula (1.1). Since the number of heterozygotes with the ith allele equals $2\bar{p}_i(1-\bar{p}_i)$ in the panmictic population and $2\bar{p}_i(1-\bar{p}_i)(1-F_i)$ in case of inbreeding, it follows from (1.1) that var $p_i = D_i = F_i\bar{p}_i(1-\bar{p}_i)$. Hence, the allele average coefficient of inbreeding can be determined as

$$\bar{F} = \sum_{i=1}^{n} \bar{p}_i F_i = \sum_{i=1}^{n} \frac{D_i}{1-\bar{p}_i} \geq 0. \tag{8.10}$$

The expectation of the homozygosity attainment time, $T(\mathbf{p})$, obeys the equation $(\mathfrak{A}T)(\mathbf{p})=-1$ and must turn into the mean time to attain homozygosity at the locus with n-1 alleles under zero concentration of one of the alleles. In case of panmixia the equation is satisfied with the function

$$\tilde{T}(\mathbf{p}) = -4N_T\sum_{i=1}^{n}(1-\bar{p}_i)\ln(1-\bar{p}_i).$$

Let us find the form of $(\mathfrak{A}\tilde{T})(\mathbf{p})$ in case of subdivision. Note first that derivatives $\partial\tilde{T}/\partial p_i^k$ do not depend on the superscripts, so that the terms with these derivatives, if summed over k, yield zero for any i, as $\Sigma_k M_{ik} = (N_1,\ldots, N_M)\|m_{ij}\|^T \mathbf{p}_i = 0$ due to vector $(N_1,\ldots, N_M)^T$ being the characteristic one with $\lambda=0$ under the hypothesis of migration equilibrium. Therefore, we can confine our considration of $\mathfrak{A}$ to the terms with second derivatives only. By means of (1.1) we find further that

$$\mathfrak{A}[-4N_T(1-\bar{p}_i)\ln(1-\bar{p}_i)] =$$

$$= -\frac{4N_T}{1-\bar{p}_i}\sum_{k=1}^{M}\frac{p_i^k(1-p_i^k)}{4N_k}\left(\frac{N_k}{N_T}\right)^2 = -\bar{p}_i + \frac{D_i}{1-\bar{p}_i}.$$

For the dependent concentration of allele A_n we have

$$\mathfrak{A}[-4N_T(1-\bar{p}_n)\ln(1-\bar{p}_n)] =$$

$$= -\frac{4N_T}{1-\bar{p}_n}\sum_{i,j=1}^{n-1}\sum_{k=1}^{M}\frac{p_i^k(\delta_{ij}-p_j^k)}{4N_k}\left(\frac{N_k}{N_T}\right)^2 = -\bar{p}_n + \frac{\mathrm{var}(1-\bar{p}_n)}{1-\bar{p}_n}$$

Finally, by taking (8.10) and the equality var$(1-\bar{p}_n) = D_n$ into account and summing up all the terms in $\tilde{T}$, we obtain

$$(\mathfrak{A}\tilde{T})(\mathbf{p}) = -1 + \sum_{i=1}^{n}\frac{D_i}{1-\bar{p}_i} = -1 + \bar{F}(\mathbf{p}). \tag{8.11}$$

Thus, in terms of a penalty on process paths, the function $\tilde{T}(\mathbf{p})$ can be represented to be the expectation of the penalty function that equals unit in each interior point of the state space (i.e. the expected time to attain homozygosity $T(\mathbf{p})$) plus the expectation of the penalty $-\bar{F}(\mathbf{p})$. Hence,

$$T(\mathbf{p}) = \tilde{T}(\mathbf{p}) + \int_0^\infty E_t\{\bar{F}(\mathbf{p}_t, \omega)\}\, dt.$$

If the random genetic drift process in a subdivided population is considered with respect to two loci, then of interest is the expectation of covariance among alleles from different loci (i.e. the coefficient of linkage disequilibrium) in the course of reaching the genetic homogeneity. In the limit as $t \to \infty$ the disequilibrium will be zero for any pair of alleles because the concentration of the gametes carrying a particular pair of alleles and the product of concentrations of those alleles in the population that is homozygous in both loci, are equal either to unit or zero simultaneously. It turns out that, under subdivision and an arbitrary pattern of migrations, the integral average disequilibrium value coincides with that for the panmictic population of the same size, provided $D^0_{i_1j_2} = \bar{D}^0_{i_1j_2}$ at the initial time moment. Here,

$$D_{i_1j_2} = \frac{1}{N_T}\sum_k (p^k_{i_1j_2} - p^k_{i_1} p^k_{j_2}) N_k = \frac{1}{N_T}\sum_k D^k_{i_1j_2} N_k ,$$
$$\bar{D}_{i_1j_2} = \bar{p}_{i_1j_2} - \bar{p}_{i_1}\bar{p}_{j_2} ,$$
$$\bar{p}_{i_1j_2} = \frac{1}{N_T}\sum_k p^k_{i_1j_2} N_k, \quad \bar{p}_{i_1} = \sum_{j_2} \bar{p}_{i_1j_2} , \quad \bar{p}_{j_2} = \sum_{i_1} \bar{p}_{i_1j_2} ,$$

N_k denotes the size of the kth of the subpopulations, which are not supposed to be equal-sized. Applying (2.1), we have

$$\frac{d}{dt} E_t\{\bar{D}_{i_1j_2}\} = -\left(\frac{1}{2N_T} + r\right) E_t\{D_{i_1j_2}\} , \tag{8.12}$$

since $\mathfrak{A}\bar{p}_{i_1j_2} = -rD_{i_1j_2}$, while, under the hypothesis of migration equilibrium in subpopulation sizes, $\mathfrak{A}\bar{p}_{i_1}\bar{p}_{j_2} = \Sigma_k D^k_{i_1j_2} N_k/(2N_T^2) = D_{i_1j_2}/(2N_T)$. We have taken here into account that the drift caused by migrations makes zero contribution, as it does in Equation (8.8), since the vector of subpopulations sizes is the characteristic one with $\lambda=0$ under the migration equilibrium hypothesis. By integrating both sides of (8.12) over t from zero to infinity and taking the equality $E_\infty\{\bar{D}_{i_1j_2}\}=0$ into account, we find that

$$\int_0^\infty E_t\{D_{i_1j_2}\}\, dt = \frac{2N_T}{1+2N_T r}\bar{D}^0_{i_1j_2} . \tag{8.13}$$

We emphasize once more the fact the index $D_{i_1j_2}$ represents the average covariance per subpopulation rather than the covariance among alleles in gametes of the system (defined as $\bar{D}_{i_1j_2}$).

Since the drift component caused by migrations contribute nothing into $\mathfrak{A}\bar{p}_{i_1j_2}$, it follows that

$$\frac{d}{dt} E_t\{\bar{x}_{i_1j_2}\} = -rE_t\{D_{i_1j_2}\} , \tag{8.14}$$

$$E_0\{\bar{x}_{i_1 j_2}\} = \bar{p}_{i_1 j_2}\,.$$

Evidently, $E_\infty\{\bar{x}_{i_1 j_2}\}$ is equal to the fixation probability $U_{i_1 j_2}$ for gamete $\Gamma_{i_1 j_2}$. Integrating (8.14) from zero to infinity with regard for (8.13) results in

$$U_{i_1 j_2} = \bar{p}_{i_1 j_2} - \frac{2N_T r}{1+2N_T r}\bar{D}^0_{i_1 j_2}\,, \tag{8.15}$$

which corresponds to the result for the panmictic population.

Coincident with the panmictic case is also the fixation probability, for instance, for the ith allele at a locus since this probability equals $E_\infty\{\bar{x}_i\}$, while application of (2.1) under migration equilibrium results in

$$\frac{d}{dt}E_t\{\bar{x}_i\}=0,\ E_0\{\bar{x}_i\}=\bar{p}_i\,, \tag{8.16}$$

which coincides with (11.7.1) under panmixia.

In case of additive selection in two alleles, T. Maruyama obtained even stronger results, yet we can not extent this approach to the case of multiple alleles. We consider first a panmictic population where one allele has a permanent selective advantage, s, before the other, the population size being equal to N. In this case the change in gene frequency x is described by the diffusion process with the drift coefficient being equal to $sp(1-p)$ and the diffusion one to $p(1-p)/(2N)$. By making the random change of time variable (see (10.7.5)–(10.7.6)) $\tau'(t,\omega)=p(1-p)/(2N)$, we obtain the diffusion process with generating operator

$$\mathfrak{A} = d^2/dp^2 + 2sN\, d/dp. \tag{8.17}$$

The new time variable τ is proportional to the fraction of heterozygotes in the population, and the mean absorption time, as well as its higher moments, are equal to the moments of integral average heterozygosity in the course of random drift until fixation of an allele. As the change of time does not change any paths of the process, the allele fixation probabilities can be found by means of (8.17).

Suppose that now considered is a subdivided population of the total size N_T invariable in time, consisting of subpopulations whose sizes $N_{t,k}$ and intensities of migration flows vary deterministically in time. Additive selection proceed in subpopulations, with a coefficient s in common, and the random mating ones are assumed to be independent. In this case the matrix of diffusion coefficients is diagonal with the entries $x^k(1-x^k)/(2N_{t,k})$, and the drift coefficients are equal to $sx^k(1-x^k)$. Denoting the fraction of heterozygotes in the total population by H, let the random change of time be defined by

$$\frac{d}{dt}\tau(t,\omega)= \sum_k x^k(1-x^k)N_{t,k}/(2N_T^2)= H/(4N_T)\,. \tag{8.18}$$

As a result, the drift and diffusion coefficients in the new time will differ from the previous ones by the multiplier $4N_T/H$. Let now the (degenerate) change of variables be made by the formula $\bar{x} = \Sigma_k x^k N_{t,k}/N_T$. The behavior of $\bar{x}$ appears to be described by a homogeneous diffusion process (in contrast to the original inhomogeneous one) whose coefficients can be defined by formulae (10.7.4). The drift vector takes on the form

$$M(\bar{x}) = \sum_k \frac{N_{t,k}}{N_T} \frac{sx^k(1-x^k)4N_T}{H} + (\| m_{ij}(t) \|^T \mathbf{x})_k \frac{4N_T}{H} = 2sN_T . \qquad (8.19)$$

since the contribution by internal migrations must not affect the total number of alleles in the population. The diffusion coefficient will equal

$$V(\bar{x}) = \sum_k \left(\frac{N_{t,k}}{N_T} \right)^2 \frac{x^k(1-x^k)}{2N_{t,k}} \frac{4N_T}{H} = 1 . \qquad (8.20)$$

So, the generating operator for the diffusion process of changes in the average concentration where the time is measured by the population heterozygosity, takes on the same form (8.17) as for the panmictic population of the same size N_T. That is why, in particular, the allele fixation probabilities and all the moments concerning the numbers of heterozygotes till absorption do not depend on a pattern of the population subdivision but coincide with the corresponding values for the case of panmixia. Due to the simplicity of operator (8.17) determining a Wiener process with a constant drift, there is no difficulties in writing down explicit expressions for these values. In particular, the fixation probability of an allele with selective advantage s is equal, as well as in (12.2.11), to $(1-\exp\{-4Nsp\})/(1-\exp\{-4Ns\})$.

13.9. Notes and Bibliography

Sections 13.1–6.

Asymptotic behavior of the random genetic drift in a subdivided population with migrations of the island type, expressed by the rate of reaching homozygosity, was studied by P. Moran, who presented the findings in his book:

Moran, P.A.P.: 1962, *Statistical Processes of Evolutionary Theory*, Clarendon Press, Oxford; Oxford Univ. Press, London, VII + 200 pp.

The Wahlund formula was presented ibidem. Its extensions to multiple alleles and two loci are given, for instance, in the papers:

Nei, M.: 1965, Variation and covariation of gene frequencies in subdivided population, *Evolution*, **19**, No. 2, pp. 256–258;

Nei, M. and Li, W.-H.: 1973, Linkage disequilibrium in subdivided populations, *Genetics*, **75**, No. 1, pp. 213–219.

The investigation of the expected heterozygosity behavior follows the note:

Passekov, V.P.: 1975, On the mean number of heterozygotes in a subdivided population. - In: *Application of Statistical Methods in Problems of Population Genetics*, issue 49. Interdept. Laboratory of Statistical Methods, Moscow State University, pp. 69–73 (in Russian);

see also:

Passekov, V.P.: 1981, The effect of genetic drift on dynamics of the genotypic and phenotypic variabilities in subdivided populations. In: Svirezhev, Y. M. and V.P. Passekov (eds.), *Mathematical Models in Ecology and Genetics*. Nauka, Moscow, pp. 148–173 (in Russian).

Section 13.7–8.

Asymptotic rate of reaching homozygosity in the model of isolation by distance with a large number of subpopulations was studied by T. Maruyama:

Maruyama, T.: 1970, Rate of decrease of genetic variability in a subdivided population, *Biometrika*, 57, No. 2, pp. 299–311.

He also studied various aspects of genetic processes in different models of subdivisions, the synopsis of results and bibliography being presented in his book:

Maruyama, T.: 1977, *Stochastic Problems in Population Genetics*, Berlin: Springer-Verlag, 254 pp.

In particular, shown in this book is the invariance of the expected integral number of heterozygotes under subdivision, including the case of additive selection too.

A model with a general pattern of migrations was considered by T. Nagylaki:

Nagylaki, T.: 1980, The strong-migration limit in geographically structured populations, *J. Math. Biol*, 9, No. 2, pp. 101–114.

An introduction to the methods of perturbation theory can be found, for instance, in the books:

Faddeev, D.K. and Faddeeva, V.N.: 1963, *Computational Methods of Linear Algebra*, W.H. Freeman, San Francisco, California,

where the first approximations of eigenvalues and eigenvectors of the perturbed matrix are considered, and

Lankaster, P.: 1969, *Theory of Matrices*, Academic Press, New York, London, 316 pp.

where the presentation is given in more detail.

Conclusion

Concluding this book, the authors would like to note that, being interested mainly in evolutionary aspects, they are obliged to have left outside its scope many other chapters of population genetics, which are penetrated with mathematical methods deeply enough. But even in the fields we have touched upon, some new ideas and new problems have aroused recently. All this needs at least a few words to be said.

We have not touched, for example, on a classical branch such as genetics of quantitative characters, with which the reader can become acquainted by two books, complementary to each other, one written by D.C. Falconer* and the other by O. Kempthorne**. This branch of genetics takes an important role not only in applied studies concerned primarily with artificial selection problems, but also in the study of evolution because selection occurs normally in morphological characters determined by genes from many loci (these complexes being often termed polygenes). Therefore, the fitness functions, which are the main characteristics of selection in the quantitative theory of evolution, depend on complex combinations of many loci and alleles, whose contributions in the total fitness of a genotype can hardly be considered additive or independent.

Another problem also arises here. Our description of an evolving population in terms of changes in its gene or genotype frequencies is relied upon assumption that the number of different genes or different genotypes in the population is not too large in comparison with that of individuals, since this is the only case which makes sense to speak of frequencies of those groups. Actually, even a mere combinatorial estimation for a number of different genotypes in the system of n loci where the gene can be in either of two states (this number equals 3^n) shows that, in real case ($n \sim 10^3 - 10^7$) the most probable is the population state where it is impossible to find a pair of individuals with identical genotypes. Therefore, to save the theory, it was necessary to 'coarsen' the real situation and to assume that identical are those genotypes which, although being distinct, but not differ too much, provided the distinction does not increase in the course of evolution.

Making up these genotype groups with simple enough laws of inheritance is, to a certain extent, arbitrary. Normally, specified are only one or two characters controlled by one or two loci, and the main selection pressure is considered to be associated just with those characters. If now we increase the number of characters (and the respective number of loci), then complexity of the description will exponentially grow, bringing

* Falconer, D.S.: 1964, Introduction to Quantitative Genetics. Edinburgh and London: Oliver and Boyd
** Kempthorne, O: 1975, An Introduction to Genetic Statistics. New York: Wiley.

about 'the curse of dimensionality' and making the problem unamenable to practical analysis.

The idea of a 'thermodynamic' approach certainly appears promising here but it is not yet clear how to implement it. The existing approaches, namely, describing the state of a population in terms of dynamics in its mean fitness, genetic variance, or in moments of the distribution of quantitative characters, lead us to disregarding the laws of inheritance by replacing them with new phenomenological concepts, such as the heritabality and so forth.

Now the problem to determine the fitness of a genotype is still far from its completion even in the most simple genetic cases. The reason is that selection pressure, determined by fitness functions and dependent on the environment, does depend on the inherent state too, i.e. on the genetic structure of the population itself. From the modelling point of view, this implies, in particular, that fitness coefficients must depend on frequencies of alleles, gametes, and genotypes. So, the assumption of constant fitness coefficients, widely used in our book, is a kind of the first approximation to real conditions.

Another difficulty that is concerned with determination of the fitness, lies in the fact this index is not 'unidimensional'. In the real nature, the evolution of a population is intimately bound up with evolution of its age structure. Naturally, the selection pressure on a genotype depends essentially on age, the same being true for its mortality, and the fecundity is also determined to a considerable extent by the ages of mating individuals. The assumptions we have widely used of additive or multiplicative patterns of fecundity have certainly the mathematical convenience, but these patterns are scarcely spread in nature. Taking, however, the age structure into account (even in the simplest, single-locus case) results in principally new and highly complicated mathematical models whose analytical techniques are quite undeveloped yet. Any progress in this direction will be not only useful but also interesting both from mathematical and genetical points of view.

Besides fitness functions, the evolution depends on other parameters too (intensities of recombinations, migrations, etc.), which are also assumed external in our models, independent of evolution itself. These parameters, however, may well be genetically determined and evolve themselves, so that there is a coevolution in the indices of recombination and migrations, mutation rates, and genetic structure of the population. Evidently, some reasonable balance must exist there among these processes, for example, between the genetically dependent rate at which new mutations spring up decreasing the mean fitness of the population*, and the rate at which the environment changes, requiring the genetic structure to be changed correspondingly to make the population 'fit', i.e. adapted, for the new conditions. The same is true for the intensity of recombinations too, which must correspond to the rate of breaking down the current adaptive complexes and setting up the new ones (polygenes or supergenes).

A highly important and interesting problem, which is left outside the limits of the present book, is the problem to test hypotheses about the pattern of evolutionary process

* Kimura, M.: 1967, On the evolutionary adjustment of spontaneous mutation rates, *Genetical Research*, 9, No. 1, pp. 25–34;
Leigh, E.C.: 1973, The evolution of mutation rates, *Genetics* Supp. 73, No. 1, pp. 1–18.

by means of particular experimental data, for instance, the data on biochemical polymorphisms in natural populations. The technique of the proper quantitative analysis is distinguished from the traditional one by more advanced methods of probability and statistics.

As it turned out, the selection pressure on all the loci under concern is not necessarily needed to account for observable cases of polymorphism. In other words, we may deal with a primarily neutral type of genetic variability (the so-called 'non-Darwinian' evolution). This gave rise to the whole non-classical trend* in modern theory of evolution (M. Kimura *et al*.). But there are no cogent reasons for rejecting the classical 'Darwinian', selection-based explanation of polymorphness.

In our opinion, each of these two trends makes too absolute just one of the components of the real evolutionary process. Actually, both of these components take their effects in phenomena observed in reality, and the question may be rather of determining quantitatively the contribution that each component makes into the general process of evolution. Developing the proper statistical techniques and designing tests for neutrality or selection presence will undoubtedly help to clarify the problem.

Genetic evolution of any population proceeds in close relation with, rather than in isolation from, the ecological evolution of a biological community that maintains the population under concern. Naturally, the genotype fitness is not only a function of its genetic composition but also depends on a complex pattern of the intra- and interspecies relations the individual bears to other ones of the community or ecosystem. In other words, there is no evolution in nature that would be 'pure' genetic, but there is a coevolution of the genetic structure of populations composing the community together with its ecological structure.

In the most simple case, this is manifested in the dependence of the fitness (as well as other model parameters) upon population sizes. We have shown that, under certain assumptions, the classical frequency models of population genetics can be regarded as a particular case of ecological genetical models with regulation by the total size. But taking into account more complicated ecological mechanisms of regulation results normally in models where dynamics of the size are not separable from those of gene frequencies, i.e. in more complicated models than the classical ones**. The further development of mathematical population genetics should apparently be under way to creation of new synthesis, i.e. genetic-ecological models.

Till recent times, the both disciplines, namely, mathematical genetics and mathematical ecology, were developing independently of each other. In ecological models (with the rare exception of some) disregarded were the genetic dynamics of populations, while in

* Experimental aspects are presented in the book:
Lewontin, R.C.: 1974, *The Genetic Basis of Evolutionary Change*, Columbia Univ. Press, New York, London, XIII+346 pp,
while the book by:
Ewens, W: 1979, *Mathematical Population Genetics*, Springer, Berlin, Heidelberg,
covers primarily mathematical aspects.
Kimura, M. 1983, *The Neutral Theory of Molecular Evolution*, Cambridge Univ. Press, Cambridge
** Slatkin, M. and Smith, J.M.: 1979, Models of coevolution, *The Quarterly Review of Biology*, **54**, No. 3, pp. 233–263.

genetic ones the pattern of intra- and interspecies relations. This was justified to some extent by the fact that genetic and ecological processes have different characteristic time scales and can be separated in the first approximation. But now many phenomena have become known which can neither be described nor accounted for by means of either ecological or genetic models alone. For example, the complete answer to the question whether a predator population is capable of controlling the population of prey, cannot be given unless the processes of mutual adaptation of prey and predator are taken into account. Meanwhile, the adaptation is a process that implies reorganization of the population genetic structure. On the other hand, numerous cases are known where a polymorphism in coloration in the population of prey is maintained by the predator, i.e. the genetic mechanism that governs the relation between frequencies of differently colored genotypes, is imbedded into the pure ecological mechanism of predation, whereby individuals of distinct coloration have different probabilities of being detected by a predator.

Even the simplest models with selection that depends on the total population size or density, show the behavior that could hardly be expected within the limits of classical, frequency models. For example, the 'chaos' springing up in the total-size dynamics of a population with non-overlapping generations, may well lead the genotype structure of the population to chaotic dynamics too.

Up to now, only first steps are made on the way to the genetic-ecological synthesis. The models, of course, become substantially complicated, but the richness of their dynamic behavior sharply increases in return, generating our certain, not unfounded hopes to account for any evolutionary phenomena observed in nature.

Finally, one more problem, whose importance is commonly recognized but whose noticeable development can be ascertained just the recent years, is the problem of evolution in spatially distributed populations. Since the population of any species occupies certain area in space and a kind of territory behavior and space migrations are observable practically in each animal population, the need for considering spatial distribution of individuals throughout the area becomes apparent in any study of evolution. But even the simplest models of spatially distributed populations run across grave difficulties in their mathematical analysis. The classical result of Fisher - Kolmogorov–Petrovsky–Piskunov on a gene wave arising along a one-dimensional homogeneous area was obtained for an extremely simplified genetic case. Taking into account more complex types of inheritance can result (even for a one-dimensional area) in a 'dissipative structure' springing up, i.e. a steady-state distribution of gene frequencies that is inhomogeneous in space. These structures can be regarded, on certain grounds, as the initial stage of new species formation. At least, they may serve as a good illustration to the phenomenon of 'patchiness' observable in nature, where the population has pronounced spatial inhomogeneity in its genetic structure despite there are no visible isolating barriers in its spatial distribution along the homogeneous area.

Even more complicated and unexpected dynamic effects might occur in going from one-dimensional problems to more complex ones for evolution of a population in a two-dimensional (not necessarily homogeneous) area. For example, owing to inhomogeneity of the medium in different directions, there might occur the dispersion of gene waves which propagate with different velocities. These waves will be non-linear due to the fundamental non-linearity in the laws of inheritance, so that the superposition principle is inapplicable for those waves. They can either suppress or enhance each other, or even some centers of activity may spring up which generate such waves but have finite existence times.

Ending our book, we emphasize that 'pure' genetic problems induce the new mathematical ones, whose investigation reveals, in turn, the new questions that can be raised before experts who are concerned with specific problems of population genetics and evolution theory. We have attempted to present a more or less systematic view of state-of-the-art in evolutionary mathematical population genetics, let the reader judge to what extent we have succeeded.

Short Glossary of Genetic Terms*

Alleles: types of the *gene* that occupies a fixed *locus* of a *chromosome*. The term 'allele genes' is used sometimes as a synonym or said to be merely the 'genes'. Roughly speaking, the alleles define an elementary character of an organism (for instance, coloration of pea seeds) controlled by heredity and governed by the *Mendel laws* of inheritance. For a *diploid* organism having a double set of each gene (whose alleles may be different however), the alleles make sense to be classified by their external manifestation in the phenotype: *dominance*, *recessiveness*, or *overdominance*.

Alleles, multiple: the *alleles* are said to be *multiple* if there are more than two types of the given *gene*.

Chromosome: an intranuclear formation consisting primarily of protein and DNA (deoxyribonucleic acid) coding hereditary information. *Genes* represent segments in the molecule of DNA; they are located linearly in a chromosome. Each chromosome of a *diploid* organism has its homologous (pair-wise) one containing the same *loci*. The sex chromosomes, unlike the autosomes, are engaged in sex determination. One of the sex chromosomes contains practically no genes.

Crossing-over: the event of regrouping (or *recombination* of) the *genes* located in the same *chromosome* because of the breakage in one or more points and exchange of segments between homologous chromosomes. In the present book, the crossing-over is meant to occur in the *meiosis*, where the *gametes* of a *diploid* organism are formed.

Diploid: the term indicating that a given individual (or cell) has a double set of each homologous *chromosomes*. One half of the set has been brought by the paternal *gamete* while the other by the maternal one.

Dominance: such an interaction of two *alleles* of a *diploid* organism whereby the *homozygote phenotype* (with respect to the dominant allele) is indistinguishable from the *heterozygote* one.

Epistasis: the mode of interaction among non-allelic *genes* which results generally speaking, in the *phenotype* of an organism (of a given genotype) that is not a mere 'sum' of the phenotypes caused by the *genotypes* at each *locus* taken separately.

Gamete: reproductive cell. The gamete of a *diploid* organism has a single (*haploid*) set of homologous *chromosomes*. In the course of fertilization, two gametes fusing together form a *zygote* from which the new organism develops.

* The purpose of the Glossary is to provide a minimum knowledge from biology that will be sufficient to understand the terms used in the text in their narrow sense (pertinent to objectives of the book). Italicized are the words that are explained in the Glossary at alphabetically respective places.

Gene: a certain segment (*locus*) in the molecule of the *chromosome* DNA, deoxiribonucleic acid, which encodes some character in the organism, e.g. a protein (a structural gene).

Genetics: a branch of biology that has to do with the study of heredity and variability.

Genotype: a set of *genes* (at a given *locus* , a group of loci, or the whole organism) of an individual.

Haploid: the term that means an organism (e.g. virus or bacterium) or cell (e.g. reproductive one) having a single set of *chromosomes*

Hemizygote: an individual that has only one *allele*, rather than a pair of alleles, located in sex *chromosomes*; a male in most cases.

Heterozygote: a *diploid* individual that carries two different *alleles* (at a *locus* under concern).

Homozygote: a *diploid* individual having two identical *alleles* (at a *locus* under concern).

Linkage: association in the inheritance of the *genes* that are located in a single *chromosome* (i.e. linkage group) and termed the linked ones. Breakage of the joint transmission of the linked genes occurs as a result of *recombination*. Non-linked genes of the parent turn out to be in a single *gamete* with probability 1/2 for a pair of genes, 1/4 for a triple, etc.

Locus: a segment in a *chromosome* where a given *gene* is located.

Meiosis: two specific divisions of the nucleus' preceding formation of the *gametes*, which result in reducing the *diploid* number of *chromosome* to its half, whereby each gamete acquires a *haploid* set of non-homologous chromosomes.

Mendel laws: statistical regularities in splitting the progeny of the two genotypically distinct individuals (in practice, of two homogeneous groups of individuals) into different types at the first and the second generations in accordance with the number of *loci* and interactions among *alleles*.

Mutation: a change in the genetic material (usually caused by the change in structure of the corresponding segment of the DNA molecule in the *chromosome*) that encodes certain character in the organism.

Overdominance: see *Superdominance*.

Panmixia: a synonym to random mating, where each individual has equal probabilities to make up a parent couple with any other individual (of the opposite sex for organisms with sexual reproduction).

Phenotype: properties (characters, features) of the organism to be an outcome of interaction between *genes* of its *genotype* and conditions of the environment in the course of development.

Polymorphism: a situation when there are more than one *genotype* of non-zero frequency simultaneously present in the population, the frequencies being not accountable by recurrent mutations.

Recessiveness: the property of one *allele* at a *locus*, relative to the other (dominant) one, whereby its presence in a *genotype* of the *diploid* organism is manifested in the *phenotype* of *homozygotes* only. The phenotype of *heterozygotes* does not differ from that of *homozygotes* with the dominant *allele*.

Recombination: a process of *gene* 'reshuffling' in the course of *gamete* formation bringing about the new combinations of genes in gametes that were absent in the parent cells. In this book the recombination is supposed to result exclusively from *crossing-over* and *segregation*.

Segregation: splitting the pair of *alleles* of a *diploid* organism (in general, independent separation of different pairs of homologous *chromosomes*) in the course of *haploid gamete* formation in *meiosis*.

Superdominance (overdominance): an interaction between two *alleles* at some *locus* of a *diploid* organism such that the character encoded by them is manifested stronger in the *heterozygote* than in any of the two *homozygotes*.

Zygote: a *diploid* cell that results from the fusion of a paternal and maternal *gametes* and marks the beginning of a new organism.

Subject index